W9-ADS-755

Intervention and Reflection
BASIC ISSUES IN MEDICAL ETHICS
Second Edition

Ronald Munson

University of Missouri–St. Louis

Wadsworth Publishing Company, Belmont, California
A division of Wadsworth, Inc.

Philosophy Editor: Kenneth King
Interior Designer: Katie Michels
Cover Designer: Michael Rogondino
Copy Editor: Winn Kalmon
Production Service: Brian K. Williams/San Francisco
Composition: Boyer & Brass

Printed in the United States of America

1 2 3 4 5 6 7 8 9 10—87 86 85 84 83

Library of Congress Cataloging in Publication Data
Main entry under title:
Intervention and reflection.

(The Wadsworth series in social philosophy)
Bibliography: p.
    1. Medical ethics—Addresses, essays, lectures.
2. Medical ethics—Problems, exercises, etc. I. Munson,
Ronald, 1939-   . II. Series.
R724.I57 1983   174'.2   82-20262
ISBN 0-534-01289-2

ISBN 0-534-01289-2

Intervention and Reflection
BASIC ISSUES IN MEDICAL ETHICS
Second Edition

Ronald Munson

University of Missouri–St. Louis

Wadsworth Publishing Company, Belmont, California
A division of Wadsworth, Inc.

Philosophy Editor: Kenneth King
Interior Designer: Katie Michels
Cover Designer: Michael Rogondino
Copy Editor: Winn Kalmon
Production Service: Brian K. Williams/San Francisco
Composition: Boyer & Brass

Printed in the United States of America

1 2 3 4 5 6 7 8 9 10—87 86 85 84 83

Library of Congress Cataloging in Publication Data
Main entry under title:
Intervention and reflection.

(The Wadsworth series in social philosophy)
Bibliography: p.
1. Medical ethics—Addresses, essays, lectures.
2. Medical ethics—Problems, exercises, etc. I. Munson,
Ronald, 1939-   . II. Series.
R724.I57 1983   174'.2   82-20262
ISBN 0-534-01289-2

ISBN 0-534-01289-2

Intervention and Reflection
BASIC ISSUES IN MEDICAL ETHICS
Second Edition

Ronald Munson
University of Missouri–St. Louis

Wadsworth Publishing Company, Belmont, California
A division of Wadsworth, Inc.

Philosophy Editor: Kenneth King
Interior Designer: Katie Michels
Cover Designer: Michael Rogondino
Copy Editor: Winn Kalmon
Production Service: Brian K. Williams/San Francisco
Composition: Boyer & Brass

Printed in the United States of America

1 2 3 4 5 6 7 8 9 10—87 86 85 84 83

Library of Congress Cataloging in Publication Data
Main entry under title:
Intervention and reflection.
(The Wadsworth series in social philosophy)
Bibliography: p.
1. Medical ethics—Addresses, essays, lectures.
2. Medical ethics—Problems, exercises, etc. I. Munson, Ronald, 1939-   . II. Series.
R724.I57 1983   174′.2   82-20262
ISBN 0-534-01289-2

ISBN 0-534-01289-2

To Miriam
''Giver of bright rings''

CONTENTS

2. TREATING OR TERMINATING: THE PROBLEM OF BIRTH DEFECTS   100

3. EUTHANASIA   142

THE READINGS

8. REPRODUCTIVE CONTROL: IN VITRO FERTILIZATION, ARTIFICIAL INSEMINATION, AND STERILIZATION

PART IV: RESOURCES

PREFACE

This is the second edition of this book, and the differences between it and the first edition are important. Yet before I discuss the changes, I want to say something about the character of the work itself.

In shaping this book, I have tried to capture both the intellectual excitement and the great seriousness now surrounding the field of medical ethics. In particular, I've done my best to convey both these aspects to students new to the field. In the choice of topics, in the chapter text, and by other means, I have tried to familiarize such readers with the issues and make them active participants in the enterprise. Whether someone is an undergraduate or graduate student, a nursing or medical student, with or without training in ethics, I think that he or she will find this a useful and engaging book.

The topics presented here are all fundamental ones in current medical ethics. They reflect the range and variety of problems that we now confront and involve the basic moral and social issues that have excited most concern. But more than this, the problems are morally serious ones that lead people to turn hopefully to philosophical consideration in search of satisfactory resolutions.

The reading selections represent current thinking about the topics and show that such consideration can be worthwhile. They reveal contemporary medical ethics at its best and are all readable and relatively nontechnical. The papers by John Arras and Andrew Jameton and J. Gay-Williams are published here for the first time. The others have been selected from the vast body of literature that has developed in the last five to ten years.

Although philosophers are strongly represented in the readings, the authors also include jurists, biologists, legal theorists, and practicing physicians and researchers. The moral problems of medicine almost always have scientific, social, legal, and economic aspects, and to deal with them sensibly we need the knowledge and perceptions of people from a variety of disciplines.

I have also opted for diversity in another way, for I have tried to see to it that opposing viewpoints are given for each major topic. Part of the intellectual excitement of medical ethics is generated by the hot controversies surrounding its issues, and to ignore these controversies would be misleading. Even worse, it would deny students the opportunity of dealing directly with proposals and arguments that may be incompatible with their own views.

The topics and readings are of crucial importance in a book of this kind. Yet I have also introduced several special features that I believe will be of help to students and will make the book more useful in class.

Most important, perhaps, is the introductory chapter "Ethical Theories and Medical Decisions." Here, among other things, I briefly sketch the principles of five major ethical theories and illustrate how they might be used to answer particular moral questions in medicine. The main purpose for doing this is to give students without a background in ethics the information they need to understand and evaluate the arguments in the readings. I hope, too, that the chapter will help prepare them for independent inquiry in medical ethics.

In each of the ten chapters of the book I try to present whatever factual information is needed to understand the moral issues that arise in actual medical practice and research. I also suggest ways in which the five moral theories might be used to resolve some of the problems. These suggestions are offered as starting points in the search for satisfactory answers. I have also included in each chapter a summary of the main line of argument in the selections, so that it is possible to identify the major themes that run through the chapter.

The Case Presentations are each based upon, or closely parallel to, an actual event or situation. They are intended to provide a focus for discussion and to illustrate how genuine moral problems arise in ordinary life. I think that they may also remind us that in dealing with medical ethics we are not engaged in some purely abstract intellectual game.

At the end of each chapter, following the readings, are several Decision Scenarios. These are brief dramatic presentations of situations in which moral questions are crucial—in which ethical decisions have to be made. The scenarios are followed by questions that ask the reader to decide what the problems are and how they might be dealt with by a particular moral theory or by principles argued for in the readings. Thus, the Decision Scenarios are, in effect, exercises in medical ethics that can direct and structure class discussion. Some of the questions, I hope, are also suitable for paper topics.

Notes and references for the introductory material in each chapter, for Case Presentations, and for Decision Scenarios begin on page 559.

Finally, I have included at the end of the book a quite extensive bibliography. It is arranged to correspond to the chapter divisions of the book, so that anyone who wants to do further reading on a particular topic should have no trouble locating appropriate works.

The opportunity to prepare a second edition has allowed me to introduce some changes that I believe substantially improve both the philosophical and pedagogical character of the book. In the interest of brevity, I shall merely list, with little discussion, the more important alterations.

Five Case Presentations have been added. Thus, half the chapters now have two substantial cases for illustration and discussion. Because the Case Pre-

sentations focus on recent events, the new additions increase both the scope and relevance of the book.

Over twenty Decision Scenarios have been added. This means that there is now a minimum of five per chapter. The extra scenarios make it possible to present a greater variety of special circumstances in which ethical problems arise. Since many of the scenarios are based on actual events, they add a sense of immediacy to the moral issues they address.

Chapter 7, "Genetics: Intervention, Control, and Research," has been much expanded and modified. More coverage is now provided for genetic screening and counseling. In addition, gene therapy, prenatal diagnosis, and selective abortion are covered for the first time. The newly written introduction to the chapter now supplies a substantial amount of information about genetic diseases and techniques for diagnosing them. Screening programs for diseases such as PKU and sickle-cell anemia are examined and the moral and social issues presented by such programs are outlined.

A wholly new chapter on reproductive control (Chapter 8) has been added. The topics covered in the chapter include in vitro fertilization, artificial insemination, and sterilization. The Case Presentation focuses on Louise Brown—the first "test-tube" baby.

Chapter 6, "Behavior Control and Psychosurgery," has been modified to put more emphasis on the problems of individual autonomy and mental illness. Chapter 9, "Competition and Allocation," has been expanded to include the issue of organ transplants. In addition, some articles within specific chapters have been replaced by ones of more interest or significance.

Information and statistics about current social practices and policies have been brought up to date. Statistics on abortion and health-care costs, recent proposals to change the Medicaid program, and new tests on the effectiveness of Laetrile are some examples of the changes made to provide current information.

The Bibliography has been both expanded and brought up to date.

Perhaps it would be appropriate to accompany my comments on this book with a few suggestions about its use in class.

There is a logic in the organization of the book. Roughly, the first topics presented (abortion, etc.) involve making individual moral decisions, while the later topics (rights to health care, etc.) require decisions about social goals and policies. But of course virtually all of the issues in medical ethics overlap and intertwine. (Abortion is a good example of this.)

For this reason, it seemed to me sensible to arrange the topics and write the introductions in a way that would make each chapter more or less independent of the others. Thus, the structure of the book does not have to be followed in teaching. Someone who wants to start with (say) human experimentation or euthanasia may do so without being faced with text or selections that presuppose familiarity with the preceding chapters.

In each chapter, I've placed the Case Presentation before the introductory text. My reason for doing so is that a case provides students with a concrete example and gives them an opportunity to appreciate the sorts of circumstances in which particular ethical issues arise. Anyone who believes it is better to discuss cases after moral issues have been talked about in a more abstract way may want to ask students to read the Case Presentation after the introductory text or the philosophical materials. The cases are written to stand alone, even when they are explicitly discussed in the selections.

Finally, a similar strategy that has much to recommend it is to ask students to read the Decision Scenarios before the selections. The questions in the scenarios can then serve as guides in reading, as flags marking important issues. Also, if the scenarios are sometimes discussed before and then after the selections are read, students are given a chance to see the ways in which their own views change.

I have tried to be helpful without being overly intrusive. Anyone who teaches medical ethics wants enough flexibility to arrange a course in the way that he or she sees fit. I have tried to offer that flexibility, while at the same time supplying students with the kind of information and support they need.

The second edition of this book, with its introductory text and other appurtenances, continues to be more ambitious than any similar work currently available. The first edition proved itself generally useful, and I have the same hope for this one. I was able to make some important changes, but I am under no illusion that the book is now perfect. (If trying always meant succeeding, there would be no adventure stories.) Accordingly, I would very much appreciate comments or suggestions from those who use the book and discover ways in which it can be improved.

Books, like people, continue to acquire debts throughout their lives. My greatest debt on behalf of this book is to those authors who allowed their works to be printed here. I hope they find no grounds for objecting to the way I have dealt with them.

I owe much to William E. Mann (University of Vermont) and to Kirk Monfort (California State University, Chico). When I was working on the first edition, their intelligent and informed criticisms and suggestions were offered to me at every step of the way. I benefited from them greatly, and they often saved me from falling victim to my own carelessness and ignorance.

Kenneth King, Wadsworth's philosophy editor, has continued to show a steady and unshakable faith in this book. Although always ready with support and recommendations, Ken, like all good editors, knows when to stay still so that the work can get done. It has been a pleasure to collaborate with him.

My colleagues James F. Doyle, Lawrence H. Davis, Robert M. Gordon, David Conway, Paul Roth, and Stephanie Ross have all helped, in various ways at various times. John Arras (University of Redlands) was generous in advising me how I might benefit from his experience in working on a similar book.

I am grateful to the publisher's reviewers for their suggestions and criticisms. Curtis Paul took on a major burden in helping prepare the bibliography, and Janiece Fister once again demonstrated her skill and capacity for hard work by typing the results. Ted Trimble offered useful advice about revisions. I am indebted to them all. And I thank Janet Berlo, Rogers Brubaker, Scott Karlan, and Kathy Rosenthal, who listened cheerfully while I talked of doom and woe and of the pains of writing prose. I am similarly grateful to Helen Doyle who suffered through a like litany of sorrows connected with second editions.

Miriam Grove Munson not only patiently endured a continuous saga of complaints, but still managed to offer much needed sympathy and encouragement. But her help was also quite practical, for she was kind enough to test the intelligibility of the introductory material and show me ways to improve it.

I hope the Academic Credit Bureau will forgive me for not itemizing all of my debts here. They are simply too numerous. Like most human beings, I hate to acknowledge responsibility for errors. But the truth is that I sometimes stubbornly refused to change direction even when kind readers warned me that I was walking into quicksand. If it swallows me up, it's my own fault.

University of Missouri—St. Louis
1982

Intervention and Reflection

ETHICAL THEORIES AND MEDICAL DECISIONS: AN INTRODUCTION

"He's stopped breathing, Doctor," the nurse said. She sounded calm and not at all hysterical. By the time Dr. Sarah Cunningham had reached Mr. Sabatini's bedside, the nurse was already providing mouth-to-mouth resuscitation. But Mr. Sabatini still had the purplish blue color of cyanosis, caused by a lack of oxygen in his blood.

Dr. Cunningham knew that if he was to survive, Mr. Sabatini would have to be given oxygen fast and placed on a respirator. But should she order this done?

Mr. Sabatini was an old man, almost ninety. So far as anyone knew, he was alone in the world and would hardly be missed when he died. His health was poor. He had congestive heart disease and was dying slowly and painfully from intestinal cancer.

Wouldn't it be a kindness to Mr. Sabatini to allow him this quick and painless death? Why condemn him to lingering on for a few extra hours or weeks?

The decision that Sarah Cunningham faces is a moral one. She has to decide whether she should take the steps that might prolong Mr. Sabatini's life or not take them and accept the consequence that he will almost surely die within minutes. She knows the medical procedures that can be employed, but she has to decide whether she should employ them.

This kind of case rivets our attention because of its immediacy and drama. But there are many other situations that arise in the context of medical practice and research that present problems that also require moral decisions. Some are equal in drama to the problem facing Dr. Cunningham, while others are not so dramatic but are of at least equal seriousness. There are far too many to catalogue, but consider this sample: Is it right for a woman to have an abortion for any reason? Should children with serious birth defects be put to death? Do people have a right to die? Does everyone have a right to medical care? Should physicians ever lie to their patients? Should people suffering from a genetic disease be allowed to have children? Can parents agree to allow their children to be used as experimental subjects?

Most of us have little tolerance for questions like these. They seem so cold and abstract. Our attitude changes, however, when we find ourselves in a position in which *we* are the decision makers. It changes, too, when we are in a position in which we must advise those who make the decisions. Or when we are on the receiving end of the decision.

But whether we view the problems abstractly or concretely, we are inclined to ask the same question: Are there any rules, standards, or principles that we can use as guides when we are faced with moral decisions? If there are, then Dr. Cunningham need not be wholly unprepared to decide whether she should order steps taken to save Mr. Sabatini. Nor need we be unprepared to decide issues like those in the questions above.

The branch of philosophy that is concerned with principles that allow us to make decisions about what is right and wrong is called *ethics* or *moral philosophy*. *Medical ethics* is specifically concerned with moral principles and decisions in the context of medical practice, policy, and research. Moral difficulties connected with medicine are so complex and important that they require special attention. Medical ethics gives them this attention, but it remains a part of the discipline of ethics. Thus, if we are to answer our question as to whether there are rules or principles to use when making moral decisions in the medical context, we must turn to general ethical theories.

In this chapter, we will discuss five major ethical theories that have been put forward by philosophers. Each of these theories represents an attempt to supply principles that we can rely on in making moral decisions. We'll consider these principles and examine how they might be applied to moral issues in the medical context. We will discuss the reasons that have been offered to persuade us to accept each theory, but we will also point out some of the difficulties that each theory presents.

Before discussing these theories, we must first deal with two serious questions. It is important to get them out of the way at the beginning because the first question raises doubt about the *need* for ethical theories in the medical context, and the second question casts doubt on the very *possibility* of getting an ethical theory that we might all accept as reliable and legitimate.

Oaths and Professional Codes of Ethics

For almost twenty-four centuries, the Oath of Hippocrates has been sworn by physicians in the Western world. It has come to serve as a symbol of the dedication and integrity that we believe physicians ought to demand of themselves. The same commitment to the highest standards of conduct is also found in the Oath of Maimonides, a thirteenth-century oath still taken by Jewish physicians.

In more recent times, a number of other oaths and codes of professional conduct have been formulated by medical organizations. Here are just a few of them: The Declaration of Geneva, the American Medical Association Principles of Medical Ethics, the Ethical and Religious Directives for Catholic Hospitals, and the International Code of Nursing Ethics.

Such formal statements play a crucially important role in health care. In expressing basic moral principles, they serve to remind physicians, nurses, and other professionals that theirs is not an ordinary calling. They are reminded that the lives and well-being of people depend on their skills, efforts, and integrity. Thus, oaths and codes of conduct encourage them to act always according to principle.

In view of the number of oaths and codes available, is there really any need for ethical theories in the medical context? Isn't it enough for physicians, nurses, and others to take an oath or to endorse a code of professional ethics?

As important as oaths and codes are, there are several quite persuasive reasons for saying that they are not enough. Not only is there a place for ethical theories in the medical context, but there is a genuine need for them.

First of all, consider that there are a variety of oaths and codes. Which one should a person accept? They are by no means equivalent to one another. The AMA Principles of Medical Ethics, for example, is silent on the issue of abortion, while the Directives for Catholic Hospitals explicitly prohibits it. It is not enough to say, "It doesn't matter which code you accept so long as you accept one." This would make the choice of a code an arbitrary matter, and this, in turn, would suggest that whether one regards abortion as right or not is an arbitrary matter. But if such matters are arbitrary, then there is no point to having a code of ethics at all.

If the choice of a code is not to be arbitrary, this means that we have to be prepared to offer sufficient reasons for choosing one over all the rest. We would want to endorse a code only when we believe that its principles are right. But to show that this is so requires that we appeal to some ethical theory and show that its principles justify those in the code or oath.

We might put this point another way by saying that the principles in codes and oaths are not self-justifying. We can always ask about each of them, "Why should we accept this rule? Why should we swear to uphold it?" It is no answer at all to say, "Just because it's a principle." The provisions in oaths and codes must be grounded in a general ethical theory. Otherwise, they are little more than high-sounding words of magic and mystery.

Second, it is quite possible that the rules expressed in a code might conflict with other moral beliefs. The Hippocratic Oath, for example, explicitly forbids both euthanasia and abortion. Yet there are many physicians who believe that these are, at least sometimes, morally permissible actions. Should they be false to their moral beliefs in order to adhere to their oath, or should they violate their oath to be true to their moral beliefs? The resolution of such a conflict requires that a person appeal to principles that are not part of the oath itself. The need for a more general set of ethical principles clearly makes itself felt in situations like this.

When the practical difficulties of applying the provisions of an oath or code are considered, it is easy to see that they cannot serve as a substitute for an ethical theory. Oaths and codes appeal strongly to our desire to have moral problems simplified and resolved in a direct, no-nonsense fashion. If we could decide what is right merely by checking a list of right actions, then who would not want to check the list?

But matters are not so easy in this world. Codes and oaths must cover a vast number of kinds of moral situations in medicine. What is more, they must be phrased in such a way that virtually no one would hesitate to subscribe to them. This means that the language of codes and oaths must be highly general. As a result, it is often difficult to determine just what the provisions prohibit or command. The Declaration of Geneva, for example, has physicians affirm that "I will maintain the utmost respect for human life, from the time of conception. . . ." Does this provision forbid abortion? Is respect for human life compatible with abortion? There is no way to answer these questions so long as we limit ourselves to the provisions of the Declaration.

Far from being able to resolve our moral difficulties by referring to a list, we must commit ourselves to a much more lengthy and difficult task. Using the principles of a general ethical theory, we must attempt to work out the details of their application to problems in the medical context. Only in this way can we hope to arrive at answers that are sufficiently precise and adequately supported.

Finally, it is worth noticing that oaths and codes sometimes contain provisions that are not moral principles at all. The most famous example of this is a section of the Hippocratic Oath that requires a physician to pledge to keep his medical knowledge secret from the general public: "I will impart knowledge of the art to my own sons and to those of my teachers, and to disciples bound by a stipulation and oath . . . but to no others."

The AMA code also contains an exclusion provision, although one of a different sort. Physicians must commit themselves to avoiding association with those who do not practice scientific healing: "A physician should practice a method of healing founded on a scientific basis; and he should not voluntarily associate professionally with anyone who violates this principle."

Such provisions are present because codes and oaths attempt to do more than provide rules of conduct. They have a social function as well, for they serve to bind groups together and affirm their commitment to certain goals. That provision of the Hippocratic Oath that pledged a physician to keep his medical knowledge secret was instrumental in making the practice of medicine the prerogative of a sort of guild, and it may well have had its origins in an economic motive. Similarly, the exclusion provision of the AMA may be seen as an effort to establish a "legitimate" medicine by excluding certain kinds of practitioners.

Such provisions are of great social importance and at times may well be justifiable. They are not, however, moral principles, and they are open to doubt or challenge on moral grounds. Is it really right for physicians to refuse to associate with Christian Science Readers or with chiropractors in ministering to the health of their patients? Even if the answer to this question is yes, arriving at the answer requires that we go beyond the range of codes and oaths and employ the principles of an ethical theory.

In summary, then, professional oaths and codes of conduct should be recognized as having a legitimate and important purpose. Not only do they bind social groups together, they express aims and aspirations of the group. In doing so, they promote integrity, dedication, and principled behavior. But codes and oaths cannot take the place of ethical theories. Indeed, the questions they raise forcefully call attention to our need for such theories.

Having determined that there is a *need* for ethical theories in a medical context, we are now free to turn our attention to the very *possibility* of developing an acceptable ethical theory.

Ethical Relativism

Ethical relativism is the view that there are no universal or absolute moral principles. Standards of right and wrong are always relative to a particular culture or society. Consequently, there is no objective basis for saying that a particular action is right or wrong independently of a specific social group.

If this view is correct, it is obvious that we will be wasting our time presenting moral theories in this chapter. If one set of principles is as legitimate as any other, we need not bother considering alternatives. Nor need we be concerned with looking for strengths and weaknesses of particular theories. In short, the whole business of philosophical ethics is called into question.

Ethical relativism has an immediate attraction for most of us. Perhaps this is due in part to the doubt and confusion we feel when we try to find ethical principles we would be willing to endorse as true. The difficulty of this task inclines us to believe that there may be no such principles. But more important, we are aware of the great diversity of cultures and societies that have flourished in different parts of the world and at different times. Even today we see diversity all around us. It would seem ignorant and arrogant of us to believe that we know, or even might know, ethical principles that are true and binding on all people.

Let's look more carefully at the support for ethical relativism. Its main defense rests on the undeniable fact that some societies consider as right various kinds of actions or practices that other societies consider to be wrong. Anthropologists and historians have repeatedly called our attention to such cultural and social differences. Some of the examples have been mentioned so often as to have become clichés. We all know of the arctic Eskimo's practice of abandoning their old people on the ice and allowing them to die of starvation and exposure. We know that in some cultures a man has an obligation to marry his brother's widow, and in some African cultures it is considered right to kill twins at their birth. Examples from history are equally numerous. Officials in seventeenth-century Europe tortured and burned to death as witches a great number of women. The officials believed their actions were morally right. During the Middle Ages, it was considered proper to drive the insane out of villages by hurling rocks at them. And so on.

It seems, then, that whether an action is regarded as right or not depends on the society judging it. Since we learn our values from our society, all of our moral judgments will reflect that society. Thus, two people from two different societies may make contradictory moral judgments. According to ethical relativism, we have no legitimate reason to say that either is wrong. To the ethical relativist this situation simply illustrates that there is no universal basis for determining what is right. Different sets of moral principles are of equal worth, and that one individual endorses one set over another is just an outcome of having been raised in a certain society or culture.

At first sight, ethical relativism seems wholly persuasive. It both appeals to our disposition to be tolerant of other societies and cultures, and it makes use of familiar facts. But there are some very good reasons for not accepting the view.

First, although societies differ in what actions are considered right, this does not necessarily establish that they hold different ethical *principles*. Some anthropologists and historians have claimed that all cultures and societies endorse principles like "Unjustified killing is wrong" and "You should not steal." Differences arise in the application of these principles for a variety of reasons. (For example, what counts as stealing in one society may not correspond exactly with what counts as stealing in another.) Also, the application of the principles may be connected with other factual or religious beliefs. Any contemporary physician who poured boiling oil into a patient's gunshot wound would be acting immorally. Yet in the sixteenth century, this was the accepted treatment because it was believed that wounds made by bullets were "venomous" due to their contact with gunpowder. Scalding oil was supposed to destroy the venom and so enhance healing. Physicians of the time accepted, as do physicians now, the principle "Do not cause unnecessary suffering." It just so happens that they wrongly believed that the suffering they caused was necessary to proper medical treatment.

Whether or not there are any universally shared moral principles is, to a great extent, an empirical question. It is one not yet settled, and there are anthropologists and historians who believe the best evidence is for the claim that there are no ethical principles universally acknowledged. Thus, our first consideration does not refute ethical relativism, but it does show that the view is open to serious doubt and is not obviously correct.

Second, even if we admit that societies often hold different ethical principles, this does not mean that there are no correct or true principles. To take a parallel case, we know that societies and cultures frequently hold different beliefs about the nature of the world and the things that are in it. This does not mean that the different beliefs are all correct or that the choice among them is arbitrary or due to upbringing.

Suppose, for example, you learn of a culture in which it is believed that wound infections are caused by moonlight. The members of your culture hold the view that infections are the result of bacterial invasions. You know that there are good reasons to regard the latter belief as true and virtually no reasons to accept the former as true. Thus, you are not very likely to say "Both beliefs are right," or "The choice between them is arbitrary," or even, "I believe what I do just because that's the way I was brought up." The members of the other culture believe, of course, that their belief is true. But believing something is true does not make it so, and we have good grounds for saying that they are wrong.

Moral principles are no different in this respect. It is at least possible in principle to persuade others to accept them as correct by providing grounds and reasons for their support. We may acknowledge that others have different principles, respect their beliefs, and be tolerant in our attitudes. At the same time, we may have grounds to reject their principles and accept others inconsistent with them. (Whether we are actually able to establish any principles as universal is a different matter.) Ethical relativism ignores the possibility of objective argument and consideration and thus ignores the possibility of establishing universal ethical principles.

Lastly, ethical relativism is contrary to our ordinary experiences and beliefs in several ways. For example, when we are faced with a moral decision like "Should I allow this patient to die?" we do not act as if any judgment is just as good as any other. We deliberate and try to decide what the *right* action is. When we face such doubt and indecision, we believe that any rational person in any culture would be faced with similar uncertainty in our circumstances. Furthermore, we would regard it as beside the point to be told that in our society the most frequent decision would be to allow the patient to die. We are not concerned with such information because we are interested in doing what is right, not just what our society considers right.

Similarly, when we make claims like "It is wrong to cause others needless pain," we are not just asserting this as a principle for our culture. We think of ourselves as offering it as one binding on all people at all times and places. We condemn the cruelty of the ancient Egyptians as much as the cruelty we saw this morning.

Other examples are possible, but these few are enough to show that moral relativism violates our ordinary concept of morality. We do not and cannot act as though ethical relativism were correct. Rather, in our ethical deliberations and assertions we are committed to the notion that ethical principles binding on all can be established as true.

In part we are inclined to adopt ethical relativism because we wish to show respect and tolerance for the moral beliefs of others. Notice, however, that a point of view that makes such tolerance a virtue is incompatible with ethical relativism. To claim that we ought to be tolerant of the beliefs of others contradicts the claim that any set of moral beliefs is as legitimate as any other. To make such a claim is to say, in effect, "This is a moral rule that is not relative, but one binding on everyone." Thus, even one who styles herself a relativist is not likely to be able to act in accordance with her own announced belief. She too acts as if at least one moral principle can be shown to be true.

Ethical relativism can be stated and defended in various qualified and sophisticated ways. We have discussed it only in its popular form, but it is this form that is the most influential. We have shown that despite its immediate appeal, there are persuasive reasons for rejecting it.

Now that we have established the need for, and possibility of, ethical theory, the road is open for us to begin our examination of particular ethical theories. We will consider five major theories: utilitarianism, Kantian ethics, the intuitionism of W. D. Ross, John Rawls's theory of justice, and the natural law theory of Roman Catholicism.

Each of these theories represents a serious effort to supply a set of moral principles that are mutually consistent, in keeping with the facts of the world, and adequate for resolving moral difficulties. Furthermore, each theory claims that its principles are not arbitrary but can be supported by considerations that make them worthy of acceptance and belief.

Our focus will be on the basic principles of each of the theories. After stating the principles and considering the nature of the support offered for them, we will then indicate how they might be applied to particular problems that arise in the medical context. Finally, we will discuss some of the objections that critics have urged against the theory.

Clearly enough, we can do little more than provide sketches of the ethical theories we will be discussing. All of them have been stated in ways much more detailed and sophisticated, and anyone who wants to know more about a particular theory should consult some of the works mentioned in the bibliography. Nevertheless, for our purposes, all we need are sketches of the theories. Using them, we will be in a position to understand the ethical issues of medicine and to argue persuasively for particular solutions to them. A little knowledge can also be a *useful* thing.

Utilitarianism

The ethical theory known as utilitarianism was given its most influential formulation in the nineteenth century by the British philosophers Jeremy Bentham (1748–1832) and John Stuart Mill (1806–1873). Bentham and Mill did not produce identical theories, but both their versions have come to be spoken of as "classical utilitarianism." Subsequent elaborations and qualifications of utilitarianism are inevitably based on the formulations of Bentham and Mill, and this prospect makes their theorizing worth careful examination.

The Principle of Utility

The foundation of utilitarianism is a single apparently simple principle. Mill calls it the "principle of utility" and states it this way: "Actions are right in proportion as they tend to promote happiness, wrong as they tend to produce the reverse of happiness."

The principle focuses attention on the *consequences* of actions, rather than upon some feature of the actions themselves. The "utility" or "usefulness" of an action is determined by the extent to which it produces happiness. Thus, no action is *in itself* right or wrong. Nor is an action right or wrong in virtue of the actor's hopes, intentions, or past actions. Consequences alone are important. Breaking a promise, lying, causing pain, or even killing a person may, under certain circumstances, be the right action to take. Under other circumstances, the action might be wrong.

We need not think of the principle as applying to just one action that we are considering. It supplies the basis for a kind of cost-benefit analysis to employ in a situation in which several lines of action are possible. Using the principle, we are supposed to consider the possible results of each of the actions. Then we are to choose the one that produces the most benefit (happiness) at the least cost (unhappiness). The action we take may produce some unhappiness, but it is the overall balance of happiness over unhappiness that the principle tells us to seek.

Suppose, for example, that a woman in a large hospital is near death: she is in a coma, an EEG shows only minimal brain function, and a respirator is required to keep her breathing. Another patient has just been brought to the hospital from the scene of an automobile accident. His kidneys have been severely damaged, and he is in need of an immediate transplant. There is a good tissue match with the woman's kidneys. Is it right to hasten her death by removing a kidney?

The principle of utility would consider the removal justified. The woman is virtually dead, while the man has a good chance of surviving. It is true that the woman's life is threatened even more by the surgery. It may, in fact, kill her. But, on balance, the kidney transplant seems likely to produce more happiness than unhappiness. In fact, it seems better than the alternative of doing nothing. For in that case, both patients are likely to die.

The principle of utility is also called the "greatest happiness principle" by Bentham and Mill. The reason for this name is clear when the principle is stated in this way: Those actions are right that produce the greatest happiness for the greatest number of people. This alternative formulation makes it obvious that in deciding how to act it is not just my happiness or the happiness of a particular person or group that must be considered. According to utilitarianism, every person is to count just as much as any other person. That is, when we are considering how we should act, everyone's interest must be considered. The right action, then, will be the one that produces the most happiness for the largest number of people.

Mill is particularly anxious that utilitarianism not be construed as no more than a sophisticated justification for crude self-interest. He stresses that in making a moral decision we must look at the situation in an objective way. We must, he says, be a "benevolent spectator," and then act in a way that will bring about the best results for all concerned. This view is summarized in a famous passage:

> The happiness which forms the utilitarian standard of what is right in conduct, is not the agent's own happiness, but that of all concerned. As between his own happiness and that of others, utilitarianism requires him to be as strictly impartial as a disinterested and benevolent spectator. In the golden rule of Jesus of Nazareth, we read the complete spirit of the ethics of utility. To do as you would be done by, and to love your neighbor as yourself, constitute the ideal perfection of utilitarian morality.

The key concept in both formulations of the principle of utility is "happiness." Bentham simply identifies happiness with pleasure—pleasure of any kind. The aim of ethics, then, is to increase the amount of pleasure in the world to the greatest possible extent. To facilitate this, Bentham recommends the use of a "calculus of pleasure and pain," in which characteristics of pleasure such as intensity, duration, and number of people affected are measured and assigned numerical values. To determine which of several possible actions is the right one, we need only determine which one receives the highest numerical score. Unfortunately, Bentham does not tell us what units to use nor how to make the measurements.

Mill also identifies happiness with pleasure, but he differs from Bentham in a major respect. Unlike Bentham, he insists that some pleasures are "higher" than others. Thus, pleasures of the intellect are superior to, say, purely sensual pleasures. This difference in the concept of pleasure can become significant in a medical context. For example, faced with the choice of using limited resources to save the life of a lathe operator or an art historian, Mill's view might assign more value to the life of the art historian. That person, Mill might say, is capable of "higher pleasures" than the lathe operator. (Of course other factors would be relevant here for Mill also.)

Both Mill and Bentham regard happiness as an intrinsic good. That is, it is something good in itself or good for its own sake. Actions, by contrast, are good only to the extent to which they tend to promote happiness. Therefore, they are only instrumentally good. Since utilitarianism determines the rightness of actions in terms of their tendency to promote the greatest happiness for the greatest number, it is considered to be a teleological ethical theory. ("Teleological" comes from the Greek word "telos," which means "end" or "goal.")

Act and Rule Utilitarianism

All utilitarians accept the principle of utility as the ultimate standard for determining the rightness of actions. But they divide into two groups over the matter of the application of the principle.

Act utilitarianism holds that the principle should be applied to particular acts in particular circumstances. *Rule utilitarianism* maintains that the principle should be used to test rules, and then the rules can be used to decide about the rightness of particular acts. Let's consider each of these views and see how they work in practice.

Suppose a physician delivers a child and finds that the child suffers from severe birth defects. The child's spine is open, the feet and legs are deformed, and there are indications of severe brain damage. What should be done? (We will leave open the question of who should decide.)

The act utilitarian holds that we must attempt to determine the consequences of the various actions that seem open to us. We might consider, for example, these possibilities: (1) give the child only the ordinary treatment that would be given to a normal child; (2) give the child special treatment for its problems; (3) give the child no treatment—allow it to die; (4) put the child to death in a painless way.

According to act utilitarianism, we must explore the potential results of each of these possibilities. We must realize, for example, that when given only ordinary treatment such a child, if it survives, will be worse off than if it had been given special treatment. Also, a child left alone and allowed to die is likely to suffer more pain than one killed by a lethal injection. We must also consider the family of the child and judge the effects that each of the possible actions may have on them. Then, too, we must take into account such matters as the potential happiness or suffering of the child (should it survive), the effect on physicians and nurses in killing the child or allowing it to die, and the cost measured in terms of happiness of long-term care for the child should it survive.

After these considerations, we should then choose the action that has the greatest utility. We should, in such cases, act in the way that will produce the most benefit for all concerned. Which of the possibilities we select will depend on the precise features of the situation: just how damaged the child is, just how good are its chances of living a normal life, just what is the character and disposition of the family, and so on. The great strength of act utilitarianism can be seen in such cases as this, for it invites us to deal with each case as a unique one. When the circumstances in another case are different, we might, without being inconsistent, choose another of the possible actions.

Act utilitarianism shows a sensitivity to specific cases, but it is not free from difficulties. Some philosophers have pointed out that there is no way we can be sure we have made the right choice of actions. We are sure to be ignorant of much relevant information. Besides, we can't know with much certainty what the results of our actions will really be. There is no way to be sure, for example, that even a severely defective infant will not recover enough to live a happier life than we might predict.

The act utilitarian can reply that acting morally doesn't mean being omniscient. We need to make a reasonable effort to get relevant information, and we can usually predict the probable consequences of our actions. Acting morally doesn't require any more than this.

Another objection to act utilitarianism is more serious than this one. Suppose a surgeon promises a patient that only he will perform an operation, yet the surgeon allows a resident to do the "opening" and "closing." All goes well and the patient never discovers that the promise was not kept. The consequences are exactly the same as they would have been had the surgeon kept his promise. From the point of view of act utilitarianism, there seems to be nothing wrong about the surgeon's failing to keep his promise. Yet our ordinary intuitions suggest that there is something wrong, for in promising, the surgeon placed himself under an obligation. Act utilitarianism seems to be unable to account for obligations in these kinds of cases. Rule utilitarianism, as we will see, can escape this difficulty.

Rule utilitarianism maintains that an action is right if it conforms to a rule of conduct that has been validated by the principle of utility. A rule like "Provide all necessary care for infants with birth defects" or "Put to death all infants with serious birth defects" would allow us to decide about the right course of action to follow in situations like that of our earlier example.

We do not have to go through the calculations involved in determining in each case whether a particular action will increase happiness. All that we have to establish is that always following a certain rule will, in general, result in a situation in which happiness is maximized and unhappiness minimized. The basic idea behind rule utilitarianism is that having a set of rules that are always observed produces the greatest social utility. That is, having everyone follow a rule in every case yields more happiness or pleasure for everybody in the long run.

An act utilitarian can agree that having rules may produce more social utility than not having them. But the act utilitarian insists that the rules be regarded as no more than general guides for action. Thus, for act utilitarianism it is perfectly legitimate to violate a rule when doing so will maximize happiness in that instance. By contrast, the rule utilitarian holds that the rules must never be violated—even though following the rules may produce more unhappiness than happiness in a particular case.

Rule utilitarianism can endorse rules like "Always keep your promises." Thus, unlike act utilitarianism, it can account for our intuition that in making a promise we are placing ourselves under an obligation. But the very fact that rule utilitarianism makes rules the basis for right actions presents difficulties for it. Clearly we should not keep a promise to meet someone for lunch when we have to choose between keeping the promise and rushing a heart-attack victim to the hospital. There always are circumstances in which it would seem wrong to follow a rule, even when we realize that *in general* greater happiness would result from following the rule all the time.

Of course rule utilitarians are not committed to endorsing general rules like "Always keep your promises." It is consistent with the view to offer quite specific rules. In fact, there seems to be no constraint on just how specific the rule might be. A rule utilitarian might, for example, offer a rule like "If an infant is born with an open spine, grossly deformed limbs, and brain damage; and if its parents have no other children and are in poor financial condition . . . , then the infant should receive no treatment." But when rules as specific as this are formulated, it becomes clear that the gap between act utilitarianism and rule utilitarianism is not great.

Utilitarianism in the Medical Context

We have already mentioned a few examples of how the principle of utility might be used to make moral decisions about medical matters. Since utilitarianism assigns no intrinsic rightness to actions or rules, we cannot say in the abstract what it would prohibit or command. We would have to construct an ethics of medicine to illustrate utilitarianism properly. We can, however, point out some of the features of utilitarianism that make it a useful theory in the medical context. (Most of the observations apply to both act and rule utilitarianism.)

Utilitarianism provides a means of testing and formulating policies. Institutions of all sizes, ranging from hospitals and research laboratories to national governments, generally take the responsibility of regulating, to some degree, medical practice and research. Usually regulation takes the form of policies expressed in laws, directives, guidelines, and codes of conduct. Such policies are intended both to ease the burden of decision making in individual cases and to encourage or discourage certain kinds of actions. The policies may be relatively minor ones like "Children under twelve are not allowed to visit patients." Or they may be major ones, such as a set of rules regulating experimentation with human subjects. But whether the policy is minor or major, what grounds are there for setting policies or for evaluating those already being followed?

Utilitarianism supplies an answer to both parts of this question. A policy is legitimate (or good) only when it promotes the greatest happiness for the greatest number of people. It must do this to an extent no less than alternate policies. Thus, to show that a policy is wrong and should be modified or replaced requires only showing that it fails this test. Similarly, in attempting to

formulate and decide upon a policy, the principle of utility tells us to consider the likely consequences of each alternative, then adopt the one that will maximize the general happiness.

In sum, utilitarianism does not require that we accept policies in any form—directives, laws, or whatever—as merely given or as intrinsically right. On the contrary, it requires us to test their worth and, in addition, stipulates the general way in which we can go about doing so.

In requiring that we decide about the rightness of actions or rules by considering their consequences, utilitarianism makes the task of evaluation easier in some respects. We need not attempt to fathom the motives of people nor try to determine whether they "really" attempted to act morally. Instead, we can ask if they acted in a reasonable and prudent manner on the basis of the information available to them and if they made a legitimate attempt to consider and weigh the likely consequences of their actions. An anesthesiologist who has not bothered to learn that a patient suffers from asthmatic spasms may not intend to harm his patient, but he may do so. So far as utilitarianism is concerned, his intention is irrelevant. By failing to acquire relevant information and causing unnecessary harm to his patient, he acted wrongly.

Utilitarianism also provides a relatively objective test that can be of considerable assistance as we make our own moral decisions. Rather than merely telling us to follow our conscience or do our duty, it enjoins us to make a reasonable effort to consider the likely results of alternatives, then to select the action that will produce the most beneficial result (the greatest total happiness) for all concerned. Granted that this test is a difficult one to put into practice and that we may always doubt whether we have calculated the results correctly, the test still seems to offer more than relatively vague injunctions about duty.

Finally, utilitarianism (including rule utilitarianism) allows us to recognize that there may be no actions of a general kind (for example, lying) that it is always right to do. Our actions (or rules for action) can be finely tailored to suit the complexities characteristic of moral decision-making in the medical context. Utilitarianism permits us to say that, in some circumstances, abortion is right, but in other circumstances it is wrong. Furthermore, this flexibility is achieved without arbitrariness, for the principle of utility always serves as the ruling standard.

These few suggestions make it clear that utilitarianism is a powerful and subtle ethical theory. It holds significant promise for resolving particular medical-moral problems and for developing policies to regulate medical practice and research.

Difficulties

Classical utilitarianism is open to a variety of objections. We shall concentrate on only one, however, for it seems to reveal a fatal flaw in the structure of the entire theory. This most serious of all objections to utilitarianism is that the principle of utility appears to justify the imposition of great suffering on a few people for the benefit of many people.

Certain kinds of human experimentation forcefully illustrate this possibility.

Suppose that an investigator is concerned with acquiring a better understanding of brain functions. He could learn a great deal by systematically destroying the brain of one person and carefully noting the results. Such a study would offer many more opportunities for increasing our knowledge of the brain than those studies that must use as subjects people who have damage to their brains in accidental ways. We may suppose that the experimenter chooses as his subject a person without education or training, without family or friends, who cannot be regarded as making much of a contribution to society. The subject will die from the experiment, but it is not unreasonable to suppose that the knowledge of the human brain gained from the experiment will improve the lives of countless numbers of people.

The principle of utility seems to make such experiments legitimate because the outcome is a greater amount of good than harm. One or a few have suffered immensely, but the many have profited to an extent that far outweighs that suffering.

Clearly what is missing from utilitarianism is a concept of *justice*. It cannot be right to increase the general happiness at the expense of one person or group. There must be some way of distributing happiness and unhappiness and avoiding exploitation.

Mill was aware that utilitarianism needs a principle of justice, but most contemporary philosophers do not believe that such a principle can be derived from the principle of utility. In their opinion, utilitarianism as an ethical theory suffers from a severe defect. Yet some philosophers, while acknowledging the defect, have still held that utilitarianism is the best substantive moral theory available.

Kant's Ethics

For utilitarianism, the rightness of an action depends upon its consequences. In stark contrast to this view is the ethical theory formulated by the German philosopher Immanuel Kant (1724–1804) in his book *Fundamental Principles of the Metaphysics of Morals*. For Kant, the consequences of an action are morally irrelevant. Rather, an action is right when it is in accordance with a rule that satisfies a principle he calls the "categorical imperative." Since this is the basic principle of Kant's ethics, we can begin our discussion with it.

The Categorical Imperative

If you decide to have an abortion and actually go through with it, it is possible to view your action as involving a rule. You can be thought of as endorsing a rule to the effect "Whenever I am in circumstances like these, then I shall have an abortion." Kant calls such a rule a "maxim." In his view, all reasoned and considered actions can be regarded as involving maxims.

The maxims in such cases are personal or subjective, but they can be thought of as being candidates for moral rules. If they pass the test imposed by the categorical imperative, then we can say that such actions are right. Furthermore, in passing the test, the maxims cease to be merely personal and subjective. They gain the status of objective rules of morality that hold for everyone.

Kant formulates the categorical imperative in this way: Act only on that maxim which you can will to be a universal law. Kant calls the principle "categorical" to distinguish it from "hypothetical" imperatives. These tell us what to do if we want to bring about certain consequences—such as happiness. A categorical imperative prescribes what we ought to do without reference to any consequences. The principle is an "imperative" because it is a command.

The test imposed on maxims by the categorical imperative is one of generalization or "universalizability." The central idea of the test is that a moral maxim is one that can be generalized to apply to all cases of the same kind. That is, you must be willing to see your rule adopted as a maxim by everyone who is in a situation similar to yours. You must be willing to see your maxim universalized, even though it may turn out on some other occasion to work to your disadvantage.

For a maxim to satisfy the categorical imperative it is not necessary that we be agreeable in some psychological sense to see it made into a universal law. Rather, the test is one that requires us to avoid inconsistency or conflict in what we will as a universal rule.

Suppose, for example, that I am a physician and I tell a patient that he has a serious illness, although I know that he doesn't. This may be to my immediate advantage, for the treatment and the supposed cure will increase my income and reputation. The maxim of my action might be phrased as, "Whenever I have a healthy patient, I shall lie to him and say that he has an illness."

Now suppose that the physician tries to generalize this maxim. In doing so, he will discover that what he is willing is the existence of a practice that has contradictory properties. It is as if he is saying, "Let there be a relationship of trust between physicians and patients, but let it not involve truth-telling." Since truth-telling is one of the features that make up trust, the physician is willing something contradictory. Thus, I can will my action in a particular case, but I can't will that my action be universal without generating a logical conflict.

Kant claims that such considerations show that it is always wrong to lie. Lying produces a contradiction in what we will. On one hand, we will that people believe what we say—that they accept our assurances and promises. But on the other hand, we will that people be free to give false assurances and make false promises. Lying thus produces a self-defeating situation, for when the maxim involved is generalized, the very framework required for lying collapses.

There are other maxims that we cannot will for subjective or psychological reasons having to do with our own self-interest. Consider a maxim like "Never show love or compassion for others." When universalized, this maxim does not result in the kind of self-defeating situation that lying does. Yet, we would not want to see it adopted as a universal law, for we may sometimes find ourselves in need of love or compassion. If we willed the maxim to be a universal law, then we would be depriving ourselves of something we desire. Our maxim made general would then run counter to our own best interest. Thus, there would be a conflict in what we will.

Another Formulation

According to Kant, there is only one categorical imperative, but it can be stated in three different ways. Each way is intended to reveal a special aspect of the principle. The second formulation, the only other we shall consider, can be stated in this way: Always act so as to treat humanity, either yourself or others, always as an end and never as only a means.

This version illustrates Kant's notion that every rational creature has a worth in itself. This worth is not conferred by being born into a society with a certain political structure, nor even by belonging to a certain biological species. The worth is inherent in the sheer possession of rationality. Rational creatures possess what Kant calls an "autonomous, self-legislating will." That is, they are able to consider the consequences of their actions, make rules for themselves, and direct their actions by those self-imposed rules. Thus, rationality confers upon everyone an intrinsic worth and dignity.

This formulation of the categorical imperative perhaps rules out some of the standards that are sometimes used to determine who is selected to receive certain medical resources (such as kidney machines) when the demand is greater than the supply. Standards that make a person's education, accomplishments, or social position relevant considerations seem contrary to this version of the categorical imperative. They violate the basic notion that each person has an inherent worth equal to that of any other person. Unlike dogs or horses, people cannot be judged on "show points."

For Kant, all of morality has its ultimate source in rationality. The categorical imperative, in any formulation, is an expression of rationality, and it is the principle that would be followed in practice by any purely rational being. Moral rules are not mere arbitrary conventions or subjective standards. They are objective truths that have their source in the rational nature of human beings.

Duty

Utilitarianism identifies the good with happiness or pleasure and makes the production of happiness the supreme principle of morality. But for Kant happiness is at best a conditional or qualified good. In his view, there is only one thing that can be said to be good in itself: a good will.

Will is what directs our actions and guides our conduct. But what makes a will a "good will"? Kant's answer is that a will becomes good when it acts purely for the sake of duty.

We act for the sake of duty (or from duty) when we act on maxims that satisfy the categorical imperative. This means, then, that it is the motive force behind our actions—the character of our will—that determines their moral character. Morality does not rest on results—such as the production of happiness—but neither does it rest on our feelings, impulses, or inclinations. An action is right, for Kant, only when it is done for the sake of duty.

Suppose that I decide to donate one of my kidneys for transplanting. If my hope is to gain approval or praise or even if I am moved by pity and a genuine wish to reduce suffering, and this is the only consideration behind my action, then the action is not morally right. By contrast, if I make the donation because I perceive it is my duty to do so, then my act is a moral one. In the first case, I may have acted *in accordance with duty* (done the same thing as duty would have required), but I did not act *from duty.*

This view of duty and its connection with morality comes close to capturing attitudes we frequently express. Consider a nurse who gives special care to a severely ill patient. Suppose you learned that the nurse was providing such extraordinary care only because he hoped that the patient or her family would reward him with a special bonus. Knowing this, it is doubtful that we would say that the nurse was performing a moral action. (Not that we would think the action was necessarily immoral.) We might even think that the nurse was being greedy or cynical.

Kant distinguishes between two types of duties: perfect and imperfect. (The distinction corresponds to the two ways in which maxims can be self-defeating when tested by the categorical imperative.) A *perfect* duty is one we must always observe, while an *imperfect* duty is one that we must observe only on some occasions. I have a perfect duty not to injure another person, but I have only an imperfect duty to show love and compassion. I must sometimes show it, but when I show it and which people I select to receive it are entirely up to me.

My duties determine what others can legitimately claim from me as a right. Some rights can be claimed as perfect rights, while others cannot. Everyone can demand of me that I do him or her no injury. But no one can tell me that I must make him or her the recipient of my love and compassion. In deciding how to discharge my imperfect duties, I am free to follow my emotions and inclinations.

For utilitarianism, an action is right when it produces what we take to be intrinsically valuable (happiness). Because actions are judged by their contributions towards achieving the goal of happiness, utilitarianism is a teleological theory. By contrast, Kant's ethics holds that it is duty alone that determines the rightness of an action. Such a theory is called "deontological," a word derived from the Greek word for "duty" or "obligation."

Kant's Ethics in the Medical Context

Four features of Kant's ethics are of particular importance in dealing with issues in medical treatment and research:

1. No matter what the consequences may be, it is always wrong to lie.

2. We must always treat people (including ourselves) as ends and not as means only.

3. An action is right when it satisfies the categorical imperative.

4. Perfect and imperfect duties give a basis for claims that certain rights should be recognized.

We can present only two brief examples of how these features can be instrumental in resolving ethical issues, but the possibilities are suggestive.

Our first application of Kant's ethics bears on medical research. The task of medical investigators would be easier if they did not have to tell hospitalized patients that they are going to be made part of a research program. Patients would then become subjects without even knowing it, and more often than not, the risk to them would be negligible. Even though no overt lying would be involved, on Kantian principles this procedure would be wrong. It would require treating people as a means only and not as an end.

Also, it would never be right for an experimenter to deceive a potential experimental subject. If an experimenter told a patient, "We would like to use this new drug on you because it might help you" and this was not really so, the experimenter would be performing a wrong action. Lying is always wrong.

Nor could the experimenter justify this deception by telling himself that the research is of such importance that it is legitimate to lie to the patient. On Kant's principles, good results never make an action morally right. Thus, for medical experimentation a patient must give voluntary and informed consent to become a subject. Otherwise, he or she is being deprived of autonomy and treated as a means only.

We may volunteer because we expect the research to bring benefits that are directly beneficial to us. But we may also volunteer even though no direct personal benefits can be expected. We may see participation in the research as an occasion for fulfilling an imperfect duty to improve human welfare.

But just as Kant's principles place restrictions on the researcher, they place limits on us as potential subjects. We have a duty to treat ourselves as ends and act so as to preserve our dignity and worth as humans. Therefore, it would not be right for us to volunteer for an experiment that threatened our lives or threatened to destroy our ability to function as autonomous rational beings without first satisfying ourselves that the experiment is legitimate and necessary.

A second application of Kant's ethics in a medical context might bear on the relationship between people as patients and those who accept responsibility for caring for them. A physician, for example, has only an imperfect duty to accept me as a patient. He has a duty to make use of his skills and talents to treat the sick, but I cannot legitimately insist on being the beneficiary. How he discharges his duty is his decision.

If, however, I am accepted as a patient, then I can make some legitimate claims. I can demand that nothing be done to cause me pointless harm because it is never right to injure a person. Furthermore, I can demand that I never be lied to or deceived. Suppose, for example, I am given a placebo (a harmless but inactive substance) and told that it is a powerful and effective medication. Or suppose that a biopsy shows that I have an inoperable form of cancer, but my physician tells me, "There's nothing seriously wrong with you." In both cases, the physician may suppose that he is deceiving me "for my own good": the placebo may be psychologically effective and make me feel better, and the lie about cancer may save me from useless worry. Yet by being deceived, I am being denied the dignity inherent in my status as a rational being. Lying is wrong, in general, but in such cases as these it also deprives me of my autonomy, of my power to make decisions and form my own opinions. As a result, such deception dehumanizes me.

As an autonomous rational being, a person is entitled to control over his or her own body. This means that medical procedures can be performed on me only with my permission. It would be wrong, for example, for my physician to have me held down and injected with a drug that I explicitly refused. It would be wrong even if the medication was needed for my "own good." I may voluntarily put myself under the care of a physician and submit to all that I am asked to submit to, but this is a decision that belongs to me alone.

In exercising control over my body, however, I also have a duty to myself. Suppose, for example, that I refuse to allow surgery to be performed on me, although I have been told it is necessary to preserve my life. Since I have a duty to preserve my life, as does every person, my refusal is morally unjustifiable. Even here, however, it is not legitimate for others to force me to "do my duty." In fact, in Kantian ethics it is impossible to force another to do his or her duty because it is not the action but the maxim involved that determines whether or not one's duty has been done.

It is obvious even from our sketchy examples that Kantian ethics is a fruitful source of principles and ideas for working out some of the specific moral difficulties of medical experimentation and practice. The absolute requirements imposed by the categorical imperative can be a source of strength and even of comfort. With utilitarianism, we must weigh alternative courses of actions by anticipating their consequences and deciding whether what we are considering doing can be justified by those results. Kant's ethics saves us from this kind of doubt and indecision: We know we must never lie, no matter what good may come of it. Furthermore, the lack of a principle of justice that is the most severe defect of utilitarianism is met by Kant's categorical imperative. When every person is to be treated as an end and never as only a means, the possibility of legitimately exploiting some for the benefit of others is wholly eliminated.

Difficulties

Kant's ethical theory is complex and controversial. It has problems of a theoretical sort that manifest themselves in practice and lead us to doubt whether the absolute rules determined by the categorical imperative can always provide a straightforward solution to our moral difficulties. We will limit ourselves to discussing just three problem areas.

First, Kant's principles supply no clear way of resolving cases in which there is a conflict of duties. I have a duty to keep my promises, and I also have a duty to help those in need. Suppose, then, that I am a physician and I have promised a colleague to attend a staff conference. Right before the conference starts, I am talking with a patient who lapses into an insulin coma. If I get involved in treating the patient, I'll have to break my promise to attend the conference. What should I do?

The answer is obvious: I should treat the patient. All our moral intuitions tell us this is what we should do. But Kant does not provide us with a clear way of answering this question. He does not rank duties and say that some take precedence over others. Rather, his view seems to be that promises should never be broken—even when the promise concerns a relatively trivial matter and the consequences of keeping it are disastrous.

Second, there are serious difficulties with the categorical imperative as a test of maxims. One of the problems concerns the subjective aspect of whether I can will a maxim to be a universal law. If I will "Never help people in need," I may live to regret it. I may find myself in need, and the maxim would work against my best interest. But suppose I am just willing to take a chance that I will never be in need? If I am willing, then I don't have to regard it as a duty to help those now in need. The categorical imperative does not seem to establish that helping others is a necessary duty, and it may fail to establish duties in all other cases involving maxims that supposedly cannot be willed for subjective reasons.

Another difficulty with the categorical imperative arises because we are free to choose how we formulate a maxim for testing. In all likelihood none of us would approve a maxim such as "Lie when it is convenient for you." But what about one like "Lie when telling the truth is likely to cause harm to another?" We would be more inclined to make this a universal law. Now consider the maxim "Whenever a physician has good reason to believe that a patient's life will be seriously threatened if he is told the truth about his condition, then the physician should lie." Virtually everyone would be willing to see this made into a universal law.

Yet these three maxims are ones that can apply to the same situation. Since Kant does not tell us how to formulate our maxims, it is clear that we can act virtually any way we choose if we are willing to describe the situation in specific detail. We might be willing to have everyone act just as we are inclined to act whenever they find themselves in *exactly* this kind of situation. The categorical imperative, then, does not seem to solve our moral problems quite as neatly as it first appears to.

A final problem area lies in Kant's notion that we have duties to rational beings or persons. Ordinarily, we have little difficulty with this commitment to persons, yet there are circumstances, particularly in the medical context, in which serious problems arise. Consider, for example, a fetus developing in its mother's womb. Is the fetus to be considered a person? The way this question is answered makes all the difference in deciding about the rightness or wrongness of abortion.

A similar difficulty is present when we consider how we are to deal with an infant with serious birth defects. Is it our duty to care for this infant and do all we can to see that it lives? If the infant is not a person, then perhaps we do not owe him the sort of treatment it would be our duty to provide a similarly afflicted adult. It's clear from these two cases that the notion of a person must be developed and clarified. Otherwise, there will be many instances in which Kant's ethics cannot be applied with the kind of definiteness and certainty he believed possible.

Another difficulty connected with Kant's concept of a rational person concerns the notion of an "autonomous self-regulating will." Under what conditions can we assume that an individual possesses such a will? Does a child, a mentally retarded person, or someone in prison? Without such a will, then in

Kant's view such an individual could not legitimately consent to be the subject of an experiment or even give permission for necessary medical treatment. This is another notion very much in need of development before Kant's principles can be relied on to resolve ethical questions in medicine.

The difficulties that we have discussed are crucial ones that require serious consideration. This does not mean, of course, that they cannot be resolved or that because of them Kant's theory is worthless. As with utilitarianism, there are some philosophers that believe the theory is the best available, despite its shortcomings. That it captures many of our intuitive beliefs about what is right (not to lie, to treat people with dignity, to act benevolently) and supplies us with a test for determining our duties (the categorical imperative) recommends it strongly as an ethical theory.

Ross's Ethics

The English philosopher W. D. Ross (b. 1877) presented an ethical theory in his book *The Right and the Good* that can be seen as an attempt to incorporate aspects of utilitarianism with aspects of Kantianism. Ross rejected entirely the utilitarian notion that an action is made right by its consequences, but he was also troubled by Kant's absolute rules. He saw that not only do such rules fail to show sensitivity to the complexities of actual situations, but there are also cases in which they conflict with one another. Like Kant, Ross is a deontologist, but with an important difference. Ross believes it is necessary to consider consequences in making a moral choice, even though he believes that it is not the results of an action that make it right.

Moral Properties and Rules

For Ross there is an unbridgeable distinction between moral and nonmoral properties. There are only two moral properties—rightness and goodness—and these cannot be replaced by, or explained in terms of, other properties. Thus, to say that an action is "right" is not at all the same as saying that it "causes pleasure" or "increases happiness," as utilitarianism claims.

At the same time, however, Ross does not deny that there is a connection between moral properties and nonmoral ones. What he denies is the possibility of establishing an identity between them. Thus, it may be right to relieve the suffering of someone, but right is not identical with relieving suffering. (More exactly put, the rightness of the action is not identical with the action's being a case of relieving suffering.)

Ross also makes clear that we must often know many nonmoral facts about a situation before we can legitimately make a moral judgment. If I see a physician injecting someone, I cannot say whether she is acting rightly without determining what she is injecting, why she is doing it, and so on. Thus, rightness is a property that is in a certain way dependent on the nonmoral properties that characterize a situation. I cannot determine whether the physician is doing the right thing or the wrong thing until I determine what the nonmoral properties are.

Ross believes that there are cases in which we have no genuine doubt about whether the property of rightness or goodness is present. The world abounds with examples of cruelty, lying, and selfishness, and in these cases we are immediately aware of the absence of rightness or goodness. But the world also abounds with examples of compassion, reliability, and generosity in which rightness and goodness are clearly present. Ross claims that our experience with such cases puts us in a position to come to know rightness and goodness with the same degree of certainty that exists when we grasp the mathematical truth that a triangle has three angles.

Furthermore, according to Ross, our experience of many individual cases puts us in a position to recognize the validity of a general statement like "It is wrong to cause needless pain." We come to see such rules in cases in much the same way in which we might come to be able to recognize the letter A after having seen it written or printed in a variety of handwritings or typefaces.

Thus, our moral intuitions can supply us with moral rules of a general kind. But Ross refuses to acknowledge these rules as absolute. For him they can serve only as guides to assist us in deciding what we should do. Ultimately, in any particular case we must rely upon our perception of what is right and good.

Thus, even with rules, we may not recognize what the right thing to do is in a given situation. We recognize, he suggests, that there is always *some* right thing to do, but what it is may be far from obvious to us. In fact, doubt about what is the right way of acting may arise just because we have rules to guide us. We become aware of the fact that there are several courses of action that we might choose, and all of them seem to be right.

Consider the problem of whether to lie to a terminally ill patient about her condition. Let us suppose that if we lie to her, we can avoid causing her at least some useless anguish. But then aren't we violating her trust in us to act morally and to speak the truth?

In such cases, we seem to have a conflict in our duties. It is because of such familiar kinds of conflicts that Ross rejects the possibility of getting absolute moral rules like "Always tell the truth" and "Always eliminate needless suffering." In cases like the one above, we cannot hold that both rules are absolute without contradicting ourselves. Ross says that we have to recognize that every rule has exceptions and must in some situations be set aside.

Actual Duties and Prima Facie Duties

If rules like "Always tell the truth" cannot be absolute, then what status can they have? When our rules come into conflict in particular situations, how are we to decide which rule applies? Ross answers this question by making use of a distinction between what is actually right and what is only prima facie right. Since we have a duty to do what is right, this distinction can be expressed as one between *actual duty* and *prima facie duty*.

An actual duty is simply what my real duty is in a situation. It is the action that, out of the various possibilities, I ought to perform. More often than not, however, I may not know what my actual duty is. In fact, for Ross, the whole problem of ethics might be said to be the problem of knowing what my actual duty is in any given situation.

"Prima facie" means "at first sight" or "on the surface." Accordingly, a prima facie duty is one that dictates what I should do when other relevant factors aren't considered. It often happens that in some given circumstance I have several prima facie duties. Take our earlier example of the terminally ill patient who asks, "Am I going to die?" I have a prima facie duty to tell her the truth, but I also have a prima facie duty to give her comfort and spare her needless suffering.

According to Ross, there is a way that we can state our moral rules so that they are absolute. We can do this by presenting them as rules of prima facie duty. Thus, I have a prima facie duty not to lie in every case in which lying is possible. Telling the truth, then, is something I ought always to try to do. Similarly, I have a prima facie duty to prevent the needless suffering of others. All things being equal, this is what I ought to try to do.

We have considered only a few simple examples of prima facie duties, but Ross is more thorough and systematic than our examples might suggest. He offers a list of prima facie duties that he considers to be binding on all moral agents. Here they are in summary form:

1. Duties of Fidelity: telling the truth, keeping actual and implicit promises, and not representing fiction as history

2. Duties of Reparation: righting the wrongs we have done to others

3. Duties of Gratitude: recognizing the services others have done for us

4. Duties of Justice: preventing a distribution of pleasure or happiness that is not in keeping with the merit of the people involved

5. Duties of Beneficence: helping to better the condition of others with respect to virtue, intelligence, or pleasure

6. Duties of Self-Improvement: bettering ourselves with respect to virtue or intelligence

7. The Duty Not to Injure Others

Ross doesn't claim that this is a complete list of the prima facie duties that we recognize. However, he does believe that the duties on the list are all ones that we acknowledge and are willing to accept as true without argument. He believes that if we simply reflect on these prima facie duties we will see that they are true. As he puts the matter:

> I . . . am claiming that we *know* them to be true. To me it seems as self-evident as anything could be, that to make a promise, for instance, is to create a moral claim on us in someone else. Many readers will perhaps say that they do *not* know this to be true. If so I certainly cannot prove it to them. I can only ask them to reflect again, in the hope that they will ultimately agree that they also know it to be true.

Notice that Ross explicitly rejects the possibility of providing us with reasons or arguments to convince us to accept his list of prima facie duties. We are merely invited to reflect on certain kinds of cases, like keeping promises, and Ross is convinced that this reflection will bring us to accept his claim that these are true duties. Ross, like other intuitionists, tries to get us to agree with his moral perceptions in much the same way as we might try to get people to agree with us about our color perceptions. We might, for example, show a paint sample to a friend and say, "Don't you think that looks blue? It does to me. Think about it for a minute."

We introduced the distinction between actual and prima facie duties to deal with those situations in which there are conflicts. The problem, as we can now state it, is this: What are we to do in a situation in which we recognize more than one prima facie duty and it is not possible for us to act in a way that will fulfill them all? We know, of course, that we should act in a way that satisfies our actual duty. But that is just our problem. What, after all, is our actual duty when our prima facie duties are in conflict?

Ross offers us two principles to deal with cases of conflicting duty. The first principle is designed to handle situations in which just two prima facie duties are in conflict. This is the principle: That act is one's duty which is in accord with the more stringent prima facie obligation.

The second principle is intended to deal with cases in which several prima facie duties are in conflict: That act is one's duty which has the greatest balance of prima facie rightness over prima facie wrongness.

Unfortunately, both these principles present problems in application. Ross does not tell us how we are to determine when an obligation is "more stringent" than another. Nor does he give us a rule for determining the "balance" of prima facie rightness over wrongness. Ultimately, according to Ross, we must simply rely upon our perceptions of the situation. There is no automatic or mechanical procedure that can be followed. If we learn the facts in the case, consider the consequences of our possible actions, and reflect on our prima facie duties, we should be able to arrive at a conclusion as to the best course of action—in Ross's view something that we as moral agents must and can do.

To return to specific cases, perhaps there is no direct way to answer the abstract question, Is the duty not to lie to a patient "more stringent" than the duty not to cause needless suffering? So much depends on the character and condition of the individual patient that an abstract determination of our duty based on "balance" or "stringency" is useless. However, knowing the patient, we should be able to perceive what the right course of action is.

Also, Ross believes that there are situations in which there are no particular difficulties about resolving the conflict between prima facie duties. For example, most of us would agree that if we can save someone from serious injury by lying, then we have more of an obligation to save someone from injury than we do to tell the truth.

Ross's Ethics in the Medical Context

Ross's moral rules are not absolute in the sense that Kant's are; consequently, as with utilitarianism, it is not possible to say in the abstract what would necessarily be prohibited or commanded. We can discuss in general, however, the advantages that Ross's theory brings to medical-moral issues. We shall mention only two for illustration.

First and most important is Ross's list of prima facie duties. The list of duties can serve an important function in the moral education of physicians, researchers, and other medical personnel. The list encourages each person responsible for patient care to reflect on the prima facie obligations that he or she has towards those people and to set aside one of those obligations only when morally certain that another obligation takes precedence.

The specific duties imposed in a prima facie way are numerous and can be expressed in terms relevant to the medical context: do not injure patients; do not distribute scarce resources in a way that fails to recognize individual worth; do not lie to patients; show patients kindness and understanding; educate patients in ways useful to them; do not hold out false hopes to patients, and so on.

Second, like utilitarianism, Ross's ethics encourages us to show sensitivity to the unique features of situations before acting. Like Kant's ethics, however, Ross's also insists that we look at the world from a particular kind of moral perspective. In arriving at decisions about what is right, we must learn the facts of the case and explore the possible consequences of our actions. Ultimately, however, we must guide our actions by attempting to do what is right, rather than by what is useful, or by what will produce happiness, or anything of the kind.

Since no action is ever justified in terms of its results, we cannot say "It's right to trick this person into becoming a research subject because the experiment may benefit thousands." Yet, we cannot say that it is always wrong for a researcher to trick a person into volunteering. Whether it is right or wrong depends on the circumstances and, at bottom, on the moral perceptions of the experimenter.

Fundamentally, then, Ross's ethics offers us the possibility of gaining the advantages of utilitarianism without ignoring the fact that there seem to be duties with an undeniable moral force behind them that cannot be accounted for by utilitarianism. Ross's ethics accommodates not only our intuitions that certain actions should be performed just because they are right but also our inclinations to pay attention to the results of actions and not just the motives behind them.

Difficulties

The advantages Ross's ethics offers over both utilitarianism and Kantianism are offset by two serious difficulties.

To begin, it simply seems false that we all grasp the same moral principles. We are well aware of the fact that beliefs that people have about what is right and about what their duties are result from the kind of education that they have had. The ability to perceive what is good or right does not appear to be something programmed into our genes. Ross does say that the principles are ones that are the convictions of "the moral consciousness of the best people." In any ordinary sense of "best," there is reason to say that such people don't always agree on moral principles. If "best" means "morally best," then Ross is close to being circular: the best people are those who acknowledge the same prima facie obligations, and those who recognize the same prima facie obligations are the best people.

Further, Ross's theory seems to be false to the facts of moral disagreements. When we disagree with someone about an ethical matter, we consider reasons for and against some position. Sometimes the disagreement results in agreement. But on Ross's view this should not be possible: I simply have my perceptions and you have yours. There seems to be no ground for discussion or resolution. When a decision is reached, it seems it can only be the arbitrary result of following one person's perceptions rather than the other's.

Few contemporary philosophers would be willing to endorse Ross's ethical theory without serious qualifications. The need for a special kind of moral perception (or "intuition") marks the theory as unacceptable for most philosophers. Yet, many would acknowledge that the theory has great value in illuminating such aspects of our moral experience as reaching decisions when there are conflicting obligations. Furthermore, at least some would acknowledge Ross's prima facie duties as constituting an adequate set of moral principles.

Rawls's Theory of Justice

In 1971 the Harvard philosopher John Rawls published a book called *A Theory of Justice.* The work has attracted a considerable amount of attention and has been described by some as the most important book in moral and social philosophy of this century.

One commentator, R. P. Wolfe, points out that Rawls attempts to develop a theory that combines the strengths of utilitarianism with those of the deontological position of Kant and Ross, while avoiding the weaknesses of each view. Utilitarianism claims outright that happiness is fundamental and suggests a direct procedure for answering ethical-social questions. But it is flawed by its lack of a principle of justice. Kant and Ross make rightness a fundamental moral notion and stress the ultimate dignity of human beings. Yet neither provides a workable method for solving problems of social morality. Clearly, Rawls's theory promises much if he can succeed in uniting the two ethical traditions we have discussed.

The Original Position and the Principles of Justice

Rawls makes use of a hypothetical device he calls "the original position" as a way of approaching the problem of establishing principles of justice. Suppose we imagine a group of people like those who make up our society. These people display the ordinary range of intelligence, talents, ambitions, convictions, and social and economic advantages. They include both sexes and members of various racial and ethnic groups.

Furthermore, suppose this group is placed behind what Rawls calls "a veil of ignorance." Assume that each person is made ignorant of his or her sex, race, natural endowments, social position, economic condition, and so on. Yet let the people remain self-interested and rational.

Rawls argues that the principles of justice chosen by such a group will be just if the conditions under which they are selected and the procedures for agreeing on them are fair. The original position, with its veil of ignorance, characterizes a state in which alternative notions of justice can be discussed freely by all. Since the ignorance of the participants means they cannot try to seek advantages for themselves, it guarantees that their eventual choice will be fair. Since the participants are assumed to be rational, they will be persuaded by the same reasons and arguments. These features of the original position lead Rawls to characterize his view as "justice as fairness."

We might imagine that some people in the original position would gamble and argue for principles that would introduce gross inequalities in their society. For example, some might argue for slavery. If these people should turn out to be masters after the veil of ignorance is stripped away, they would gain immensely. But if they turn out to be slaves, then they would lose immensely. However, since the veil of ignorance keeps them from knowing their actual positions in society, it would not be rational for them to endorse a principle that might condemn them to the bottom of the social order.

Given the uncertainties of the original situation, there is a better strategy that these rational people would choose. In the economic discipline known as game theory, this strategy is called "maximin." When we choose in uncertain situations, this strategy directs us to select from the alternatives the one whose worst possible outcome is better than the worst possible outcome of the other alternatives. (If you don't know whether you're going to be a slave, you shouldn't approve a set of principles that permits slavery when you have other options.)

Acting in accordance with this strategy, Rawls argues that people in the original position would agree on the following two principles of justice:

1. Each person is to have an equal right to the most extensive total system of equal basic liberties compatible with a similar system of liberty for all.

2. Social and economic inequalities are to be arranged so that they are both: (a) to the greatest benefit of the least advantaged . . . , and (b) attached to offices and positions open to all under conditions of fair equality of opportunity.

For Rawls, these two principles are taken to govern the distribution of all social goods: liberty, property, wealth, and social privilege. The first principle has priority. It guarantees a system of equal liberty for all. Furthermore, because of its priority, it explicitly prohibits the bartering away of liberty for social or economic benefits. (A person cannot sell the right to vote, for example.)

The second principle governs the distribution of social goods other than liberty. According to Rawls, it is simply a fact about the world that some people are born with greater wealth than others or into advantageous social positions. *In themselves* such differences among people are neither just nor unjust. But in a just society such differences can be tolerated only when they can be shown to benefit everyone and to benefit, in particular, those who have the fewest advantages. A just society is not one in which everyone is equal, but it is one in which inequalities must be demonstrated to be legitimate. Furthermore, there must be a genuine opportunity for acquiring membership in a group that enjoys special benefits. Those not qualified to enter medical schools because of past discrimination in education, for example, can claim a right for special preparation to qualify them.

Rawls argues that these two principles are ones that are required to establish a just society. Furthermore, in distributing liberty and social goods, the principles guarantee the worth and self-respect of the individual. People are free to pursue their own conception of the good and fashion their own lives. Ultimately, the only constraints placed on them as members of society are those expressed in the principles of justice.

Yet Rawls also acknowledges that those in the original position would recognize that we have duties both to ourselves and to others. They would, for example, want to take measures to see that their interests are protected if they should meet with disabling accidents, become seriously mentally disturbed, and so on. Thus, Rawls approves a form of paternalism: others should act for us when we are unable to act for ourselves. When our preferences are known to them, those acting for us should attempt to follow what we would wish. Otherwise, they should act for us as they would act for themselves if they were viewing our situation from the standpoint of the original position. Paternalism is thus a duty to ourselves that would be recognized by those in the original position.

Rawls is also aware of the need for principles that bind and guide individuals as moral decision makers. He claims that those in the original position would reach agreement on principles for such notions as fairness in our dealings with others, fidelity, respect for persons, and beneficence. From these principles we gain some of our obligations to one another.

But, Rawls claims, there are also "natural duties" that would be recognized by those in the original position. Among those Rawls mentions are (1) the duty of justice—supporting and complying with just institutions; (2) the duty of helping others in need or jeopardy; (3) the duty not to harm or injure another; (4) the duty to keep our promises.

For the most part, these are duties that hold between or among people. They are only some of the duties that would be offered by those in the original position as unconditional duties. Thus, Rawls in effect endorses virtually the same duties as those that Ross presents as prima facie duties. Rawls realizes that the problem of conflicts of duty was left unsolved by Ross and so perceives the need for assigning priorities to duties—ranking them as higher and lower. Rawls believes that a full system of principles worked out from the original position would include rules for ranking duties. Rawls's primary concern, however, is with justice in social institutions, and he does not attempt to establish any rules for ranking.

Rawls's Theory of Justice in the Medical Context

Rawls's "natural duties" are virtually the same as Ross's prima facie duties. Consequently, most of what we said earlier about prima facie duties and moral decision making applies to Rawls.

Rawls endorses the legitimacy of paternalism although he does not attempt to specify detailed principles to justify individual cases. He does tell us that we

should consider the preferences of others when they are known to us and when we are in a situation in which we must act for them because they are unable to act for themselves. For example, suppose we know that a person approves of electro-convulsive therapy (shock treatments or ECT) for the treatment of severe depression. If that person should become so depressed as to be unable to reach a decision about his own treatment, then we would be justified in seeing to it that he received ECT.

To take a similar case, suppose you are a surgeon and have a patient who has expressed to you her wish to avoid numerous operations that may prolong her life six months or so but will ultimately be unable to restore her to health. If in operating you learned that she has a form of uterine cancer that had spread through her lower extremities and in your best judgment nothing could be done to restore her to health, then it would be your duty to her to allow her to die as she chooses. Repeated operations would be contrary to her concept of her own good.

The most important question to explore in connection with Rawls is how the two principles of justice might apply to the social institutions and practices that involve medical care and research.

Most obviously, Rawls's principles repair utilitarianism's flaw with respect to human experimentation. It would never be right, on Rawls's view, to exploit one group of people or even one person for the benefit of others. Thus, experiments in which people are forced to be subjects or are tricked into participating are ruled out. They involve a violation of basic liberties of individuals and of the absolute respect for persons that the principles of justice require. A person has a right to decide what risks she is willing to take with her own life and health. Thus, voluntary consent is required before someone can legitimately become a research subject. However, society might decide to reward research volunteers with money, honors, or social privileges to encourage participation in research, and this is a perfectly legitimate practice so long as it brings benefits (ideally) to everyone and the possibility of gaining the rewards of participation is open to all.

In the area of allocation of social resources in the training of medical personnel (physicians, nurses, therapists, and so on), one may conclude that such investments are justified only if the withdrawal of the support would work to the disadvantage of those already most disadvantaged. Public money may be spent in the form of scholarships and institutional grants to educate personnel, who may then derive great social and economic benefits from their education. But for Rawls the inequality that is produced is not necessarily unjust. Society can invest its resources in this way if it brings benefits to those most in need of them.

The implication of this position seems to be that everyone is entitled to health care. Whether a person can pay for such care or not, the inequalities of the health-care system can be justified only if those in most need can benefit from them. In effect, Rawls's principles seem to call for a reform in our system.

Rawls's principles, particularly the second, can also be used to restrict access to certain kinds of health care. In general, individuals may spend their money any way they wish to seek their notions of what is good. Thus, if someone wants cosmetic surgery to change the shape of his chin and has the money to pay a surgeon, then he may have it done. But if medical facilities or personnel should become overburdened and unable to provide needed care for the more seriously afflicted, then the society would be obligated to forbid cosmetic surgery. By doing this it would then increase the net access to needed health care by all members of society. The rich wanting cosmetic surgery would not be permitted to exploit the poor needing basic health care.

These are just a few of the possible implications that Rawls's theory has for medical research and practice. It seems likely that more and more applications of the theory will be worked out in detail in the future.

Difficulties

Rawls's theory is currently the subject of much discussion in philosophy. The debate is often highly technical, and a great number of objections have been raised. At present, however, there are no objections that would be acknowledged as legitimate by all critics. Rather than attempt to summarize the debate, we shall simply point to two aspects of Rawls's theory that have been acknowledged as difficulties.

One criticism is connected with the original position and its veil of ignorance. Rawls does not permit those in the original position to know anything of their own purposes, plans, or interests—of their conception of the good. They do not know whether they prefer tennis to Tennyson, pleasures of the mind over pleasures of the body. They are allowed to consider only those goods—self-respect, wealth, social position—that Rawls puts before them. Thus, critics have said, Rawls has excluded morally-relevant knowledge. It is impossible to see how people could agree on principles to regulate their lives when they are so ignorant of their desires and purposes. Rawls seems to have biased the original position in his favor, and this calls into question his claim that the original position is a fair and reasonable way of arriving at principles of justice.

A second criticism focuses on whether Rawls's theory is really as different from utilitarianism as it appears to be. Rawls's theory may well permit inequalities of treatment under certain conditions in the same way as the principle of utility permits them. The principles of justice that were stated earlier apply, Rawls says, only when liberty can be effectively established and maintained. Rawls is very unclear about when a situation may be regarded as one of this kind. When it is not, his principles of justice are ones of a "general conception." Under this conception, liberties of individuals can be restricted, provided that the restrictions are for the benefit of all. It is possible to imagine, then, circumstances in which we might force individuals to become experimental subjects both for their own benefit and for that of others. We might, for example, require that all cigarette smokers participate in experiments intended to acquire knowledge about lung and heart damage. Since everyone would benefit, directly or indirectly, from such knowledge, forcing their participation would be legitimate. Thus, under the general conception of justice, the difference between

Rawls's principles and the principle of utility may, in practice, become vanishingly small.

Natural Law Ethics and Moral Theology

The general view that moral principles are objective truths that can be discovered in the nature of things by reason and reflection is called "natural law theory." The basic idea of the theory was expressed succinctly by Cicero (106–43 B.C.): "Law is the highest reason, implanted in Nature, which commands what ought to be done and forbids the opposite. This reason, when firmly fixed and fully developed in the human mind, is Law."

Natural law theory has been immensely influential on the development of moral and political theories. With the possible exception of utilitarianism, all the ethical theories we have discussed can be seen as indebted to the natural law tradition. The reliance upon reason as a means of settling upon or establishing ethical principles and the value attributed to human freedom and dignity by virtue of human rationality are just two of the threads of the natural law tradition that are woven into the particular theories we have discussed.

But our major concern here is neither with natural law theory in general nor with its history in ethical formulations. Rather, we shall focus on some of the aspects of natural law theory as interpreted in the moral theology of Roman Catholicism. More than any other group, the Roman Catholic Church has devoted careful attention to the moral issues in medicine. Its doctrines, based on its interpretation of natural law, have exerted great influence on our laws, institutions, and practices. Thus, whether one accepts the doctrines or not, it is important to understand them.

Purposes, Reason, and the Moral Law as Interpreted by Roman Catholicism

The natural law theory of Roman Catholicism was given its most influential formulation in the thirteenth century by St. Thomas Aquinas (1225–1274). Contemporary versions of the theory are mostly elaborations and interpretations of Aquinas's basic statement. Thus, an understanding of Aquinas's views is important for grasping the philosophical principles that underlie the Catholic position on such issues as abortion.

Aquinas was writing at a time in which a great number of the texts of Aristotle (384–322 B.C.) were becoming available in the West, and Aquinas's philosophical theories incorporated many of Aristotle's principles. A fundamental notion borrowed by Aquinas is the view that the universe is organized in a teleological way. That is, the universe is regarded as being structured in such a way that all things in it have a goal or purpose. Thus, when conditions are right, a tadpole will develop into a frog. In its growth and change, the tadpole is following "the law of its nature." It is achieving its goal.

Humans have a material nature, just as a tadpole does, and in their own growth and development they too follow a law of their material nature. But

Aquinas stresses that humans also possess a trait that no other creature possesses—reason. Thus, the full development of human potentialities—the fulfillment of human purpose—requires that we follow the direction of the law of reason, as well as being subjected to the laws of material human nature.

For Aquinas, reason is the source of the moral law. Reason is practical in its operation, for it directs our actions so that we can bring about certain results. In giving us directions, reason imposes obligations on us, the obligations to bring about the results that it specifies. But Aquinas says that reason cannot just arbitrarily set goals for us. Reason directs us towards our good as the goal of our action, and what that good is, is discoverable within our nature. Thus, in its operation reason recognizes the basic principle: "Good is to be done and evil avoided."

But this principle is purely formal or empty of content. To make it a practical principle we must consider what the human good is. According to Aquinas, the human good is that which is suitable or proper to human nature. It is what is "built into" human nature in the way that, in a sense, a frog is already "built into" a tadpole. Thus, the good is that to which we are directed by our natural inclinations as both physical and rational creatures.

Like other creatures, we have a natural inclination to preserve our lives; consequently, reason imposes on us an obligation to care for our health, not to kill ourselves, and not to put ourselves in positions in which we might be killed. We realize through reason that others have a rational nature like ours, and we see that we are bound to treat them with the same dignity and respect that we accord ourselves. Furthermore, when we see that humans require a society to make their full development possible, we realize that we have an obligation to support laws and practices that make society possible.

Thus, for example, as we have a natural inclination to propagate our species (viewed as a "natural" good), reason places on us an obligation not to thwart or pervert this inclination. As a consequence, to fulfill this obligation within society, reason supports the institution of marriage.

Reason also finds in our nature grounds for procedural principles. For example, because everyone has an inclination to preserve his life and well-being, no one should be forced to testify against himself. Similarly, because all individuals are self-interested, no one should be permitted to be a judge in his own case.

Physical inclinations, under the direction of reason, point us towards our natural good. But, according to Aquinas, reason itself can also be a source of inclinations. For example, Aquinas says that reason is the source of our natural inclination to seek the truth, particularly the truth about the existence and nature of God.

Just from the few examples we have considered, it should be clear how Aquinas believed it was possible to discover in human nature natural goods. Relying upon these as goals or purposes to be achieved, reason would then work out the practical way of achieving them. Thus, through the subtle application of reason, it should be possible to establish a body of moral principles and rules. These are the doctrines of natural law.

Because natural law is founded on human nature, which is regarded as unchangeable, Aquinas regards natural law itself as unchangeable. Moreover, it is seen as the same for all people, at all times, and in all societies. Even those without knowledge of God can, through the operation of reason, recognize their natural obligations.

For Aquinas and for Roman Catholicism, this view of natural law is just one aspect of a broader theological framework. The teleological organization of the universe is attributed to the planning of a creator—goals or purposes are or-dained by God. Furthermore, although natural law is discoverable in the uni-verse, its ultimate source is divine wisdom and God's eternal law. Everyone who is rational is capable of grasping natural law. But because passions and irrational inclinations may corrupt human nature and because some people lack the abilities or time to work out the demands of natural law, God also chose to reveal our duties to us in explicit ways. The major source of revelation, of course, is taken to be the Biblical scriptures.

Natural law, scriptural revelation, the interpretation of the scriptures by the Church, Church tradition, and the teachings of the Church are regarded in Roman Catholicism as the sources of moral ideals and principles. By guiding one's life by them, one can develop the rational and moral part of one's nature and move towards the goal of achieving the sort of perfection that is suitable for humans.

This general moral-theological point of view is the source for particular Roman Catholic doctrines that have special relevance to medicine. We shall consider just two of the most important principles.

The principle of double effect. A particular kind of moral conflict arises when we are faced with a situation in which the performance of an action will produce both good and bad effects. On the basis of the good effect, it seems it is our duty to perform the action; but on the basis of the bad effect, it seems our duty not to perform it.

Let's assume that the death of a fetus is in itself a bad effect and consider a case like the following: A woman who is three months pregnant is found to have a cancerous uterus. If the woman's life is to be saved, the uterus must be removed at once. But if the uterus is removed, then the life of the unborn child will be lost. Should the operation be performed?

The principle of double effect is intended to help in the resolution of these kinds of conflicts. Basically, the principle holds that such an action should be performed only if the intention is to bring about the good effect and the bad effect will be an unintended or indirect consequence. More specifically, four conditions must be satisfied:

1. The action itself must be morally indifferent or morally good.

2. The bad effect must not be the means by which the good effect is achieved.

3. The motive must be the achievement of the good effect only.

4. The good effect must be at least equivalent in importance to the bad effect.

Are these conditions satisfied in the case that we mentioned? The operation itself, if this is considered to be the action, is at least morally indifferent. That is, in itself it is neither good nor bad. That takes care of the first condition. If the mother's life is to be saved, it will not be *by means of* killing the fetus. It will be by means of removing the cancerous uterus. Thus, the second condition is met. The motive of the surgeon, we may suppose, is not the death of the fetus but saving the life of the woman. If so, then the third condition is satisfied. Finally, since two lives are at stake, the good effect (saving the life of the woman) is at least equal to the bad effect (the death of the fetus). The fourth condition is thus met. Under ordinary conditions, then, these conditions would be considered satisfied and such an operation would be morally justified.

The principle of double effect is most often mentioned in a medical context in cases of abortion. But in fact, it has a much wider range of application in medical ethics. It bears on cases of contraception, sterilization, organ transplants, and the use of extraordinary measures to maintain life.

The principle of totality. The principle of totality can be expressed in this way: An individual has a right to dispose of his organs or to destroy their capacity to function only to the extent that the general well-being of the whole body demands it. Thus, it is clear that we have a natural obligation to preserve our lives, but on the Roman Catholic view, we also have a duty to preserve the integrity of our bodies. This duty is based on the belief that each of our organs was designed by God to play a role in maintaining the functional integrity of our bodies, that each has a place in the divine plan. As we are the custodians of our bodies, not their owners, it is our duty to care for them as part of a trust.

The principle of totality has implications for a great number of medical procedures. Strictly speaking, even cosmetic surgery is morally right only when it is required to maintain or assure the normal functioning of the rest of the body. More important, procedures that are typically employed for contraceptive purposes—vasectomies and tubal ligations—are ruled out. After all, such procedures involve "mutilation" and the destruction of the capacity of the organs of reproduction to function properly. The principle of totality thus also forbids the sterilization of the mentally retarded.

Applications of Roman Catholic Moral-Theological Viewpoints in the Medical Context

Roman Catholic ethicists and moral theologians have written on numerous aspects of medical ethics and developed a body of widely-accepted doctrine. We shall consider only four topics.

First, the application of the principle of double effect and the principle of totality have definite consequences in the area of medical experimentation. Since we hold our bodies in trust, we are responsible for assessing the degree of risk present in an experiment in which we are asked to participate as a subject. Thus, we need to be fully informed of the nature of the experiment and the risks that it holds for us. If after obtaining this knowledge, we decide to give our consent, it must be freely given and not be the result of deception or coercion.

Because human experimentation carries with it the possibility of injury or death, the principle of double effect and its four strictures apply. If available scientific evidence indicates that a sick person may benefit from participating in an experiment, then the experiment is morally justifiable. If, however, the evidence indicates that the chances of helping that person are slight and he or she may die or be gravely injured, then the experiment is not justified. In general, the likelihood of a person's benefitting from the experiment must exceed the danger of that person's suffering greater losses.

A person who is incurably ill may volunteer to be an experimental subject, even though she or he cannot reasonably expect personal gain in the form of improved health. The good that is hoped for is good for others, in the form of increased medical knowledge. Even here, however, there are constraints imposed by the principle of double effect. There must be no likelihood that the experiment will seriously injure, and the probable value of the knowledge expected to result must balance the risk run by the patient. Not even the incurably ill can be made subjects of trivial experiments.

The good sought by healthy volunteers is also the good of others. The same restrictions mentioned in connection with the incurably ill also apply to experimenting on healthy people. Additionally, the principle of totality places constraints on what a person may volunteer to do with his or her body. No healthy person may submit to an experiment that involves the probability of serious injury, impaired health, mutilation, or death.

A second medical topic addressed by Roman Catholic theologians is whether "ordinary" or "extraordinary" measures are to be taken in the preservation of human life. While it is believed that natural law and divine law impose on us a moral obligation to preserve our lives, Catholic moralists have interpreted this obligation as requiring that we rely upon only ordinary means. In the medical profession, the phrase "ordinary means" is used to refer to medical procedures that are standard or orthodox, in contrast with those that are untried or experimental. But from the viewpoint of Catholic ethics, "ordinary" used in the medical context applies to "all medicines, treatments, and operations which offer a reasonable hope of benefit for the patient and which can be obtained and used without excessive expense, pain, or other inconvenience." Thus, by contrast, extraordinary means are those that offer the patient no reasonable hope and whose use involves serious hardships for the patient or others.

Medical measures that would save the life of a patient but subject her to years of pain or would produce in her severe physical or mental incapacities are considered extraordinary ones. A patient or her family are under no obligations to choose them, and physicians are under a positive obligation not to encourage their choice.

The third medical topic for consideration is euthanasia. In the Roman Catholic ethical view, euthanasia in all forms is considered to be immoral. It is presumed to be a direct violation of God's dominion over creation and the human obligation to preserve life. The Ethical Directives for Catholic Hospitals is explicit on the matter of taking a life:

> The direct killing of any innocent person, even at his own request, is always
> morally wrong. Any procedure whose sole immediate effect is the death of a
> human being is a direct killing. . . . Euthanasia ("mercy killing") in all its forms

is forbidden. . . . The failure to supply the ordinary means of preserving life is equivalent to euthanasia.

According to this view, it is wrong to allow babies suffering from serious birth defects to die. If they can be saved by ordinary means, there is an obligation to do so. It is also wrong to act to terminate the lives of those hopelessly ill, either by taking steps to bring about their deaths or by failing to take steps to maintain their lives by ordinary means.

It is never permissible to hasten the death of a person as a direct intention. It is, however, permissible to administer drugs that alleviate pain. The principle of double effect suggests that giving such drugs is a morally justifiable action even though the drugs may indirectly hasten the death of a person.

Lastly, we may inquire how Roman Catholicism views abortion. According to the Roman Catholic view, from the moment of conception, the conceptus (later, the fetus) is considered to be a person with all the rights of a person. For this reason, direct abortion at any stage of pregnancy is regarded as morally wrong. Abortion is "direct" when it results from a procedure "whose sole immediate effect is the termination of pregnancy." This means that what is generally referred to as therapeutic abortion, in which an abortion is performed to safeguard the life or health of the woman, is considered wrong. For example, a woman with serious heart disease who becomes pregnant cannot morally justify an abortion on the grounds that the pregnancy is a serious threat to her life. Even when the ultimate aim is to save the life of the woman, direct abortion is wrong.

We have already seen, however, that the principle of double effect permits the performance of an action that may result in the death of an unborn child if the action satisfies the four criteria for applying the principle. Thus, *indirect* abortion is considered to be morally permissible. That is, the abortion must be the outcome of some action (for example, removal of a cancerous uterus) that is performed for the direct and total purpose of treating a pathological condition affecting the woman. The end sought in direct abortion is the destruction of life, but the end sought in indirect abortion is the preservation of life.

Difficulties

Our discussion has centered on the natural law theory of ethics as it has been interpreted in Roman Catholic theology. Thus, there are two possible types of difficulties: those associated with natural law ethics in its own right and those associated with its incorporation into theology. The theological difficulties go beyond the scope of our aims and interests. We shall restrict ourselves to considering the basic difficulty that faces natural law theory as formulated by Aquinas. Since it is this formulation that has been used in Roman Catholic moral theology, we shall be raising a problem for it in an indirect way.

The fundamental difficulty with Aquinas's argument for natural law is caused by the assumption, borrowed from Aristotle, that the universe is organized in a teleological fashion. (This is the assumption that every kind of thing has a goal or purpose.) This assumption is essential to Aquinas's ethical theory, for he identifies the good of a thing with its natural mode of operation. Without the assumption, we are faced with the great diversity and moral indifference of nature. Inclinations, even when shared by all humans, are no more than inclinations. There are no grounds for considering them "goods," and they have no moral status. The universe is bereft of natural values.

Yet, there are many reasons to consider this assumption false. Physics surrendered the notion of a teleological organization in the world as long ago as the seventeenth century—the rejection of Aristotle's physics also entailed the rejection of Aristotle's teleological view of the world. This left biology as the major source of arguments in favor of teleology. But contemporary evolutionary theory shows that the apparent purposive character of evolutionary change can be accounted for by the operation of natural selection on random mutations. Also, the development and growth of organisms can be explained by the presence of genetic information that controls the processes. The tadpole develops into a frog because evolution has produced a genetic program that directs the sequence of complicated chemical changes. Thus, there seems to be no adequate grounds for asserting that the teleological organization of nature is anything more than apparent.

Science and "reason alone" do not support teleology. It can be endorsed only if one is willing to assume that any apparent teleological organization is the product of a divine plan. Yet, because all apparent teleology can be explained in nonteleological ways, this assumption seems neither necessary nor legitimate.

Without its foundation of teleology, Aquinas's theory of natural law ethics seems to collapse. This is not to say, of course, that some other natural law theory, one not requiring the assumption of teleology, might not be persuasively defended.

Retrospect

We began by asking whether there are any standards or principles that can be used as guides when we are faced with moral decisions. The survey of ethical theories that this question prompted was not exhaustive, but it was adequate to show that serious and systematic attempts have been made to supply such principles. Utilitarianism offers us the principle of utility, which is grounded on the claim that all people seek happiness. Kant argues for the categorical imperative as a test for maxims and locates its source in reason alone. Ross rejects the utilitarian view that happiness or pleasure can be identified with rightness, yet cannot accept the Kantian notion that moral rules are absolute. He compromises by distinguishing between actual and prima facie duties and making our moral intuitions the ultimate guide in particular cases. Rawls attempts to preserve the strengths both of utilitarianism and of the Kant-Ross view by arguing that, under a veil of ignorance, certain principles would be chosen by all reasonable people. Finally, the natural law theory asserts that reason can discover the principles of conduct in nature. Incorporated in Roman Catholic theology, the general principle "Do good and avoid evil" is interpreted as a collection of moral rules with both a natural and divine basis.

Each theory we have considered offers principles that we can rely on in guiding our actions, formulating social policies, and judging the actions of others. But this in itself may be seen as a problem. Having too many theories may be just as confusing and unhelpful as having none. Additionally, each theory seems to suffer from weaknesses and flaws so that even if we find the theory basically plausible, we may have serious doubts about accepting it. Perhaps the whole enterprise of trying to formulate and defend moral principles should be abandoned as one doomed to disappointment and failure.

Such an attitude is understandable, but there are good reasons for not acting on the suggestion. That an ethical theory is open to objections is not necessarily grounds for dismissing it or for giving up the attempt to establish a satisfactory theory. The world is complicated, and the relations of people with one another are subtle and tangled. It is not surprising that we do not have a single ethical theory that compels everyone's belief and is acknowledged as correct and adequate.

The very diversity of theories is an acknowledgement of the complexities of life. The most satisfactory of ethical theories can hardly be more than a rough guide for action. Theories often point to areas of moral experience that are slighted or misconstrued by competing theories. Competition among theories can thus lead to refinements and improvements. Most contemporary philosophers, for example, would probably agree that Rawls's ethical-social theory is superior to the original forms of utilitarianism and Kantianism to which it is strongly indebted.

With respect to diversity of theories and acknowledged weaknesses in particular theories, ethics is not so different from science. Controversies over competing theories in psychology and sociology are proverbial, but the situation is quite similar in developing areas of physics and biology. Even those theories that are accepted as fundamentally correct, such as evolutionary theory and quantum mechanics, are generally recognized as being incomplete or unsatisfactory in important ways. Here, too, the complexities of the world must be struggled with, and total success cannot be guaranteed.

Another feature of scientific practice is also illuminating for ethics. It is acknowledged in the sciences that it is better to have a theory with known weaknesses than no theory at all. Even an imperfect theory can guide research, serve as a basis for prediction, and provide understanding. The theory can be used to good effect even while efforts are being made to improve it.

Similar considerations suggest that it is better to have moral principles than try to do without them. Such principles identify the relevant factors in situations in which we must make decisions. They serve as the basis for deliberation and as guides for action. Furthermore, by acting on principle, rather than on impulse or inclination, we make our actions more defensible; that is, we are in a position to provide explanations and reasons for our actions. In situations in which much hangs on our decisions, as is often the case in medical matters, being able to justify our decisions is of great importance. Most important, the principles of a moral theory give us a perspective other than that of immediate self-interest. They invite us to weigh the effects of our actions on others and to consider whether we are willing to endorse the action or its consequences. They even encourage us to put ourselves in the position of others who may be affected.

The moral principles that we follow may not be ones that belong to an explicit theory. They may simply underlie our behavior and condition it so that we ourselves are not conscious of their influence. A morally good person is not necessarily one who self-consciously holds a moral theory. Yet there are advantages to having an explicit theory. Free from the pressures of circumstance, we can make a deliberate effort to formulate principles. We can consider alternative theories, examine consequences, and search for weaknesses and shortcomings. In the end, we can hope to arrive at an ethical theory that is rationally persuasive and defensible.

Despite a diversity of competing theories and despite the fact that no theory is free of difficulties, it is still worthwhile to try to formulate and defend ethical principles. Choosing an ethical theory is ultimately a matter of individual judgment. This is not to say that the choice is arbitrary—that any one of the theories we have considered is just as good as any other. Judgment is individual because after considering the reasons and arguments in favor of a theory and after honestly confronting its weaknesses, then one must simply decide for one's self whether to accept the theory.

A major task of this chapter has been to provide information about several important ethical theories. One aim in doing this was to make it easier to follow the arguments and discussions in the selections that make up the major part of this book. Another and ultimately more serious aim has been to call attention to principles you may wish to consider accepting. From this standpoint, the problems and issues presented in the selections offer test cases for moral principles. You may find that some of the theories we have discussed are inadequate to deal with certain moral issues in the medical context, although they may seem satisfactory in more common or simpler cases. Other theories may appear to give definite answers to medical-moral problems, but you may find that they rest on assumptions that it does not appear reasonable to accept. Such a dialectical process of claim and criticism is slow and frustrating. Yet, it offers the best hope of settling on principles that we can accept with confidence and employ without misgivings.

Moral issues in the domain of medical practice and research are, at the present, largely unsettled and even unexplored. Although there is hardly a topic on which moral consensus exists, the demands of practical decision-making generate a force that presses us for immediate solutions. In such a situation, we cannot afford to try to settle all doubts about moral principles in an abstract way and only then apply them to problems in medicine. The dialectical process must be made practical. Formulating and testing principles must go on at the same time as we are actually making moral decisions. We must do our best to discover the principles of aerodynamics while staying aloft!

To a considerable extent, that is what this book is about. Positions are taken and defended by the authors. But they, too, are aware that they are participating in a search for a satisfactory resolution to the problems they discuss, and few, if any, would regard their solutions as beyond criticism. For the moment, medical ethics is an area in which there are more legitimate questions than there are satisfactory answers.

Part I
TERMINATION

1
ABORTION AND INFANTICIDE

CASE PRESENTATION
The Ordeal of Alice Wilson

Late in the afternoon on a September day, twelve-year-old Alice Wilson (as we will call her) was walking the eight blocks home from the public school she attended. She liked the walk, for the south St. Louis neighborhood she lived in was a generally pleasant place. Large, turn-of-the-century brick houses predominated, and the streets were lined with leafy sycamore trees.

But, like many urban areas, the neighborhood showed signs of decay. Several houses were abandoned, their windows boarded up with unpainted plywood. The streets were littered, and once well-tended front lawns were often hardly more than scraggly patches of weeds.

At the corner of Grand and Hervy, Alice left the well-traveled sidewalk through the business district and crossed the street to Shaw Park. By walking through the park, rather than around it, she could cut the distance to her house almost by half. She wouldn't dare go through the park after dark, but on that bright afternoon the park seemed beautiful and safe. She had walked through the park dozens of times, both alone and with her friends, and had never had any trouble.

That day was different. Alice stayed on the main asphalt path leading across the park and passed by the first picnic area. Then, just beyond that area, she was attacked by three teen-aged males. They were older and larger than Alice, and she had never seen them before. One grabbed her from behind and put his hand over her mouth so she couldn't scream. Another said they would kill her if she didn't keep quiet. They dragged her off the path and into a place surrounded by bushes. Then all three of them raped her.

Afterwards, the boys ran from the park, leaving Alice crying on the ground. She eventually recovered enough to dress herself and walk the rest of the way home. When her mother came home from work, Alice told her what had happened. Because Alice seemed to be basically unhurt, except for being frightened and distraught, Mrs. Wilson decided that Alice didn't need medical attention. Alice's father was dead so Mrs. Wilson was responsible for making decisions about her welfare.

Alice went back to school and resumed her normal life. But about a week later she developed a high fever and vaginal pains and discharges. Mrs. Wilson was sufficiently alarmed to take her daughter to the clinic of nearby South General Hospital.

After a physical examination and laboratory tests, Dr. Charles Kranski, a resident at South General working at the clinic, first talked with Alice, then presented the results to Mrs. Wilson. He explained that Alice was in generally good health, but the chances were quite high that she had been infected with gonorrhea as a result of the sexual assault. It would be necessary to wait for a culture to grow to be certain; meanwhile, Alice would be treated with a course of penicillin.

The most troubling news, however, was that Alice was pregnant from the rape. That would be an unfortunate thing to happen for any rape victim, but in Alice's case it was particularly terrible. Dr. Kranski explained that although Alice was old enough to conceive a child, she was not really old enough to have one. She was simply not sufficiently developed physiologically to undergo pregnancy. She might well have a spontaneous abortion, a miscarriage, but if she did not, the chances were very good that attempting to have the child might kill her.

Dr. Kranski told Mrs. Wilson that he had discussed Alice's case with two obstetricians and they both agreed with him that the only reasonable course of action was for Alice to have an abortion as soon as possible. In fact, Dr. Kranski said, as soon as the venereal disease was controlled, he would like to schedule Alice for an abortion for therapeutic reasons. He had already explained the situation to Alice, he said, and she agreed to the abortion. But because she was still a minor, it was necessary to have Mrs. Wilson's consent before the operation could be performed.

To Dr. Kranski's surprise, Mrs. Wilson told him that she would not give her consent. "I belong to the Church of the Spiritual Life," she said. "We follow the commandment 'Thou shall not kill.'"

Thinking that she had not understood the implications of Alice's pregnancy, Dr. Kranski again expained that Alice would probably die unless she had an abortion. Because of Alice's youth and small size, he said, the developing fetus would severely compress her internal organs and perhaps rupture them. If that happened, she would probably bleed to death. Even if that did not happen, she might suffer irreversible liver or kidney damage.

Mrs. Wilson remained totally unmoved. "God will save my daughter's life, if He wants it saved," she said. "And God will abort the child she's carrying, if He wants it aborted."

Dr. Kranski gave up his attempt to secure Mrs. Wilson's approval for the abortion. Later, he explained the situation to the director of the clinic, Dr. Saul Mendlovitz. Dr. Mendlovitz took up the matter with the legal staff of South General Hospital, and it was decided to seek a court order permitting the abortion.

The appropriate legal steps were taken, and after a court hearing, at which Mrs. Wilson was represented by a state-appointed attorney, South General Hospital was granted permission to take necessary medical steps to save the life of Alice Wilson. No appeal was filed.

Despite her mother's continued personal opposition, Alice Wilson received an abortion.

Introduction

Not many years ago most Americans considered abortion a crime so disgusting that it was hardly mentioned in public. Back-alley abortionists with dirty hands and unclean instruments were real enough, but they were also used in cautionary tales to warn women against being tempted into the crime. Abortion was the dramatic stuff of novels and movies portraying girls in trouble or women pushed to the brink. To choose to have an abortion was to choose to be degraded.

Times have changed somewhat. Abortion is now legal in the United States and has gained acceptance from a large part of the population. Yet controversy over the legitimacy of abortion continues to flare. Indeed, no other topic in medical ethics has attracted more attention or so polarized public opinion. The reason is understandable. In the abortion question, major moral, legal, and social issues are intertwined to form a problem of great subtlety and complexity.

Before focusing on some of the specific issues raised by abortion, we would do well to have in hand some of the relevant factual information about human developmental biology and the techniques of abortion.

Human Development and Abortion

Fertilization occurs when an ovum is penetrated by a sperm cell and the nuclei of the two unite to form a single cell containing forty-six chromosomes. This normally occurs in the Fallopian tube (or oviduct), a narrow tube leading from the ovary into the uterus (womb). The fertilized ovum or zygote continues its passage down the Fallopian tube, and during its two to three day passage, the zygote undergoes a number of cell divisions that increase its size. (Rarely, the zygote does not descend but continues to develop in the Fallopian tube. Because the tube is so small, the pregnancy usually has to be terminated surgically.) After reaching the uterus, a pear-shaped organ, the zygote (or conceptus) floats free in the intrauterine fluid. Here it develops into a blastocyst, a ball of cells surrounding a fluid-filled cavity.

By the end of the second week, the blastocyst becomes embedded in the wall of the uterus. At this point and until the end of the eighth week, it is known as an embryo. During the fourth and fifth weeks, organ systems begin to develop, and the external features take on a definite human shape.

During the eighth week, brain activity usually becomes detectable. At this time, the embryo comes to be known as a fetus. Birth generally occurs about nine months after fertilization. It is customary to divide this time into three three-month periods or trimesters. At present, pregnancy cannot be diagnosed with certainty by ordinary methods until ten to fourteen days after a woman has missed her menstrual period.

Abortion is the termination of pregnancy. It can occur because of internal biochemical factors or as a result of physical injury to the woman. Terminations from such causes are usually referred to as "spontaneous abortion," but they are also commonly called miscarriages.

Abortion can also be a deliberate process resulting from human intervention. The methods used in contemporary medicine depend to a great extent on the stage of the pregnancy. The earliest intervention involves the use of drugs (the morning-after pill) to prevent the embedding of the blastocyst in the uterine wall. Subsequent intervention during the first trimester (up to about twelve weeks) commonly employs one of two techniques. The first of the two is uterine or vacuum aspiration. The cervix, the narrow outer opening of the uterus, is dilated (widened) by instruments. Then a small tube is inserted into the uterus, and its contents are emptied by suction. The second commonly used procedure is dilation and curettage. The cervix is dilated and its contents are gently scraped out by the use of a curette, a spoon-shaped surgical instrument.

After sixteen weeks, when the fetus is too large to make the other methods practical, the most common abortion technique is saline injection. The fluid in the membrane-sac (amnion) surrounding the fetus is withdrawn through a hollow needle and replaced by a solution of salt and water. This induces a miscarriage.

A second method, hysterotomy, is a surgical procedure in which the fetus is removed from the uterus through an incision. The procedure is the same as that known as Caesarean section and is rarely performed for the purpose of abortion.

These facts about pregnancy and abortion put us in a position to move on and discuss some of the moral problems connected with them. We shall not be able to untangle the skein of issues wrapped around the abortion question. We shall only attempt to state a few of the more serious ones and to indicate the lines of argument that have been offered to support positions that have been taken with respect to them. Afterwards, we will sketch out some possible responses that might be offered on the basis of the ethical theories we considered in the introductory chapter. Finally, we will present summary statements of the views taken by the authors of the selections that make up the bulk of this chapter.

The Status of the Fetus

It is absolutely crucial for the application of the principles of any moral theory that we have a settled opinion about the objects and subjects of morality. Although principles are generally stated with respect to rational individuals, every theory recognizes that there are people who in fact cannot be considered rational agents. For example, mental and physical incapacities may diminish or destroy rationality. But ethical theories generally recognize that we still have duties to people who are so incapacitated.

The basic problem that this raises is: Who or what is to be considered a person? Are there characteristics that we can point to and say that it is by virtue of possessing these characteristics that an individual must be considered a person and thus accorded moral treatment?

The abortion issue raises this question most particularly with regard to the fetus. (We will use the term "fetus," for the moment, to refer to the developing organism at any stage.) Just what is the status of the fetus in the world? We must find a satisfactory answer to this question, some writers have suggested, before we can resolve the general moral problem of abortion. The first question, then, is not one of ethics but of what is usually called metaethics. That is, it is one concerning the application of a moral theory. Or it might be said to be one of metaphysics, for it concerns the position we are willing to assign the fetus in our view of the world.

Let's consider the possible consequences of answering this question one way or the other. First, if a fetus is a person, then it has a serious claim to life. We must assert the claim on its behalf, for like an unconscious person, the fetus is unable to do so. The claim of the fetus as a person must be given weight and respect in deliberating about any action that would terminate its life. Perhaps only circumstances as extreme as a threat to the life of the mother would justify abortion.

Assuming that the fetus is a person, then an abortion would be a case of killing and not something to be undertaken without reasons sufficient to over-ride the fetus's claim to life. In effect, only conditions of the same sort as would justify our killing an adult person (for example, self-defense) would justify our killing a fetus. Thus, the moral burden in every case would be to demonstrate that abortion is not a case of wrongful killing.

By contrast, if a fetus is *not* a person in a morally relevant sense, then abortion need not be considered a case of killing equivalent to the killing of an adult human. On one view, it might be said that abortion is, at most, the preventing of a possible person. Thus, the issues raised may not be unique moral problems, for then they would resemble those of contraception or voluntary sexual abstinence.

On another view, it could be argued that since a fetus is not a person, an abortion is not essentially different from an appendectomy. According to this way of thinking, a fetus is no more than a complicated clump of organic material, and its removal involves no serious moral difficulty.

On a third view, it could be argued that even though the fetus is not a person, it is a *potential* person, and this is a significant and morally-relevant property. The fetus's very potentiality makes it unique and distinguishes it from a diseased appendix or a cyst or any other kind of organic material. Thus, because the fetus can become a person, abortion does present a moral problem. A fetus can be destroyed only for serious reasons. Thus, preventing a person from coming into existence must be justified to an extent comparable to the justification required for killing a person. (Some have suggested that the justification does not have to be identical because the fetus is only a potential person. The justifications we might present for killing a person would thus serve only as a guide for those that might justify abortion.)

So far we have used the word "fetus," and this usage tends to obscure the fact that human development is a process with many stages. Perhaps it is only in the later stages that the entity that is developing becomes a person. But exactly when might this happen?

The differences between a fertilized ovum and a fully-developed baby just a few minutes before birth are considerable. The ovum or the blastocyst seems just so much tissue. But the embryo and the fetus present more serious claims to being persons. Should abortion be allowed until the fetus becomes visibly human, or until the fetus shows heartbeat and brain waves, or until the fetus can live outside the uterus (becomes viable)?

The process of development is continuous, and so far it has proved impossible to find differences between stages that can be generally accepted as morally relevant. Some writers on abortion have suggested that it is useless to look for such differences because any place where the line is drawn will be arbitrary. Others have claimed that it is possible to draw the line by relying on criteria that can be rationally defended. A few have even argued that a reasonable set of criteria for determining who shall be considered a person might even deny the status to infants.

Duties and Rights of Women

Is it a woman's moral duty to nurture and to carry to term an unwanted child? Pregnancies resulting from rape and incest are the kinds of dramatic cases frequently mentioned to emphasize the seriousness of the burden imposed on women. But the question is also important when the conditions surrounding the pregnancy are more ordinary.

Suppose that a woman becomes pregnant unintentionally and decides that having a child will be harmful to her career or to her way of life. Or suppose that she already has several children and does not believe that she can afford to care for another. Does a woman have a moral duty to see to it that the developing child comes to be born?

Some philosophers (Judith J. Thomson, for example) have suggested that even if we grant that the fetus is a person, its claim to life cannot be given unconditional precedence over the woman's claim to control her own life. She is entitled to her own autonomy and the right to arrange her life in accordance with her own concept of the good. It would be wrong for her to destroy the fetus for a trivial reason, but legitimate and adequate reasons for taking the life of the fetus might be offered.

Others, by contrast, have argued that when a woman becomes pregnant she assumes an obligation for the life of the fetus. It is, after all, completely dependent on her for its continued existence. She has no more right to take its life in order to seek her own best interest than she has to murder someone whose death may bring benefits to her.

Therapeutic Abortion

Abortion is sometimes required in order to save the life of the mother or in order to provide her with medical treatment that may correct some life-threatening condition. Abortion performed for such a purpose is ordinarily regarded as a case of self-defense. For this reason, it is almost universally considered to be morally unobjectionable. (Strictly speaking, the Roman Catholic view condemns abortion in all of its forms. It does approve of providing medical treatment for the mother, even if this results in the death of the fetus. But the death of the fetus must never be intended.)

If the principle of preserving the life and health of the mother is taken to be one that justifies abortion, then what conditions fall under that principle? If a woman has cancer of the uterus and her life can be saved only by an operation that will result in the death of the fetus, then this clearly falls under the principle. But what about psychological conditions? Is a woman's mental health relevant to deciding whether an abortion is justified? What if a psychiatrist believes that a woman cannot face the physical rigors of pregnancy or bear the psychological stresses that go along with it without developing severe psychiatric symptoms? Would such a judgment be sufficient to morally justify an abortion? Or is the matter of psychological health irrelevant to the abortion issue?

Consider, too, the welfare of the fetus. Suppose prenatal tests show that the developing child suffers from serious abnormalities or there are other good reasons to believe that the child is severely defective. (This was the case of the "thalidomide babies.") Is abortion for the purpose of preventing the birth of such children justifiable?

It might be argued that it is not, for a defective fetus has as much right to its life as a defective person. We do not, after all, consider it legitimate to kill people who become seriously injured or suffer from diseases that render them helpless. Rather, we care for them and work to improve their lives—at least we ought to.

Someone might argue, however, that abortion in such cases is not only justifiable, but it is a duty. (See, for example, the article by H. T. Engelhardt in Chapter 2.) It is our duty to kill the fetus to spare the person that it will become a life of unhappiness and suffering. We might even be said to be acknowledging the dignity of the fetus by doing what it might do for itself if it could, what any rational creature would do. Destroying such a fetus would spare future pain to the individual and his or her family and save society from an enormous investment. Thus, not only would we be justified in killing such a fetus, we have a positive obligation to do so.

In this chapter, we will not deal explicitly with the issues that are raised by attempting to decide whether it is justifiable to terminate the life of a defective fetus. Because such issues are directly connected with prenatal genetic diagnosis and treatment, we will discuss them more fully in Chapter 7. Nonetheless, in considering the general question of the legitimacy of abortion, it is important to keep such special considerations in mind.

Abortion and the Law

Abortion in our society has been a legal issue as well as a moral issue. Until the Supreme Court decision in *Roe* v. *Wade*, nontherapeutic abortion was illegal in virtually all states. And even now there are groups lobbying strongly for a Constitutional amendment that would protect a fetus's "right to life" and prohibit elective abortion.

The rightness or wrongness of abortion is a moral matter, one whose issues can be resolved only by appealing to a moral theory. Different theories may yield incompatible answers, and even individuals who accept the same theory may arrive at different conclusions.

Such a state of affairs raises the question of whether the moral convictions or conclusions of some people should be embodied in laws that govern the lives of all people in the society. The question can be put succinctly in this way: Should the moral beliefs of some people serve as the basis for laws that will impose those beliefs on everyone?

There is no straightforward way of answering this general question. To some extent, the moral beliefs that are at issue are a relevant consideration. So too are the political principles that we are willing to accept as ones basic to our society. Every ethical theory recognizes that there is a scope of action that must be left to individuals as moral agents acting freely on the basis of their own understanding and perceptions. Laws requiring the expression of benevolence or gratitude, for example, seem peculiarly inappropriate.

Yet, one of the major aims of a government is to protect through its laws the rights of its citizens. Consequently, a society must have just laws that recognize and enforce those rights. In a very real way, then, the moral theory that we hold and the conclusions arrived at on the basis of it will determine whether we believe that certain types of laws are justified. They are justified when they protect the rights recognized in our moral theories—when political rights reflect moral rights. (See the introduction to Chapter 10 for a fuller discussion of moral rights and their relation to political rights.)

An ethical theory that accords the status of a person to a fetus is likely to claim also that the laws of the society should recognize the rights of the fetus. A theory that does not grant the fetus this position is not likely to regard laws forbidding abortion as justifiable.

Ethical Theories: Abortion and Infanticide

Theories like those of Kant, Ross, and Rawls attribute to individuals autonomy or self-direction. An individual is entitled to control his or her own life, and it seems reasonable to extend this principle to apply to one's own body. If this is done, then a woman should have the right to determine whether or not she wishes to have a child. If she is pregnant with an unwanted child, then no matter how she came to be pregnant, then she might legitimately decide on an abortion. Utilitarianism also suggests this answer. In the absence of other considerations, if it seems likely that having a child will produce more unhappiness than an abortion would, then an abortion would be justifiable.

If the fetus is considered to be a person, however, the situation is different for some theories. The Roman Catholic view holds that the fetus is an innocent person and that direct abortion is never justifiable. Even if the pregnancy is due to rape, the fetus cannot be held at fault and made to suffer through its death. Even though she may not wish to have the child, it is the mother's duty to preserve the life of the fetus.

For deontological theories like those of Kant and Ross, the situation becomes more complicated. If the fetus is a person, then it has an inherent dignity and worth. It is an innocent life which cannot be destroyed except for the weightiest moral reasons. Those reasons may include the interests and wishes of the woman, but deontological theories provide no clear answer as to how those are to be weighed.

By contrast, for utilitarianism, even if the fetus is considered a person, the principle of utility may still justify an abortion. Killing a person is not, for utilitarianism, inherently wrong. (Yet, it is also compatible with rule utilitarianism to argue that permitting elective abortion as a matter of policy would produce more unhappiness than forbidding abortion altogether. Thus, utilitarianism does not offer a definite answer to the abortion issue.)

As we have already seen, both utilitarianism and deontological theories can be used to justify therapeutic abortion. When the mother's life or health is at stake, then the situation is one of self-defense. Both Kant and Ross recognize that we each have a right to protect ourselves, even if it means taking the life of another person. For utilitarianism, preserving one's life is justifiable, for being alive is a necessary condition for all forms of happiness.

We have also indicated that abortion "for the sake of the fetus" can be justified by both utilitarianism and deontological theories. If by killing the fetus we can spare it a life of suffering, minimize the sufferings of its family, and preserve the resources of the society, then abortion is legitimate on utilitarian grounds. In the terms of Kant and Ross, destroying the fetus might be a way of recognizing its dignity. If we assume that it is a person, then by sparing it a life of indignity and pain, we are treating it in the way that a rational being would want to be treated.

The legitimacy of laws forbidding abortion is an issue that utilitarianism would resolve by considering their effects. If such laws promote the general happiness of the society, then they are justifiable. Otherwise, they are not. In general, Kant, Ross, Rawls, and natural law theory recognize intrinsic human worth and regard it as legitimate to have laws protecting that worth even if those holding this view are only a minority of the society. Thus, laws discriminating against blacks and women, for example, would be considered unjust on the basis of these theories. Laws enforcing equality, by contrast, would be considered just.

But what about fetuses? The Roman Catholic interpretation of natural law would regard the case as exactly the same. As full human persons, they are entitled to have their rights protected by law. Those who fail to recognize this are guilty of moral failure, and laws permitting abortion are the moral equivalent of laws permitting murder.

For Kant and other deontologists, the matter is less clear. So long as there is substantial doubt about the status of the fetus, it is not certain that it is legitimate to demand that the rights of fetuses be recognized and protected by law. It is clear that whether or not the fetus is considered a person is most often taken as the crucial issue in the abortion controversy.

The Selections

All the issues we have discussed previously are dealt with in the selections in this chapter. Yet it is the last issue, the status of the fetus as a person, that dominates concern. In *Roe v. Wade* the U.S. Supreme Court declared unconstitutional a Texas statute that restricted legal abortions to cases in which the life of the mother was threatened. The decision implied that all such state laws regulating abortion were unconstitutional. In effect, then, the decision made abortion legal in the United States.

The reasoning behind the decision rested, in part, on the right of a woman to act for her own health and well-being as part of a more general right of privacy. The Court also considered the question of the legitimate limits of state interference to protect a woman's health and to protect the life of a fetus. The Court refused to recognize the fetus as a "person in the full sense" or to grant the right of the state to act on its behalf until the time (around the twenty-eighth week) that it can live outside the mother's body.

The ruling laid down three guidelines for regulating abortion: (1) until the end of the first trimester, the abortion decision is a medical one that must be left to the woman and her physician; (2) after the end of the first trimester, the state may regulate the abortion procedure in ways reasonably related to maternal health; (3) after the fetus is viable, the state may regulate or even prohibit abortion, except where it is necessary to preserve the life or health of the mother.

The Court faced the line-drawing problem and drew the line at viability. John T. Noonan, in our second reading, "An Almost Absolute Value in History," avoids the difficulty the problem poses by making the moment of fertilization the stage at which the developing organism becomes a person. Noonan reviews the distinctions used by abortion proponents (viability, experience, quickening, attitudes of adults towards the fetus, social viability) and concludes that they are all illegitimate. By contrast, he argues that conception is the decisive moment of humanization—for it is then that the new being receives the genetic code of its parents.

The basic principle that should govern our attitude towards the fetus, Noonan claims, is the theological and humanistic one: Do not injure your fellow man without a reason. Thus, once the humanity of the fetus is perceived, abortion is never right except in "self-defense." With the exception of saving the mother's life then, abortion is immoral because it "violates the rational humanist tenet of the quality of human lives."

Like Noonan, Michael Tooley in his "Abortion and Infanticide" conceives the basic issue in abortion to be the question of what properties a thing must possess to have a serious right to life. He argues that the conditions are as follows: (1) the capacity to have the concept of a continuing subject of experiences; (2) the capacity to envisage a future; (3) to be or have been a continuing subject of experiences; (4) to possess or have possessed self-consciousness; (5) to possess or have possessed the capacity for self-consciousness.

Tooley's defense of these requirements is based on an analysis of the concept of a right and an account of the conditions under which an individual's rights can be violated. One of the consequences of Tooley's way of dealing with the line-drawing problem is that the line may be drawn after birth and so make both abortion and infanticide legitimate. Tooley faces this consequence squarely and attempts to show that traditional views that involve a rejection of his requirements for being a person are untenable. He claims that either they appeal to unacceptable moral principles or they fail to deal with basic moral principles.

Judith Jarvis Thomson in her very influential "A Defense of Abortion" avoids the problem of determining when the fetus becomes a person. For the sake of argument only, she grants the conservative view that the fetus is a person from the moment of conception. She points out, however, that the conservative argument using this claim as a premise actually involves an additional unstated premise. The argument typically runs: The fetus is an innocent person; therefore, killing a fetus is always wrong. The argument requires that we assume that killing an innocent person is always wrong. But, Thomson claims, killing an innocent person is sometimes allowable. This is most clearly so when self-defense requires it.

Using several moral analogies, Thomson goes on to attempt to show that a fetus's right to life does not consist in the right not to be killed, but in the right not to be killed unjustly. The fetus's claim to life is not an absolute one which must always be granted unconditional precedence over the interests of its mother. Thus, abortion is not always permissible, but neither is it always impermissible. When the reasons for having an abortion are trivial, then abortion is not legitimate. When the reasons are serious and involve the health or welfare of the woman, then abortion is justifiable.

In the last selection in this chapter, "Abortion and the Concept of a Person," Jane English argues that both the conservative view (represented by Noonan) and the liberal view (represented by Tooley) on abortion are mistaken. The conservatives maintain that since human life begins at conception, abortion is wrong because it is murder. But English claims that not all killings of humans, even innocent ones, are murder. Furthermore, she claims that liberals are also wrong in arguing that since a fetus does not become a person until birth, then a woman may do whatever she pleases with her own body. You cannot do as you please with your own body if it affects other persons adversely. What is more, if a fetus is not a person, this does not imply that you can do with it as you wish. Animals are not persons, for example, yet we are not free to torture them.

English identifies the concept of a person as the central issue in the abortion debate. She examines the concept of a person and concludes that no sharp line can be drawn. She also argues that if a fetus is a person, abortion is still justifiable in many cases. And if a fetus is not a person, killing it is still wrong in many cases. Her general conclusion is that our concept of a person cannot and need not bear the weight that the abortion controversy has placed on it.

Clearly, the Supreme Court decision did not resolve the philosophical difficulties posed by abortion. Making abortion legal did not necessarily make it moral. Making the end of the first trimester the beginning of legitimate state control is pragmatically useful, but it does not provide a satisfactory answer to the question of whether the fetus is a person.

Noonan's conservative view that the moment of conception is also the beginning of a person has a powerful simplicity, but because the differences between a fertilized ovum and an about-to-be-born baby are so great, it too seems arbitrary. It does violence to our perceptions that potentiality (the genetic code of DNA) is very different from actuality (a child), that a blueprint and a pile of building materials is very different from a house.

By contrast, Tooley's criteria have the shocking results of making it legitimate to kill young children. His arguments must be accepted as wholly persuasive to overcome our intuitions that such an act is morally wrong, that a child is really all that different from an adult. Furthermore, he leaves unsettled the crucial question of when his criteria are to be considered satisfied.

Thomson makes no effort to deal with criteria that would allow us to decide whether a fetus is a person. She does, however, call to our attention the important notion that we are sometimes justified in causing the death of an innocent person. This offers a means of considering the permissibility of abortion in a case-by-case way, without our having to secure agreement on the question of the status of the fetus.

Perhaps English is right in her claim that no concept of a person can be formulated as clear, correct, and adequate and that we do not even need such a concept to resolve the abortion question. Yet there are many other questions in which the concept of a person is of essential relevance in deciding whether our moral principles apply. Perhaps we should try to settle the issue in dealing with abortion so that we will have the tools to deal with other issues. What shall we say about children born with severe brain damage or people condemned to life in a comatose, vegetative state?

The social problems of abortion show no signs of being resolved. At the present, about a million legal abortions are performed every year in the United States—one abortion for every three live births. About one-quarter of them are paid for with tax money in the form of Medicaid payments.

In 1980 the Supreme Court ruled that the federal government was under no obligation to fund abortions for the poor under the Medicaid program. Because Medicaid is presently both a state and federally funded program, fourteen states, accounting for 75 percent of the women eligible for Medicaid, chose to continue to finance elective abortions with state funds. In those states, nearly 98 percent of the women seeking an abortion obtained one. In states providing no funding, about 20 percent of women wanting abortions were forced to continue their pregnancies. Those who secured abortions obtained money from private sources to pay for both legal abortions and (in 4 percent of the cases) illegal ones.

If recent proposals are put into effect, full responsibility for financing the Medicaid program will be assumed by the federal government. This means that states that currently pay for abortions with state-contributed Medicaid funds would have to create their own programs for funding abortions for the poor. Most political observers believe that it is unlikely that many such programs would ever be established.

The effect of this is likely to be that women with financial means will have no difficulty obtaining abortions, while those without money will either have to bear children they do not want or have to take their chances with back-alley abortionists whose services they can afford. Yet should those who consider abortion a form of murder have to pay for the operation that commits it?

This is just one of the moral dilemmas that we can hope to see satisfactorily resolved in the future.

United States Supreme Court Decision in *Roe* v. *Wade*

Background Note: A pregnant single woman, Roe, brought a class-action suit against Wade, the District Attorney of Dallas County. Roe challenged the constitutionality of the Texas criminal abortion laws, which prohibited procuring or performing an abortion except on medical advice for the purpose of saving the mother's life. A three-judge District Court ruled that the abortion statutes were void,

This selection is taken from the text of the decision reprinted in Robert L. Perkins, ed., Abortion: Pro and Con. *Cambridge, Massachusetts: Schenkman Publishing Company, 1974, pp. 213–225.*

and Wade appealed directly to the Supreme Court. By seven to two the Court ruled in favor of Roe, and Justice Blackmun delivered the majority opinion. That opinion is abridged here and citations to other cases omitted. The decision was handed down on January 22, 1973.

Three reasons have been advanced to explain historically the enactment of criminal abortion laws in the 19th century and to justify their continued existence.

It has been argued occasionally that these laws were the product of a Victorian social concern to discourage illicit sexual conduct. Texas, however, does not advance this justification in the present case, and it appears that no court or commentator has taken the argument seriously. The appellants and *amici* contend, moreover, that this is not a proper state purpose at all and suggest that, if it were, the Texas statutes are overbroad in protecting it since the law fails to distinguish between married and unwed mothers.

A second reason is concerned with abortion as a medical procedure. When most criminal abortion laws were first enacted, the procedure was a hazardous one for the woman. This was particularly true prior to the development of antisepsis. Antiseptic techniques, of course, were based on discoveries by Lister, Pasteur, and others first announced in 1867, but were not generally accepted and employed until about the turn of the century. Abortion mortality was high. Even after 1900, and perhaps until as late as the development of antibiotics in the 1940's, standard modern techniques such as dilation and curettage were not nearly so safe as they are today. Thus it has been argued that a State's real concern in enacting a criminal abortion law was to protect the pregnant woman, that is, to restrain her from submitting to a procedure that placed her life in serious jeopardy.

Modern medical techniques have altered this situation. Appellants and various *amici* refer to medical data indicating that abortion in early pregnancy, that is, prior to the end of first trimester, although not without its risk, is now relatively safe. Mortality rates for women undergoing early abortions, where the procedure is legal, appear to be as low as or lower than the rates for normal childbirth. Consequently, any interest of the State in protecting the woman from an inherently hazardous procedure, except when it would be equally dangerous for her to forego it, has largely disappeared. Of course, important state interests in the area of health and medical standards do remain. The state has a legitimate interest in

seeing to it that abortion, like any other medical procedure, is performed under circumstances that insure maximum safety for the patient. This interest obviously extends at least to the performing physician and his staff, to the facilities involved, to the availability of after-care, and to adequate provision for any complication or emergency that might arise. The prevalence of high mortality rates at illegal "abortion mills" strengthens, rather than weakens, the State's interest in regulating the conditions under which abortions are performed. Moreover, the risk to the woman increases as her pregnancy continues. Thus the State retains a definite interest in protecting the woman's own health and safety when an abortion is proposed at a late stage of pregnancy.

The third reason is the State's interest—some phrase it in terms of duty—in protecting prenatal life. Some of the argument for this justification rests on the theory that a new human life is present from the moment of conception. The State's interest and general obligation to protect life then extends, it is argued, to prenatal life. Only when the life of the pregnant mother herself is at stake, balanced against the life she carries within her, should the interest of the embryo or fetus not prevail. Logically, of course, a legitimate state interest in this area need not stand or fall on acceptance of the belief that life begins at conception or at some other point prior to live birth. In assessing the State's interest, recognition may be given to the less rigid claim that as long as at least *potential* life is involved, the State may assert interests beyond the protection of the pregnant woman alone.

Parties challenging state abortion laws have sharply disputed in some courts the contention that a purpose of these laws, when enacted, was to protect prenatal life. Pointing to the absence of legislative history to support the contention, they claim that most state laws were designed solely to protect the woman. Because medical advances have lessened this concern, at least with respect to abortion in early pregnancy, they argue that with respect to such abortions the laws can no longer be justified by any state interest. There is some scholarly support for this view of original purpose. The few state courts called upon to interpret their laws in the late 19th and early 20th centuries did focus on the State's interest in protecting the woman's health rather than in preserving the embryo and fetus. Proponents of this view point out that in many States, including Texas, by statute or judicial interpretation, the pregnant woman herself could not be prosecuted for self-abortion or for cooperating in an abortion performed upon her by another. They claim that adoption of the "quickening" distinction through received common law and state statutes tacitly recognizes the greater health hazards inherent in late abortion and impliedly repudiates the theory that life begins at conception.

It is with these interests, and the weight to be attached to them, that this case is concerned.

The Constitution does not explicitly mention any right of privacy. In a line of decisions, however, going back perhaps as far as *Union Pacific R. Co.* v. *Botsford*, 141 U.S. 250, 251 (1891), the Court has recognized that a right of personal privacy, or a guarantee of certain areas or zones of privacy, does exist under the Constitution. In varying contexts the Court or individual Justices have indeed found at least the roots of that right in the First Amendment, in the Fourth and Fifth Amendments, in the penumbras of the Bill of Rights, in the Ninth Amendment, or in the concept of liberty guaranteed by the first section of the Fourteenth Amendment. These decisions make it clear that only personal rights that can be deemed "fundamental" or "implicit in the concept of ordered liberty" are included in this guarantee of personal privacy. They also make it clear that the right has some extension to activities relating to marriage, procreation, contraception, family relationships, and child rearing and education.

This right of privacy, whether it be founded in the Fourteenth Amendment's concept of personal liberty and restrictions upon state action, as we feel it is, or, as the District Court determined, in the Ninth Amendment's reservation of rights to the people, is broad enough to encompass a woman's decision whether or not to terminate her pregnancy. The detriment that the State would impose upon the pregnant woman by denying this choice altogether is apparent. Specific and direct harm medically diagnosable even in early pregnancy may be involved. Maternity, or additional offspring, may force upon the woman a distressful life and future. Psychological harm may be imminent. Mental and physical health may be taxed by child care. There is also the distress, for all concerned, associated with the unwanted child, and there is the problem of bringing a child into a family already unable, psychologically and otherwise, to care for it. In other cases, as in this one, the additional difficulties and continuing stigma of unwed motherhood may be involved. All these are factors the woman and her responsible physician necessarily will consider in consultation.

On the basis of elements such as these, appellants and some *amici* argue that the woman's right is absolute and that she is entitled to terminate her pregnancy at whatever time, in whatever way, and for whatever reason she alone chooses. With these we do not agree. Appellants' arguments that Texas either has no valid interest at all in regulating the abortion decision, or no interest strong enough to support any limitation upon the woman's sole determination, is unpersuasive. The Court's decisions recognizing a right of privacy also acknowledge that some state regulation in areas protected by that right is appropriate. As noted above, a state may properly assert important interests in safeguarding health, in maintaining medical standards, and in protecting potential life. At some point in pregnancy, these respective interests become sufficiently compelling to sustain regulation of the factors that govern the abortion decision. The privacy right involved, therefore, cannot be said to be absolute. In fact, it is not clear to us that the claim asserted by some *amici* that one has an unlimited right to do with one's body as one pleases bears a close relationship to the right of privacy previously articulated in the Court's decisions. The Court has refused to recognize an unlimited right of this kind in the past.

We therefore conclude that the right of personal privacy includes the abortion decision, but that this right is not unqualified and must be considered against important state interests in regulation.

We note that those federal and state courts that have recently considered abortion law challenges have reached the same conclusion. A majority, in addition to the District Court in the present case, have held state laws unconstitutional, at least in part, because of vagueness or because of overbreadth and abridgement of rights.

Although the results are divided, most of these courts have agreed that the right of privacy, however based, is broad enough to cover the abortion decision; that the right, nonetheless, is not absolute and is subject to some limitations; and

that at some point the state interests as to protection of health, medical standards, and prenatal life, become dominant. We agree with this approach.

Where certain "fundamental rights" are involved, the Court has held that regulation limiting these rights may be justified only by a "compelling state interest" . . . and that legislative enactments must be narrowly drawn to express only the legitimate state interests at stake.

In the recent abortion cases courts have recognized these principles. Those striking down state laws have generally scrutinized the State's interest in protecting health and potential life and have concluded that neither interest justified broad limitations on the reasons for which a physician and his pregnant patient might decide that she should have an abortion in the early stages of pregnancy. Courts sustaining state laws have held that the State's determinations to protect health or prenatal life are dominant and constitutionally justifiable.

The District Court held that the appellee failed to meet his burden of demonstrating that the Texas statute's infringement upon Roe's rights was necessary to support a compelling state interest, and that, although the defendant presented "several compelling justifications for state presence in the area of abortions," the statutes outstripped these justifications and swept "far beyond any areas of compelling state interest." Appellant and appellee both contest that holding. Appellant, as has been indicated, claims an absolute right that bars any state imposition of criminal penalties in the area. Appellee argues that the State's determination to recognize and protect prenatal life from and after conception constitutes a compelling state interest. As noted above, we do not agree fully with either formulation.

A. The appellee and certain *amici* argue that the fetus is a "person" within the language and meaning of the Fourteenth Amendment. In support of this they outline at length and in detail the well-known facts of fetal development. If this suggestion of personhood is established, the appellant's case, of course, collapses, for the fetus' right to life is then guaranteed specifically by the Amendment. The appellant conceded as much on reargument. On the other hand, the appellee conceded on reargument that no case could be cited that holds that a fetus is a person within the meaning of the Fourteenth Amendment.

The Constitution does not define "person" in so many words. Section 1 of the Fourteenth Amendment contains three references to "person." . . . But in nearly all these instances, the use of the word is such that it has application only postnatally. None indicates, with any assurance, that it has any possible prenatal application.

All this, together with our observation, *supra*, that throughout the major portion of the 19th century prevailing legal abortion practices were far freer than they are today, persuades us that the word "person," as used in the Fourteenth Amendment, does not include the unborn. . . .

B. The pregnant woman cannot be isolated in her privacy. She carries an embryo and, later, a fetus, if one accepts the medical definitions of the developing young in the human uterus. See Dorland's Illustrated Medical Dictionary, 478–479, 547 (24th ed. 1965). The situation therefore is inherently different from marital intimacy, or bedroom possession of obscene material, or marriage, or procreation, or education, with which *Eisenstadt, Giswold, Stanley, Loving, Skinner, Pierce,* and *Meyer* were respectively concerned. As we have intimated above, it is reasonable and appropriate for a State to decide that at some point in time another interest, that of health of the mother or that of potential human life, becomes significantly involved. The woman's privacy is no longer sole and any right of privacy she possesses must be measured accordingly.

Texas urges that, apart from the Fourteenth Amendment, life begins at conception and is present throughout pregnancy, and that, therefore, the State has a compelling interest in protecting that life from and after conception. We need not resolve the difficult question of when life begins. When those trained in the respective disciplines of medicine, philosophy, and theology are unable to arrive at any consensus, the judiciary, at this point in the development of man's knowledge, is not in a position to speculate as to the answer.

It should be sufficient to note briefly the wide divergence of thinking on this most sensitive and difficult question. There has always been strong support for the view that life does not begin until live birth. This was the belief of the Stoics. It appears to be the predominant, though not the unanimous, attitude of the Jewish faith. It may be taken to represent also the position of a large segment of the Protestant community, insofar as that can be ascertained; organized groups that have taken a formal position on the abortion issue have generally regarded abortion as a matter for the conscience of the individual and her family. As we have noted, the common law found greater significance in quickening. Physicians and their scientific colleagues have regarded that event with less interest and have tended to focus either upon conception or upon live birth or upon the interim point at which the fetus becomes "viable," that is, potentially able to live outside the mother's womb, albeit with artificial aid. Viability is usually placed at about seven months (28 weeks) but may occur earlier, even at 24 weeks. The Aristotelian theory of "mediate animation," that held sway throughout the Middle Ages and the Renaissance in Europe, continued to be official Roman Catholic dogma until the 19th century, despite opposition to this "ensoulment" theory from those in the Church who would recognize the existence of life from the moment of conception. The latter is now, of course, the official belief of the Catholic Church. As one of the briefs *amicus* discloses, this is a view strongly held by many non-Catholics as well, and by many physicians. Substantial problems for precise definition of this view are posed, however, by new embryological data that purport to indicate that conception is a "process" over time, rather than an event, and by new medical techniques such as menstrual extraction, the "morning-after" pill, implantation of embryos, artificial insemination, and even artificial wombs.

In areas other than criminal abortion the law has been reluctant to endorse any theory that life, as we recognize it, begins before live birth or to accord legal rights to the unborn except in narrowly defined situations and except when the rights are contingent upon live birth. For example, the traditional rule of tort law had denied recovery for prenatal injuries even though the child was born alive. That rule has been changed in almost every jurisdiction. In most States recovery is said to be permitted only if the fetus was viable, or at least quick, when the injuries were sustained, though few courts have squarely so held. In a recent development, generally opposed by the commentators, some States permit the parents of a stillborn child to maintain an action for wrongful death because of prenatal injuries. Such an action, however, would appear to be one to vindicate the parents' interest and is thus consistent with the view that the fetus, at most, represents only the potentiality of life. Similarly, unborn children have

been recognized as acquiring rights or interests by way of inheritance or other devolution of property, and have been represented by guardians *ad litem*. Perfection of the interests involved, again, has generally been contingent upon live birth. In short, the unborn have never been recognized in the law as persons in the whole sense.

In view of all this, we do not agree that, by adopting one theory of life, Texas may override the rights of the pregnant woman that are at stake. We repeat, however, that the State does have an important and legitimate interest in preserving and protecting the health of the pregnant woman, whether she be a resident of the State or a nonresident who seeks medical consultation and treatment there, and that it has still *another* important and legitimate interest in protecting the potentiality of human life. These interests are separate and distinct. Each grows in substantiality as the woman approaches term and, at a point during pregnancy, each becomes "compelling."

With respect to the State's important and legitimate interest in the health of the mother, the "compelling" point, in the light of present medical knowledge, is at approximately the end of the first trimester. This is so because of the now established medical fact . . . that until the end of the first trimester mortality in abortion is less than mortality in normal childbirth. It follows that, from and after this point, a State may regulate the abortion procedure to the extent that the regulation reasonably relates to the preservation and protection of maternal health. Examples of permissible state regulation in this area are requirements as to the qualifications of the person who is to perform the abortion; as to the licensure of that person; as to the facility in which the procedure is to be performed, that is, whether it must be a hospital or may be a clinic or some other place of less-than-hospital status; as to the licensing of the facility; and the like.

This means, on the other hand, that, for the period of pregnancy prior to this "compelling" point, the attending physician, in consultation with his patient, is free to determine, without regulation by the State, that in his medical judgment the patient's pregnancy should be terminated. If that decision is reached, the judgment may be effectuated by an abortion free of interference by the State.

With respect to the State's important and

legitimate interest in potential life, the "compelling" point is at viability. This is so because the fetus then presumably has the capability of meaningful life outside the mother's womb. State regulation protective of fetal life after viability thus has both logical and biological justifications. If the State is interested in protecting fetal life after viability, it may go so far as to proscribe abortion during that period except when it is necessary to preserve the life or health of the mother.

Measured against these standards, Art. 1196 of the Texas Penal Code, in restricting legal abortions to those "procured or attempted by medical advice for the purpose of saving the life of the mother," sweeps too broadly. The statute makes no distinction between abortions performed early in pregnancy and those performed later, and it limits to a single reason, "saving" the mother's life, the legal justification for the procedure. The statute, therefore, cannot survive the constitutional attack made upon it here. . . .

To summarize and to repeat:

1. A state criminal abortion statute of the current Texas type, that excepts from criminality only a *life saving* procedure on behalf of the mother, without regard to pregnancy stage and without recognition of the other interests involved, is violative of the Due Process Clause of the Fourteenth Amendment.

   a. For the stage prior to approximately the end of the first trimester, the abortion decision and its effectuation must be left to the medical judgment of the pregnant woman's attending physician.

   b. For the stage subsequent to approximately the end of the first trimester, the State, in promoting its interest in the health of the mother, may, if it chooses, regulate the abortion procedure in ways that are reasonably related to maternal health.

   c. For the stage subsequent to viability the State, in promoting its interest in the potentiality of human life, may, if it chooses, regulate, and even proscribe, abortion except where it is necessary, in appropriate medical judgment, for the preservation of the life or health of the mother.

2. The State may define the term "physician" . . . to mean only a physician currently licensed by the State, and may proscribe any abortion by a person who is not a physician as so defined. . . .

This holding, we feel, is consistent with the relative weights of the respective interests involved, with the lessons and example of medical and legal history, with the lenity of the common law, and with the demands of the profound problems of the present day. The decision leaves the State free to place increasing restrictions on abortion as the period of pregnancy lengthens, so long as those restrictions are tailored to the recognized state interests. The decision vindicates the right of the physician to administer medical treatment according to his professional judgment up to the points where important state interests provide compelling justifications for intervention. Up to those points the abortion decision in all its aspects is inherently, and primarily, a medical decision, and basic responsibility for it must rest with the physician. If an individual practitioner abuses the privilege of exercising proper medical judgment, the usual remedies, judicial and intra-professional, are available. . . .

An Almost Absolute Value in History

John T. Noonan, Jr.

The most fundamental question involved in the long history of thought on abortion is: How do you determine the humanity of a being? To phrase the question that way is to put in comprehensive humanistic terms what the theologians either dealt with as an explicitly theological question under the

Reprinted by permission of the author and publisher from John T. Noonan, Jr., editor, The Morality of Abortion: Legal and Historical Perspectives, *pp. 51–59. Cambridge, Mass.: Harvard University Press. Copyright © 1970 by the President and Fellows of Harvard College.*

heading of "ensoulment" or dealt with implicitly in their treatment of abortion. The Christian position as it originated did not depend on a narrow theological or philosophical concept. It had no relation to theories of infant baptism.[1] It appealed to no special theory of instantaneous ensoulment. It took the world's view on ensoulment as that view changed from Aristotle to Zacchia. There was, indeed, theological influence affecting the theory of ensoulment finally adopted, and, of course, ensoulment itself was a theological concept, so that the position was always explained in theological terms. But the theological notion of ensoulment could easily be translated into humanistic language by substituting "human" for "rational soul"; the problem of knowing when a man is a man is common to theology and humanism.

If one steps outside the specific categories used by the theologians, the answer they gave can be analyzed as a refusal to discriminate among human beings on the basis of their varying potentialities. Once conceived, the being was recognized as man because he had man's potential. The criterion for humanity, thus, was simple and all-embracing: if you are conceived by human parents, you are human.

The strength of this position may be tested by a review of some of the other distinctions offered in the contemporary controversy over legalizing abortion. Perhaps the most popular distinction is in terms of viability. Before an age of so many months, the fetus is not viable, that is, it cannot be removed from the mother's womb and live apart from her. To that extent, the life of the fetus is absolutely dependent on the life of the mother. This dependence is made the basis of denying recognition to its humanity.

There are difficulties with this distinction. One is that the perfection of artificial incubation may make the fetus viable at any time: it may be removed and artificially sustained. Experiments with animals already show that such a procedure is possible. This hypothetical extreme case relates to an actual difficulty: there is considerable elasticity to the idea of viability. Mere length of life is not an exact measure. The viability of the fetus depends on the extent of its anatomical and functional development. The weight and length of the fetus are better guides to the state of its development than age, but weight and length vary. Moreover, different racial groups have different ages at which their fetuses are viable. Some evidence, for example, suggests that Negro fetuses mature more quickly than white fetuses. If viability is the norm, the standard would vary with race and with many individual circumstances.

The most important objection to this approach is that dependence is not ended by viability. The fetus is still absolutely dependent on someone's care in order to continue existence; indeed a child of one or three or even five years of age is absolutely dependent on another's care for existence; uncared for, the older fetus or the younger child will die as surely as the early fetus detached from the mother. The unsubstantial lessening in dependence at viability does not seem to signify any special acquisition of humanity.

A second distinction has been attempted in terms of experience. A being who has had experience, has lived and suffered, who possesses memories, is more human than one who has not. Humanity depends on formation by experience. The fetus is thus "unformed" in the most basic human sense.

This distinction is not serviceable for the embryo which is already experiencing and reacting. The embryo is responsive to touch after eight weeks and at least at that point is experiencing. At an earlier stage the zygote is certainly alive and responding to its environment. The distinction may also be challenged by the rare case where aphasia has erased adult memory: has it erased humanity? More fundamentally, this distinction leaves even the older fetus or the younger child to be treated as an unformed inhuman thing. Finally, it is not clear why experience as such confers humanity. It could be argued that certain central experiences such as loving or learning are necessary to make a man human. But then human beings who have failed to love or to learn might be excluded from the class called man.

A third distinction is made by appeal to the sentiments of adults. If a fetus dies, the grief of the parents is not the grief they would have for a living child. The fetus is an unnamed "it" till birth, and is not perceived as personality until at least the fourth month of existence when movements in the womb manifest a vigorous presence demanding joyful recognition by the parents.

Yet feeling is notoriously an unsure guide to the humanity of others. Many groups of humans have had difficulty in feeling that persons of another tongue, color, religion, sex, are as human as they. Apart from reactions to alien groups, we

mourn the loss of a ten-year-old boy more than the loss of his one-day-old brother or his 90-year-old grandfather. The difference felt and the grief expressed vary with the potentialities extinguished, or the experience wiped out; they do not seem to point to any substantial difference in the humanity of baby, boy, or grandfather.

Distinctions are also made in terms of sensation by the parents. The embryo is felt within the womb only after about the fourth month. The embryo is seen only at birth. What can be neither seen nor felt is different from what is tangible. If the fetus cannot be seen or touched at all, it cannot be perceived as man.

Yet experience shows that sight is even more untrustworthy than feeling in determining humanity. By sight, color became an appropriate index for saying who was a man, and the evil of racial discrimination was given foundation. Nor can touch provide the test; a being confined by sickness, "out of touch" with others, does not thereby seem to lose his humanity. To the extent that touch still has appeal as a criterion, it appears to be a survival of the old English idea of "quickening"—a possible mistranslation of the Latin *animatus* used in the canon law. To that extent touch as a criterion seems to be dependent on the Aristotelian notion of ensoulment, and to fall when this notion is discarded.

Finally, a distinction is sought in social visibility. The fetus is not socially perceived as human. It cannot communicate with others. Thus, both subjectively and objectively, it is not a member of society. As moral rules are rules for the behavior of members of society to each other, they cannot be made for behavior toward what is not yet a member. Excluded from the society of men, the fetus is excluded from the humanity of men.[2]

By force of the argument from the consequences, this distinction is to be rejected. It is more subtle than that founded on an appeal to physical sensation, but it is equally dangerous in its implications. If humanity depends on social recognition, individuals or whole groups may be dehumanized by being denied any status in their society. Such a fate is fictionally portrayed in *1984* and has actually been the lot of many men in many societies. In the Roman empire, for example, condemnation to slavery meant the practical denial of most human rights; in the Chinese Communist world, landlords have been classified as enemies of the people and so treated as nonpersons by the

state. Humanity does not depend on social recognition, though often the failure of society to recognize the prisoner, the alien, the heterodox as human has led to the destruction of human beings. Anyone conceived by a man and a woman is human. Recognition of this condition by society follows a real event in the objective order, however imperfect and halting the recognition. Any attempt to limit humanity to exclude some group runs the risk of furnishing authority and precedent for excluding other groups in the name of the consciousness or perception of the controlling group in the society.

A philosopher may reject the appeal to the humanity of the fetus because he views "humanity" as a secular view of the soul and because he doubts the existence of anything real and objective which can be identified as humanity. One answer to such a philosopher is to ask how he reasons about moral questions without supposing that there is a sense in which he and the others of whom he speaks are human. Whatever group is taken as the society which determines who may be killed is thereby taken as human. A second answer is to ask if he does not believe that there is a right and wrong way of deciding moral questions. If there is such a difference, experience may be appealed to: to decide who is human on the basis of the sentiment of a given society has led to consequences which rational men would characterize as monstrous.

The rejection of the attempted distinctions based on viability and visibility, experience and feeling, may be buttressed by the following considerations: Moral judgments often rest on distinctions, but if the distinctions are not to appear arbitrary *fiat*, they should relate to some real difference in probabilities. There is a kind of continuity in all life, but the earlier stages of the elements of human life possess tiny probabilities of development. Consider for example, the spermatozoa in any normal ejaculate: There are about 200,000,000 in any single ejaculate, of which one has a chance of developing into a zygote. Consider the oocytes which may become ova: there are 100,000 to 1,000,000 oocytes in a female infant, of which a maximum of 390 are ovulated. But once spermatozoon and ovum meet and the conceptus is formed, such studies as have been made show that roughly in only 20 percent of the cases will spontaneous abortion occur. In other words, the chances are about 4 out of 5 that this new being will develop.

At this stage in the life of the being there is a sharp shift in probabilities, an immense jump in potentialities. To make a distinction between the rights of spermatozoa and the rights of the fertilized ovum is to respond to an enormous shift in possibilities. For about twenty days after conception the egg may split to form twins or combine with another egg to form a chimera, but the probability of either event happening is very small.

It may be asked, What does a change in biological probabilities have to do with establishing humanity? The argument from probabilities is not aimed at establishing humanity but at establishing an objective discontinuity which may be taken into account in moral discourse. As life itself is a matter of probabilities, as most moral reasoning is an estimate of probabilities, so it seems in accord with the structure of reality and the nature of moral thought to found a moral judgment on the change in probabilities at conception. The appeal to probabilities is the most commonsensical of arguments, to a greater or smaller degree all of us base our actions on probabilities, and in morals, as in law, prudence and negligence are often measured by the account one has taken of the probabilities. If the chance is 200,000,000 to 1 that the movement in the bushes into which you shoot is a man's, I doubt if many persons would hold you careless in shooting; but if the chances are 4 out of 5 that the movement is a human being's, few would acquit you of blame. Would the argument be different if only one out of ten children conceived came to term? Of course this argument would be different. This argument is an appeal to probabilities that actually exist, not to any and all state of affairs which may be imagined.

The probabilities as they do exist do not show the humanity of the embryo in the sense of a demonstration in logic any more than the probabilities of the movement in the bush being a man demonstrate beyond all doubt that the being is a man. The appeal is a "buttressing" consideration, showing the plausibility of the standard adopted. The argument focuses on the decisional factor in any moral judgment and assumes that part of the business of a moralist is drawing lines. One evidence of the nonarbitrary character of the line drawn is the difference of probabilities on either side of it. If a spermatozoon is destroyed, one destroys a being which had a chance of far less than 1 in 200 million of developing into a reasoning being, possessed of

the genetic code, a heart and other organs, and capable of pain. If a fetus is destroyed, one destroys a being already possessed of the genetic code, organs, and sensitivity to pain, and one which had an 80 percent chance of developing further into a baby outside the womb who, in time, would reason.

The positive argument for conception as the decisive moment of humanization is that at conception the new being receives the genetic code. It is this genetic information which determines his characteristics, which is the biological carrier of the possibility of human wisdom, which makes him a self-evolving being. A being with a human genetic code is man.

This review of current controversy over the humanity of the fetus emphasizes what a fundamental question the theologians resolved in asserting the inviolability of the fetus. To regard the fetus as possessed of equal rights with other humans was not, however, to decide every case where abortion might be employed. It did decide the case where the argument was that the fetus should be aborted for its own good. To say a being was human was to say it had a destiny to decide for itself which could not be taken from it by another man's decision. But human beings with equal rights often come in conflict with each other, and some decision must be made as whose claims are to prevail. Cases of conflict involving the fetus are different only in two respects: the total inability of the fetus to speak for itself and the fact that the right of the fetus regularly at stake is the right to life itself.

The approach taken by the theologians to these conflicts was articulated in terms of "direct" and "indirect." Again, to look at what they were doing from outside their categories, they may be said to have been drawing lines or "balancing values." "Direct" and "indirect" are spatial metaphors; "line-drawing" is another. "To weigh" or "to balance" values is a metaphor of a more complicated mathematical sort hinting at the process which goes on in moral judgments. All the metaphors suggest that, in the moral judgments made, comparisons were necessary, that no value completely controlled. The principle of double effect was no doctrine fallen from heaven, but a method of analysis appropriate where two relative values were being compared. In Catholic moral theology, as it developed, life even of the innocent was not taken as an absolute. Judgments on acts affecting life issued from a process of weighing. In the weighing, the fetus was always given a value greater than zero, always a value separate and independent from its parents. This valuation was crucial and fundamental in all Christian thought on the subject and marked it off from any approach which considered that only the parents' interests needed to be considered.

Even with the fetus weighed as human, one interest could be weighed as equal or superior: that of the mother in her own life. The casuists between 1450 and 1895 were willing to weigh this interest as superior. Since 1895, that interest was given decisive weight only in the two special cases of the cancerous uterus and the ectopic pregnancy. In both of these cases the fetus itself had little chance of survival even if the abortion were not performed. As the balance was once struck in favor of the mother whenever her life was endangered, it could be so struck again. The balance reached between 1895 and 1930 attempted prudentially and pastorally to forestall a multitude of exceptions for interests less than life.

The perception of the humanity of the fetus and the weighing of fetal rights against other human rights constituted the work of the moral analysts. But what spirit animated their abstract judgments? For the Christian community it was the injunction of Scripture to love your neighbor as yourself. The fetus as human was a neighbor; his life had parity with one's own. The commandment gave life to what otherwise would have been only rational calculation.

The commandment could be put in humanistic as well as theological terms: Do not injure your fellow man without reason. In these terms, once the humanity of the fetus is perceived, abortion is never right except in self-defense. When life must be taken to save life, reason alone cannot say that a mother must prefer a child's life to her own. With this exception, now of great rarity, abortion violates the rational humanist tenet of the equality of human lives.

For Christians the commandment to love had received a special imprint in that the exemplar proposed of love was the love of the Lord for his disciples. In the light given by this example, self-sacrifice carried to the point of death seemed in the extreme situations not without meaning. In the less extreme cases, preference for one's own interests to the life of another seemed to express cruelty or selfishness irreconcilable with the demands of love.

Notes

1. According to Glanville Williams (*The Sanctity of Human Life*, p. 193), "The historical reason for the Catholic objection to abortion is the same as for the Christian Church's historical opposition to infanticide: the horror of bringing about the death of an unbaptized child." This statement is made without any citation of evidence. [As previously argued], desire to administer baptism could, in the Middle Ages, even be urged as a reason for procuring an abortion. It is highly regrettable that the American Law Institute was apparently misled by Williams' account and repeated after him the same baseless statement. See American Law Institute, *Model Penal Code: Tentative Draft No. 9* (1959), p. 148, n. 12.

2. Thomas Aquinas gave an analogous reason against baptizing a fetus in the womb: "As long as it exists in the womb of the mother, it cannot be subject to the operation of the ministers of the Church as it is not known to men" (*In sententias Petri Lombardi* 4.6 1.1.2).

Abortion and Infanticide

Michael Tooley

This essay deals with the question of the morality of abortion and infanticide.[1] The fundamental ethical objection traditionally advanced against these practices rests on the contention that human fetuses and infants have a right to life. It is this claim which will be the focus of attention here. The

Michael Tooley, "Abortion and Infanticide," Philosophy & Public Affairs, *Vol. 2, no. 1 (Fall 1972).*

basic issue to be discussed, then, is what properties a thing must possess in order to have a serious right to life. My approach will be to set out and defend a basic moral principle specifying a condition an organism must satisfy if it is to have a serious right to life. It will be seen that this condition is not satisfied by human fetuses and infants, and thus that they do not have a right to life. So unless there are other substantial objections to abortion and infanticide, one is forced to conclude that these practices are morally acceptable ones. In contrast, it may turn out that our treatment of adult members of other species—cats, dogs, polar bears—is morally indefensible. For it is quite possible that such animals do possess properties that endow them with a right to life.

I. Abortion and Infanticide

One reason the question of the morality of infanticide is worth examining is that it seems very difficult to formulate a completely satisfactory liberal position on abortion without coming to grips with the infanticide issue. The problem the liberal encounters is essentially that of specifying a cutoff point which is not arbitrary: at what stage in the development of a human being does it cease to be morally permissible to destroy it? It is important to be clear about the difficulty here. The conservative's objection is not that since there is a continuous line of development from a zygote to a newborn baby, one must conclude that if it is seriously wrong to destroy a newborn baby it is also seriously wrong to destroy a zygote or any intermediate stage in the development of a human being. His point is rather that if one says it is wrong to destroy a newborn baby but not a zygote or some intermediate stage in the development of a human being, one should be prepared to point to a *morally relevant* difference between a newborn baby and the earlier stage in the development of a human being.

Precisely the same difficulty can, of course, be raised for a person who holds that infanticide is morally permissible. The conservative will ask what morally relevant differences there are between an adult human being and a newborn baby. What makes it morally permissible to destroy a baby, but wrong to kill an adult? So the challenge remains. But I will argue that in this case there is an extremely plausible answer.

Reflecting on the morality of infanticide forces one to face up to this challenge. In the case of abortion a number of events—quickening or viability, for instance—might be taken as cutoff points, and it is easy to overlook the fact that none of these events involves any morally significant change in the developing human. In contrast, if one is going to defend infanticide, one has to get very clear about what makes something a person, what gives something a right to life.

One of the interesting ways in which the abortion issue differs from most other moral issues is that the plausible positions on abortion appear to be extreme positions. For if a human fetus is a person, one is inclined to say that, in general, one would be justified in killing it only to save the life of the mother.[2] Such is the extreme conservative position.[3] On the other hand, if the fetus is not a person, how can it be seriously wrong to destroy it? Why would one need to point to special circumstances to justify such action? The upshot is that there is no room for a moderate position on the issue of abortion such as one finds, for example, in the Model Penal Code recommendations.[4]

Aside from the light it may shed on the abortion question, the issue of infanticide is both interesting and important in its own right. The theoretical interest has been mentioned: it forces one to face up to the question of what makes something a person. The practical importance need not be labored. Most people would prefer to raise children who do not suffer from gross deformities or from severe physical, emotional, or intellectual handicaps. If it could be shown that there is no moral objection to infanticide the happiness of society could be significantly and justifiably increased.

Infanticide is also of interest because of the strong emotions it arouses. The typical reaction to infanticide is like the reaction to incest or cannibalism, or the reaction of previous generations to masturbation or oral sex. The response, rather than appealing to carefully formulated moral principles, is primarily visceral. When philosophers themselves respond in this way, offering no arguments, and dismissing infanticide out of hand, it is reasonable to suspect that one is dealing with a taboo rather than with a rational prohibition.[5] I shall attempt to show that this is in fact the case.

II. Terminology: "Person" versus "Human Being"

How is the term "person" to be interpreted? I shall treat the concept of a person as a purely moral concept, free of all descriptive content. Specifically, in my usage, the sentence "X is a person" will be synonymous with the sentence "X has a (serious) moral right to life."

This usage diverges slightly from what is perhaps the more common way of interpreting the term "person" when it is employed as a purely moral term, where to say that X is a person is to say that X has rights. If everything that had rights had a right to life, these interpretations would be extensionally equivalent. But I am inclined to think that it does not follow from acceptable moral principles that whatever has any rights at all has a right to life. My reason is this. Given the choice between being killed and being tortured for an hour, most adult humans would surely choose the latter. So it seems plausible to say it is worse to kill an adult human being than it is to torture him for an hour. In contrast, it seems to me that while it is not seriously wrong to kill a newborn kitten, it is seriously wrong to torture one for an hour. This *suggests* that newborn kittens may have a right not to be tortured without having a serious right to life. For it seems to be true that an individual has a right to something whenever it is the case that, if he wants that thing, it would be wrong for others to deprive him of it. Then if it is wrong to inflict a certain sensation upon a kitten if it doesn't want to experience that sensation, it will follow that the kitten has a right not to have sensation inflicted upon it.[6] I shall return to this example later. My point here is merely that it provides some reason for holding that it does not follow from acceptable moral principles that if something has any rights at all, it has a serious right to life.

There has been a tendency in recent discussions of abortion to use expressions such as "person" and "human being" interchangeably. B. A. Brody, for example, refers to the difficulty of determining "whether destroying the fetus constitutes the taking of a human life," and suggests it is very plausible that "the taking of a human life is an action that has bad consequences for him whose life is being taken."[7] When Brody refers to something as a human life he apparently construes this as entailing that the thing is a person. For if every living organism belonging to the species homo sapiens counted as a human life, there would be no difficulty in determining whether a fetus inside a human mother was a human life.

The same tendency is found in Judith Jarvis Thomson's article, which opens with the statement: "Most opposition to abortion relies on the premise that the fetus is a human being, a person, from the moment of conception."[8] The same is true of Roger Wertheimer, who explicitly says: "First off I should note that the expressions 'a human life,' 'a human being,' 'a person' are virtually interchangeable in this context."[9]

The tendency to use expressions like "person" and "human being" interchangeably is an unfortunate one. For one thing, it tends to lend covert support to antiabortionist positions. Given such usage, one who holds a liberal view of abortion is put in the position of maintaining that fetuses, at least up to a certain point, are not human beings. Even philosophers are led astray by this usage. Thus Wertheimer says that "except for monstrosities, every member of our species is indubitably a person, a human being, at the very latest at birth."[10] Is it really *indubitable* that newborn babies are persons? Surely this is a wild contention. Wertheimer is falling prey to the confusion naturally engendered by the practice of using "person" and "human being" interchangeably. Another example of this is provided by Thomson: "I am inclined to think also that we shall probably have to agree that the fetus has already become a human person well before birth. Indeed, it comes as a surprise when one first learns how early in its life it begins to acquire human characteristics. By the tenth week, for example, it already has a face, arms and legs, fingers and toes; it has internal organs, and brain activity is detectable."[11] But what do such physiological characteristics have to do with the question of whether the organism is a person? Thomson, partly, I think, because of the unfortunate use of terminology, does not even raise this question. As a result she virtually takes it for granted that there are some cases in which abortion is "positively indecent."[12]

There is a second reason why using "person" and "human being" interchangeably is unhappy philosophically. If one says that the dispute between pro- and anti-abortionists centers on whether the fetus is a human, it is natural to conclude that it is essentially a disagreement about certain facts, a disagreement about what properties a fetus possesses. Thus Wertheimer says that "if one insists on using the raggy fact-value distinction, then one ought to say that the dispute is over a matter of fact in the sense in which it is a fact that the Negro slaves were human beings."[13] I shall argue that the two cases are not parallel, and that in the case of abortion what is primarily at stake is what moral principles one should accept. If one says that the central issue between conservatives and liberals in the abortion question is whether the fetus is a person, it is clear that the dispute may be either about what properties a thing must have in order to be a person, in order to have a right to life—a moral question—or about whether a fetus at a given stage of development as a matter of fact possesses the properties in question. The temptation to suppose that the disagreement must be a factual one is removed.

It should now be clear why the common practice of using expressions such as "person" and "human being" interchangeably in discussions of abortion is unfortunate. It would perhaps be best to avoid the term "human" altogether, employing instead some expression that is more naturally interpreted as referring to a certain type of biological organism characterized in physiological terms, such as "member of the species Homo sapiens." My own approach will be to use the term "human" only in contexts where it is not philosophically dangerous.

III. The Basic Issue: When Is a Member of the Species Homo Sapiens a Person?

Settling the issue of the morality of abortion and infanticide will involve answering the following questions: What properties must something have to be a person, i.e., to have a serious right to life? At what point in the development of a member of the species Homo sapiens does the organism possess the properties that make it a person? The first question raises a moral issue. To answer it is to decide what basic[14] moral principles involving the ascription of a right to life one ought to accept. The second question raises a purely factual issue, since the properties in question are properties of a purely descriptive sort.

Some writers seem quite pessimistic about the

possibility of resolving the question of the morality of abortion. Indeed, some have gone so far as to suggest that the question of whether the fetus is a person is in principle unanswerable: "we seem to be stuck with the indeterminateness of the fetus' humanity."[15] An understanding of some of the sources of this pessimism will, I think, help us to tackle the problem. Let us begin by considering the similarity a number of people have noted between the issue of abortion and the issue of Negro slavery. The question here is why it should be more difficult to decide whether abortion and infanticide are acceptable than it was to decide whether slavery was acceptable. The answer seems to be that in the case of slavery there are moral principles of a quite uncontroversial sort that settle the issue. Thus most people would agree to some such principle as the following: No organism that has experiences, that is capable of thought and of using language, and that has harmed no one, should be made a slave. In the case of abortion, on the other hand, conditions that are generally agreed to be sufficient grounds for ascribing a right to life to something do not suffice to settle the issue. It is easy to specify other, purportedly sufficient conditions that will settle the issue, but no one has been successful in putting forward considerations that will convince others to accept those additional moral principles.

I do not share the general pessimism about the possibility of resolving the issue of abortion and infanticide because I believe it is possible to point to a very plausible moral principle dealing with the question of *necessary* conditions for something's having a right to life, where the conditions in question will provide an answer to the question of the permissibility of abortion and infanticide.

There is a second cause of pessimism that should be noted before proceeding. It is tied up with the fact that the development of an organism is one of gradual and continuous change. Given this continuity, how is one to draw a line at one point and declare it permissible to destroy a member of Homo sapiens up to, but not beyond, that point? Won't there be an arbitrariness about any point that is chosen? I will return to this worry shortly. It does not present a serious difficulty once the basic moral principles relevant to the ascription of a right to life to an individual are established.

Let us turn now to the first and most fundamental question: What properties must something have in order to be a person, i.e., to have a serious right to life? The claim I wish to defend is this: An organism possesses a serious right to life only if it possesses the concept of a self as a continuing subject of experiences and other mental states, and believes that it is itself such a continuing entity.

My basic argument in support of this claim, which I will call the self-consciousness requirement, will be clearest, I think, if I first offer a simplified version of the argument, and then consider a modification that seems desirable. The simplified version of my argument is this. To ascribe a right to an individual is to assert something about the prima facie obligations of other individuals to act, or to refrain from acting, in certain ways. However, the obligations in question are conditional ones, being dependent upon the existence of certain desires of the individual to whom the right is ascribed. Thus if an individual asks one to destroy something to which he has a right, one does not violate his right to that thing if one proceeds to destroy it. This suggests the following analysis: "A has a right to X" is roughly synonymous with "If A desires X, then others are under a prima facie obligation to refrain from actions that would deprive him of it."[16]

Although this analysis is initially plausible, there are reasons for thinking it not entirely correct. I will consider these later. Even here, however, some expansion is necessary, since there are features of the concept of a right that are important in the present context, and that ought to be dealt with more explicitly. In particular, it seems to be a conceptual truth that things that lack consciousness, such as ordinary machines, cannot have rights. Does this conceptual truth follow from the above analysis of the concept of a right? The answer depends on how the term "desire" is interpreted. If one adopts a completely behavioristic interpretation of "desire," so that a machine that searches for an electrical outlet in order to get its batteries recharged is described as having a desire to be recharged, then it will not follow from this analysis that objects that lack consciousness cannot have rights. On the other hand, if "desire" is interpreted in such a way that desires are states necessarily standing in some sort of relationship to states of consciousness, it will follow from the analysis that a machine that is not capable of being conscious, and consequently of having desires, cannot have any rights. I think those who defend analyses of the concept of a right along the lines of this one do have in mind an interpretation of the term "desire" that involves reference to something more than behavioral dispositions. However, rather than relying on this, it seems preferable to make such an interpretation explicit. The following analysis is a natural way of doing that: "A has a right to X" is roughly synonymous with "A is the sort of thing that is a subject of experiences and other mental states, A is capable of desiring X, and if A does desire X, then others are under a prima facie obligation to refrain from actions that would deprive him of it."

The next step in the argument is basically a matter of applying this analysis to the concept of a right to life. Unfortunately the expression "right to life" is not entirely a happy one, since it suggests that the right in question concerns the continued existence of a biological organism. That this is incorrect can be brought out by considering possible ways of violating an individual's right to life. Suppose, for example, that by some technology of the future the brain of an adult human were to be completely reprogrammed, so that the organism wound up with memories (or rather, apparent memories), beliefs, attitudes, and personality traits completely different from those associated with it before it was subjected to reprogramming. In such a case one would surely say that an individual had been destroyed, that an adult human's right to life had been violated, even though no biological organism had been killed. This example shows that the expression "right to life" is misleading, since what one is really concerned about is not just the continued existence of a biological organism, but the right of a subject of experiences and other mental states to continue to exist.

Given this more precise description of the right with which we are here concerned, we are now in a position to apply the analysis of the concept of a right stated above. When we do so we find that the statement "A has a right to continue to exist as a subject of experiences and other mental states" is roughly synonymous with the statement "A is a subject of experiences and other mental states, A is capable of desiring to continue to exist as a subject of experiences and other mental states, and if A does desire to continue to exist as such an entity, then others are under a prima facie obligation not to prevent him from doing so.''

The final stage in the argument is simply a matter of asking what must be the case if something is to be capable of having a desire to continue existing as a subject of experiences and other mental states. The basic point here is that the desires a thing can have are limited by the concepts it possesses. For the fundamental way of describing a given desire is as a desire that a certain proposition be true.[17] Then, since one cannot desire that a certain proposition be true unless one understands it, and since one cannot understand it without possessing the concepts involved in it, it follows that the desires one can have are limited by the concepts one possesses. Applying this to the present case results in the conclusion that an entity cannot be the sort of thing that can desire that a subject of experiences and other mental states exist unless it possesses the concept of such a subject. Moreover, an entity cannot desire that it itself *continue* existing as a subject of experiences and other mental states unless it believes that it is now such a subject. This completes the justification of the claim that it is a necessary condition of something's having a serious right to life that it possess the concept of a self as a continuing subject of experiences, and that it believe that it is itself such an entity.

Let us now consider a modification in the above argument that seems desirable. This modification concerns the crucial conceptual claim advanced about the relationship between ascription of rights and ascription of the corresponding desires. Certain situations suggest that there may be exceptions to the claim that if a person doesn't desire something, one cannot violate his right to it. There are three types of situations that call this claim into question: (i) situations in which an individual's desires reflect a state of emotional disturbance; (ii) situations in which a previously conscious individual is temporarily unconscious; (iii) situations in which an individual's desires have been distorted by conditioning or by indoctrination.

As an example of the first, consider a case in which an adult human falls into a state of depression which his psychiatrist recognizes as temporary. While in the state he tells people he wishes he were dead. His psychiatrist, accepting the view that there can be no violation of an individual's right to life unless the individual has a desire to live, decides to let his patient have his way and kills him. Or consider a related case in which one person gives another a drug that produces a state of temporary depression; the recipient expresses a wish that he were dead. The person who administered the drug then kills him. Doesn't one want to say in both these cases that the agent did something seriously wrong in killing the other person? And isn't the reason the action was seriously wrong in each case the fact that it violated the individual's right to life? If so, the right to life cannot be linked with a desire to live in the way claimed above.

The second set of situations are ones in which an individual is unconscious for some reason— that is, he is sleeping, or drugged, or in a temporary coma. Does an individual in such a state have any desires? People do sometimes say that an unconscious individual wants something, but it might be argued that if such talk is not to be simply false it must be interpreted as actually referring to the desires the individual *would* have if he were now conscious. Consequently, if the analysis of the concept of a right proposed above were correct, it would follow that one does not violate an individual's right if one takes his car, or kills him, while he is asleep.

Finally, consider situations in which an individual's desires have been distorted, either by inculcation of irrational beliefs or by direct conditioning. Thus an individual may permit someone to kill him because he has been convinced that if he allows himself to be sacrificed to the gods he will be gloriously rewarded in a life to come. Or an individual may be enslaved after first having been conditioned to desire a life of slavery. Doesn't one want to say that in the former case an individual's right to life has been violated, and in the latter his right to freedom?

Situations such as these strongly suggest that even if an individual doesn't want something, it is still possible to violate his right to it. Some modification of the earlier account of the concept of a right thus seems in order. The analysis given covers, I believe, the paradigmatic cases of violation of an individual's rights, but there are other, secondary cases where one also wants to say that someone's right has been violated which are not included.

Precisely how the revised analysis should be formulated is unclear. Here it will be sufficient merely to say that, in view of the above, an individual's right to X can be violated not only when he desires X, but also when he *would* now desire X were it not for one of the following: (i) he is in an emotionally unbalanced state; (ii) he is temporarily unconscious; (iii) he has been conditioned to desire the absence of X.

The critical point now is that, even given this extension of the conditions under which an individual's right to something can be violated, it is still true that one's right to something can be violated only when one has the conceptual capability of desiring the thing in question. For example, an individual who would now desire not to be a slave if he weren't emotionally unbalanced, or if he weren't temporarily unconscious, or if he hadn't previously been conditioned to want to be a slave, must possess the concepts involved in the desire not to be a slave. Since it is really only the conceptual capability presupposed by the desire to continue existing as a subject of experiences and other mental states, and not the desire itself, that enters into the above argument, the modification required in the account of the conditions under which an individual's rights can be violated does not undercut my defense of the self-consciousness requirement.[18]

To sum up, my argument has been that having a right to life presupposes that one is capable of desiring to continue existing as a subject of experiences and other mental states. This in turn presupposes both that one has the concept of such a continuing entity and that one believes that one is oneself such an entity. So an entity that lacks such a consciousness of itself as a continuing subject of mental states does not have a right to life.

It would be natural to ask at this point whether satisfaction of this requirement is not only necessary but also sufficient to ensure that a thing has a right to life. I am inclined to an affirmative answer. However, the issue is not urgent in the present context, since as long as the requirement is in fact a necessary one we have the basis of an adequate defense of abortion and infanticide. If an organism must satisfy some other condition before it has a serious right to life, the result will merely be that the interval during which infanticide is morally permissible may be somewhat longer. Although the point at which an organism first achieves self-consciousness and hence the capacity of desiring to continue existing as a subject of experiences and other mental states may be a theoretically incorrect cutoff point, it is at least a morally safe one: any error it involves is on the side of caution.

IV. Some Critical Comments on Alternative Proposals

I now want to compare the line of demarcation I am proposing with the cutoff points traditionally advanced in discussions of abortion. My fundamental claim will be that none of these cutoff points can be defended by appeal to plausible, basic moral principles. The main suggestions as to the point past which it is seriously wrong to destroy something that will develop into an adult member of the species Homo sapiens are these: (a) conception; (b) the attainment of human form; (c) the achievement of the ability to move about spontaneously; (d) viability; (e) birth.[19] The corresponding moral principles suggested by these cutoff points are as follows: (1) It is seriously wrong to kill an organism, from a zygote on, that belongs to the species Homo sapiens. (2) It is seriously wrong to kill an organism that belongs to Homo sapiens and that has achieved human form. (3) It is seriously wrong to kill an organism that is a member of Homo sapiens and that is capable of spontaneous movement. (4) It is seriously wrong to kill an organism that belongs to Homo sapiens and that is capable of existing outside the womb. (5) It is seriously wrong to kill an organism that is a member of Homo sapiens that is no longer in the womb.

My first comment is that it would not do *simply* to omit the reference to membership in the species Homo sapiens from the above principles, with the exception of principle (2). For then the principles would be applicable to animals in general, and one would be forced to conclude that it was seriously wrong to abort a cat fetus, or that it was seriously wrong to abort a motile cat fetus, and so on.

The second and crucial comment is that none of the five principles given above can plausibly be viewed as a *basic* moral principle. To accept any of them as such would be akin to accepting as a basic moral principle the proposition that it is morally permissible to enslave black members of the species Homo sapiens but not white members. Why should it be seriously wrong to kill an unborn member of the species Homo sapiens but not seriously wrong to kill an unborn kitten? Difference in species is not per se a morally relevant difference. If one holds that it is seriously wrong to kill an unborn member of the species Homo sapiens but not an unborn kitten, one should be prepared to point to some property that is morally significant and that is possessed by unborn members of Homo sapiens but not by unborn kittens. Similarly, such a property must be identified if one believes it seriously wrong to kill unborn members of Homo sapiens that have achieved viability but not seriously wrong to kill unborn kittens that have achieved that state.

What property might account for such a difference? That is to say, what *basic* moral principles might a person who accepts one of these five principles appeal to in support of his secondary moral judgment? Why should events such as the achievement of human form, or the achievement of the ability to move about, or the achievement of viability, or birth serve to endow something with a right to life? What the liberal must do is to show that these events involve changes, or are associated with changes, that are morally relevant.

Let us now consider reasons why the events involved in cutoff points (b) through (e) are not morally relevant, beginning with the last two: viability and birth. The fact that an organism is not physiologically dependent upon another organism, or is capable of such physiological independence, is surely irrelevant to whether the organism has a right to life. In defense of this contention, consider a speculative case where a fetus is able to learn a language while in the womb. One would surely not say that the fetus had no right to life until it emerged from the womb, or until it was capable of existing outside the womb. A less speculative example is the case of Siamese twins who have learned to speak. One doesn't want to say that since one of the twins would die were the two to be separated, it therefore has no right to life. Consequently it seems difficult to disagree with the conservative's claim that an organism which lacks a right to life before birth or before becoming viable cannot acquire this right immediately upon birth or upon becoming viable.

This does not, however, completely rule out viability as a line of demarcation. For instead of defending viability as a cutoff point on the ground that only then does a fetus acquire a right to life, it is possible to argue rather that when one organism is physiologically dependent upon another, the former's right to life may conflict with the latter's right to use its body as it will, and moreover, that the latter's right to do what it wants with its body may often take precedence over the other organism's right to life. Thomson has defended this view: "I am arguing only that having a right to life does not guarantee having either a right to the use of or a right to be allowed continued use of another person's body—even if one needs it for life itself. So the right to life will not serve the opponents of abortion in the very simple and clear way in which they seem to have thought it would."[20] I believe that Thomson is right in contending that philosophers have been altogether too casual in assuming that if one grants the fetus a serious right to life, one must accept a conservative position on abortion.[21] I also think the only defense of viability as a cutoff point which has any hope of success at all is one based on the considerations she advances. I doubt very much, however, that this defense of abortion is ultimately tenable. I think that one can grant even stronger assumptions than those made by Thomson and still argue persuasively for a semiconservative view. What I have in mind is this. Let it be granted, for the sake of argument, that a woman's right to free her body of parasites which will inhibit her freedom of action and possibly impair her health is stronger than the parasite's right to life, and is so even if the parasite has as much right to life as an adult human. One can still argue that abortion ought not to be permitted. For if A's right is stronger than B's, and it is impossible to satisfy both, it does not follow that A's should be satisfied rather than B's. It may be possible to compensate A if his right isn't satisfied, but impossible to compensate B if his right isn't satisfied. In such a case the best thing to do may be to satisfy B's claim and to compensate A. Abortion may be a case in point. If the fetus has a right to life and the right is not satisfied, there is certainly no way the fetus can be compensated. On the other hand, if the woman's right to rid her body of harmful and annoying parasites is not satisfied, she can be compensated. Thus it would seem that the just thing to do would be to prohibit abortion, but to compensate women for the burden of carrying a parasite to term. Then, however, we are back at a (modified) conservative position.[22] Our conclusion must be that it appears unlikely there is any satisfactory defense either of viability or of birth as cutoff points.

Let us now consider the third suggested line of demarcation, the achievement of the power to move about spontaneously. It might be argued that acquiring this power is a morally relevant event on the grounds that there is a connection between the concept of an agent and the concept of a person, and being motile is an indication that a thing is an agent.[23]

It is difficult to respond to this suggestion unless it is made more specific. Given that one's interest here is in defending a certain cutoff point, it is natural to interpret the proposal as suggesting that motility is a necessary condition of an organism's having a right to life. But this won't do, because one certainly wants to ascribe a right to life to adult humans who are completely paralyzed. Maybe the suggestion is rather that motility is a sufficient condition of something's having a right to life. However, it is clear that motility alone is not sufficient, since this would imply that all animals, and also certain machines, have a right to life. Perhaps, then, the most reasonable interpretation of the claim is that motility together with some other property is a sufficient condition of something's having a right to life, where the other property will have to be a property possessed by unborn members of the species Homo sapiens but not by unborn members of other familiar species.

The central question, then, is what this other property is. Until one is told, it is very difficult to evaluate either the moral claim that motility together with that property is a sufficient basis for ascribing to an organism a right to life or the factual claim that a motile human fetus possesses that property while a motile fetus belonging to some other species does not. A conservative would presumably reject motility as a cutoff point by arguing that whether an organism has a right to life depends only upon its potentialities, which are

of course not changed by its becoming motile. If, on the other hand, one favors a liberal view of abortion, I think that one can attack this third suggested cutoff point, in its unspecified form, only by determining what properties are necessary, or what properties sufficient, for an individual to have a right to life. Thus I would base my rejection of motility as a cutoff point on my claim, defended above, that a necessary condition of an organism's possessing a right to life is that it conceive of itself as a continuing subject of experiences and other mental states.

The second suggested cutoff point—the development of a recognizably human form—can be dismissed fairly quickly. I have already remarked that membership in a particular species is not itself a morally relevant property. For it is obvious that if we encountered other "rational animals," such as Martians, the fact that their physiological makeup was very different from our own would not be grounds for denying them a right to life.[24] Similarly, it is clear that the development of human form is not in itself a morally relevant event. Nor do there seem to be any grounds for holding that there is some other change, associated with this event, that is morally relevant. The appeal of this second cutoff point is, I think, purely emotional.

The overall conclusion seems to be that it is very difficult to defend the cutoff points traditionally advanced by those who advocate either a moderate or a liberal position on abortion. The reason is that there do not seem to be any basic moral principles one can appeal to in support of the cutoff points in question. We must now consider whether the conservative is any better off.

V. Refutation of the Conservative Position

Many have felt that the conservative's position is more defensible than the liberal's because the conservative can point to the gradual and continuous development of an organism as it changes from a zygote to an adult human being. He is then in a position to argue that it is morally arbitrary for the liberal to draw a line at some point in this continuous process and to say that abortion is permissible before, but not after, that particular point. The liberal's reply would presumably be that the emphasis upon the continuity of the process is misleading. What the conservative is really doing is simply challenging the liberal to specify the properties a thing must have in order to be a person, and to show that the developing organism does acquire the properties at the point selected by the liberal. The liberal may then reply that the difficulty he has meeting this challenge should not be taken as grounds for rejecting his position. For the conservative cannot meet this challenge either; the conservative is equally unable to say what properties something must have if it is to have a right to life.

Although this rejoinder does not dispose of the conservative's argument, it is not without bite. For defenders of the view that abortion is always wrong have failed to face up to the question of the basic moral principles on which their position rests. They have been content to assert the wrongness of killing any organism, from a zygote on, if that organism is a member of the species Homo sapiens. But they have overlooked the point that this cannot be an acceptable *basic* moral principle, since difference in species is not in itself a morally relevant difference. The conservative can reply, however, that it is possible to defend his position—but not the liberal's—*without* getting clear about the properties a thing must possess if it is to have a right to life. The conservative's defense will rest upon the following two claims: first, that there is a property, even if one is unable to specify what it is, that (i) is possessed by adult humans, and (ii) endows any organism possessing it with a serious right to life. Second, that if there are properties which satisfy (i) and (ii) above, at least one of those properties will be such that any organism potentially possessing that property has a serious right to life even now, simply by virtue of that potentiality, where an organism possesses a property potentially if it will come to have that property in the normal course of its development. The second claim—which I shall refer to as the potentiality principle—is critical to the conservative's defense. Because of it he is able to defend his position without deciding what properties a thing must possess in order to have a right to life. It is enough to know that adult members of Homo sapiens do have such a right. For then one can conclude that any organism which belongs to the species Homo sapiens, from a zygote on, must also have a right to life by virtue of the potentiality principle.

The liberal, by contrast, cannot mount a comparable argument. He cannot defend his position without offering at least a partial answer to the question of what properties a thing must possess in order to have a right to life.

The importance of the potentiality principle, however, goes beyond the fact that it provides support for the conservative's position. If the principle is unacceptable, then so is his position. For if the conservative cannot defend the view that an organism's having certain potentialities is sufficient grounds for ascribing to it a right to life, his claim that a fetus which is a member of Homo sapiens has a right to life can be attacked as follows. The reason an adult member of Homo sapiens has a right to life, but an infant ape does not, is that there are certain psychological properties which the former possesses and the latter lacks. Now, even if one is unsure exactly what these psychological properties are, it is clear that an organism in the early stages of development from a zygote into an adult member of Homo sapiens does not possess these properties. One need merely compare a human fetus with an ape fetus. What mental states does the former enjoy that the latter does not? Surely it is reasonable to hold that there are no significant differences in their respective mental lives—assuming that one wishes to ascribe any mental states at all to such organisms. (Does a zygote have a mental life? Does it have experiences? Or beliefs? Or desires?) There are, of course, physiological differences, but these are not in themselves morally significant. *If* one held that potentialities were relevant to the ascription of a right to life, one could argue that the physiological differences, though not morally significant in themselves, are morally significant by virtue of their causal consequences: they will lead to later psychological differences that are morally relevant, and for this reason the physiological differences are themselves morally significant. But if the potentiality principle is not available, this line of argument cannot be used, and there will then be no differences between a human fetus and an ape fetus that the conservative can use as grounds for ascribing a serious right to life to the former but not to the latter.

It is therefore tempting to conclude that the conservative view of abortion is acceptable if and only if the potentiality principle is acceptable. But to say that the conservative position can be defended if the potentiality principle is acceptable is to assume that the argument is over once it is granted that the fetus has a right to life, and, as was noted above, Thomson has shown that there are serious grounds for questioning this assumption. In any case, the important point here is that the conservative position on abortion is acceptable *only if* the potentiality principle is sound.

One way to attack the potentiality principle is simply to argue in support of the self-consciousness requirement—the claim that only an organism that conceives of itself as a continuing subject of experiences has a right to life. For this requirement, when taken together with the claim that there is at least one property, possessed by adult humans, such that any organism possessing it has a serious right to life, entails the denial of the potentiality principle. Or at least this is so if we add the uncontroversial empirical claim that an organism that will in the normal course of events develop into an adult human does not from the very beginning of its existence possess a concept of a continuing subject of experiences together with a belief that it is itself such an entity.

I think it best, however, to scrutinize the potentiality principle itself, and not to base one's case against it simply on the self-consciousness requirement. Perhaps the first point to note is that the potentiality principle should not be confused with principles such as the following: the value of an object is related to the value of the things into which it can develop. This "valuation principle" is rather vague. There are ways of making it more precise, but we need not consider these here. Suppose now that one were to speak not of a right to life, but of the value of life. It would then be easy to make the mistake of thinking that the valuation principle was relevant to the potentiality principle—indeed, that it entailed it. But an individual's right to life is not based on the value of his life. To say that the world would be better off if it contained fewer people is not to say that it would be right to achieve such a better world by killing some of the present inhabitants. *If* having a right to life were a matter of a thing's value, then a thing's potentialities, being connected with its expected value, would clearly be relevant to the question of what rights it had. Conversely, once one realizes that a thing's rights are not a matter of its value, I think it becomes clear that an organism's potentialities are irrelevant to the question of whether it has a right to life.

But let us now turn to the task of finding a direct refutation of the potentiality principle. The basic issue is this. Is there any property J which satisfies the following conditions: (1) There is a property K such that any individual possessing property K has a right to life, and there is a scientific law L to the effect that any organism possessing property J will in the normal course of events come to possess property K at some later time. (2) Given the relationship between property J and property K just described, anything possessing property J has a right to life. (3) If property J were not related to property K in the way indicated, it would not be the case that anything possessing property J thereby had a right to life. In short, the question is whether there is a property J that bestows a right to life on an organism *only because* J stands in a certain causal relationship to a second property K, which is such that anything possessing that property ipso facto has a right to life.

My argument turns upon the following critical principle: Let C be a causal process that normally leads to outcome E. Let A be an action that initiates process C, and B be an action involving a minimal expenditure of energy that stops process C before outcome E occurs. Assume further that actions A and B do not have any other consequences, and that E is the only morally significant outcome of process C. Then there is no moral difference between intentionally performing action B and intentionally refraining from performing action A, assuming identical motivation in both cases. This principle, which I shall refer to as the moral symmetry principle with respect to action and inaction, would be rejected by some philosophers. They would argue that there is an important distinction to be drawn between "what we owe people in the form of aid and what we owe them in the way of non-interference,"[25] and that the latter, "negative duties," are duties that it is more serious to neglect than the former, "positive" ones. This view arises from an intuitive response to examples such as the following. Even if it is wrong not to send food to starving people in other parts of the world, it is more wrong still to kill someone. And isn't the conclusion, then, that one's obligation to refrain from killing someone is a more serious obligation than one's obligation to save lives?

I want to argue that this is not the correct conclusion. I think it is tempting to draw this conclusion if one fails to consider the motivation that is likely to be associated with the respective actions. If someone performs an action he knows will kill someone else, this will usually be grounds for concluding that he wanted to kill the person in question. In contrast, failing to help someone may indicate only apathy, laziness, selfishness, or an amoral outlook: the fact that a person knowingly allows another to die will not normally be grounds for concluding that he desired that person's death. Someone who knowingly kills another is more likely to be seriously defective from a moral point of view than someone who fails to save another's life.

If we are not to be led to false conclusions by our intuitions about certain cases, we must explicitly assume identical motivations in the two situations. Compare, for example, the following: (1) Jones sees that Smith will be killed by a bomb unless he warns him. Jones's reaction is: "How lucky, it will save me the trouble of killing Smith myself." So Jones allows Smith to be killed by the bomb, even though he could easily have warned him. (2) Jones wants Smith dead, and therefore shoots him. Is one to say there is a significant difference between the wrongness of Jones's behavior in these two cases? Surely not. This shows the mistake of drawing a distinction between positive duties and negative duties and holding that the latter impose stricter obligations than the former. The difference in our intuitions about situations that involve giving aid to others and corresponding situations that involve not interfering with others is to be explained by reference to probable differences in the motivations operating in the two situations, and not by reference to a distinction between positive and negative duties. For once it is specified that the motivation is the same in the two situations, we realize that inaction is as wrong in the one case as action is in the other.

There is another point that may be relevant. Action involves effort, while inaction usually does not. It usually does not require any effort on my part to refrain from killing someone, but saving someone's life will require an expenditure of energy. One must then ask how large a sacrifice a person is morally required to make to save the life of another. If the sacrifice of time and energy is quite large it may be that one is not morally obliged to save the life of another in that situation. Superficial reflection upon such cases might easily lead us to introduce the distinction between positive and negative duties, but again it is clear that this would be a mistake. The point is not that one has a greater duty to refrain from killing others than to perform positive actions that will save them. It is rather that positive actions require effort, and this means that in deciding what to do a person has to take into account his own right to do what he wants with his life, and not only the other person's right to life. To avoid this confusion, we should confine ourselves to comparisons between situations in which the positive action involves minimal effort.

The moral symmetry principle, as formulated above, explicitly takes these two factors into account. It applies only to pairs of situations in which the motivations are identical and the positive action involves minimal effort. Without these restrictions, the principle would be open to serious objection; with them, it seems perfectly acceptable. For the central objection to it rests on the claim that we must distinguish positive from negative duties and recognize that negative duties impose stronger obligations than positive ones. I have tried to show how this claim derives from an unsound account of our moral intuitions about certain situations.

My argument against the potentiality principle can now be stated. Suppose at some future time a chemical were to be discovered which when injected into the brain of a kitten would cause the kitten to develop into a cat possessing a brain of the sort possessed by humans, and consequently into a cat having all the psychological capabilities characteristic of adult humans. Such cats would be able to think, to use language, and so on. Now it would surely be morally indefensible in such a situation to ascribe a serious right to life to members of the species Homo sapiens without also ascribing it to cats that have undergone such a process of development: there would be no morally significant differences.

Secondly, it would not be seriously wrong to refrain from injecting a newborn kitten with the special chemical, and to kill it instead. The fact that one could initiate a causal process that would transform a kitten into an entity that would eventually possess properties such that anything possessing them ipso facto has a serious right to life does not mean that the kitten has a serious right to life even before it has been subjected to the process of injection and transformation. The possibility of transforming kittens into persons will not make it any more wrong to kill newborn kittens than it is now.

Thirdly, in view of the symmetry principle, if it is not seriously wrong to refrain from initiating such a causal process, neither is it seriously wrong to interfere with such a process. Suppose a kitten is accidentally injected with the chemical. As long as it has not yet developed those properties that in themselves endow something with a right to life, there cannot be anything wrong with interfering with the causal process and preventing the development of the properties in question. Such interference might be accomplished either by injecting the kitten with some "neutralizing" chemical or simply by killing it.

But if it is not seriously wrong to destroy an injected kitten which will naturally develop the properties that bestow a right to life, neither can it be seriously wrong to destroy a member of Homo sapiens which lacks such properties, but will naturally come to have them. The potentialities are the same in both cases. The only difference is that in the case of a human fetus the potentialities have been present from the beginning of the organism's development, while in the case of the kitten they have been present only from the time it was injected with the special chemical. This difference in the time at which the potentialities were acquired is a morally irrelevant difference.

It should be emphasized that I am not here assuming that a human fetus does not possess properties which in themselves, and irrespective of their causal relationships to other properties, provide grounds for ascribing a right to life to whatever possesses them. The point is merely that if it is seriously wrong to kill something, the reason cannot be that the thing will later acquire properties that in themselves provide something with a right to life.

Finally, it is reasonable to believe that there are properties possessed by adult members of Homo sapiens which establish their right to life, and also that any normal human fetus will come to possess those properties shared by adult humans. But it has just been shown that if it is wrong to kill a human fetus, it cannot be because of its potentialities. One is therefore forced to conclude that the conservative's potentiality principle is false.

In short, anyone who wants to defend the potentiality principle must either argue against the moral symmetry principle or hold that in a world in which kittens could be transformed into "rational animals" it would be seriously wrong to kill newborn kittens. It is hard to believe there is much to be said for the latter moral claim. Consequently one expects the conservative's rejoinder to be directed against the symmetry principle. While I have not attempted to provide a thorough defense of that principle, I have tried to show that what seems to be the most important objection to it—the one that appeals to a distinction between positive and negative duties—is based on a superficial analysis of our moral intuitions. I believe that a more thorough examination of the symmetry principle would show it to be sound. If so, we should reject the potentiality principle, and the conservative position on abortion as well.

VI. Summary and Conclusions

Let us return now to my basic claim, the self-consciousness requirement: An organism possesses a serious right to life only if it possesses the concept of a self as a continuing subject of experiences and other mental states, and believes that it is itself such a continuing entity. My defense of this claim has been twofold. I have offered a direct argument in support of it, and I have tried to show that traditional conservative and liberal views on abortion and infanticide, which involve a rejection of it, are unsound. I now want to mention one final reason why my claim should be accepted. Consider the example mentioned in section II—that of killing, as opposed to torturing, newborn kittens. I suggested there that while in the case of adult humans most people would consider it worse to kill an individual than to torture him for an hour, we do not usually view the killing of a newborn kitten as morally outrageous, although we would regard someone who tortured a newborn kitten for an hour as heinously evil. I pointed out that a possible conclusion that might be drawn from this is that newborn kittens have a right not to be tortured, but do not have a serious right to life. If this is the correct conclusion, how is one to explain it? One merit of the self-consciousness requirement is that it provides an explanation of this situation. The reason a newborn kitten does not have a right to life is explained by the fact that it does not possess the concept of a self. But how is one to explain the kitten's having a right not to be tortured? The answer is that a desire not to suffer pain can be ascribed to something without assuming that it has any concept of a continuing self. For while something that lacks the concept of a self cannot desire that a self not suffer, it can desire that a given sensation not exist. The state desired—the absence of a particular sensation, or of sensations of a certain sort—can be described in a purely phenomenalistic language, and hence without the concept of a continuing self. So long as the newborn kitten possesses the relevant phenomenal concepts, it can truly be said to desire that a certain sensation not exist. So we can ascribe to it a right not to be tortured even though, since it lacks the concept of a continuing self, we cannot ascribe to it a right to life.

This completes my discussion of the basic moral principles involved in the issue of abortion and infanticide. But I want to comment upon an important factual question, namely, at what point an organism comes to possess the concept of a self as a continuing subject of experiences and other mental states, together with the belief that it is itself such a continuing entity. This is obviously a matter for detailed psychological investigation, but everyday observation makes it perfectly clear, I believe, that a newborn baby does not possess the concept of a continuing self, any more than a newborn kitten possesses such a concept. If so, infanticide during a time interval shortly after birth must be morally acceptable.

But where is the line to be drawn? What is the cutoff point? If one maintained, as some philosophers have, that an individual possesses concepts only if he can express these concepts in language, it would be a matter of everyday observation whether or not a given organism possessed the concept of a continuing self. Infanticide would then be permissible up to the time an organism learned how to use certain expressions. However, I think the claim that acquisition of concepts is dependent on acquisition of language is mistaken. For example, one wants to ascribe mental states of a conceptual sort—such as beliefs and desires—to organisms that are incapable of learning a language. This issue of prelinguistic understanding is clearly outside the scope of this discussion. My point is simply that *if* an organism can acquire

concepts without thereby acquiring a way of expressing those concepts linguistically, the question of whether a given organism possesses the concept of a self as a continuing subject of experiences and other mental states, together with the belief that it is itself such a continuing entity, may be a question that requires fairly subtle experimental techniques to answer.

If this view of the matter is roughly correct, there are two worries one is left with at the level of practical moral decisions, one of which may turn out to be deeply disturbing. The lesser worry is where the line is to be drawn in the case of infanticide. It is not troubling because there is no serious need to know the exact point at which a human infant acquires a right to life. For in the vast majority of cases in which infanticide is desirable, its desirability will be apparent within a short time after birth. Since it is virtually certain that an infant at such a stage of its development does not possess the concept of a continuing self, and thus does not possess a serious right to life, there is excellent reason to believe that infanticide is morally permissible in most cases where it is otherwise desirable. The practical moral problem can thus be satisfactorily handled by choosing some period of time, such as a week after birth, as the interval during which infanticide will be permitted. This interval could then be modified once psychologists have established the point at which a human organism comes to believe that it is a continuing subject of experiences and other mental states.

The troubling worry is whether adult animals belonging to species other than Homo sapiens may not also possess a serious right to life. For once one says that an organism can possess the concept of a continuing self, together with the belief that it is itself such an entity, without having any way of expressing that concept and that belief linguistically, one has to face up to the question of whether animals may not possess properties that bestow a serious right to life upon them. The suggestion itself is a familiar one, and one that most of us are accustomed to dismiss very casually. The line of thought advanced here suggests that this attitude may turn out to be tragically mistaken. Once one reflects upon the question of the *basic* moral principles involved in the ascription of a right to life to organisms, one may find himself driven to conclude that our everyday treatment of animals is morally indefensible, and that we are in fact murdering innocent persons.

Notes

1. I am grateful to a number of people, particularly the Editors of *Philosophy & Public Affairs*, Rodelia Hapke, and Walter Kaufmann, for their helpful comments. It should not, of course, be inferred that they share the views expressed in this paper.

2. Judith Jarvis Thomson has argued with great force and ingenuity that this conclusion is mistaken. I will comment on her argument later. [See Judith Jarvis Thomson, "A Defense of Abortion." reprinted as next selection.]

3. While this is the position conservatives tend to hold, it is not clear that it is the position they ought to hold. For if the fetus is a person it is far from clear that it is permissible to destroy it to save the mother. Two moral principles lend support to the view that it is the fetus which should live. First, other things being equal, should not one give something to a person who has had less rather than to a person who has had more? The mother has had a chance to live, while the fetus has not. The choice is thus between giving the mother more of an opportunity to live while giving the fetus none at all and giving the fetus an opportunity to enjoy life while not giving the mother a further opportunity to do so. Surely fairness requires the latter. Secondly, since the fetus has a greater life expectancy than the mother, one is in effect distributing more goods by choosing the life of the fetus over the life of the mother.

    The position I am here recommending to the conservative should not be confused with the official Catholic position. The Catholic Church holds that it is seriously wrong to kill a fetus directly even if failure to do so will result in the death of *both* the mother and the fetus. This perverse value judgment is not part of the conservative's position.

4. Section 230.3 of the American Law Institute's *Model Penal Code* (Philadelphia, 1962). There is some interesting, though at times confused, discussion of the proposed code in *Model Penal Code—Tentative Draft No. 9* (Philadelphia, 1959), pp. 146–162.

5. A clear example of such an unwillingness to entertain seriously the possibility that moral judgments widely accepted in one's own society may nevertheless be incorrect is provided by Roger Wertheimer's superficial dismissal of infanticide on pages 25–26. [See Roger Wertheimer, "Understanding the Abortion Argument," *Philosophy and Public Affairs* 1 (1971): 67–95.

Reprinted in Marshall Cohen *et al.* ed., *The Rights and Wrongs of Abortion*. Princeton, N.J.: Princeton University Press, 1974, pp. 23–51. Page references are to the reprint.]

6. Compare the discussion of the concept of a right offered by Richard B. Brandt in his *Ethical Theory* (Englewood Cliffs, N.J., 1959), pp. 434–441. As Brandt points out, some philosophers have maintained that only things that can *claim* rights can have rights. I agree with Brandt's view that "inability to claim does not destroy the right" (p. 440).

7. B. A. Brody, "Abortion and the Law," *Journal of Philosophy*, LXVIII, no. 12 (17 June 1971): 357–369. See pp. 357–358.

8. P. 3.

9. P. 25.

10. *Ibid.*

11. Pp. 3–4.

12. P. 21.

13. P. 34.

14. A moral principle accepted by a person is *basic for him* if and only if his acceptance of it is not dependent upon any of his (nonmoral) factual beliefs. That is, no change in his factual beliefs would cause him to abandon the principle in question.

15. Wertheimer, p. 44.

16. Again, compare the analysis defended by Brandt in *Ethical Theory*, pp. 434–441.

17. In everyday life one often speaks of desiring things, such as an apple or a newspaper. Such talk is elliptical, the context together with one's ordinary beliefs serving to make it clear that one wants to eat the apple and read the newspaper. To say that what one desires is that a certain proposition be true should not be construed as involving any particular ontological commitment. The point is merely that it is sentences such as "John wants it to be the case that he is eating an apple in the next few minutes" that provide a completely explicit description of a person's desires. If one fails to use such sentences one can be badly misled about what concepts are presupposed by a particular desire.

18. There are, however, situations other than those discussed here which might seem to count against the claim that a person cannot have a right unless he is conceptually capable of having the corresponding desire. Can't a young child, for example, have a right to an estate, even though he may not be conceptually capable of wanting the estate? It is clear that such situations have to be carefully considered if one is to arrive at a satisfactory account of the concept of a right. My

inclination is to say that the correct description is not that the child now has a right to the estate, but that he will come to have such a right when he is mature, and that in the meantime no one else has a right to the estate. My reason for saying that the child does not now have a right to the estate is that he cannot now do things with the estate, such as selling it or giving it away, that he will be able to do later on.

19. Another frequent suggestion as to the cutoff point not listed here is quickening. I omit it because it seems clear that if abortion after quickening is wrong, its wrongness must be tied up with the motility of the fetus, not with the mother's awareness of the fetus' ability to move about.

20. P. 12.

21. A good example of a failure to probe this issue is provided by Brody's "Abortion and the Law."

22. Admittedly the modification is a substantial one, since given a society that refused to compensate women, a woman who had an abortion would not be doing anything wrong.

23. Compare Wertheimer's remarks, p. 35.

24. This requires qualification. If their central nervous systems were radically different from ours, it might be thought that one would not be justified in ascribing to them mental states of an experiential sort. And then, since it seems to be a conceptual truth that only things having experiential states can have rights, one would be forced to conclude that one was not justified in ascribing any rights to them.

25. Philippa Foot, "The Problem of Abortion and the Doctrine of the Double Effect," *The Oxford Review* 5 (1967): 5–15. See the discussion on pp. 11ff.

A Defense of Abortion[1]

Judith Jarvis Thomson

Most opposition to abortion relies on the premise that the fetus is a human being, a person, from the moment of conception. The premise is argued for, but, as I think, not well. Take, for example, the most common argument. We are asked to notice that the development of a human being from conception through birth into childhood is continuous; then it is said that to draw a line, to choose a point in this development and say "before this point the thing is not a person, after this point it is a person" is to make an arbitrary choice, a choice for which in the nature of things no good reason can be given. It is concluded that the fetus is, or anyway that we had better say it is, a person from the moment of conception. But this conclusion does not follow. Similar things might be said about the development of an acorn into an oak tree, and it does not follow that acorns are oak trees, or that we had better say they are. Arguments of this form are sometimes called "slippery slope arguments"—the phrase is perhaps self-explanatory—and it is dismaying that opponents of abortion rely on them so heavily and uncritically.

I am inclined to agree, however, that the prospects for "drawing a line" in the development of the fetus look dim. I am inclined to think also that we shall probably have to agree that the fetus has already become a human person well before birth. Indeed, it comes as a surprise when one first learns how early in its life it begins to acquire human characteristics. By the tenth week, for example, it already has a face, arms and legs, fingers and toes; it has internal organs, and brain activity is detectable.[2] On the other hand, I think that the premise is false, that the fetus is not a person from the moment of conception. A newly fertilized ovum, a newly implanted clump of cells, is no more a person than an acorn is an oak tree. But I shall not discuss any of this. For it seems to me to be of great interest to ask what happens if, for the sake of argument, we allow the premise. How, precisely, are we supposed to get from there to the conclusion that abortion is morally impermissible? Opponents of abortion commonly spend most of their time establishing that the fetus is a person, and hardly any time explaining the step from there to the impermissibility of abortion. Perhaps they

Judith Jarvis Thomson, "A Defense of Abortion," Philosophy & Public Affairs, *Vol. 1, no. 1 (Fall 1971).*
Copyright © 1971 by Princeton University Press. Reprinted by permission of Princeton University Press.

think the step too simple and obvious to require much comment. Or perhaps instead they are simply being economical in argument. Many of those who defend abortion rely on the premise that the fetus is not a person, but only a bit of tissue that will become a person at birth; and why pay out more arguments than you have to? Whatever the explanation, I suggest that the step they take is neither easy nor obvious, that it calls for closer examination than it is commonly given, and that when we do give it this closer examination we shall feel inclined to reject it.

I propose, then, that we grant that the fetus is a person from the moment of conception. How does the argument go from here? Something like this, I take it. Every person has a right to life. So the fetus has a right to life. No doubt the mother has a right to decide what shall happen in and to her body; everyone would grant that. But surely a person's right to life is stronger and more stringent than the mother's right to decide what happens in and to her body, and so outweighs it. So the fetus may not be killed; an abortion may not be performed.

It sounds plausible. But now let me ask you to imagine this. You wake up in the morning and find yourself back to back in bed with an unconscious violinist. A famous unconscious violinist. He has been found to have a fatal kidney ailment, and the Society of Music Lovers has canvassed all the available medical records and found that you alone have the right blood type to help. They have therefore kidnapped you, and last night the violinist's circulatory system was plugged into yours, so that your kidneys can be used to extract poisons from his blood as well as your own. The director of the hospital now tells you, "Look, we're sorry the Society of Music Lovers did this to you—we would never have permitted it if we had known. But still, they did it, and the violinist now is plugged into you. To unplug you would be to kill him. But never mind, it's only for nine months. By then he will have recovered from his ailment, and can safely be unplugged from you." Is it morally incumbent on you to accede to this situation? No doubt it would be very nice of you if you did, a great kindness. But do you *have* to accede to it? What if it were not nine months, but nine years? Or longer still? What if the director of the hospital says, "Tough luck, I agree, but you've now got to stay in bed, with the violinist plugged into you, for the rest of your life. Because remember this. All

persons have a right to life, and violinists are persons. Granted you have a right to decide what happens in and to your body, but a person's right to life outweighs your right to decide what happens in and to your body. So you cannot ever be unplugged from him." I imagine you would regard this as outrageous, which suggests that something really is wrong with that plausible-sounding argument I mentioned a moment ago.

In this case, of course, you were kidnapped; you didn't volunteer for the operation that plugged the violinist into your kidneys. Can those who oppose abortion on the ground I mentioned make an exception for a pregnancy due to rape? Certainly. They can say that persons have a right to life only if they didn't come into existence because of rape; or they can say that all persons have a right to life, but that some have less of a right to life than others, in particular, that those who came into existence because of rape have less. But these statements have a rather unpleasant sound. Surely the question of whether you have a right to life at all, or how much of it you have, shouldn't turn on the question of whether or not you are a product of a rape. And in fact the people who oppose abortion on the ground I mentioned do not make this distinction, and hence do not make an exception in case of rape.

Nor do they make an exception for a case in which the mother has to spend the nine months of her pregnancy in bed. They would agree that would be a great pity, and hard on the mother; but all the same, all persons have a right to life, the fetus is a person, and so on. I suspect, in fact, that they would not make an exception for a case in which, miraculously enough, the pregnancy went on for nine years, or even the rest of the mother's life.

Some won't even make an exception for a case in which continuation of the pregnancy is likely to shorten the mother's life; they regard abortion as impermissible even to save the mother's life. Such cases are nowadays very rare, and many opponents of abortion do not accept this extreme view. All the same, it is a good place to begin: a number of points of interest come out in respect to it.

1.

Let us call the view that abortion is impermissible even to save the mother's life "the extreme view." I want to suggest first that it does not issue from the argument I mentioned earlier without the addition of some fairly powerful premises. Suppose a woman has become pregnant, and now learns that she has a cardiac condition such that she will die if she carries the baby to term. What may be done for her? The fetus, being a person, has a right to life, but as the mother is a person too, so has she a right to life. Presumably they have an equal right to life. How is it supposed to come out that an abortion may not be performed? If mother and child have an equal right to life, shouldn't we perhaps flip a coin? Or should we add to the mother's right to life her right to decide what happens in and to her body. which everybody seems to be ready to grant—the sum of her rights now outweighing the fetus's right to life?

The most familiar argument here is the following. We are told that performing the abortion would be directly killing[3] the child, whereas doing nothing would not be killing the mother, but only letting her die. Moreover, in killing the child, one would be killing an innocent person, for the child has committed no crime, and is not aiming at his mother's death. And then there are a variety of ways in which this might be continued. (1) But as directly killing an innocent person is always and absolutely impermissible, an abortion may not be performed. Or, (2) as directly killing an innocent person is murder, and murder is always and absolutely impermissible, an abortion may not be performed.[4] Or, (3) as one's duty to refrain from directly killing an innocent person is more stringent than one's duty to keep a person from dying, an abortion may not be performed. Or, (4) if one's only options are directly killing an innocent person or letting a person die, one must prefer letting the person die, and thus an abortion may not be performed.[5]

Some people seem to have thought that these are not further premises which must be added if the conclusion is to be reached, but that they follow from the very fact that an innocent person has a right to life.[6] But this seems to me to be a mistake, and perhaps the simplest way to show this is to bring out that while we must certainly grant that innocent persons have a right to life, the theses in (1) through (4) are all false. Take (2), for example. If directly killing an innocent person is murder, and thus is impermissible, then the mother's directly killing the innocent person inside her is murder, and thus is impermissible. But

it cannot seriously be thought to be murder if the mother performs an abortion on herself to save her life. It cannot seriously be said that she *must* refrain, that she *must* sit passively by and wait for her death. Let us look again at the case of you and the violinist. There you are, in bed with the violinist, and the director of the hospital says to you, "It's all most distressing, and I deeply sympathize, but you see this is putting an additional strain on your kidneys, and you'll be dead within the month. But you *have* to stay where you are all the same. Because unplugging you would be directly killing an innocent violinist, and that's murder, and that's impermissible." If anything in the world is true, it is that you do not commit murder, you do not do what is impermissible, if you reach around to your back and unplug yourself from that violinist to save your life.

The main focus of attention in writings on abortion has been on what a third party may or may not do in answer to a request from a woman for an abortion. This is in a way understandable. Things being as they are, there isn't much a woman can safely do to abort herself. So the question asked is what a third party may do, and what the mother may do, if it is mentioned at all, is deduced, almost as an afterthought, from what it is concluded that third parties may do. But it seems to me that to treat the matter in this way is to refuse to grant to the mother that very status of person which is so firmly insisted on for the fetus. For we cannot simply read off what a person may do from what a third party may do. Suppose you find yourself trapped in a tiny house with a growing child. I mean a very tiny house, and a rapidly growing child—you are already up against the wall of the house and in a few minutes you'll be crushed to death. The child on the other hand won't be crushed to death if nothing is done to stop him from growing he'll be hurt, but in the end he'll simply burst open the house and walk out a free man. Now I could well understand it if a bystander were to say, "There's nothing we can do for you. We cannot choose between your life and his, we cannot be the ones to decide who is to live, we cannot intervene." But it cannot be concluded that you too can do nothing, that you cannot attack it to save your life. However innocent the child may be, you do not have to wait passively while it crushes you to death. Perhaps a pregnant woman is vaguely felt to have the status of house,

to which we don't allow the right of self-defense. But if the woman houses the child, it should be remembered that she is a person who houses it.

I should perhaps stop to say explicitly that I am not claiming that people have a right to do anything whatever to save their lives. I think, rather, that there are drastic limits to the right of self-defense. If someone threatens you with death unless you torture someone else to death, I think you have not the right, even to save your life, to do so. But the case under consideration here is very different. In our case there are only two people involved, one whose life is threatened, and one who threatens it. Both are innocent: the one who is threatened is not threatened because of any fault, the one who threatens does not threaten because of any fault. For this reason we may feel that we bystanders cannot intervene. But the person threatened can.

In sum, a woman surely can defend her life against the threat to it posed by the unborn child, even if doing so involves its death. And this shows not merely that the theses in (1) through (4) are false; it shows also that the extreme view of abortion is false, and so we need not canvass any other possible ways of arriving at it from the argument I mentioned at the outset.

2.

The extreme view could of course be weakened to say that while abortion is permissible to save the mother's life, it may not be performed by a third party, but only by the mother herself. But this cannot be right either. For what we have to keep in mind is that the mother and the unborn child are not like two tenants in a small house which has, by an unfortunate mistake, been rented to both: the mother *owns* the house. The fact that she does adds to the offensiveness of deducing that the mother can do nothing from the supposition that third parties can do nothing. But it does more than this: it casts a bright light on the supposition that third parties can do nothing. Certainly it lets us see that a third party who says "I cannot choose between you" is fooling himself if he thinks this is impartiality. If Jones has found and fastened on a certain coat, which he needs to keep him from freezing, but which Smith also needs to keep him from freezing, then it is not impartiality that says "I cannot choose between

you" when Smith owns the coat. Women have said again and again "This body is *my* body!" and they have reason to feel angry, reason to feel that it has been like shouting into the wind. Smith, after all, is hardly likely to bless us if we say to him, "Of course it's your coat, anybody would grant that it is. But no one may choose between you and Jones who is to have it."

We should really ask what it is that says "no one may choose" in the face of the fact that the body that houses the child is the mother's body. It may be simply a failure to appreciate this fact. But it may be something more interesting, namely the sense that one has a right to refuse to lay hands on people, even where it would be just and fair to do so, even where justice seems to require that somebody do so. Thus justice might call for somebody to get Smith's coat back from Jones, and yet you have a right to refuse to be the one to lay hands on Jones, a right to refuse to do physical violence to him. This, I think, must be granted. But then what should be said is not "no one may choose," but only "*I* cannot choose," and indeed not even this, but "*I* will not *act*," leaving it open that somebody else can or should, and in particular that anyone in a position of authority, with the job of securing people's rights, both can and should. So this is no difficulty. I have not been arguing that any given third party must accede to the mother's request that he perform an abortion to save her life, but only that he may.

I suppose that in some views of human life the mother's body is only on loan to her, the loan not being one which gives her any prior claim to it. One who held this view might well think it impartiality to say "I cannot choose." But I shall simply ignore this possibility. My own view is that if a human being has any just, prior claim to anything at all, he has a just, prior claim to his own body. And perhaps this needn't be argued for here anyway, since, as I mentioned, the arguments against abortion we are looking at do grant that the woman has a right to decide what happens in and to her body.

But although they do grant it, I have tried to show that they do not take seriously what is done in granting it. I suggest the same thing will reappear even more clearly when we turn away from cases in which the mother's life is at stake, and attend, as I propose we now do, to the vastly more common cases in which a woman wants an abortion for some less weighty reason than preserving her own life.

3.

Where the mother's life is not at stake, the argument I mentioned at the outset seems to have a much stronger pull. "Everyone has a right to life, so the unborn person has a right to life." And isn't the child's right to life weightier than anything other than the mother's own right to life, which she might put forward as ground for an abortion?

This argument treats the right to life as if it were unproblematic. It is not, and this seems to me to be precisely the source of the mistake.

For we should now, at long last, ask what it comes to, to have a right to life. In some views having a right to life includes having a right to be given at least the bare minimum one needs for continued life. But suppose that what in fact *is* the bare minimum a man needs for continued life is something he has no right at all to be given? If I am sick unto death, and the only thing that will save my life is the touch of Henry Fonda's cool hand on my fevered brow, then all the same, I have no right to be given the touch of Henry Fonda's cool hand on my fevered brow. It would be frightfully nice of him to fly in from the West Coast to provide it. It would be less nice, though no doubt well meant, if my friends flew out to the West Coast and carried Henry Fonda back with them. But I have no right at all against anybody that he should do this for me. Or again, to return to the story I told earlier, the fact that for continued life that violinist needs the continued use of your kidneys does not establish that he has a right to be given the continued use of your kidneys. He certainly has no right against you that *you* should give him continued use of your kidneys. For nobody has any right to use your kidneys unless you give him this right—if you do allow him to go on using your kidneys, this is a kindness on your part, and not something he can claim from you as his due. Nor has he any right against anybody else that *they* should give him continued use of your kidneys. Certainly he had no right against the Society of Music Lovers that they should plug him into you in the first place. And if you now start to unplug yourself, having learned that you will otherwise have to spend nine years in bed with him, there is nobody in the world who must try to prevent you, in order to see to it that he is given something he has a right to be given.

Some people are rather stricter about the right to life. In their view, it does not include the right to be given anything, but amounts to, and only to, the right not to be killed by anybody. But here a related difficulty arises. If everybody is to refrain from killing that violinist, then everybody must refrain from doing a great many different sorts of things. Everybody must refrain from slitting his throat, everybody must refrain from shooting him—and everybody must refrain from unplugging you from him. But does he have a right against everybody that they shall refrain from unplugging you from him? To refrain from doing this is to allow him to continue to use your kidneys. It could be argued that he has a right against us that *we* should allow him to continue to use your kidneys. That is, while he had no right against us that we should give him the use of your kidneys, it might be argued that he anyway has a right against us that we shall not now intervene and deprive him of the use of your kidneys. I shall come back to third-party interventions later. But certainly the violinist has no right against you that *you* shall allow him to continue to use your kidneys. As I said, if you do allow him to use them, it is a kindness on your part, and not something you owe him.

The difficulty I point to here is not peculiar to the right of life. It reappears in connection with all the other natural rights, and it is something which an adequate account of rights must deal with. For present purposes it is enough just to draw attention to it. But I would stress that I am not arguing that people do not have a right to life—quite to the contrary, it seems to me that the primary control we must place on the acceptability of an account of rights is that it should turn out in that account to be a truth that all persons have a right to life. I am arguing only that having a right to life does not guarantee having either a right to be given the use of or a right to be allowed continued use of another person's body—even if one needs it for life itself. So the right to life will not serve the opponents of abortion in the very simple and clear way in which they seem to have thought it would.

4.

There is another way to bring out the difficulty. In the most ordinary sort of case, to deprive someone of what he has a right to is to treat him unjustly. Suppose a boy and his small brother are

jointly given a box of chocolates for Christmas. If the older boy takes the box and refuses to give his brother any of the chocolates, he is unjust to him, for the brother has been given a right to half of them. But suppose that, having learned that otherwise it means nine years in bed with that violinist, you unplug yourself from him. You surely are not being unjust to him, for you gave him no right to use your kidneys, and no one else can have given him any such right. But we have to notice that in unplugging yourself, you are killing him; and violinists, like everybody else, have a right to life, and thus in the view we were considering just now, the right not to be killed. So here you do what he supposedly has a right you shall not do, but you do not act unjustly to him in doing it.

The emendation which may be made at this point is this: the right to life consists not in the right not to be killed, but rather in the right not to be killed unjustly. This runs a risk of circularity, but never mind: it would enable us to square the fact that the violinist has a right to life with the fact that you do not act unjustly toward him in unplugging yourself, thereby killing him. For if you do not kill him unjustly, you do not violate his right to life, and so it is no wonder you do him no injustice.

But if this emendation is accepted, the gap in the argument against abortion stares us plainly in the face: it is by no means enough to show that the fetus is a person, and to remind us that all persons have a right to life—we need to be shown also that killing the fetus violates its right to life, i.e., that abortion is unjust killing. And is it?

I suppose we may take it as a datum that in a case of pregnancy due to rape the mother has not given the unborn person a right to the use of her body for food and shelter. Indeed, in what pregnancy could it be supposed that the mother has given the unborn person such a right? It is not as if there were unborn persons drifting about the world, to whom a woman who wants a child says "I invite you in."

But it might be argued that there are other ways one can have acquired a right to the use of another person's body than by having been invited to use it by that person. Suppose a woman voluntarily indulges in intercourse, knowing of the chance it will issue in pregnancy, and then she does become pregnant; is she not in part responsible for the presence, in fact the very existence, of the unborn person inside? No doubt she did not

invite it in. But doesn't her partial responsibility for its being there itself give it a right to the use of her body?[7] If so, then her aborting it would be more like the boys taking away the chocolates, and less like your unplugging yourself from the violinist—doing so would be depriving it of what it does have a right to, and thus would be doing it an injustice.

And then, too, it might be asked whether or not she can kill it even to save her own life: If she voluntarily called it into existence, how can she now kill it, even in self-defense?

The first thing to be said about this is that it is something new. Opponents of abortion have been so concerned to make out the independence of the fetus, in order to establish that it has a right to life, just as its mother does, that they have tended to overlook the possible support they might gain from making out that the fetus is *dependent* on the mother, in order to establish that she has a special kind of responsibility for it, a responsibility that gives it rights against her which are not possessed by any independent person—such as an ailing violinist who is a stranger to her.

On the other hand, this argument would give the unborn person a right to its mother's body only if her pregnancy resulted from a voluntary act, undertaken in full knowledge of the chance a pregnancy might result from it. It would leave out entirely the unborn person whose existence is due to rape. Pending the availability of some further argument, then, we would be left with the conclusion that unborn persons whose existence is due to rape have no right to the use of their mothers' bodies, and thus that aborting them is not depriving them of anything they have a right to and hence is not unjust killing.

And we should also notice that it is not at all plain that this argument really does go even as far as it purports to. For there are cases and cases, and the details make a difference. If the room is stuffy, and I therefore open a window to air it, and a burglar climbs in, it would be absurd to say, "Ah, now he can stay, she's given him a right to the use of her house—for she is partially responsible for his presence there, having voluntarily done what enabled him to get in, in full knowledge that there are such things as burglars, and that burglars burgle." It would be still more absurd to say this if I had had bars installed outside my windows, precisely to prevent burglars from getting in, and a burglar got in only because of a defect in the bars.

It remains equally absurd if we imagine it is not a burglar who climbs in, but an innocent person who blunders or falls in. Again, suppose it were like this: people-seeds drift about in the air like pollen, and if you open your windows, one may drift in and take root in your carpets or upholstery. You don't want children, so you fix up your windows with fine mesh screens, the very best you can buy. As can happen, however, and on very, very rare occasions does happen, one of the screens is defective; and a seed drifts in and takes root. Does the person-plant who now develops have a right to the use of your house? Surely not— despite the fact that you voluntarily opened your windows, you knowingly kept carpets and upholstered furniture, and you knew that screens were sometimes defective. Someone may argue that you are responsible for its rooting, that it does have a right to your house, because after all you *could* have lived out your life with bare floors and furniture, or with sealed windows and doors. But this won't do—for by the same token anyone can avoid a pregnancy due to rape by having a hysterectomy, or anyway by never leaving home without a (reliable!) army.

It seems to me that the argument we are looking at can establish at most that there are *some* cases in which the unborn person has a right to the use of its mother's body, and therefore *some* cases in which abortion is unjust killing. There is room for much discussion and argument as to precisely which, if any. But I think we should sidestep this issue and leave it open, for at any rate the argument certainly does not establish that all abortion is unjust killing.

5.

There is room for yet another argument here, however. We surely must all grant that there may be cases in which it would be morally indecent to detach a person from your body at the cost of his life. Suppose you learn that what the violinist needs is not nine years of your life, but only one hour: all you need do to save his life is to spend one hour in that bed with him. Suppose also that letting him use your kidneys for that one hour would not affect your health in the slightest. Admittedly you were kidnapped. Admittedly you did not give anyone permission to plug him into you. Nevertheless it seems to me plain you *ought* to allow him to use your kidneys for that hour—it would be indecent to refuse.

Again, suppose pregnancy lasted only an hour, and constituted no threat to life or health. And suppose that a woman becomes pregnant as a result of rape. Admittedly she did not voluntarily do anything to bring about the existence of a child. Admittedly she did nothing at all which would give the unborn person a right to the use of her body. All the same it might well be said, as in the newly amended violinist story, that she *ought* to allow it to remain for that hour—that it would be indecent in her to refuse.

Now some people are inclined to use the term "right" in such a way that it follows from the fact that you ought to allow a person to use your body for the hour he needs, that he has a right to use your body for the hour he needs, even though he has not been given that right by any person or act. They may say that it follows also that if you refuse, you act unjustly toward him. This use of the term is perhaps so common that it cannot be called wrong; nevertheless it seems to me to be an unfortunate loosening of what we would do better to keep a tight rein on. Suppose that box of chocolates I mentioned earlier had not been given to both boys jointly, but was given only to the older boy. There he sits, stolidly eating his way through the box, his small brother watching enviously. Here we are likely to say, "You ought not to be so mean. You ought to give your brother some of those chocolates." My own view is that it just does not follow from the truth of this that the brother has any right to any of the chocolates. If the boy refuses to give his brother any, he is greedy, stingy, callous—but not unjust. I suppose that the people I have in mind will say it does follow that the brother has a right to some of the chocolates, and thus that the boy does act unjustly if he refuses to give his brother any. But the effect of saying this is to obscure what we should keep distinct, namely the difference between the boy's refusal in this case and the boy's refusal in the earlier case, in which the box was given to both boys jointly, and in which the small brother thus had what was from any point of view clear title to half.

A further objection to so using the term "right" that from the fact that A ought to do a thing for B, it follows that B has a right against A that A do it for him, is that it is going to make the question of whether or not a man has a right to a thing turn on how easy it is to provide him with it; and this seems not merely unfortunate, but morally unacceptable. Take the case of Henry Fonda again. I said earlier that I had no right to the touch of his cool hand on my fevered brow, even though I needed it to save my life. I said it would be frightfully nice of him to fly in from the West Coast to provide me with it, but that I had no right against him that he should do so. But suppose he isn't on the West Coast. Suppose he has only to walk across the room, place a hand briefly on my brow—and lo, my life is saved. Then surely he ought to do it, it would be indecent to refuse. Is it to be said, "Ah, well, it follows that in this case she has a right to the touch of his hand on her brow, and so it would be an injustice in him to refuse"? So that I have a right to it when it is easy for him to provide it, though no right when it's hard? It's rather a shocking idea that anyone's rights should fade away and disappear as it gets harder and harder to accord them to him.

So my own view is that even though you ought to let the violinist use your kidneys for the one hour he needs, we should not conclude that he has a right to do so—we should say that if you refuse, you are, like the boy who owns all the chocolates and will give none away, self-centered and callous, indecent in fact, but not unjust. And similarly, that even supposing a case in which a woman pregnant due to rape ought to allow the unborn person to use her body for the hour he needs, we should not conclude that he has a right to do so; we should conclude that she is self-centered, callous, indecent, but not unjust, if she refuses. The complaints are no less grave; they are just different. However, there is no need to insist on this point. If anyone does wish to deduce "he has a right" from "you ought," then all the same he must surely grant that there are cases in which it is not morally required of you that you allow that violinist to use your kidneys, and in which he does not have a right to use them, and in which you do not do him an injustice if you refuse. And so also for mother and unborn child. Except in such cases as the unborn person has a right to demand it— and we were leaving open the possibility that there may be such cases—nobody is morally *required* to make large sacrifices, of health, of all other interests and concerns, of all other duties and commitments, for nine years, or even for nine months, in order to keep another person alive.

6.

We have in fact to distinguish between two kinds of Samaritan: the Good Samaritan and what we might call the Minimally Decent Samaritan. The story of the Good Samaritan, you will remember, goes like this:

> A certain man went down from Jerusalem to Jericho, and fell among thieves, which stripped him of his raiment, and wounded him, and departed, leaving him half dead.
>
> And by chance there came down a certain priest that way: and when he saw him, he passed by on the other side.
>
> And likewise a Levite, when he was at the place, came and looked on him, and passed by on the other side.
>
> But a certain Samaritan, as he journeyed, came where he was; and when he saw him he had compassion on him.
>
> And went to him, and bound up his wounds, pouring in oil and wine, and set him on his own beast, and brought him to an inn, and took care of him.
>
> And on the morrow, when he departed, he took out two pence, and gave them to the host, and said unto him, "Take care of him; and whatsoever thou spendest more, when I come again, I will repay thee." (Luke 10:30–35)

The Good Samaritan went out of his way, at some cost to himself, to help one in need of it. We are not told what the options were, that is, whether or not the priest and the Levite could have helped by doing less than the Good Samaritan did, but assuming they could have, then the fact they did nothing at all shows they were not even Minimally Decent Samaritans, not because they were not Samaritans, but because they were not even minimally decent.

These things are a matter of degree, of course, but there is a difference, and it comes out perhaps most clearly in the story of Kitty Genovese, who, as you will remember, was murdered while thirty-eight people watched or listened, and did nothing at all to help her. A Good Samaritan would have rushed out to give direct assistance against the murderer. Or perhaps we had better allow that it would have been a Splendid Samaritan who did this, on the ground that it would have involved a risk of death for himself. But the thirty-eight not only did not do this, they did not even trouble to pick up a phone to call the police. Minimally Decent Samaritanism would call for doing at least that, and their not having done it was monstrous.

After telling the story of the Good Samaritan, Jesus said, "Go, and do thou likewise." Perhaps he meant that we are morally required to act as the Good Samaritan did. Perhaps he was urging people to do more than is morally required of them. At all events it seems plain that it was not morally required of any of the thirty-eight that he rush out to give direct assistance at the risk of his own life, and that it is not morally required of anyone that he give long stretches of his life—nine years or nine months—to sustaining the life of a person who has no special right (we were leaving open the possibility of this) to demand it.

Indeed, with one rather striking class of exceptions, no one in any country in the world is *legally* required to do anywhere near as much as this for anyone else. The class of exceptions is obvious. My main concern here is not the state of the law in respect to abortion, but it is worth drawing attention to the fact that in no state in this country is any man compelled by law to be even a Minimally Decent Samaritan to any person; there is no law under which charges could be brought against the thirty-eight who stood by while Kitty Genovese died. By contrast, in most states in this country women are compelled by law to be not merely Minimally Decent Samaritans, but Good Samaritans to unborn persons inside them. This doesn't by itself settle anything one way or the other, because it may well be argued that there should be laws in this country—as there are in many European countries—compelling at least Minimally Decent Samaritanism.[8] But it does show that there is a gross injustice in the existing state of the law. And it shows also that the groups currently working against liberalization of abortion laws, in fact working toward having it declared unconstitutional for a state to permit abortion, had better start working for the adoption of Good Samaritan laws generally, or earn the charge that they are acting in bad faith.

I should think, myself, that Minimally Decent Samaritan laws would be one thing, Good Samaritan laws quite another, and in fact highly improper. But we are not here concerned with the law. What we should ask is not whether anybody should be compelled by law to be a Good Samaritan, but whether we must accede to a situation in which somebody is being compelled—by nature,

perhaps—to be a Good Samaritan. We have, in other words, to look now at third-party interventions. I have been arguing that no person is morally required to make large sacrifices to sustain the life of another who has no right to demand them, and this even where the sacrifices do not include life itself; we are not morally required to be Good Samaritans or anyway Very Good Samaritans to one another. But what if a man cannot extricate himself from such a situation? What if he appeals to us to extricate him? It seems to me plain that there are cases in which we can, cases in which a good Samaritan would extricate him. There you are, you were kidnapped, and nine years in bed with that violinist lie ahead of you. You have your own life to lead. You are sorry, but you simply cannot see giving up so much of your life to the sustaining of his. You cannot extricate yourself, and ask us to do so. I should have thought that— in light of his having no right to the use of your body—it was obvious that we do not have to accede to your being forced to give up so much. We can do what you ask. There is no injustice to the violinist in our doing so.

7.

Following the lead of the opponents of abortion, I have throughout been speaking of the fetus merely as a person, and what I have been asking is whether or not the argument we began with, which proceeds only from the fetus's being a person, really does establish its conclusion. I have argued that it does not.

But of course there are arguments and arguments, and it may be said that I have simply fastened on the wrong one. It may be said that what is important is not merely the fact that the fetus is a person, but that it is a person for whom the woman has a special kind of responsibility issuing from the fact that she is its mother. And it might be argued that all my analogies are therefore irrelevant—for you do not have that special kind of responsibility for that violinist, Henry Fonda does not have that special kind of responsibility for me. And our attention might be drawn to the fact that men and women both *are* compelled by law to provide support for their children.

I have in effect dealt (briefly) with this argument in section 4 above; but a (still briefer) recapitulation now may be in order. Surely we do not

have any such "special responsibility" for a person unless we have assumed it, explicitly or implicitly. If a set of parents do not try to prevent pregnancy, do not obtain an abortion, but rather take it home with them, then they have assumed responsibility for it, they have given it rights, and they cannot *now* withdraw support from it at the cost of its life because they now find it difficult to go on providing for it. But if they have taken all reasonable precautions against having a child, they do not simply by virtue of their biological relationship to the child who comes into existence have a special responsibility for it. They may wish to assume responsibility for it, or they may not wish to. And I am suggesting that if assuming responsibility for it would require large sacrifices, then they may refuse. A Good Samaritan would not refuse—or anyway, a Splendid Samaritan, if the sacrifices that had to be made were enormous. But then so would a Good Samaritan assume responsibility for that violinist; so would Henry Fonda, if he is a Good Samaritan, fly in from the West Coast and assume responsibility for me.

8.

My argument will be found unsatisfactory on two counts by many of those who want to regard abortion as morally permissible. First, while I do argue that abortion is not impermissible, I do not argue that it is always permissible. There may well be cases in which carrying the child to term requires only Minimally Decent Samaritanism of the mother, and this is a standard we must not fall below. I am inclined to think it a merit of my account precisely that it does *not* give a general yes or a general no. It allows for and supports our sense that, for example, a sick and desperately frightened fourteen-year-old schoolgirl, pregnant due to rape, may of *course* choose abortion, and that any law which rules this out is an insane law. And it also allows for and supports our sense that in other cases resort to abortion is even positively indecent. It would be indecent in the woman to request an abortion, and indecent in a doctor to perform it, if she is in her seventh month, and wants the abortion just to avoid the nuisance of postponing a trip abroad. The very fact that the arguments I have been drawing attention to treat all cases of abortion, or even all cases of abortion in which the mother's life is not at stake, as morally

on a par ought to have made them suspect at the outset.

Second, while I am arguing for the permissibility of abortion in some cases, I am not arguing for the right to secure the death of the unborn child. It is easy to confuse these two things in that up to a certain point in the life of the fetus it is not able to survive outside the mother's body; hence removing it from her body guarantees its death. But they are importantly different. I have argued that you are not morally required to spend nine months in bed, sustaining the life of that violinist; but to say this is by no means to say that if, when you unplug yourself, there is a miracle and he survives, you then have a right to turn round and slit his throat. You may detach yourself even if this costs him his life; you have no right to be guaranteed his death, by some other means, if unplugging yourself does not kill him. There are some people who will feel dissatisfied by this feature of my argument. A woman may be utterly devastated by the thought of a child, a bit of herself, put out for adoption and never seen or heard of again. She may therefore want not merely that the child be detached from her, but more, that it die. Some opponents of abortion are inclined to regard this as beneath contempt—thereby showing insensitivity to what is surely a powerful source of despair. All the same, I agree that the desire for the child's death is not one which anybody may gratify, should it turn out to be possible to detach the child alive.

At this place, however, it should be remembered that we have only been pretending throughout that the fetus is a human being from the moment of conception. A very early abortion is surely not the killing of a person, and so is not dealt with by anything I have said here.

Notes

1.   I am very much indebted to James Thomson for discussion, criticism, and many helpful suggestions.

2.   Daniel Callahan, *Abortion: Law, Choice and Morality* (New York, 1970), p. 373. This book gives a fascinating survey of the available information on abortion. The Jewish tradition is surveyed in David M. Feldman, *Birth Control in Jewish Law* (New York, 1968). part 5, the Catholic tradition in John T. Noonan, Jr., "An Almost Absolute Value

in History," in *The Morality of Abortion*, ed. John T. Noonan, Jr. (Cambridge, Mass., 1970).

3. The term "direct" in the arguments I refer to is a technical one. Roughly, what is meant by "direct killing" is either killing as an end in itself, or killing as a means to some end, for example, the end of saving someone else's life. See note 6, below, for an example of its use.

4. Cf. *Encyclical Letter of Pope Pius XI on Christian Marriage*, St. Paul Editions (Boston, n.d.), p. 32: "However much we may pity the mother whose health and even life is gravely imperiled in the performance of the duty allotted to her by nature, nevertheless what could ever be a sufficient reason for excusing in any way the direct murder of the innocent? This is precisely what we are dealing with here." Noonan (*The Morality of Abortion*, p. 43) reads this as follows: "What cause can ever avail to excuse in any way the direct killing of the innocent? For it is a question of that."

5. The thesis in (4) is in an interesting way weaker than those in (1), (2), and (3): they rule out abortion even in cases in which both mother *and* child will die if the abortion is not performed. By contrast, one who held the view expressed in (4)

could consistently say that one needn't prefer letting two persons die to killing one.

6. Cf. the following passage from Pius XII, *Address to the Italian Catholic Society of Midwives*: "The baby in the maternal breast has the right to life immediately from God.—Hence there is no man, no human authority, no science, no medical, eugenic, social, economic or moral 'indication' which can establish or grant a valid juridical ground for a direct deliberate disposition of an innocent human life, that is a disposition which looks to its destruction either as an end or as a means to another end perhaps in itself not illicit.—The baby, still not born, is a man in the same degree and for the same reason as the mother" (quoted in Noonan, *The Morality of Abortion*, p. 45).

7. The need for a discussion of this argument was brought home to me by members of the Society for Ethical and Legal Philosophy, to whom this paper was originally presented.

8. For a discussion of the difficulties involved, and a survey of the European experience with such laws, see *The Good Samaritan and the Law*, ed. James M. Ratcliffe (New York, 1966).

Abortion and the Concept of a Person

Jane English

The abortion debate rages on. Yet the two most popular positions seem to be clearly mistaken. Conservatives maintain that a human life begins at conception and that therefore abortion must be wrong because it is murder. But not all killings of humans are murders. Most notably, self defense may justify even the killing of an innocent person.

Liberals, on the other hand, are just as mistaken in their argument that since a fetus does not become a person until birth, a woman may do whatever she pleases in and to her own body. First, you cannot do as you please with your own body if it affects other people adversely.[1] Second, if a fetus is not a person, that does not imply that

you can do to it anything you wish. Animals, for example, are not persons, yet to kill or torture them for no reason at all is wrong.

At the center of the storm has been the issue of just when it is between ovulation and adulthood that a person appears on the scene. Conservatives draw the line at conception, liberals at birth. In this paper I first examine our concept of a person and conclude that no single criterion can capture the concept of a person and no sharp line can be drawn. Next I argue that if a fetus is person, abortion is still justifiable in many cases; and if a fetus is not a person, killing it is still wrong in many cases. To a large extent, these two solutions

This article is reprinted from the Canadian Journal of Philosophy, *5, no. 2 (October 1975) by permission of the Canadian Association for Publishing in Philosophy.*

are in agreement. I conclude that our concept of a person cannot and need not bear the weight that the abortion controversy has thrust upon it.

I

The several factions in the abortion argument have drawn battle lines around various proposed criteria for determining what is and what is not a person. For example, Mary Anne Warren[2] lists five features (capacities for reasoning, self-awareness, complex communication, etc.) as her criteria for personhood and argues for the permissibility of abortion because a fetus falls outside this concept. Baruch Brody[3] uses brain waves. Michael Tooley[4] picks having-a-concept-of-self as his criterion and concludes that infanticide and abortion are justifiable, while the killing of adult animals is not. On the other side, Paul Ramsey[5] claims a certain gene structure is the defining characteristic. John Noonan[6] prefers conceived-of-humans and presents counterexamples to various other candidate criteria. For instance, he argues against viability as the criterion because the newborn and infirm would then be non-persons, since they cannot live without the aid of others. He rejects any criterion that calls upon the sorts of sentiments a being can evoke in adults on the grounds that this would allow us to exclude other races as non-persons if we could just view them sufficiently unsentimentally.

These approaches are typical: foes of abortion propose sufficient conditions for personhood which fetuses satisfy, while friends of abortion counter with necessary conditions for personhood which fetuses lack. But these both presuppose that the concept of a person can be captured in a straightjacket of necessary and/or sufficient conditions.[7] Rather, "person" is a cluster of features, of which rationality, having a self-concept and being conceived of humans are only part.

What is typical of persons? Within our concept of a person we include, first, certain biological factors: descended from humans, having a certain genetic make-up, having a head, hands, arms, eyes, capable of locomotion, breathing, eating, sleeping. There are psychological factors: sentience, perception, having a concept of self and of one's own interests and desires, the ability to use tools, the ability to use language or symbol systems, the ability to joke, to be angry, to doubt. There are rationality factors: the ability to reason and draw conclusions, the ability to generalize and to learn from past experience, the ability to sacrifice present interests for greater gains in the future. There are social factors: the ability to work in groups and respond to peer pressures, the ability to recognize and consider as valuable the interests of others, seeing oneself as one among "other minds," the ability to sympathize, encourage, love, the ability to evoke from others the responses of sympathy, encouragement, love, the ability to work with others for mutual advantage. Then there are legal factors: being subject to the law and protected by it, having the ability to sue and enter contracts, being counted in the census, having a name and citizenship, the ability to own property, inherit, and so forth.

Now the point is not that this list is incomplete, or that you can find counterinstances to each of its points. People typically exhibit rationality, for instance, but someone who was irrational would not thereby fail to qualify as a person. On the other hand, something could exhibit the majority of these features and still fail to be a person, as an advanced robot might. There is no single core of necessary and sufficient features which we can draw upon with the assurance that they constitute what really makes a person; there are only features that are more or less typical.

This is not to say that no necessary or sufficient conditions can be given. Being alive is a necessary condition for being a person, and being a U.S. Senator is sufficient. But rather than falling inside a sufficient condition or outside a necessary one, a fetus lies in the penumbra region where our concept of a person is not so simple. For this reason I think a conclusive answer to the question whether a fetus is a person is unattainable.

Here we might note a family of simple fallacies that proceed by stating a necessary condition for personhood and showing that a fetus has that characteristic. This is a form of the fallacy of affirming the consequent. For example, some have mistakenly reasoned from the premise that a fetus is human (after all, it is a human fetus rather than, say, a canine fetus), to the conclusion that it is a human. Adding an equivocation on 'being', we get the fallacious argument that since a fetus is something both living and human, it is a human being.

Nonetheless, it does seem clear that a fetus has very few of the above family of characteristics, whereas a newborn baby exhibits a much larger proportion of them—and a two-year-old has even more. Note that one traditional anti-abortion argument has centered on pointing out the many ways in which a fetus resembles a baby. They emphasize its development ("It already has ten fingers . . .") without mentioning its dissimilarities to adults (it still has gills and a tail). They also try to evoke the sort of sympathy on our part that we only feel toward other persons ("Never to laugh . . . or feel the sunshine?"). This all seems to be a relevant way to argue, since its purpose is to persuade us that a fetus satisfies so many of the important features on the list that it ought to be treated as a person. Also note that a fetus near the time of birth satisfies many more of these factors than a fetus in the early months of development. This could provide reason for making distinctions among the different stages of pregnancy, as the U.S. Supreme Court has done.[8]

Historically, the time at which a person has been said to come into existence has varied widely. Muslims date personhood from fourteen days after conception. Some medievals followed Aristotle in placing ensoulment at forty days after conception for a male fetus and eighty days for a female fetus.[9] In European common law since the Seventeenth Century, abortion was considered the killing of a person only after quickening, the time when a pregnant woman first feels the fetus move on its own. Nor is this variety of opinions surprising. Biologically, a human being develops gradually. We shouldn't expect there to be any specific time or sharp dividing point when a person appears on the scene.

For these reasons I believe our concept of a person is not sharp or decisive enough to bear the weight of a solution to the abortion controversy. To use it to solve that problem is to clarify *obscurum per obscurius*.

II

Next let us consider what follows if a fetus is a person after all. Judith Jarvis Thomson's landmark article, "A Defense of Abortion,"[10] correctly points out that some additional argumentation is needed at this point in the conservative argument to bridge the gap between the premise that a fetus is an innocent person and the conclusion that killing it is always wrong. To arrive at this conclusion, we would need the additional premise that killing an innocent person is always wrong. But killing an innocent person is sometimes permissible, most notably in self defense. Some examples may help draw out our intuitions or ordinary judgments about self defense.

Suppose a mad scientist, for instance, hypnotized innocent people to jump out of the bushes and attack innocent passers-by with knives. If you are so attacked, we agree you have a right to kill the attacker in self defense, if killing him is the only way to protect your life or to save yourself from serious injury. It does not seem to matter here that the attacker is not malicious but himself an innocent pawn, for your killing of him is not done in a spirit of retribution but only in self defense.

How severe an injury may you inflict in self defense? In part this depends upon the severity of the injury to be avoided: you may not shoot someone merely to avoid having your clothes torn. This might lead one to the mistaken conclusion that the defense may only equal the threatened injury in severity; that to avoid death you may kill, but to avoid a black eye you may only inflict a black eye or the equivalent. Rather, our laws and customs seem to say that you may create an injury somewhat, but not enormously, greater than the injury to be avoided. To fend off an attack whose outcome would be as serious as rape, a severe beating or the loss of a finger, you may shoot; to avoid having your clothes torn, you may blacken an eye.

Aside from this, the injury you may inflict should only be the minimum necessary to deter or incapacitate the attacker. Even if you know he intends to kill you, you are not justified in shooting him if you could equally well save yourself by the simple expedient of running away. Self defense is for the purpose of avoiding harms rather than equalizing harms.

Some cases of pregnancy present a parallel situation. Though the fetus is itself innocent, it may pose a threat to the pregnant woman's well-being, life prospects or health, mental or physical. If the pregnancy presents a slight threat to her interests, it seems self defense cannot justify abortion. But if the threat is on a par with a serious beating or the loss of a finger, she may kill the fetus that poses such a threat, even if it is an innocent person. If a lesser harm to the fetus could have the same defensive effect, killing it would not be justified. It is unfortunate that the only way to free the woman from the pregnancy entails the death of the fetus (except in very late stages of pregnancy). Thus a self defense model supports Thomson's point that the woman has a right only to be freed from the fetus, not a right to demand its death.[11]

The self defense model is most helpful when we take the pregnant woman's point of view. In the pre-Thomson literature, abortion is often framed as a question for a third party: do you, a doctor, have a right to choose between the life of the woman and that of the fetus? Some have claimed that if you were a passer-by who witnessed a struggle between the innocent hypnotized attacker and his equally innocent victim, you would have no reason to kill either in defense of the other. They have concluded that the self defense model implies that a woman may attempt to abort herself, but that a doctor should not assist her. I think the position of the third party is somewhat more complex. We do feel some inclination to intervene on behalf of the victim rather than the attacker, other things equal. But if both parties are innocent, other factors come into consideration. You would rush to the aid of your husband whether he was attacker or attackee. If a hypnotized famous violinist were attacking a skid row bum, we would try to save the individual who is of more value to society. These considerations would tend to support abortion in some cases.

But suppose you are a frail senior citizen who wishes to avoid being knifed by one of these innocent hypnotics, so you have hired a bodyguard to accompany you. If you are attacked, it is clear we believe that the bodyguard, acting as your agent, has a right to kill the attacker to save you from a serious beating. Your rights of self defense are transferred to your agent. I suggest that we should similarly view the doctor as the pregnant woman's agent in carrying out a defense she is physically incapable of accomplishing herself.

Thanks to modern technology, the cases are rare in which a pregnancy poses as clear a threat to a woman's bodily health as an attacker brandish-ing a switchblade. How does self defense fare when more subtle, complex and long-range harms are involved?

To consider a somewhat fanciful example, suppose you are a highly trained surgeon when you are kidnapped by the hypnotic attacker. He says he does not intend to harm you but to take you back to the mad scientist who, it turns out, plans to hypnotize you to have a permanent mental block against all your knowledge of medicine. This would automatically destroy your career which would in turn have a serious adverse impact on your family, your personal relationships and your happiness. It seems to me that if the only way you can avoid this outcome is to shoot the innocent attacker, you are justified in so doing. You are defending yourself from a drastic injury to your life prospects. I think it is no exaggeration to claim that unwanted pregnancies (most obviously among teenagers) often have such adverse life-long consequences as the surgeon's loss of livelihood.

Several parallels arise between various views on abortion and the self defense model. Let's suppose further that these hypnotized attackers only operate at night, so that it is well known that they can be avoided completely by the consider-able inconvenience of never leaving your house after dark. One view is that since you could stay home at night, therefore if you go out and are selected by one of these hypnotized people, you have no right to defend yourself. This parallels the view that abstinence is the only acceptable way to avoid pregnancy. Others might hold that you ought to take along some defense such as Mace which will deter the hypnotized person without killing him, but that if this defense fails, you are obliged to submit to the resulting injury, no matter how severe it is. This parallels the view that contraception is all right but abortion is always wrong, even in cases of contraceptive failure.

A third view is that you may kill the hypnotized person only if he will actually kill you, but not if he will only injure you. This is like the position that abortion is permissible only if it is required to save a woman's life. Finally we have the view that it is all right to kill the attacker, even if only to avoid a very slight inconvenience to yourself and even if you knowingly walked down the very street where all these incidents have been taking place without taking along any Mace or protective escort. If we assume that a fetus is a person, this is the analogue of the view that abortion is always justifiable, "on demand."

The self defense model allows us to see an important difference that exists between abortion and infanticide, even if a fetus is a person from conception. Many have argued that the only way to justify abortion without justifying infanticide would be to find some characteristic of personhood that is acquired at birth. Michael Tooley, for one, claims infanticide is justifiable because the really significant characteristics of person are acquired some time after birth. But all such approaches look to characteristics of the developing human and ignore the relation between the fetus and the woman. What if, after birth, the presence of an infant or the need to support it posed a grave threat to the woman's sanity or life prospects? She could escape this threat by the simple expedient of running away. So a solution that does not entail the death of the infant is available. Before birth, such solutions are not available because of the biological dependence of the fetus on the woman. Birth is the crucial point not because of any characteristics the fetus gains, but because after birth the woman can defend herself by a means less drastic than killing the infant. Hence self defense can be used to justify abortion without necessarily thereby justifying infanticide.

III

On the other hand, supposing a fetus is not after all a person, would abortion always be morally permissible? Some opponents of abortion seem worried that if a fetus is not a full-fledged person, then we are justified in treating it in any way at all. However, this does not follow. Non-persons do get some consideration in our moral code, though of course they do not have the same rights as persons have (and in general they do not have moral responsibilities), and though their interests may be overridden by the interests of persons. Still, we cannot just treat them in any way at all.

Treatment of animals is a case in point. It is wrong to torture dogs for fun or to kill wild birds for no reason at all. It is wrong Period, even though dogs and birds do not have the same rights persons do. However, few people think it is wrong to use dogs as experimental animals, causing them considerable suffering in some cases, provided that the resulting research will probably bring discoveries of great benefit to people. And most of us think it all right to kill birds for food or to protect our crops. People's rights are different from the consideration we give to animals, then, for it is wrong to experiment on people, even if others might later benefit a great deal as a result of their suffering. You might volunteer to be a subject, but this would be supererogatory; you certainly have a right to refuse to be a medical guinea pig.

But how do we decide what you may or may not do to non-persons? This is a difficult problem, one for which I believe no adequate account exists. You do not want to say, for instance, that torturing dogs is all right whenever the sum of its effects on people is good—when it doesn't warp the sensibilities of the torturer so much that he mistreats people. If that were the case, it would be all right to torture dogs if you did it in private, or if the torturer lived on a desert island or died soon afterward, so that his actions had no effect on people. This is an inadequate account, because whatever moral consideration animals get, it has to be indefeasible, too. It will have to be a general proscription of certain actions, not merely a weighing of the impact on people on a case-by-case basis.

Rather, we need to distinguish two levels on which consequences of actions can be taken into account in moral reasoning. The traditional objections to Utilitarianism focus on the fact that it operates solely on the first level, taking all the consequences into account in particular cases only. Thus Utilitarianism is open to "desert island" and "lifeboat" counterexamples because these cases are rigged to make the consequences of actions severely limited.

Rawls's theory could be described as a teleological sort of theory, but with teleology operating on a higher level.[12] In choosing the principles to regulate society from the original position, his hypothetical choosers make their decision on the basis of the total consequences of various systems. Furthermore, they are constrained to choose a general set of rules which people can readily learn and apply. An ethical theory must operate by generating a set of sympathies and attitudes toward others which reinforces the functioning of that set of moral principles. Our prohibition against killing people operates by means of certain moral sentiments including sympathy, compassion and guilt. But if these attitudes are to form a coherent set, they carry us further: we tend to perform supererogatory actions, and we tend to feel similar compassion toward person-like non-persons.

It is crucial that psychological facts play a role here. Our psychological constitution makes it the case that for our ethical theory to work, it must prohibit certain treatment of non-persons which are significantly person-like. If our moral rules allowed people to treat some person-like non-persons in ways we do not want people to be treated, this would undermine the system of sympathies and attitudes that makes the ethical system work. For this reason, we would choose in the original position to make mistreatment of some sorts of animals wrong in general (not just wrong in the cases with public impact), even though animals are not themselves parties in the original position. Thus it makes sense that it is those animals whose appearance and behavior are most like those of people that get the most consideration in our moral scheme.

It is because of "coherence of attitudes," I think, that the similarity of a fetus to a baby is very significant. A fetus one week before birth is so much like a newborn baby in our psychological space that we cannot allow any cavalier treatment of the former while expecting full sympathy and nurturative support for the latter. Thus, I think that anti-abortion forces are indeed giving their strongest arguments when they point to the similarities between a fetus and a baby, and when they try to evoke our emotional attachment to and sympathy for the fetus. An early horror story from New York about nurses who were expected to alternate between caring for six-week premature infants and disposing of viable 24-week aborted fetuses is just that—a horror story. These beings are so much alike that no one can be asked to draw a distinction and treat them so very differently.

Remember, however, that in the early weeks after conception, a fetus is very much unlike a person. It is hard to develop these feelings for a set of genes which doesn't yet have a head, hands, beating heart, response to touch or the ability to move by itself. Thus it seems to me that the alleged "slippery slope" between conception and birth is not so very slippery. In the early stages of pregnancy, abortion can hardly be compared to murder for psychological reasons, but in the latest stages it is psychologically akin to murder.

Another source of similarity is the bodily continuity between fetus and adult. Bodies play a surprisingly central role in our attitudes toward persons. One has only to think of the philosophical literature on how far physical identity suffices for personal identity or Wittgenstein's remark that the best picture of the human soul is the human body. Even after death, when all agree the body is no longer a person, we still observe elaborate customs of respect for the human body; like people who torture dogs, necrophiliacs are not to be trusted with people.[13] So it is appropriate that we show respect to a fetus as the body continuous with the body of a person. This is a degree of resemblance to persons that animals cannot rival.

Michael Tooley also utilizes a parallel with animals. He claims that it is always permissible to drown newborn kittens and draws conclusions about infanticide.[14] But it is only permissible to drown kittens when their survival would cause some hardship. Perhaps it would be a burden to feed and house six more cats or to find other homes for them. The alternative of letting them starve produces even more suffering than the drowning. Since the kittens get their rights secondhand, so to speak, *via* the need for coherence in our attitudes, their interests are often overridden by the interests of full-fledged persons. But if their survival would be no inconvenience to people at all, then it is wrong to drown them, *contra* Tooley.

Tooley's conclusions about abortion are wrong for the same reason. Even if a fetus is not a person, abortion is not always permissible, because of the resemblance of a fetus to a person. I agree with Thomson that it would be wrong for a woman who is seven months pregnant to have an abortion just to avoid having to postpone a trip to Europe. In the early months of pregnancy when the fetus hardly resembles a baby at all, then, abortion is permissible whenever it is in the interests of the pregnant woman or her family. The reasons would only need to outweigh the pain and inconvenience of the abortion itself. In the middle months, when the fetus comes to resemble a person, abortion would be justifiable only when the continuation of the pregnancy or the birth of the child would cause harms—physical, psychological, economic or social—to the woman. In the late months of pregnancy, even on our current assumption that a fetus is not a person, abortion seems to be wrong except to save a woman from significant injury or death.

The Supreme Court has recognized similar gradations in the alleged slippery slope stretching between conception and birth. To this point, the present paper has been a discussion of the moral status of abortion only, not its legal status. In view of the great physical, financial and sometimes psychological costs of abortion, perhaps the legal arrangement most compatible with the proposed moral solution would be the absence of restrictions, that is, so-called abortion "on demand."

So I conclude, first, that application of our concept of a person will not suffice to settle the abortion issue. After all, the biological development of a human being is gradual. Second, whether a fetus is a person or not, abortion is justifiable early in pregnancy to avoid modest harms and seldom justifiable late in pregnancy except to avoid significant injury or death.

Notes

I am deeply indebted to Larry Crocker and Arthur Kuflik for their constructive comments.

1. We also have paternalistic laws which keep us from harming our own bodies even when no one else is affected. Ironically, anti-abortion laws were originally designed to protect pregnant women from a dangerous but tempting procedure.

2. Mary Anne Warren, "On the Moral and Legal Status of Abortion," *Monist* 5 (1973), p. 55.

3. Baruch Brody, "Fetal Humanity and the Theory of Essentialism," in Robert Baker and Frederick Elliston (eds.), *Philosophy and Sex* (Buffalo, N.Y., 1975).

4. Michael Tooley, "Abortion and Infanticide," *Philosophy and Public Affairs* 1 (1971). [See above, pp. 61–76.]

5. Paul Ramsey, "The Morality of Abortion," in James Rachels, ed., *Moral Problems* (New York, 1971).

6. John Noonan, "Abortion and the Catholic Church: a Summary History," *Natural Law Forum* 12 (1967), pp. 125–131.

7. Wittgenstein has argued against the possibility of so capturing the concept of a game, *Philosophical Investigations* (New York, 1958), §66–71.

8. Not because the fetus is partly a person and so has some of the rights of persons but rather because of the rights of person-like non-persons. This I discuss in part III below.

9. Aristotle himself was concerned, however, with the different question of when the soul takes form. For historical data, see Jimmye Kimmey, "How the Abortion Laws Happened," *Ms.* 1 (April, 1973), pp. 48ff and John Noonan, *loc. cit.*

10. J. J. Thomson, "A Defense of Abortion," *Philosophy and Public Affairs* 1 (1971).

11. *Ibid.*, p. 52. [See p. 88.]

12. John Rawls, *A Theory of Justice* (Cambridge, Mass., 1971), §§ 3–4.

13. On the other hand, if they can be trusted with people, then our moral customs are mistaken. It all depends on the facts of psychology.

14. *Op. cit.*, pp. 40, 60–61.

CASE RETROSPECTIVE
Mrs. Sherri Finkbine and the Thalidomide Tragedy

Background Note: The following case concerns an event that took place before the U.S. Supreme Court decision in Roe v. Wade was handed down in 1973. That decision had the effect of legalizing abortion in the United States. Before the decision, most state laws permitted abortion only for the purpose of saving the life of the mother. The case presented here illustrates the kinds of problems faced by many women who sought an abortion for other reasons.

In 1962 Mrs. Sherri Finkbine was the mother of four normal children and was pregnant. Her health was good, but she was having some trouble sleeping.

Rather than talking with her doctor, she simply took some of the tranquilizers that her husband had brought back from a trip to Europe. The tranquilizers were widely used there, and, like aspirin, they could simply be bought over the counter.

Subsequently, Mrs. Finkbine read an article that told of the great increase in the number of deformed children being born in Europe. Some of the children's arms and legs failed to develop or developed only in malformed ways; others were blind and deaf or had seriously defective internal organs. The birth defects had been traced to the use in pregnancy of a supposedly harmless and widely-used tranquilizer. Its active ingredient was thalidomide.

Mrs. Finkbine was worried enough to ask her doctor to find out if the pills she had been taking contained thalidomide. They did. When he learned this, her doctor told her, "The odds are so against you that I am recommending termination of pregnancy." He explained that getting approval for an abortion should not be difficult. She had good medical reasons and all she had to do was to explain them to the three-member medical board of Phoenix.

Mrs. Finkbine agreed with her doctor's advice. But then she began to think that maybe it was her duty to inform other women who may have been taking thalidomide about its disastrous consequences. She called a local newspaper and told her story to the editor. He agreed not to use her name, but on a front page, bordered in black, he used the headline "BABY-DEFORMING DRUG MAY COST WOMAN HER CHILD HERE."

The story was picked up by the wire services, and it was not long before Mrs. Finkbine's identity became known. The medical board had already approved her request for an abortion, but because of the great publicity her case received, they canceled their approval. The State of Arizona abortion statute legally sanctioned abortion only when it was required to save the life of the mother. The board was afraid that their decision might be challenged in court and that the decision could not stand up to the challenge.

Mrs. Finkbine became the object of a great outpouring of antiabortion feelings. *Il Osservatore Romano*, the official Vatican newspaper, condemned Mrs. Finkbine and her husband as murderers. Although she received some letters of support, others were abusive. One writer said: "I hope someone takes the other four children and strangles them, because it is all the same thing." Another wrote from the perspective of the fetus: "Mommy, please dear Mommy, let me live. Please, please, I want to live. Let me love you, let me see the light of day, let me smell a rose, let me sing a song, let me look into your face, let me say Mommy."

Although Mrs. Finkbine tried to obtain a legal abortion outside her own state, she was unable to do so. Eventually, she went to Sweden. After a rigorous investigation by a medical board, Mrs. Finkbine was given an abortion in a Swedish hospital.

Mrs. Finkbine saw her own problem as solved at last. But she continued to have sympathy with those thousands of potential parents of thalidomide children who lacked the money to follow the course of action she had been forced to take by abortion laws she considered to be restrictive and inhumane.

Decision Scenario 1

Ruth Perkins is twenty-four years old, and her husband Carl Freedon is four years older. Both are employed, Ruth as a junior executive for Laporte Gas Transmission and Carl as a librarian at the San Antonio Free Library. Their combined income is over forty-thousand dollars a year.

Perkins and Freedon live up to their income. They have an eleven-room house with a tennis court in a high-priced San Antonio suburb, both dress well, and Carl is a modest collector of sports cars (three MG-TDs). Both like to travel and try to get out of the country at least twice a year—Europe for a month in the summer and Mexico or the Caribbean for a couple of weeks during the winter.

Perkins and Freedon have no children. They agreed when they were married that children would not be a part of their plan for life together. They were distressed when Ruth became pregnant, and at first refused to face the problem. They worried about it for several months, considering arguments for and against abortion. At last they decided that Ruth should have an abortion.

"I don't see why I have to go through with this interview," Ruth said to the woman at the Morton Hospital Counseling Center.

"It's required of all who request an abortion," the counselor explained. "We think it's better for a person to be sure about what she is doing so she won't regret it later."

"My husband and I are certain," Ruth said. "A child doesn't fit in at all with our life style. We go out a lot and we like to do things. A child would just get in the way."

"A child can offer many pleasures," the woman said.

"I don't doubt it. If some want them, that's fine with me. We don't. Besides, we both have careers that we're devoted to. I'm not about to quit my job to take care of a child, and the same is true of my husband."

"How long have you been pregnant?"

Ruth looked embarrassed. "Almost six months," she said. "Carl and I weren't sure what we wanted to do at first. It took a while for us to get used to the idea."

"You don't think you waited too long?"

"That's stupid," Ruth said. She could hardly keep her voice under control. "I didn't mean that personally. But Carl and I have a right to live our lives the way we want. So far as we are concerned a six-month fetus is not a person. If we want to get rid of it, that's our business."

"Would you feel the same if it were a child already born?"

"I might," Ruth said. "I mean, a baby doesn't have much personality or anything does it?"

"I take it you're certain you want the abortion."

"Absolutely. My husband and I think it's the right thing for us. If others think we're wrong . . . well, it's their right to think what they please."

How might Tooley's arguments be used to support Perkins's position?

Could a utilitarian consider abortion justified in this case?

Would English consider the harm to Perkins and Freedon sufficient to justify the decision to have an abortion?

Do you believe Perkins is right about a six-month fetus not being a person? If not, why not?

If a person believes abortion is a kind of murder, can she legitimately endorse the tolerant position taken by Perkins?

Decision Scenario 2

It happened after a concert. Sixteen-year-old Mary Pluski had gone with three of her friends to hear the Bee-Gees at Chicago's new Blanton Auditorium. After the concert, in a crowd estimated at eleven thousand, Mary became separated from the other three girls. She decided that the best thing to do was to meet them at the car.

But when she got to the eight-story parking building, Mary realized she wasn't sure what level they had parked on. She thought it might be somewhere in the middle so she started looking on the fourth floor. While she was walking down the aisles of cars, two men in their early twenties, one white and the other black, stopped her and asked if she was having some kind of trouble.

Mary explained the situation to them, and one of the men suggested that they get his car and drive around inside the parking building. Mary hesitated, but both seemed so polite and genuinely concerned to help that she decided to go with them.

Once they were in the car, however, the situation changed. They drove out of the building and towards the south side. Mary pleaded with them to let her out of the car, but they refused. They threatened her with violence if she called for help or tried to escape from the car. Then, some seven miles from the auditorium, the driver stopped the car in a dark area behind a vacant building. Mary was then raped by both men.

Mary was treated at Allenworth Hospital and released into the custody of her parents. She filed a complaint with the police, but her troubles were not yet over. Two weeks after she missed her menstrual period, tests showed that Mary was pregnant.

"How do you feel about having this child?" asked Sarah Ruben, the Pluski family physician.

"I hate the idea," Mary said. "I feel guilty about it, though. I mean, it's not the child's fault."

"Let me ask a delicate question," said Dr. Ruben. "I know from what you've told me before that you and your boyfriend have been having sex. Can you be sure this pregnancy is not really the result of that?"

Mary shook her head. "Not really. I use my diaphragm, but I know it doesn't give a hundred percent guarantee."

"That's right. Now, does it make any difference to you who the father might be, so far as a decision about terminating the pregnancy is concerned?"

"If I were sure that it was Bob, I guess the problem would be even harder," Mary said.

"There are some tests we can use to give us that information," Dr. Ruben said. "But that would mean waiting for the embryo to develop into a fetus. It would be easier and safer to terminate the pregnancy now."

Mary started crying. "I don't want a child," she said. "I don't want any child. I don't care who's the father, it was forced on me and I want to get rid of it."

"I'll make the arrangements," said Dr. Ruben.

Would Thomson's position recognize abortion here as a form of self-defense?

Would Noonan consider abortion immoral in this case?

Suppose the fetus is a person; Would the maxim in this case satisfy the categorical imperative?

Does Mary's uncertainty about the father add any special moral difficulties?

Decision Scenario 3

"I don't want no more children," Mrs. Hinson said. "I've already got five, and I can't look after them the way they should be looked after. My husband's been gone three years. I don't know where he is but I know he ain't coming back."

After two years as a psychiatric social worker, David Rossum found Mrs. Hinson's situation familiar. He looked around the small living room. It was clean but crowded with broken second-hand furniture. Cheap dime-store metal frames lined the top of the television set. Children smiled in the blurry color snapshots.

"You're sure you're pregnant?" Rossum asked.

"The doctor at the clinic told me so," Mrs. Hinson said. "He gave me a paper to prove it. But I'm already on the welfare and the ADC. I can't do right by my children if I have another one to take care of."

"And you can't count on the father of this child to help you?"

"I can't count on him for nothing," said Mrs. Hinson. "I don't even see him anymore."

"So what do you want to do?" Rossum asked. He knew the answer, but the main part of his job was just listening.

"I want an abortion. That's what I want. But the people at the clinic, they told me I'd have to talk to you people first. If you won't say it's okay they won't do it, because there won't be nobody to pay for it."

"That's right," Rossum said. "You've got to have an authorization from our agency for any kind of special medical procedure of a nonemergency kind."

Suppose that you are David Rossum. On what grounds would you authorize (or refuse to authorize) Mrs. Hinson's request? If you were opposed to all abortions on moral grounds, ought you to allow this to influence your decision?

Does the reasoning in the Supreme Court decision (Roe v. Wade) apply in this case?

Do Rawls's principles of justice suggest a legitimate social policy to cover such cases?

Does the principle of utility?

If the fetus is a person, are there sufficient reasons for considering abortion here a case of justified killing?

Decision Scenario 4

Clare Macwurter was twenty-two years old chronologically, but mentally she remained a child. As a result of her mother's prolonged and difficult labor, Clare had been deprived of an adequate blood-oxygen supply during her birth. The consequence was that she suffered irreversible brain damage.

Clare enjoyed life and was generally a happy person. She couldn't read, but she liked listening to music and watching television, although she could rarely understand the stories. She was physically attractive and, with the help of her parents, she could care for herself.

Clare was also interested in sex. When she was seventeen, she and a fellow student at the special school they attended had been caught having intercourse. Clare's parents had been told about the incident, but after Clare left the school the following year, they took no special precautions to ensure that Clare would not become sexually involved with anyone. After all, she stayed at home with her mother every day, and, besides, it was a matter they didn't much like to think about.

The Macwurters were both surprised and upset when Clare became pregnant. At first they couldn't imagine how it could have happened. Then they recalled that on several occasions Clare had been sent to stay at the house of Mr. Macwurter's brother and his wife while Mrs. Macwurter went shopping.

John Macwurter at first denied that he had anything to do with Clare's pregnancy. But during the course of a long and painful conversation with his brother, he admitted that he had sexual relations with Clare.

"I wasn't wholly to blame," John Macwurter said. "I mean, I know I shouldn't have done it. But still, she was interested in it, too. I didn't really rape her. Nothing like that."

The Macwurters were at a loss about what they should do. The physician they consulted told them that Clare would probably have a perfectly normal baby. But of course Clare couldn't really take care of herself, much less a baby. She was simply unfit to be a mother. Mrs. Macwurter, for her part, was not eager to assume the additional responsibilities of caring for another child. Mr. Macwurter would be eligible to retire in four more years, and the couple had been looking forward to selling their house and moving back to the small town in Oklahoma where they had first met and then married. The money they had managed to save, plus insurance and a sale of their property, would permit them to place Clare in a long-term care facility after their deaths. Being responsible for another child would both ruin their plans and jeopardize Clare's future well-being.

"I never thought I would say such a thing," Mrs. Macwurter told her husband, "but I think we should arrange for Clare to have an abortion."

"That's killing," Mr. Macwurter said.

"I'm not so sure it is. I don't really know. But even if it is, I think it's the best thing to do."

Mrs. Macwurter made the arrangements with Clare's physician for an abortion to be performed. When Mr. Macwurter asked his brother to pay for the operation, John Macwurter refused. He explained that he was opposed to abortion and so it would not be right for him to provide money to be used in that way.

> *Can the reasoning in* Roe *v.* Wade *be applied in this case? After all, the person involved is not mentally competent and cannot be expected to exercise any right of privacy.*
>
> *Could Thomson's defense of abortion be employed here to show that the proposed abortion is permissible?*
>
> *Why would Noonan oppose abortion here? What alternatives might he recommend? What if it were likely that the baby would be defective? Would this alter the situation for Noonan?*
>
> *Do the considerations Tooley offers to determine when a member of our species is to count as a person require that we think of Clare Macwurter as not being a person in a morally relevant sense?*

Decision Scenario 5

Daniel Bocker was worried. The message his secretary had taken merely said, "Go to see Dr. Tai at 3:30 today." He hadn't been asked if 3:30 was convenient for him, and he hadn't been given a reason for coming in.

Mr. Bocker knew it would have to do with his wife Mary. She had been suffering a lot of pain during her pregnancy, and the preceding week she had been examined by a specialist that Dr. Tai, her gynecologist, had sent her to see. The specialist had performed a thorough examination and taken blood, tissue, and urine samples, but he had told Mary nothing.

"Thank you for coming in," Dr. Tai said. "I want to talk to you before I talk to your wife, because I need your help."

"The tests showed something bad, didn't they?" Mr. Bocker said. "Something is wrong with the baby."

"The baby is fine, but there is something wrong with your wife, something very seriously wrong. She has what we call uterine neoplasia."

"Is that cancer?"

"Yes it is," said Dr. Tai. "But I don't want either of you to panic about it. It's not at a very advanced stage, and at the moment it's localized. If an operation is performed very soon, then she has a good chance to make a full recovery. The standard figures show about 80 percent success."

"But what about the baby?"

"The pregnancy will have to be terminated," Dr. Tai said. "And I should tell you that your wife will not be able to have children after the operation."

Mr. Bocker sat quietly for a moment. He had always wanted children; for him a family without children was not a family at all. He and Mary had talked about having at least three, and the one she was pregnant with now was the first.

"Is it possible to save the baby?" he asked Dr. Tai.

"Mrs. Bocker is only in her fourth month; there is no chance the child could survive outside her body."

"But what if she didn't have the operation? Would the baby be normal?"

"Probably so, but the longer we wait to perform the operation, the worse your wife's chances become. I don't want to seem to tell you what to do, but my advice is for your wife to have an abortion and to undergo the operation as soon as it is reasonably possible."

"But she might recover, even if she had the child and then had the operation, might't she?"

"It's possible, but her chances of recovery are much less. I don't know what the exact figures would be, but she would be running a terrible risk."

Mr. Bocker understood what Dr. Tai was saying, but he also understood what he wanted.

"I'm not going to encourage Mary to have an abortion," he said. "I want her to have a child, and I think she wants that, too."

"What if she wants to have a better chance to live? I think the decision is really hers. After all, it's her life that is at stake."

"But it's not just her decision," Mr. Bocker said. "It's a family decision, hers and mine. I'm not going to agree to an abortion, even if she does want one. I'm going to try to get her to take the extra risk and have the child before she has the operation."

"I think that's the cruelist, most immoral thing I've ever heard," Dr. Tai said.

Would the doctrine of double effect justify taking steps to treat Mrs. Bocker's illness, even at the cost of terminating her pregnancy?

Would both Noonan and Thomson see the situation as one in which considerations of self-defense are relevant?

It is sometimes said that the father of a child also has a right to decide whether an abortion is to be performed. Would Daniel Bocker be justified in urging his wife to take the risk of having the child?

Does the categorical imperative have any relevance in determining whether an abortion is morally right in this case?

2

TREATING OR TERMINATING:
THE PROBLEM OF BIRTH DEFECTS

CASE PRESENTATION
Baby Owens: Down's Syndrome and Duodenal Atresia

On a chill December evening in 1976 Dr. Joan Owens pushed through the plateglass doors of Midwestern Medical Center and walked over to the admitting desk. Dr. Owens was a physician in private practice and regularly visited Midwestern to attend to her patients.

But this night was different. Dr. Owens was coming to the hospital to be admitted as a patient. She was pregnant, and shortly after nine o'clock she began having periodic uterine contractions. Dr. Owens recognized them as the beginnings of labor pains. She was sure of this not only because of her medical knowledge but also because the pains followed the same pattern they had before her other three children were born.

While her husband, Phillip, parked the car, Dr. Owens went through the formalities of admission. She was not particularly worried, for the birth of her other children had been quite normal and uneventful. But the pains were coming more frequently now, and she was relieved when she completed the admission process and was taken to her room. Phillip came with her, bringing her small blue suitcase of personal belongings.

At eleven-thirty that evening, Dr. Owens gave birth to a four-and-a-half pound baby girl. The plastic bracelet fastened around her wrist identified her as Baby Owens and listed her patient number as 23-764-2509.

Dr. Owens was groggy from exhaustion and from the medication she had received. But when the baby was shown to her, she saw at once that it was not normal. The baby's head was misshapen and the skin around her eyes strangely formed. Dr. Owens recognized that her daughter had Down's syndrome.

"Clarence," she called to her obstetrician. "Is the baby mongoloid?"

"We'll talk about it after your recovery," Dr. Clarence Ziner said.

"Tell me now," said Dr. Owens. "Examine it!"

Dr. Ziner made a hasty examination of the child. He had already seen that Dr. Owens was right and was doing no more than making doubly certain. A more careful examination would have to be made later.

When Dr. Ziner confirmed Joan Owens's suspicion, she did not hesitate to say what she was thinking. "Get rid of it," she told Dr. Ziner. "I don't want a mongoloid child."

Dr. Ziner tried to be soothing. "Just sleep for a while now," he told her. "We'll talk about it later."

Four hours later, a little after five in the morning and before it was fully light, Joan Owens woke up. Phillip was with her, and he had more bad news to tell. A more detailed examination had shown that the child's small intestine had failed to develop properly and was closed off in one place—the condition known as duodenal atresia. It could be corrected by a relatively simple surgical procedure, but until surgery was performed, the child could not be fed. Phillip had refused to consent to the operation until he had talked to his wife.

Joan Owens had not changed her mind: she did not want the child. "It wouldn't be fair to the other children to raise them with a mongoloid," she told Phillip. "It would take all of our time, and we wouldn't be able to give David, Sean, and Melinda the love and attention they need."

"I'm willing to do whatever you think best," Phillip said. "But what can we do?"

"Let the child die," Joan said. "If we don't consent to the surgery, the baby will die soon. And that's what we have to let happen."

Phillip put in a call for Dr. Ziner, and when he arrived in Joan's room, they told him of their decision. He was not pleased with it.

"The surgery has very low risk," he said. "The baby's life can almost certainly be saved. We can't tell how retarded she'll be, but most DS children get along quite well with help from their families. The whole family will grow to love her."

"I know," Joan said. "And I don't want that to happen. I don't want us to center our lives around a defective child. Phillip and I and our other children will be forced to lose out on many of life's pleasures and possibilities."

"We've made up our minds," Phillip said. "We don't want the surgery."

"I'm not sure the matter is as simple as that," Dr. Ziner said. "I'm not sure we can legally just let the baby die. I'll have to talk to the Director and the hospital attorney."

At six in the morning, Dr. Ziner called Dr. Felix Entraglo, the Director of Midwestern Medical Center, and Issac Putnam, the head of the center's legal staff. They agreed to meet at nine o'clock to talk over the problem presented to them by the Owenses.

They met for two hours. It was Putnam's opinion that the hospital would not be legally liable if Baby Owens were allowed to die because her parents refused to give consent for necessary surgery.

"What about getting a court order requiring surgery?" Dr. Entraglo asked. "That's the sort of thing we do when an infant requires a blood transfusion or immunization and his parents' religious beliefs make them refuse consent."

"This case is not exactly parallel," said Mr. Putnam. "Here we're talking about getting a court to force parents to allow surgery to save the life of a defective infant. The infant will still be defective after the surgery, and I think a court would be reluctant to make a family undergo significant emotional and financial hardships when the parents have seriously deliberated about the matter and decided against surgery."

"But doesn't the child have some claim in this situation?" Dr. Ziner asked.

"That's not clear," said Mr. Putnam. "In general we assume that parents will act for the sake of their child's welfare, and when they are reluctant to do so, we look to the courts to act for the child's welfare. But in a situation like this . . . who can say? Is the Owens baby really a person in any legal or moral sense?"

"I think I can understand why a court would hesitate to order surgery," said Dr. Entraglo. "What sort of life would it be for a family when they had been pressured into accepting a child they didn't want. It would turn a family into a cauldron of guilt and resentment mixed in with love and concern. In this case, the lives of five normal people would be profoundly altered for the worse."

"So we just stand by and let the baby die?" asked Dr. Ziner.

"I'm afraid so," Dr. Entraglo said.

It took twelve days for Baby Owens to die. Her lips and throat were moistened with water to lessen her suffering, and in a small disused room set apart from the rooms of patients, she was allowed to starve to death.

Many nurses and physicians thought it was wrong that Baby Owens was forced to die such a lingering death. Some thought it was wrong for her to have to die at all, but such a protracted death seemed needlessly cruel. Yet they were cautioned by Dr. Entraglo that anything done to shorten the baby's life would probably constitute a criminal action. Thus, fear of being charged with a crime kept the staff from administering any medication to Baby Owens.

The burden of caring for the dying baby fell on the nurses in the obstetrics ward. The physicians avoided the child entirely, and it was the nurses who had to see to it that she received her water and was turned in her bed. This was the source of much resentment among the nursing staff, and a few nurses refused to have anything to do with the dying child. Most kept their ministrations to an absolute minimum.

But one nurse, Sara Ann Moberly, was determined to make Baby Owens's last days as comfortable as possible. She held the baby, rocked her, and talked soothingly to her when she cried. Doing all for the baby that she could do soothed Sara Ann as well.

But even Sara Ann was glad when Baby Owens died. "It was a relief to me," she said. "I almost couldn't bear the frustration of just sitting there day after day and doing nothing that could really help her."

Note: I have made this case wholly fictional. But for discussions of a similar actual case, see the citations in Notes and References.

Introduction

If we could speak of nature in human terms, we would often say that it is cruel and pitiless. Nowhere does it seem more heartless than in the case of babies born into the world with severe physical defects and deformities. The birth of such a child transforms an occasion of expected joy into one of immense sadness. It forces the child's parents to make a momentous decision at a time they are least prepared to reason clearly: Shall they insist that everything be done to save the child's life? Or shall they request that the child be allowed an easeful death?

Nor can physicians and nurses escape the burden that the birth of such a child delivers. Committed to saving lives, can they condone the death of that child? What shall the physician say to the parents when they turn to him for advice? No one involved in the situation can escape the moral agonies that it brings.

To see more clearly what the precise moral issues are in such cases, we need to consider some of the factual details that may be involved in them. We need also to mention other kinds of moral considerations that may be relevant to deciding how a defective newborn child is to be dealt with by those who have the responsibility to decide.

Genetic and Congenital Defects

The development of a child to the point of birth is an unimaginably complicated process, and there are many ways in which it can go wrong. Two kinds of errors are most frequently responsible for producing defective children.

1. *Genetic defects*. The program of information that is coded into DNA (the genetic material) may be in some way abnormal because of the occurrence of a mutation. Consequently, when the DNA blueprint is "read" and its instructions followed, the child that develops will have defects. The defective gene may have been inherited or it may be due to a new mutation.

2. *Congenital defects*. "Congenital" means only "present at birth," and since genetic defects have results that are present at birth, the term is misleading. Ordinarily, however, the phrase is used to designate errors that result during the developmental process. The defect, then, is not in the original blueprint (genes) but either results from genetic damage or from the reading of the blueprint. The manufacture and assembly of the materials that constitute the child's development are affected.

We know that many factors can influence fetal development. Radiation (such as x rays), drugs (such as thalidomide), chemicals (such as mercury), and nutritional deficiencies can all cause changes in an otherwise normal process. Also, biological disease agents, such as certain viruses or spirochetes, may intervene in development. They may alter the machinery of the cells, interfere with the formation of tissues, and defeat the carefully programmed process that leads to a normal child.

Genetic defects are inherited; they are the outcome of the genetic endowment of the child. A carrier of defective genes who has children can pass on the genes. Congenital defects are not inherited and cannot be passed on. This point is of great theoretical and practical importance. With proper genetic counseling, individuals belonging to families in which certain diseases "run" can assess the risk that their children might inherit defects. Also, some genetic diseases can be diagnosed before birth. In a procedure known as amniocentesis, fluid is withdrawn from the uterus and cells from the developing embryo are examined for genetic abnormalities. If they are present, the woman may decide to have an abortion rather than give birth to a defective child. A recognition of defects that are developmental can lead to efforts to eliminate the defects by controlling the factors responsible for them.

Once the defective child is born, the medical and moral problems are immediate. Let us consider now some of the defects commonly found in newborn children. Our focus will be on what they are rather than on what caused them, for so far as the moral issue is concerned in a particular case, how the child came to be defective is of no importance.

Down's syndrome.   This is a genetic disease first identified in 1866 by the English physician J. L. H. Down. Normally, humans have twenty-three pairs of chromosomes, but Down's syndrome results from the presence of an extra chromosome. The condition is called Trisomy-21, for instead of a twenty-first pair of chromosomes, the affected person has a twenty-first *triple*. (Less often, the syndrome is produced when the string of chromosomes gets twisted and chromosome pair number 21 sticks to number 15.)

In ways not wholly understood, the normal process of development is altered by this extra chromosome. The child is born with retardation and various physical abnormalities. Typically, these are relatively minor and include such features as a broad skull, a large tongue, and an upward slant of the eyelids. It is this last feature that led to the name "mongolism" for the condition.

Down's syndrome occurs in about one of every thousand births. There is no cure for it—no way to compensate for the abnormality of the development process. Those with the defect generally have an IQ of about 50–80 and usually require the care and help of others. They can be taught easy tasks, and despite their defect, those with Down's syndrome usually seem to be quite happy people.

Spina bifida.   Spina bifida is a general name for birth defects that involve an opening in the spine. In development, the spine of the child fails to fuse properly, and often the open vertebrae permit the membrane covering the spinal cord to protrude to the outside. The membrane sometimes forms a bulging, thin sac that contains spinal fluid and nerve tissue. When nerve tissue is present, the condition is called myelomeningocele. This form of spina bifida is a very severe one.

Complications arising from spina bifida must often be treated surgically. The initial condition, the opening in the spine, must be closed up. In severe cases, the sac is removed and the nerve tissue inside is placed within the spinal canal. Normal skin is then grafted over the area. The danger of an infection of the meninges (meningitis) is great; thus, treatment with antibiotic drugs is also necessary.

Furthermore, a child with spina bifida is also likely to require orthopedic operations to attempt to correct the deformities of the legs and feet that occur because of muscle weakness and lack of muscular control due to nerve damage. The bones of such children are thin and brittle and fractures are frequent.

A child born with spina bifida is virtually always paralyzed to some extent. Generally, the paralysis is below the waist. Because of the nerve damage, the child will have limited sensation in the lower part of the body. This means that he will have no control over his bladder or bowels. The lack of bladder control may result in infection of the bladder, urinary tract, and kidneys, because the undischarged urine may serve as a breeding place for microorganisms. Surgery may help with the problem of lack of control of the bladder and bowels.

Spina bifida occurs in between one and ten per 1,000 births. For reasons not understood, the rate in white families of low socioeconomic status is three times higher than that in families of higher socioeconomic status. The rate in the black population is less than half of that in the white population.

Spina bifida is almost always accompanied by hydrocephaly.

Hydrocephaly.   This term literally means "water on the brain." When, for whatever reasons, the flow of fluid through the spinal canal is blocked, the cerebrospinal fluid produced within the brain cannot escape. Pressure build-up from the fluid can cause brain damage, and if it is not released, the child will die. Although hydrocephaly is frequently the result of spina bifida, it can have several causes and can develop late in a child's life.

Treatment requires surgically inserting a thin tube or shunt to drain the fluid from the skull to the heart or abdomen where it can be absorbed. The operation can save the baby's life, but physical and mental damage is frequent. Placing the shunt and getting it to work properly are difficult tasks that may require many operations. If hydrocephaly accompanies spina bifida (and it almost always does), it is treated first.

Anencephaly.   This term means literally "without brain." In this condition, the brain is partially or almost totally absent. The defect is related to spina bifida, for in some forms the bones of the skull are not completely formed and leave an opening through which brain material bulges to the outside.

In some cases, death is a virtual certainty. Other cases can be dealt with in much the same way as is spina bifida. Ordinarily, the individual is so severely retarded that he has minimum control over bodily movements and functions. There is never hope for improvement by any known means.

Esophageal atresia.   In medical terms, an atresia is the closing of a normal opening or canal. The esophagus is the muscular tube that extends from the back of the throat to the stomach. Sometimes the tube forms without an opening, or it does not completely develop so that it does not extend to the stomach. The condition must be corrected by surgery in order that the child may get food into its stomach. The chances of success in such surgery are very high.

Duodenal atresia.   The duodenum is the upper part of the small intestine. Food from the stomach empties into it. When the duodenum is closed off, food cannot pass through and be digested. Surgery can repair this condition and is successful in most cases.

The birth defects we have singled out for special mention are those that are currently the source of major moral problems. Those correctable by standard surgical procedures present no special moral difficulties. But they are often involved with other defects, such as Down's syndrome, that make them important factors in moral deliberations.

Ethical Theories and the Problem of Birth Defects

A great number of serious moral issues are raised by defective newborns. Should they be given only ordinary care or should special efforts be made to save their lives? Should they be given no care and allowed to die? Should they be killed in a merciful manner? Who should decide what is in the interest of the child? Might acting in the interest of the child require not acting to save the child's life?

A more basic question that cuts even deeper than these concerns the status of the newborn. It is virtually the same as the question raised in Chapter 1 about the fetus. Namely, are severely defective newborns persons? It might be argued that some infants are so severely impaired that they should not be considered persons in a relevant moral sense. Not only do they lack the capacity to function, but they lack even the potentiality for ordinary psychological and social development. In this respect, they are worse off than most maturing fetuses.

If this view is accepted, then the principles of our moral theories do not require that we act to preserve the lives of defective newborns. We might, considering their origin, be disposed to show them some consideration and treat them benevolently—perhaps in the same way we might deal with animals that are in a similarly hopeless condition. We might kill them or allow them to die as a demonstration of our compassion.

One major difficulty with this view is that it is not at all clear which defective infants could legitimately be considered nonpersons. Birth defects vary widely in severity, and unless one is prepared to endorse infanticide generally, it is necessary to have defensible criteria for distinguishing among newborns. Also, one must defend a general concept of person that would make it reasonable to regard human offspring as occupying a different status. (See Michael Tooley's article in Chapter 1 for such an attempt.)

By contrast, it might be claimed that the fact that a newborn is a human progeny is sufficient to consider it a person. Assuming that this is so, the question becomes, "How ought we to treat a severely defective infant person?" Just because they are infants, defective newborns cannot express wishes, make claims, or enter into deliberations. All that is done concerning them must be done by others.

A utilitarian might decide that the social and personal cost (the suffering of the infant, the anguish of the parents and family, the monetary cost to society) of saving the life of such an infant is greater than the social and personal benefits that can be expected. Accordingly, such a child should not be allowed to live, and it should be killed as painlessly as possible to minimize its suffering. Yet a rule utilitarian might claim, on the contrary, that the rule "Save every child where possible" would, in the long run, produce more utility than disutility.

The position of Roman Catholicism is that even the most defective newborn is a human person. Yet this view does not require that extraordinary means be used to save the life of such a child. The suffering of the family, great expense, and the need for multiple operations would be reasons for providing only ordinary care. Ordinary care does not mean that every standard medical procedure that might help should be followed. It means only that the defective newborn should receive care of the same type provided for a normal infant. It would be immoral to kill the child or to cause its death by withholding all care.

If the infant is a person, then Kant would regard it as possessing an inherent dignity and value. But the infant in its condition lacks the capacity to reason and to express its will. How, then, should we, acting as its agents, treat it? Kant's principles provide no clear-cut answer. The infant does not threaten our own existence, and we have no grounds for killing it. But, it could be argued, we should allow the child to die. We can imaginatively put ourselves in the place of the infant. Although it would be morally wrong to will our own death (which would involve a self-defeating maxim), we might express our autonomy and rationality by choosing to refuse treatment that would prolong a painful and hopeless life. If this is so, then we might act in this way on behalf of the defective child. We might allow the child to die. Indeed, it may be our duty to do so. A similar line of argument from Ross's viewpoint might lead us to decide that, although we have a prima facie duty to preserve the child's life, our actual duty is to allow it to die.

Another basic question remains: Who is to make the decision about how a defective newborn is to be treated? One might argue that no individual should make the decision. The infant is not the "property" of anyone, but it is dependent on its parents and physicians. Because they have the highest concern for its welfare and the most knowledge about its conditions and prospects, they are the ones who have the primary responsibility for deciding its fate. If there is reason to believe that they are not acting in a responsible manner, then it becomes the responsibility of the courts to guarantee that the interests of the infant are served. In practice, this has usually meant ordering that the life of the infant be saved. A society with laws conforming to Rawls's social and ethical principles, however, might dictate another set of arrangements. Those in the original position might decide that permitting the deaths of defective newborns would better serve the interests of justice and demonstrate respect for human worth than requiring that every life be saved.

The Selections

John A. Robertson in his essay, "Examination of Arguments in Favor of Withholding Ordinary Medical Care from Defective Infants," defends a conservative natural-law position in criticizing two arguments in favor of withholding "necessary but ordinary" medical care from defective infants. He rejects the claim made by Tooley that infants are not persons and argues that, on the contrary, there is no nonarbitrary consideration that requires us to protect the past realization of conceptual capability but not its potential realization.

The second argument that Robertson considers is one to the effect that we have no obligation to treat defective newborns when the cost of doing so greatly outweighs the benefits (a utilitarian argument). In criticism, Robertson claims that we have no way of judging this. Life itself may be of sufficient worth to a defective person to offset his or her suffering, and the suffering and cost to society are not sufficient to justify withholding care.

Contrary to Robertson, H. T. Engelhardt in "Ethical Issues in Aiding the Death of Young Children" contends that children are not persons in the full sense. They must exist in and through their families. Thus parents, in conference with a physician who provides information, are the appropriate ones to decide whether to treat a defective newborn when (1) there is not only little likelihood of a full human life, but also there is the likelihood of suffering if the life is prolonged, or (2) when the cost of prolonging the life is very great.

Engelhardt further argues that it is reasonable to speak of a *duty* not to treat a defective infant when this will only prolong a painful life or would only lead to a painful death. He bases his claim on the legal notion of a "wrongful life." This notion suggests that there are cases in which nonexistence would be better than existence under the conditions in which a person must live. Life can thus be seen as an injury, rather than as a gift.

In their essay on infanticide R. S. Duff and A. G. M. Campbell are concerned less with abstract philosophical arguments and more with making recommendations about dealing with actual cases in which decisions must be made. They claim that, in practice, there are two "philosophies" of deciding how the severely defective are to be dealt with. The first is disease-oriented and regards death as the worst possible event. This view encourages the development of medical technology, but its application frequently dehumanizes patients and worsens suffering. The second view is person-oriented and regards some severely compromised living patterns as worse than death. It would protect persons from the indignities of pointless treatment or the cruelties of hopeless disease. (This view would support active euthanasia were euthanasia legal.) Because defective infants are unable to participate in the decision making, the application of this view becomes especially problematic.

In deciding which approach to take in a given case, Duff and Campbell argue that, in the case of infants, the family and the physician are the best judges. They must be trusted with more freedom to change or to ignore commonly accepted principles if these conflict with the values of the family. For this reason, Duff and Campbell are in favor of permitting families to decide to allow defective infants to die or be put to death.

In 1973 Duff and Campbell, in another article, shocked the public by reporting that during a thirty-month period forty-three infants at the Yale-New Haven Hospital had been permitted to die. Each of the children suffered from one or more severe birth defects. Although the staff of the hospital took no steps to end the lives of the infants, treatment was withheld from them.

Such decisions had been made for years in hospitals throughout the world. Sometimes they were made by physicians acting alone and sometimes by physicians in consultation with families. But almost never had the situation been discussed openly and publicly.

Now there is more openness about the whole complex of moral and human problems presented by defective newborns. There is a greater willingness to consider the possibility that saving the life of a child might not be the right act to perform, that it may even be our duty to assist the child's dying. In any case, the time of covert decisions and half-guilty conferences has passed. The issues are there, they are known to be there, and they must be faced.

Examination of Arguments in Favor of Withholding Ordinary Medical Care from Defective Infants
John A. Robertson

This [selection] considers two arguments in favor of withholding necessary but ordinary medical care from defective infants, and concludes that neither is persuasive. . . .

1. Defective Infants Are Not Persons

Children born with congenital malformations may lack human form and the possibility of ordinary, psychosocial development. In many cases mental retardation is or will be so profound, and physical incapacity so great, that the term "persons" or "humanly alive"[1] have odd or questionable meaning when applied to them. In these cases the infant's physical and mental defects are so severe that they will never know anything but a vegetative existence, with no discernible personality, sense of self, or capacity to interact with others.[2] Withholding ordinary medical care in such cases, one may argue, is justified on the ground that these infants are not persons or human beings in the ordinary or legal sense of the term, and therefore do not possess the right of care that persons possess.

Central to this argument is the idea that living products of the human uterus can be classified into offspring that are persons, and those that are not. Conception and birth by human parents does not automatically endow one with personhood and its accompanying rights. Some other characteristic or feature must be present in the organism for personhood to vest,[3] and this the defective infant arguably lacks. Lacking that property, an organism is not a person or deserving to be treated as such.

Before considering what "morally significant features" might distinguish persons from nonpersons, and examining the relevance of such features

to the case of the defective infant, we must face an initial objection to this line of inquiry. The objection questions the need for any distinction among human offspring because of

> the monumental misuse of the concept of 'humanity' in so many practices of discrimination and atrocity throughout history. Slavery, witchhunts and wars have all been justified by their perpetrators on the grounds that they held their victims to be less than fully human. The insane and the criminal have for long periods been deprived of the most basic necessities for similar reasons, and been excluded from society. . . .
>
> . . . Even when entered upon with the best of intentions, and in the most guarded manner, the enterprise of basing the protection of human life upon such criteria and definitions is dangerous. To question someone's humanity or personhood is a first step to mistreatment and killing.[4]

Hence, according to this view, human parentage is a necessary and sufficient condition for personhood, whatever the characteristics of the offspring, because qualifying criteria inevitably lead to abuse and untold suffering to beings who are unquestionably human. Moreover, the human species is sufficiently different from other sentient species that assigning its members greater rights on birth alone is not arbitrary.

This objection is indeed powerful. The treatment accorded slaves in the United States, the

Reprinted by permission of the publisher from "Involuntary Euthanasia of Defective Newborns: A Legal Analysis," Stanford Law Review 27 (1975): 246–261. Copyright 1975 by the Board of Trustees of the Leland Stanford Junior University. Editor's Note: The footnotes in this essay have been renumbered.

Nazi denial of personal status to non-Aryans, and countless other incidents, testify that man's inhumanity to man is indeed greatest when a putative nonperson is involved.[5] Arguably, however, a distinction based on gross physical form, profound mental incapacity, and the very existence of personality or selfhood, besides having an empirical basis in the monstrosities and mutations known to have been born to women[6] is a basic and fundamental one. Rather than distinguishing among the particular characteristics that persons might attain through the contingencies of race, culture, and class, it merely separates out those who lack the potential for assuming any personal characteristics beyond breathing and consciousness.

This reply narrows the issue: should such creatures be cared for, protected, or regarded as "ordinary" humans? If such treatment is not warranted, they may be treated as nonpersons. The arguments supporting care in all circumstances are based on the view that all living creatures are sacred, contain a spark of the divine, and should be so regarded. Moreover, indentifying those human offspring unworthy of care is a difficult task and will inevitably take a toll on those whose humanity cannot seriously be questioned. At this point the argument becomes metaphysical or religious and immune to resolution by empirical evidence, not unlike the controversy over whether a fetus is a person.[7] It should be noted, however, that recognizing all human offspring as persons, like recognizing the fetus to be a person,[8] does not conclude the treatment issue.[9]

Although this debate can be resolved only by reference to religious or moral beliefs, a procedural solution may reasonably be considered. Since reasonable people can agree that we ordinarily regard human offspring as persons, and further, that defining categories of exclusion is likely to pose special dangers of abuse, a reasonable solution is to presume that all living human offspring are persons. This rule would be subject to exception only if it can be shown beyond a reasonable doubt that certain offspring will never possess the minimal properties that reasonable persons ordinarily associate with human personality. If this burden cannot be satisfied, then the presumption of personhood obtains.

For this purpose I will address only one of the many properties proposed as a necessary condition of personhood—the capacity for having a sense of self—and consider whether its advocates present a cogent account of the nonhuman. Since other accounts may be more convincingly articulated, this discussion will neither exhaust nor conclude the issue. But it will illuminate the strengths and weaknesses of the personhood argument and enable us to evaluate its application to defective infants.

Michael Tooley has recently argued that a human offspring lacking the capacity for a sense of self lacks the rights to life or equal treatment possessed by other persons.[10] In considering the morality of abortion and infanticide, Tooley considers "what properties a thing must possess in order to have a serious right to life,"[11] and he concludes that:

> [h]aving a right to life presupposes that one is capable of desiring to continue existing as a subject of experiences and other mental states. This in turn presupposes both that one has the concept of such a continuing entity and that one believes that one is oneself such an entity. So an entity that lacks such a consciousness of itself as a continuing subject of mental states does not have a right to life.[12]

However, this account is at first glance too narrow, for it appears to exclude all those who do not presently have a desire "to continue existing as a subject of experiences and other mental states." The sleeping or unconscious individual, the deranged, the conditioned, and the suicidal do not have such desires, though they might have had them or could have them in the future. Accordingly, Tooley emphasizes the capability of entertaining such desires, rather than their actual existence.[13] But it is difficult to distinguish the capability for such desires in an unconscious, conditioned, or emotionally disturbed person from the capability existing in a fetus or infant. In all cases the capability is a future one; it will arise only if certain events occur, such as normal growth and development in the case of the infant, and removal of the disability in the other cases. The infant, in fact, might realize its capability[14] long before disabled adults recover emotional balance or consciousness.

To meet this objection, Tooley argues that the significance of the capability in question is not solely its future realization (for fetuses and infants will ordinarily realize it), but also its previous existence and exercise.[15] He seems to say that once the conceptual capability has been realized, one's right to desire continued existence permanently vests, even though the present capability for desiring does not exist, and may be lost for substantial periods or permanently. Yet, what nonarbitrary reasons require that we protect the past realization of conceptual capability but not its potential realization in the future? As a reward for its past realization? To mark our reverence and honor for someone who has realized that state? Tooley is silent on this point.

Another difficulty is Tooley's ambiguity concerning the permanently deranged, comatose, or conditioned. Often he phrases his argument in terms of a temporary suspension of the capability of conceptual thought.[16] One wonders what he would say of someone permanently deranged, or with massive brain damage, or in a prolonged coma. If he seriously means that the past existence of a desire for life vests these cases with the right to life, then it is indeed difficult to distinguish the comatose or deranged from the infant profoundly retarded at birth. Neither will ever possess the conceptual capability to desire to be a continuing subject of experiences. A distinction based on reward or desert seems arbitrary, and protection of life applies equally well in both cases. Would Tooley avoid this problem by holding that the permanently comatose and deranged lose their rights after a certain point because conceptual capacity will never be regained? This would permit killing (or at least withholding of care) from the insane and comatose—doubtless an unappealing prospect.[17] Moreover, we do not ordinarily think of the insane, and possibly the comatose, as losing personhood before their death. Although their personality or identity may be said to change, presumably for the worse, or become fragmented or minimal, we still regard them as specific persons. If a "self" in some minimal sense exists here then the profoundly retarded, who at least is conscious, also may be considered a self, albeit a minimal one. Thus, one may argue that Tooley fails to provide a convincing account of criteria distinguishing persons and nonpersons. He both excludes beings we ordinarily think of as persons—infants, deranged, conditioned, possibly the comatose—and fails to articulate criteria that convincingly distinguish the nonhuman.[18] But, even if we were to accept Tooley's distinction that beings lacking the

potential for desire and a sense of self are not persons who are owed the duty to be treated by ordinary medical means, this would not appear to be very helpful in deciding whether to treat the newborn with physical or mental defects. Few infants, it would seem, would fall into this class.[19] First, those suffering from malformations, however gross, that do not affect mental capabilities would not fit the class of nonpersons. Second, frequently even the most severe cases of mental retardation cannot be reliably determined until a much later period;[20] care thus could not justifiably be withheld in the neonatal period, although this principle would permit nontreatment at the time when nonpersonality is clearly established.[21] Finally, the only group of defective newborns who would clearly qualify as nonpersons is anencephalics, who altogether lack a brain, or those so severely brain-damaged that it is immediately clear that a sense of self or personality can never develop. Mongols, myelomeningoceles, and other defective infants from whom ordinary care is now routinely withheld would not qualify as nonpersons. Thus, even the most coherent and cogent criteria of humanity are only marginally helpful in the situation of the defective infant. We must therefore consider whether treatment can be withheld on grounds other than the claim that such infants are not persons.

2. No Obligation to Treat Exists When the Costs of Maintaining Life Greatly Outweigh the Benefits

If we reject the argument that defective newborns are not persons, the question remains whether circumstances exist in which the consequences of treatment as compared with nontreatment are so undesirable that the omission of care is justified. As we have seen, the doctrine of necessity permits one to violate the criminal law when essential to prevent the occurrence of a greater evil.[22] The circumstances, however, when the death of a nonconsenting person is a lesser evil than his continuing life are narrowly circumscribed, and do not include withholding care from defective infants.[23] Yet many parents and physicians deeply committed to the loving care of the newborn think that treating severely defective infants causes more harm than good, thereby justifying the withholding of ordinary care.[34] In their view the suffering and diminished quality of the child's life do not justify the social and economic costs of treatment. This claim has a growing commonsense appeal, but it assumes that the utility or quality of one's life can be measured and compared with other lives, and that health resources may legitimately be allocated to produce the greatest personal utility. This argument will now be analyzed from the perspective of the defective patient and others affected by his care.

a. The Quality of the Defective Infant's Life

Comparisons of relative worth among persons, or between persons and other interests, raise moral and methodological issues that make any argument that relies on such comparisons extremely vulnerable. Thus the strongest claim for not treating the defective newborn is that treatment seriously harms the infant's own interests, whatever may be the effects on others. When maintaining his life involves great physical and psychosocial suffering for the patient, a reasonable person might conclude that such a life is not worth living. Presumably the patient, if fully informed and able to communicate, would agree. One then would be morally justified in withholding lifesaving treatment if such action served to advance the best interests of the patient.[25]

Congenital malformations impair development in several ways that lead to the judgment that deformed retarded infants are "a burden to themselves."[26] One is the severe physical pain, much of it resulting from repeated surgery that defective infants will suffer.[27] Defective children also are likely to develop other pathological features, leading to repeated fractures, dislocations, surgery, malfunctions, and other sources of pain. The shunt, for example, inserted to relieve hydrocephalus, a common problem in defective children, often becomes clogged, necessitating frequent surgical interventions.[28]

Pain, however, may be intermittent and manageable with analgesics. Since many infants and adults experience great pain, and many defective infants do not, pain alone, if not totally unmanageable, does not sufficiently show that a life is so worthless that death is preferable. More important are the psychosocial deficits resulting from the child's handicaps. Many defective children never can walk even with prosthesis,

never interact with normal children, never appreciate growth, adolescence, or the fulfillment of education and employment, and seldom are even able to care for themselves. In cases of severe retardation, they may be left with a vegetative existence in a crib, incapable of choice or the most minimal response to stimuli. Parents or others may reject them, and much of their time will be spent in hospitals, in surgery, or fighting the many illnesses that beset them. Can it be said that such a life is worth living?

There are two possible responses to the quality-of-life argument. One is to accept its premises but to question the degree of suffering in particular cases, and thus restrict the justification for death to the most extreme cases. The absence of opportunities for schooling, career, and interaction may be the fault of social attitudes and the failings of healthy persons, rather than a necessary result of congenital malformations. Psychosocial suffering occurs because healthy, normal persons reject or refuse to relate to the defective, or hurry them to poorly funded institutions. Most nonambulatory, mentally retarded persons can be trained for satisfying roles. One cannot assume that a nonproductive existence is necessarily unhappy; even social rejection and nonacceptance can be mitigated.[29] Moreover, the psychosocial ills of the handicapped often do not differ in kind from those experienced by many persons. With training and care, growth, development, and a full range of experiences are possible for most people with physical and mental handicaps. Thus, the claim that death is a far better fate than life cannot in most cases be sustained.

This response, however, avoids meeting the quality-of-life argument on its strongest grounds. Even if many defective infants can experience growth, interaction, and most human satisfactions if nurtured, treated, and trained, some infants are so severely retarded or grossly deformed that their response to love and care, in fact their capacity to be conscious, is always minimal. Although mongoloid and nonambulatory spina bifida children may experience an existence we would hesitate to adjudge worse than death, the profoundly retarded, nonambulatory, blind, deaf infant who will spend his few years in the back-ward cribs of a state institution is clearly a different matter.

To repudiate the quality-of-life argument,

therefore, requires a defense of treatment in even these extreme cases. Such a defense would question the validity of any surrogate or proxy judgments of the worth or quality of life when the wishes of the person in question cannot be ascertained. The essence of the quality-of-life argument is a proxy's judgment that no reasonable person can prefer the pain, suffering, and loneliness of, for example, life in a crib at an IQ level of 20, to an immediate, painless death.

But in what sense can the proxy validly conclude that a person with different wants, needs, and interests, if able to speak, would agree that such a life were worse than death? At the start one must be skeptical of the proxy's claim to objective disinterestedness. If the proxy is also the parent or physician, as has been the case in pediatric euthanasia, the impact of treatment on the proxy's interests, rather than solely on those of the child, may influence his assessment. But even if the proxy were truly neutral and committed only to caring for the child, the problem of egocentricity and knowing another's mind remains. Compared with the situation and life prospects of a "reasonable man," the child's potential quality of life indeed appears dim. Yet a standard based on healthy, ordinary development may be entirely inappropriate to this situation. One who has never known the pleasures of mental operation, ambulation, and social interaction surely does not suffer from their loss as much as one who has. While one who has known these capacities may prefer death to a life without them, we have no assurance that the handicapped person, with no point of comparison, would agree. Life, and life alone, whatever its limitations, might be of sufficient worth to him.[30]

One should also be hesitant to accept proxy assessments of quality-of-life because the margin of error in such predictions may be very great. For instance, while one expert argues that by a purely clinical assessment he can accurately forecast the minimum degree of future handicap an individual will experience,[31] such forecasting is not infallible,[32] and risks denying care to infants whose disability might otherwise permit a reasonably acceptable quality-of-life. Thus given the problems in ascertaining another's wishes, the proxy's bias to personal or culturally relative interests, and the unreliability of predictive criteria, the quality-of-life argument is open to serious question. Its

strongest appeal arises in the case of a grossly deformed, retarded, institutionalized child, or one with incessant unmanageable pain, where continued life is itself torture. But these cases are few, and cast doubt on the utility of any such judgment. Even if the judgment occasionally may be defensible, the potential danger of quality-of-life assessments may be a compelling reason for rejecting this rationale for withholding treatment.[33]

b. The Suffering of Others

In addition to the infant's own suffering, one who argues that the harm of treatment justifies violation of the defective infant's right to life usually relies on the psychological, social, and economic costs of maintaining his existence to family and society. In their view the minimal benefit of treatment to persons incapable of full social and physical development does not justify the burdens that care of the defective infant imposes on parents, siblings, health professionals, and other patients. Matson, a noted pediatric neurosurgeon, states:

> [I]t is the doctor's and the community's responsibility to provide [custodial] care and to minimize suffering; but, at the same time, it is also their responsibility not to prolong such individual, familial, and community suffering unnecessarily, and not to carry out multiple procedures and prolonged, expensive, acute hospitalization in an infant whose chance for acceptable growth and development is negligible.[34]

Such a frankly utilitarian argument raises problems. It assumes that because of the greatly curtailed orbit of his existence, the costs or suffering of others is greater than the benefit of life to the child. This judgment, however, requires a coherent way of measuring and comparing interpersonal utilities, a logical-practical problem that utilitarianism has never surmounted.[35] But even if such comparisons could reliably show a net loss from treatment, the fact remains that the child must sacrifice his life to benefit others. If the life of one individual, however useless, may be sacrificed for the benefit of any person, however useful, or for the benefit of any number of persons, then we have acknowledged the principle that rational utility may justify any outcome.[36] As many philosophers have demonstrated, utilitarianism can always permit the sacrifice of one life for other interests, given the appropriate arrangement of utilities on the balance sheet.[37] In the absence of principled grounds for such a decision, the social equation involved in mandating direct, involuntary euthanasia[38] becomes a difference of degree, not kind, and we reach the point where protection of life depends solely on social judgments of utility.

These objections may well be determinative.[39] But if we temporarily bracket them and examine the extent to which care of the defective infant subjects others to suffering, the claim that inordinate suffering outweighs the infant's interest in life is rarely plausible. In this regard we must examine the impact of caring for defective infants on the family, health professions, and society-at-large.

The Family. The psychological impact and crisis created by birth of a defective infant is devastating.[40] Not only is the mother denied the normal tension release from the stresses of pregnancy,[41] but both parents feel a crushing blow to their dignity, self-esteem and self-confidence.[42] In a very short time, they feel grief for the loss of the normal expected child, anger at fate, numbness, disgust, waves of helplessness, and disbelief.[43] Most feel personal blame for the defect, or blame their spouse. Adding to the shock is fear that social position and mobility are permanently endangered.[44] The transformation of a "joyously awaited experience into one of catastrophe and profound psychological threat[45] often will reactivate unresolved maturational conflicts. The chances for social pathology—divorce, somatic complaints, nervous and mental disorders—increase and hard-won adjustment patterns may be permanently damaged.[46]

The initial reactions of guilt, grief, anger, and loss, however, cannot be the true measure of family suffering caused by care of a defective infant, because these costs are present whether or not the parents choose treatment. Rather, the question is to what degree treatment imposes psychic and other costs greater than would occur if the child were not treated. The claim that care is more costly rests largely on the view that parents and family suffer inordinately from nurturing such a child.

Indeed, if the child is treated and accepted at home, difficult and demanding adjustments must be made. Parents must learn how to care for a disabled child, confront financial and psychological uncertainty, meet the needs of other siblings, and work through their own conflicting feelings. Mothering demands are greater than with a normal child, particularly if medical care and hospitalization are frequently required.[47] Counseling or professional support may be nonexistent or difficult to obtain.[48] Younger siblings may react with hostility and guilt, older with shame and anger.[49] Often the normal feedback of child growth that renders the turmoil of childrearing worthwhile develops more slowly or not at all. Family resources can be depleted (especially if medical care is needed), consumption patterns altered, or standards of living modified.[50] Housing may have to be found closer to a hospital, and plans for further children changed.[51] Finally, the anxieties, guilt, and grief present at birth may threaten to recur or become chronic.[52]

Yet, although we must recognize the burdens and frustrations of raising a defective infant, it does not necessarily follow that these costs require nontreatment, or even institutionalization. Individual and group counseling can substantially alleviate anxiety, guilt, and frustration, and enable parents to cope with underlying conflicts triggered by the birth and the adaptations required.[53] Counseling also can reduce psychological pressures on siblings, who can be taught to recognize and accept their own possibly hostile feelings and the difficult position of their parents. They may even be taught to help their parents care for the child.[54]

The impact of increased financial costs also may vary.[55] In families with high income or adequate health insurance, the financial costs are manageable. In others, state assistance may be available.[56] If severe financial problems arise or pathological adjustments are likely, institutionalization, although undesirable for the child, remains an option.[57] Finally, in many cases, the experience of living through a crisis is a deepening and enriching one, accelerating personality maturation, and giving one a new sensitivity to the needs of spouse, siblings, and others. As one parent of a defective child states: "In the last months I have come closer to people and can understand them more. I have met them more deeply. I did not know there were so many people with troubles in the world."[58]

Thus, while social attitudes regard the

handicapped child as an unmitigated disaster, in reality the problem may not be insurmountable, and often may not differ from life's other vicissitudes. Suffering there is, but seldom is it so overwhelming or so imminent that the only alternative is death of the child.[59]

Health professionals. Physicians and nurses also suffer when parents give birth to a defective child, although, of course, not to the degree of the parents. To the obstetrician or general practitioner the defective birth may be a blow to his professional identity. He has the difficult task of informing the parents of the defects, explaining their causes, and dealing with the parents' resulting emotional shock. Often he feels guilty for failing to produce a normal baby.[60] In addition, the parents may project anger or hostility on the physician, questioning his professional competence or seeking the services of other doctors.[61] The physician also may feel that his expertise and training are misused when employed to maintain the life of an infant whose chances for a productive existence are so diminished. By neglecting other patients, he may feel that he is prolonging rather than alleviating suffering.

Nurses, too, suffer role strain from care of the defective newborn. Intensive-care-unit nurses may work with only one or two babies at a time. They face the daily ordeals of care—the progress and relapses—and often must deal with anxious parents who are themselves grieving or ambivalent toward the child. The situation may trigger a nurse's own ambivalence about death and mothering, in a context in which she is actively working to keep alive a child whose life prospects seem minimal.[62]

Thus, the effects of care on physicians and nurses are not trivial, and must be intelligently confronted in medical education or in management of a pediatric unit. Yet to state them is to make clear that they can but weigh lightly in the decision of whether to treat a defective newborn. Compared with the situation of the parents, these burdens seem insignificant, are short term, and most likely do not evoke such profound emotions. In any case, these difficulties are hazards of the profession—caring for the sick and dying will always produce strain. Hence, on these grounds alone it is difficult to argue that a defective person may be denied the right to life.

Society. Care of the defective newborn also imposes societal costs, the utility of which is questioned when the infant's expected quality-of-life is so poor. Medical resources that can be used by infants with a better prognosis, or throughout the health-care system generally, are consumed in providing expensive surgical and intensive-care services to infants who may be severely retarded, never lead active lives, and die in a few months or years. Institutionalization imposes costs on taxpayers and reduces the resources available for those who might better benefit from it,[63] while reducing further the quality of life experienced by the institutionalized defective.

One answer to these concerns is to question the impact of the costs of caring for defective newborns. Precise data showing the costs to taxpayers or the trade-offs with health and other expenditures do not exist. Nor would ceasing to care for the defective necessarily lead to a reallocation within the health budget that would produce net savings in suffering or life;[64] in fact, the released resources might not be reallocated for health at all.[65] In any case, the trade-offs within the health budget may well be small. With advances in prenatal diagnosis of genetic disorders, many deformed infants who would formerly require care will be aborted beforehand.[66] Then, too, it is not clear that the most technical and expensive procedures always constitute the best treatment for certain malformations.[67] When compared with the almost seven percent of the GNP now spent on health,[68] the money in the defense budget, or tax revenues generally, the public resources required to keep defective newborns alive seem marginal, and arguably worth the commitment to life that such expenditures reinforce. Moreover, as the Supreme Court recently recognized,[69] conservation of the taxpayer's purse does not justify serious infringement of fundamental rights. Given legal and ethical norms against sacrificing the lives of nonconsenting others, and the imprecisions in diagnosis and prediction concerning the eventual outcomes of medical care,[70] the social-cost argument does not compel nontreatment of defective newborns.[71]

Notes

1. Commentary, *The Ethics of Surgery in Newborn Infants*, 8 CLINICAL PEDIATRICS 251 (1969); *cf.* Grunberg, *Who Lives and Dies?*, N.Y. Times, Apr. 22, 1974, at 35, col. 2.

2. *Id.* While the proposition appears to draw some support from Bracton's statement in a noncriminal context that a monster is not a human being, "Quia partus monstruosus est cum non nascatur ut homo," *cited* in G. WILLIAMS, THE SANCTITY OF LIFE AND THE CRIMINAL LAW 20–21 (1957), no case has ever held that a live human offspring is not a human being because of certain physical or mental deficits, and therefore may be killed. *See* G. WILLIAMS, *supra*, at 20–24. The state, in the exercise of its *parens patriae* power to protect persons incapacitated by infancy, neglect, or mental incompetence, recognizes that many "persons" incapable of leading an ordinary or normal life are nevertheless persons with rights and interests to be protected. *See, e.g.,* Herr, *Retarded Children and the Law: Enforcing the Constitutional Rights of the Mentally Retarded*, 23 SYR. L. REV. 995 (1972). Even a slave was protected by the law of homicide even though incapable of full social interaction. *See, e.g.,* Fields v. State, 1 Yager's Rep. 156 (Tenn. 1829). Thus, a judge in Maine recently had little difficulty in concluding that a deformed child with multiple anomalies and brain damage was "at the moment of live birth . . . a human being entitled to the fullest protection of the law." Maine Medical Center v. Houle, No. 74–145, at 4 (Super. Ct., Cumberland Cty., Feb. 14, 1974).

3. *See* Tooley, *Abortion and Infanticide*, 2 PHIL. & PUB. AFFAIRS 37, 51 (1972).

4. Bok, *Ethical Problems of Abortion*, 2 HASTINGS CENTER STUDIES, Jan. 1974, at 33, 41.

5. *See* Alexander, *Medical Science under Dictatorship*, 241 NEW ENG. J. MED. 39 (1949).

6. T. BECK & J. BECK, ELEMENTS OF MEDICAL JURISPRUDENCE 422 (11th ed. 1960).

7. *See* Tribe, *Foreword—Toward a Model of Roles in the Due Process of Life and Law*, HARV. L. REV. 1, 18–20 (1973).

8. *See* Thomson, *A Defense of Abortion*, 1 PHIL. AND PUB. AFFAIRS 47 (1971).

9. *See* notes [22–71] *infra* and accompanying text.

10. Tooley, *supra* note [3] at 49.

11. *Id.* at 37.

12. *Id.* at 49.

13. *Id.* at 50.

14. Tooley concedes that the infant attains this capacity in the first year of life, though further research is necessary to identify the exact time. *Id.* at 64.

15. *Correspondence*, 2 PHIL. & PUB. AFFAIRS 419 (1973).

16. *Id.* at 421–23.

17. A somewhat similar approach to the definition of personhood by Richard McCormick also fails to cogently distinguish the case of the deranged. McCormick argues that if the potential for human relationships "is simply nonexistent or would be utterly submerged and undeveloped in the mere struggle to survive, that life has achieved its potential" and ordinary care need not be provided. McCormick, *To Save or Let Die—The Dilemma of Modern Medicine*, 229 J.A.M.A. 172, 175 (1974). But would we sanction withholding antibiotics from an insane person suffering a serious infection simply because his capacity to enter into human relationships had become minimal?

18. John Rawls makes a similar argument for the proposition that not all human offspring are entitled to "equal basic rights" of liberty or "the guarantees of justice," *see* J. RAWLS, A THEORY OF JUSTICE 504–10 (1971), and is equally unsuccessful in articulating convincing criteria. His argument arises in the course of a discussion of the features of human beings which entitle them, as opposed to plants, animals, and machines, to be treated in accordance with the principles of justice. To be owed or entitled to equal justice one must possess a certain capacity not present in all human organisms. The capacity is moral personality: "Moral persons are distinguished by two features: First, they are capable of having (and are assumed to have) a conception of their good (as expressed by a rational plan of life); and second they are capable of having (and are assumed to acquire) a sense of justice, a normally effective desire to apply and to act upon the principles of justice, at least to a certain minimum degree." *Id.* at 505. Moral personality qualifies one to be treated with justice, because the principles of justice are derived from the choices which moral persons in the original position desiring to maximize their own (but unknown) good would make; "We use the characterization of the person in the original position to single out the kinds of beings to whom the principles chosen apply. After all, the parties are thought of as adopting those criteria to regulate their common institutions and their conduct toward one another: and the description of their nature enters into the reasoning by which these principles are selected. Thus equal justice is owed to those who have the capacity to take part in and to act in accordance with the public understanding of the initial situation." *Id.*

    Rawls, unlike Tooley, accepts the potential rather than present or soon-to-be-assumed capability for moral personality, which includes infants and those "who could take part in the initial agreement, were it not for fortuitous circumstances. . . ." *Id.* at 504. Although he is hesitant in describing moral personality as both a necessary and sufficient condition for justice, he does distinguish those "who have lost their realized capacity temporarily through misfortune, accident, or mental stress" from those "more or less permanently deprived of moral personality," who "may present a difficulty." *Id.* at 510. However, even if creatures lacking this capacity are not entitled to strict justice, "it does not follow that there are no requirements at all in regard to them, [n]or in our relations with the natural order. Certainly it is wrong to be cruel to animals and the destruction of a whole species can be a great evil. The capacity for feelings of pleasure and pain and for the forms of life of which animals are capable clearly imposes duties of compassion and humanity in their case." *Id.* at 512.

Rawls' position, however, is not strictly necessary for the "natural completion of justice as fairness." While Rawls needs to distinguish human claims from those of machines, plants, and animals, such a distinction can stand without dividing human organisms into two classes—the privileged and nonprivileged to enjoy justice. The need for persons in the original position to have certain capacities does not necessarily entail that the principles chosen apply only to those blessed in the natural lottery with the capacity to choose in the original position. Surely those whose capacity for justice or a life plan has been ended by accident or mental disturbance do not lose equal liberty. Why then should incapacity at birth disqualify one? If I understand Rawls correctly those in the original position would protect themselves against such a contingency by deriving principles which apply to all human offspring, whatever their capacity for a sense of justice or a life plan at any stage of life. Thus Rawls' statement that "[t]hose who can give justice are owed justice," *id.* at 510, need not exclude those who by accident or natural infirmity are incapable of giving justice.

19. Warkany, for example, reports the incidence of anencephaly, the absence of all or most of an infant's brain, as approximately 1 in 1,000 for children born in hospital wards, but notes that "remarkable variations have been reported from different areas." J. WARKANY, [*Congenital Malformations,* (1971)], at 189.

20. *Id.* at 39.

21. But other factors might lead to treatment at this later point in time. For example, if care and nurturing occur immediately after birth, a strong mother-child bond is built, which might prevent mothers from deciding to withhold care when a serious defect is discovered weeks later. Barnett, Leiderman, Globstein & Klaus, *Neonatal Separation: The Maternal Side of Interactional Deprivation,* 45 PEDIATRICS 197,

197–99 (1970); Kennel & Klaus, *Care of the Mother of the High Risk Infant,* 14 CLIN. OBSTET. & GYNECOL. 926, 930–36 (1971).

22. *See* notes 157–64 and accompanying text [in the original].

23. *See* notes 169–80 and accompanying text [in the original].

24. See Duff and Campbell, *Moral and Ethical Dilemmas in the Special-Care Nursery,* 289 NEW ENG. J. MED. 890 (1973).

25. The perspective that the mere saving of life is not enough unless the lives are "worth saving" is well represented in the medical literature. Lorber, in discussing the process of selecting spina bifida infants for treatment, states: "Severe degree of paralysis is the most generally adopted reason for withholding treatment, but incontinence, severe hydrocephalus, gross deformities and social conditions are also taken into account. . . . There is no doubt that the future quality of life of many patients with myelomeningocele depends at least partly on the speed, efficiency and comprehensiveness of treatment from birth onwards—and often throughout their lives. Nevertheless, there are large numbers who are so severely handicapped at birth that those who survive are bound to suffer from a combination of major physical defects. In addition, many will be retarded in spite of everything that can be done for them. It is not necessary to enumerate all that this means to the patient, the family and the community in terms of suffering, deprivation, anxiety, frustration, family stress and financial cost. The large majority surviving at present have yet to reach the most difficult period of adolescence and young adult life and the problems of love, marriage and employment." Lorber, [*Results of Treatment of Myelomeningocele,* DEVELOP. MED. & CHILD NEURO. 13 (1971): 279–303], at 279, *citing* Rickham & Mawdsley, "The Effect of Early Operation on the Survival of Spina Bifida Cystica," *Develop. Med. & Child Neurol.* 20 (Supp. 11, 1966) at 20. He summarizes the results of treating 524 cases of myelomeningocele on an unselected basis: "In summary, at the most 7 per cent of those admitted have less than grossly crippling disabilities and may be considered to have a quality of life not inconsistent with self-respect, earning capacity, happiness and even marriage. The next 20 per cent are also of normal intelligence and some may be able to earn their living in sheltered employment, but their lives are full of illness and operations. They are severely handicapped and are unlikely to live a full life-span. They are at a risk of sudden death from shunt complications or are likely to die

of renal failure at an early age. The next 14 per cent are even more severely handicapped because they are retarded. They are unlikely to earn their living and their opportunities in life will be severely restricted. They will always be totally dependent on others." *Id.* at 286. He concludes that "[i]t is unlikely that many would wish to save a life which will consist of a long succession of operations, hospital admissions and other deprivations, or if the end result will be a combination of gross physical defects with retarded intellectual development." *Id.* at 300.

26. Smith & Smith, *Selection for Treatment in Spina Bifida Cystica,* 4 BRIT. MED. J. 189, 195 (1973).

27. *See* Lorber, *supra* note [25], at 284.

28. Ames & Schut, *Results of Treatment of 171 Consecutive Myelomeningoceles—1963 to 1968,* 52 PEDIATRICS 466, 469 (1972); Shurtleff & Foltz, *A Comparative Study of Meningomyelocele Repair or Cerebrospinal Fluid Shunt As Primary Treatment in Ninety Children,* DEVELOP. MED. & CHILD NEURO. 57 (Supp. 13, 1967).

29. *See* E. GOFFMAN, STIGMA: NOTES ON THE MANAGEMENT OF SPOILED IDENTITY 57–129 (1963).

30. *Cf.* Gleitman v. Cosgrove, 49 N.J. 22, 227 A.2d 689 (1967). The court denied plaintiff's right to collect damages for being born with deformities when a defendant physician was allegedly negligent in informing the plaintiff's mother of rubella, which would have led her to seek an abortion. The court stated: "It is basic to the human condition to seek life and hold on to it however heavily burdened. If Jeffrey could have been asked as to whether his life should be snuffed out before his full term of gestation could run its course, our felt intuition of human nature tells us he would almost surely choose life with defects as against no life at all." *Id.* at 30, 227 A.2d at 693.

Similarly, in the case of *In re* Hudson, 13 Wash. 2d. 673, 126 P.2d 765 (1942), a child was held not to be neglected when her parent refused to consent to life-endangering surgery to correct a gross deformity that made normal development and interaction impossible: "As we read the evidence, it is admitted by all concerned that . . . the child may not survive the ordeal of amputation; nevertheless, every one except the child's mother is willing, desirous, that the child be required to undergo the operation. Implicit in their position is their opinion that it would be preferable that the child die instead of going through life handicapped by the enlarged, deformed left arm. That may be to some today the humane, and in the future it may be the generally accepted, view. However, we have not advanced or retrograded to the stage where, in the name of mercy, we may lawfully decide that one shall be deprived of life rather than continue to exist crippled or burdened with some abnormality. That right of decision is a prerogative of the Creator." *Id.* at 684, 126 P.2d at 771. *See also* Cooke, [*Whose Suffering?* J. OF PEDIATRICS 80 (1971)], at 906–08.

31. *See* Lorber, *supra* note [25], at 299.

32. In Lorber's series, 20% of 110 infants "with major adverse criteria at birth were of normal intellectual development at 2–4 years of age, though all [had] severe physical handicaps and their life expectation [was] short." *Id.* at 300. Moreover, other researchers question the adequacy of Lorber's selection criteria. Ames and Schut, for example, in a report on unselected treatment cases of myelomeningocele find "it is not always possible to determine potential at birth," and report success with infants that Lorber would not have selected. *See* Ames & Schut, *supra* note [28], at 469–70.

33. If this judgment is to be made, it is essential that the circumstances in which nontreatment may be said to be in a patient's best interests be specified beforehand by an authoritative body, and that procedures which assure that a particular case falls within such criteria be followed. *See* notes 272–77 and accompanying text [in the original].

34. Matson, *Surgical Treatment of Myelomeningocele,* 42 PEDIATRICS 225, 226 (1968).

35. J. RAWLS, *supra* note [18], at 90–91.

36. *Cf.* Silving, *Euthanasia: A Study in Comparative Criminal Law,* 103, U. PA. L. REV. 350, 356 (1954).

37. *See, e.g.,* J. RAWLS, *supra* note [18], at 22–27.

38. Alexander, *supra* note [5], at 39.

39. The New Jersey Supreme Court, for example, would clearly reject a balancing test in such situations. *See* Gleitman v. Cosgrove, 49 N.J. 22, 227 A.2d 689 (1967).

40. "The experience of learning that your child is defective immediately after birth can still be categorized among the most painful and stigmatizing experiences of modern people. It is as if the parents' raison d'etre were called into question before an imagined parental bar of justice and an ontological blow dealt to their hopes of continuing their identities." Fletcher, [*Attitudes Towards Defective Newborns,* HASTINGS CENTER STUDIES 2 (1974)], at 34.

41. *See* Goodman, [*Continuing Treatment of Parents with Congenitally Defective Infants,* SOCIAL WORK 9, no. 1, at 92]. *See generally* Kennel & Klaus, *supra* note [21].

42. Bentovim, *Emotional Disturbances of Handicapped Pre-School Children and Their Families—Attitudes to the Child,* 3 BRIT. MED. J. 579, 580 (1972); Giannini & Goodman, *Counseling Families During the Crisis Reaction to Mongolism,* 67 AM. J. MENTAL DEFICIENCY

740, 740–741 (1962); Goodman, *supra* note [41]; Mandelbaum & Wheeler, *The Meaning of A Defective Child to Parents*, 41 SOCIAL CASEWORK 360 (1960); Schild, *Counselling with Parents of Retarded Children Living at Home*, 9 SOCIAL WORK 86 (1964); Zachary, *Ethical and Social Aspects of Treatment of Spina Bifida*, THE LANCET, Aug. 3, 1968, at 274–75.

43. *See* note [42], *supra*.

44. *See* Giannini & Goodman, *supra* note [42], at 743.

45. Goodman, *supra* note [41], at 92.

46. *Id.* at 93.

47. *See* Hunt, *Implications of the Treatment of Myelomeningocele for the Child and his Family*, THE LANCET, Dec. 8, 1973, at 1308, 1309–10; Zachary, *supra* note [42], at 275.

48. Hunt, *supra* note [47], at 1310.

49. *Id.* at 1309; Bentovim, *supra* note [42], at 581.

50. Zachary, *supra* note [42], at 275.

51. Hunt, *supra* note [47], at 1310.

52. "At each stage there may be a fresh feeling of loss: the precarious balance is once more shattered, rage, depression, rejecting feelings, fear of battering, strain, somatic aches and pains, may be the result. Problems such as financial difficulties, poor housing, marital strain, pressure from siblings can compound such problems. Social life can be severely restricted and the handicapped child then has to cope with the additional handicap of a withdrawn, preoccupied, depressed, angry and hopeless parent, as well as the effect of the handicap itself." Bentovim, *supra* note [42], at 581.

53. *See, e.g.*, Cohen [*The Impact of the Handicapped Child on the Family*, SOCIAL CASEWORK 43 (1962): 137]; Giannini & Goodman, *supra* note [42]; Schild, *supra* note [42], at 86.

54. *See* citations in note [53] *supra*.

55. The financial impact of caring for the defective child is difficult to estimate and varies with the seriousness of the defect, the resultant medical costs, health insurance coverage, and state assistance programs. For example, it may cost the parents of a child born with spina bifida from $5,000 to more than $40,000 to pay for the necessary operations, hospital care, medication, doctor's checkups, and braces. Interview with Peggy Miezio, Wis. Spina Bifida Ass'n, Aug. 24, 1974.

Since almost 180 million Americans in 1971 were covered by some form of health insurance, HEALTH INSURANCE INSTITUTE, 1972–73 SOURCE BOOK OF HEALTH INSURANCE DATA 19 (1972), many parents find that insurance covers at least some of the costs. Until recently many policies excluded coverage for disorders commencing before the age of 15 days, and thus did not cover such congenital disorders as spina bifida, Down's syndrome, or cystic fibrosis. *See, e.g.*, Kissil v. Beneficial Nat'l Life Ins., 64 N.J. 555, 319 A.2d 67 (1974). Recently, several states have passed legislation requiring health insurance policies to cover newborn children from the day of birth. *See, e.g.*, CAL. INS. CODE § 10119 (West 1972). In addition, even if the policy lawfully excludes coverage of deformed newborns, indications are that in many cases, because of "social pressures," insurance companies cover newborn infants from the day of birth. Interview with Roy Anderson, Office of Comm'r of Ins. Madison, Wis., Aug. 22, 1974.

In addition to the availability of coverage, two other problems face parents of defective newborns. One is the limits of such coverage. If the medical expenses of the child are high, and the coverage limits of the policy low, parents may have to resort to use of savings or income, or seek state aid. Second, even if a parent were covered by a group policy, the coverage does not transfer if the primary insured leaves the business from which he obtained his policy. Availability of insurance coverage depends on "insurability," and as it is virtually impossible for a family to obtain new coverage for a handicapped child after birth, the families are, in effect, "locked into" their group policy, with a resulting decrease in mobility.

For families with inadequate or no insurance coverage and who lack the means to absorb high expenditures for care of a deformed newborn, the availability of state assistance becomes crucial. In general, fairly adequate state aid is available to parents who do not wish to institutionalize their child. In California, for example, the state Crippled Children Services offers extensive aid for families with deformed children. When a deformed child requires medical attention that the parents are unable to afford, the parents, hospital, or family doctor may contact the local health department, which will then determine if the child is "medically eligible" for the services of the Crippled Children Department. A diagnostic evaluation of the child's condition is performed and an estimate is made of the cost of care. The Crippled Children Services then determines if the family is financially eligible for aid. An allowable income level is set according to several factors, and below a certain level (presently $6,300 for a family of four), all expenses are paid by the state. Above this level, the families pay an amount not greater than one-half of the difference between their income and the cost-of-living allowance level. Hospital expenses, medication, braces, nursing care–all the needs of the deformed child–are provided, and the only limit on aid is the agency's budget. Telephone interview with Darleen Gibben, State Crippled Children Services, Sacramento, Cal., Aug. 22, 1974.

For retarded children without serious physical defects, state aid, whether the child is institutionalized or not, is available depending on parental income. Telephone interview with Robert Baldo, Regional Center for Developmentally Disabled, Sacramento, Cal., Aug. 22, 1974.

Similar systems of aid for both physical and mental handicaps, and special education needs, are available in Illinois, Telephone interview with Dr. Graham Blanton, Director of Developmental Disabilities, Dep't of Mental Health and Developmental Disabilities, Springfield, Ill., Aug. 22, 1974; and in Wisconsin, Telephone interview with Elie Asleson, Bureau of Handicapped Children, Dep't of Health and Social Services, Madison, Wis., Aug. 27, 1974; and presumably in other states, since much of the state budget for these services is federally funded.

Although the data is too incomplete to conclude that care of a defective newborn will never severely drain a family's financial resources, it seems clear that the impact can be cushioned or minimized by institutionalization of the child, health insurance, or state aid. Obviously, if legislative policy remains committed to the value of life, a strong argument may be made that the taxpayers as a whole rather than individual families or insurance holders should bear the cost of care.

I am indebted to Marsha Peckham for clarification of the financial issues involved in the care of the defective newborn.

56. *See* note [55] *supra.*

57. Moreover, parental rights and obligations can be terminated. *See* note 37 [in the original].

58. *Quoted in* Johns, *Family Reactions to the Birth of a Child with a Congenital Abnormality,* 26 OBSTET. & GYNECOL. SURVEY 635, 637 (1971).

59. Since parents and physicians now view treatment and acceptance of a defective child as discretionary with the parents, acceptance may be viewed as a gift on the part of the parents to the child. Because of the child's defects, however, the debt or obligation owed to the donor by the recipient of a gift cannot be repaid, and few substitutions for that debt seem available. Given the frequency with which families donate organs to ailing members, it may be that the defective infant situation is not structured to maximize the chance of parental giftgiving. *See* R. FOX & J. SWAYZE, THE COURAGE TO FAIL: A SOCIAL VIEW OF ORGAN TRANSPLANTS AND DIALYSIS 20–27 (1974).

60. Kennel & Klaus, *supra* note [21], at 946. This is particularly true if a physician identifies with the family and its values. "The physician may feel a sense of having failed the family with whom he has a relationship—and his own emotions and feelings come into play—seemingly to a greater extent than with lower class families. His recommendations may be influenced unconsciously by his discomfort with the situation and his strong desire to 'save' the family." Giannini & Goodman, *supra* note [42], at 744.

61. Cohen, *supra* note [53], at 138.

62. Author's observations at conference concerning treatment of a defective newborn at St. Mary's Hospital, Madison, Wis., Apr. 15, 1974.

63. "It may be true that further advances should improve the outlook for many, but unfortunately the basic defect is usually so severe that the children will always be severely handicapped in spite of any advances which can be foreseen today. Meanwhile it may be best to concentrate our therapeutic efforts on those who can truly benefit from treatment. If all the most severe cases are treated, the pressure of work will be such that adequate time cannot be devoted to the less severely affected who would benefit most." Lorber, *supra* note [25], at 300.

64. For example, the resources instead might be used to increase physicians' salaries or the profits of drug or medical supply industries.

65. Resources presently consumed in the care of the defective may have been appropriated for that purpose only, and if not so utilized, will be withdrawn.

66. For instance, amniocentesis carried out on pregnant women over 35—the most risky age for Down's syndrome—should reduce the incidence of mongolism and the attendant problems of care. *Cf.* Smith, *On Letting Some Babies Die,* HASTINGS CENTER STUDIES, Vol. 2, No. 2, at 37, 45 (1974).

67. *See* Ames & Schut, *supra* note [28], at 467–70, which emphasizes the counseling and shunting of spina bifida babies rather than more elaborate and expensive intervention. *See also* C. FRIED, [AN ANATOMY OF VALUES (1970)], at 200–06.

68. Mechanic, *Problems in the Future Organization of Medical Practice,* 35 LAW & CONTEMP. PROB. 233, 234 (1970).

69. Memorial Hosp. v. Maricopa County, 415 U.S. 250 (1974).

70. *See* note [32] *supra* and accompanying text.

71. Moreover, although the case is unlikely to arise in medically developed nations, imagine, for example, that two myelomeningocele infants both need a

shunt, orthopedic surgery, and other services, but resources are so limited that either complete care can be given to one and custodial care to the other, or both can be given only minimal care. Complete care for Baby *A* would lead to ambulation and normal intelligence, while complete care for Baby *B* would still leave him severely retarded and nonambulatory. Minimal care for both would leave both nonambulatory and retarded. Or suppose that resources would permit only one surgical procedure to correct duodenal atresia, but both a Down's syndrome and a normal baby need the operation. In either situation one may argue that physicians should be able to allocate scarce medical resources on the basis of their perception of which allocation will produce the most "good." Presumably, an outcome where the normal infant survives would be chosen. However, one may question whether, in situations of scarcity, distributive justice is satisfied by anything but a random or a first-come-first-served allocation, or an allocation system indifferent to the personal characteristics of each infant. To allocate health resources on the basis of prospective quality of life or social utility would raise in all but a few extreme cases the difficult task of (1) determining and measuring quality, and (2) specifying criteria for a nonarbitrary conclusion that

quality X is better than quality Y. As David Smith observes: "Such an approach leads one to think that the ideal result is either a 'perfect' baby or a dead baby. And the root problems of this way of looking at the issue are that both the human rights of defectives and the imperfection of all babies are glossed over." Smith, *supra* note [66], at 46 (footnote omitted).

Thus, one may argue that even here qualitative or utilitarian judgments are out of place, for these depend on nonobjective, culturally relative standards of quality. The lot of some is improved by making others worse off, yet the reasons for preferring one group are not compelling on nonarbitrary grounds. Unless one were willing to accept the principle that medical decisionmakers may opt to maximize social utility when limited resources require a selection among patients, then the defective newborn could not be denied treatment because of his defects alone. Fortunately, this dilemma, which arose frequently when hemodialysis resources were in short supply, does not yet seem to have arisen in the case of defective newborns. *See* C. FRIED, *supra* note [67], at 200–06; Katz, *Process Design for Selection of Hemodialysis and Organ Transplant Recipients*, 22 BUFF. L. REV. 373 (1973).

Ethical Issues in Aiding the Death of Young Children

H. Tristram Engelhardt, Jr.

Euthanasia in the pediatric age group involves a constellation of issues that are materially different from those of adult euthanasia.[1] The difference lies in the somewhat obvious fact that infants and young children are not able to decide about their own futures and thus are not persons in the same sense that normal adults are. While adults usually decide their own fate, others decide on behalf of young children. Although one can argue that euthanasia is or should be a personal right, the sense of such an argument is obscure with respect to children. Young children do not have any personal rights, at least none that they can exercise on their own behalf with regard to the manner of their life and death. As a result, euthanasia of

young children raises special questions concerning the standing of the rights of children, the status of parental rights, the obligations of adults to prevent the suffering of children, and the possible effects on society of allowing or expediting the death of seriously defective infants.

What I will refer to as the euthanasia of infants and young children might be termed by others infanticide, while some cases might be termed the withholding of extraordinary life-prolonging treatment.[2] One needs a term that will encompass both death that results from active intervention and death that ensues when one simply ceases further therapy.[3] In using such a term, one must recognize that death is often not directly but only

This article first appeared in the book Beneficient Euthanasia, *edited by Marvin Kohl, published by Prometheus Books, Buffalo, N.Y., 1975, and is reprinted by permission.*

obliquely intended. That is, one often intends only to treat no further, not actually to have death follow, even though one knows death will follow.[4]

Finally, one must realize that deaths as the result of withholding treatment constitute a significant proportion of neonatal deaths. For example, as high as 14 percent of children in one hospital have been identified as dying after a decision was made not to treat further, the presumption being that the children would have lived longer had treatment been offered.[5]

Even popular magazines have presented accounts of parental decisions not to pursue treatment.[6] These decisions often involve a choice between expensive treatment with little chance of achieving a full, normal life for the child and "letting nature take its course," with the child dying as a result of its defects. As this suggests, many of these problems are products of medical progress. Such children in the past would have died. The quandaries are in a sense an embarrassment of riches; now that one *can* treat such defective children, *must* one treat them? And, if one need not treat such defective children, may one expedite their death?

I will here briefly examine some of these issues. First, I will review differences that contrast the euthanasia of adults to euthanasia of children. Second, I will review the issue of the rights of parents and the status of children. Third, I will suggest a new notion, the concept of the "injury of continued existence," and draw out some of its implications with respect to a duty to prevent suffering. Finally, I will outline some important questions that remain unanswered even if the foregoing issues can be settled. In all, I hope more to display the issues involved in a difficult question than to advance a particular set of answers to particular dilemmas.

For the purpose of this paper, I will presume that adult euthanasia can be justified by an appeal to freedom. In the face of imminent death, one is usually choosing between a more painful and more protracted dying and a less painful or less protracted dying, in circumstances where either choice makes little difference with regard to the discharge of social duties and responsibilities. In the case of suicide, we might argue that, in general, social duties (for example, the duty to support one's family) restrain one from taking one's own life. But in the face of imminent death and in the presence of the pain and deterioration

of a fatal disease, such duties are usually impossible to discharge and are thus rendered moot. One can, for example, picture an extreme case of an adult with a widely disseminated carcinoma, including metastases to the brain, who because of severe pain and debilitation is no longer capable of discharging any social duties. In these and similar circumstances, euthanasia becomes the issue of the right to control one's own body, even to the point of seeking assistance in suicide. Euthanasia is, as such, the issue of assisted suicide, the universalization of a maxim that all persons should be free, *in extremis*, to decide with regard to the circumstances of their death.

Further, the choice of positive euthanasia could be defended as the more rational choice: the choice of a less painful death and the affirmation of the value of a rational life. In so choosing, one would be acting to set limits to one's life in order not to live when pain and physical and mental deterioration make further rational life impossible. The choice to end one's life can be understood as a noncontradictory willing of a smaller set of states of existence for oneself, a set that would not include a painful death. As such, it would not involve a desire to destroy oneself. That is, adult euthanasia can be construed as an affirmation of the rationality and autonomy of the self.[7]

The remarks above focus on the active or positive euthanasia of adults. But they hold as well concerning what is often called passive or negative euthanasia, the refusal of life-prolonging therapy. In such cases, the patient's refusal of life-prolonging therapy is seen to be a right that derives from personal freedom, or at least from a zone of privacy into which there are no good grounds for social intervention.[8]

Again, none of these considerations apply directly to the euthanasia of young children, because they cannot participate in such decisions. Whatever else pediatric, in particular neonatal, euthanasia involves, it surely involves issues different from those of adult euthanasia. Since infants and small children cannot commit suicide, their right to assisted suicide is difficult to pose. The difference between the euthanasia of young children and that of adults resides in the difference between children and adults. The difference, in fact, raises the troublesome question of whether young children are persons, or at least whether they are persons in the sense in which adults are. Answering that question will resolve in part at

least the right of others to decide whether a young child should live or die and whether he should receive life-prolonging treatment.

The Status of Children

Adults belong to themselves in the sense that they are rational and free and therefore responsible for their actions. Adults are *sui juris*. Young children, though, are neither self-possessed nor responsible. While adults exist in and for themselves, as self-directive and self-conscious beings, young children, especially newborn infants, exist for their families and those who love them. They are not, nor can they in any sense be, responsible for themselves. If being a person is to be a responsible agent, a bearer of rights and duties, children are not persons in a strict sense. They are, rather, persons in a social sense: others must act on their behalf and bear responsibility for them. They are, as it were, entities defined by their place in social roles (for example, mother-child, family-child) rather than beings that define themselves as persons, that is, in and through themselves. Young children live as persons in and through the care of those who are responsible for them, and those responsible for them exercise the children's rights on their behalf. In this sense children belong to families in ways that most adults do not. They exist in and through their family and society.

Treating young children with respect has, then, a sense different from treating adults with respect. One can respect neither a newborn infant's or very young child's wishes nor its freedom. In fact, a newborn infant or young child is more an entity that is valued highly because it will grow to be a person and because it plays a social role as if it were a person.[9] That is, a small child is treated as if it were a person in social roles such as mother-child and family-child relationships, though strictly speaking the child is in no way capable of claiming or being responsible for the rights imputed to it. All the rights and duties of the child are exercised and "held in trust" by others for a future time and for a person yet to develop.

Medical decisions to treat or not to treat a neonate or small child often turn on the probability and cost of achieving that future status—a developed personal life. The usual practice of letting anencephalic children (who congenitally lack all or most of the brain) die can be understood as a decision based on the absence of the possibility of achieving a personal life. The practice of refusing treatment to at least some children born with meningomyelocele can be justified through a similar, but more utilitarian, calculus. In the case of anencephalic children one might argue that care for them as persons is futile since they will never be persons. In the case of a child with meningomyelocele, one might argue that when the cost of cure would likely be very high and the probable lifestyle open to attainment very truncated, there is not a positive duty to make a large investment of money and suffering. One should note that the cost here must include not only financial costs but also the anxiety and suffering that prolonged and uncertain treatment of the child would cause the parents.

This further raises the issue of the scope of positive duties not only when there is no person present in a strict sense, but when the likelihood of a full human life is also very uncertain. Clinical and parental judgment may and should be guided by the expected lifestyle and the cost (in parental and societal pain and money) of its attainment. The decision about treatment, however, belongs properly to the parents because the child belongs to them in a sense that it does not belong to anyone else, even to itself. The care and raising of the child falls to the parents, and when considerable cost and little prospect of reasonable success are present, the parents may properly decide against life-prolonging treatment.

The physician's role is to present sufficient information in a usable form to the parents to aid them in making a decision. The accent is on the absence of a positive duty to treat in the presence of severe inconvenience (costs) to the parents; treatment that is very costly is not obligatory. What is suggested here is a general notion that there is never a duty to engage in extraordinary treatment and that "extraordinary" can be defined in terms of costs. This argument concerns children (1) whose future quality of life is likely to be seriously compromised and (2) whose present treatment would be very costly. The issue is that of the circumstances under which parents would not be obliged to take on severe burdens on behalf of their children or those circumstances under which society would not be so obliged. The argument should hold as well for those cases where the expected future life would surely be of normal quality, though its attainment would be extremely costly. The fact of little likelihood of success in attaining a normal life for the child makes decisions to do without treatment more plausible because the hope of success is even more remote and therefore the burden borne by parents or society becomes in that sense more extraordinary. But very high costs themselves could be a sufficient criterion, though in actual cases judgments in that regard would be very difficult when a normal life could be expected.[10]

The decisions in these matters correctly lie in the hands of the parents, because it is primarily in terms of the family that children exist and develop—until children become persons strictly, they are persons in virtue of their social roles. As long as parents do not unjustifiably neglect the humans in those roles so that the value and purpose of that role (that is, child) stands to be eroded (thus endangering other children), society need not intervene. In short, parents may decide for or against the treatment of their severely deformed children.

However, society has a right to intervene and protect children for whom parents refuse care (including treatment) when such care does not constitute a severe burden and when it is likely that the child could be brought to a good quality of life. Obviously, "severe burden" and "good quality of life" will be difficult to define and their meanings will vary, just as it is always difficult to say when grains of sand dropped on a table constitute a heap. At most, though, society need only intervene when the grains clearly do not constitute a heap, that is, when it is clear that the burden is light and the chance of a good quality of life for the child is high. A small child's dependence on his parents is so essential that society need intervene only when the absence of intervention would lead to the role "child" being undermined. Society must value mother-child and family-child relationships and should intervene only in cases where (1) neglect is unreasonable and therefore would undermine respect and care for children, or (2) where societal intervention would prevent children from suffering unnecessary pain.[11]

The Injury of Continued Existence

But there is another viewpoint that must be considered: that of the child or even the person that the child might become. It might be argued that the child has a right not to have its life prolonged. The idea that forcing existence on a child could be wrong is a difficult notion, which, if true, would serve to amplify the foregoing argument. Such an argument would allow the construal of the issue in terms of the perspective of the child, that is, in terms of a duty not to treat in circumstances where treatment would only prolong suffering. In particular, it would at least give a framework for a decision to stop treatment in cases where, though the costs of treatment are not high, the child's existence would be characterized by severe pain and deprivation.

A basis for speaking of continuing existence as an injury to the child is suggested by the proposed legal concept of "wrongful life." A number of suits have been initiated in the United States and in other countries on the grounds that life or existence itself is, under certain circumstances, a tort or injury to the living person.[12] Although thus far all such suits have ultimately failed, some have succeeded in their initial stages. Two examples may be instructive. In each case the ability to receive recompense for the injury (the tort) presupposed the existence of the individual, whose existence was itself the injury. In one case a suit was initiated on behalf of a child against his father alleging that his father's siring him out of wedlock was an injury to the child.[13] In another case a suit on behalf of a child born of an inmate of a state mental hospital impregnated by rape in that institution was brought against the state of New York.[14] The suit was brought on the grounds that being born with such historical antecedents was itself an injury for which recovery was due. Both cases presupposed that nonexistence would have been preferable to the conditions under which the person born was forced to live.

The suits for tort for wrongful life raise the issue not only of when it would be preferable not to have been born but also of when it would be *wrong* to cause a person to be born. This implies that someone should have judged that it would have been preferable for the child never to have had existence, never to have been in the position to judge that the particular circumstances of life were intolerable.[15] Further, it implies that the person's existence under those circumstances should have been prevented and that, not having been prevented, life was not a gift but an injury. The concept of tort for wrongful life raises an issue concerning the responsibility for giving another person existence, namely, the notion that giving life is not always necessarily a good and justifiable action. Instead, in certain circumstances, so it has been argued, one may have a duty *not* to give existence to another person. This concept involves the claim that certain qualities of life have a negative value, making life an injury, not a gift; it involves, in short, a concept of human accountability and responsibility for human life. It contrasts with the notion that life is a gift of God and thus similar to other "acts of God" (that is, events for which no man is accountable). The concept thus signals the fact that humans can now control reproduction and that where rational control is possible humans are accountable. That is, the expansion of human capabilities has resulted in an expansion of human responsibilities such that one must now decide when and under what circumstances persons will come into existence.

The concept of tort for wrongful life is transferable in part to the painfully compromised existence of children who can only have their life prolonged for a short, painful, and marginal existence. The concept suggests that allowing life to be prolonged under such circumstances would itself be an injury of the person whose painful and severely compromised existence would be made to continue. In fact, it suggests that there is a duty not to prolong life if it can be determined to have a substantial negative value for the person involved.[16] Such issues are moot in the case of adults, who can and should decide for themselves. But small children cannot make such a choice. For them it is an issue of justifying prolonging life under circumstances of painful and compromised existence. Or, put differently, such cases indicate the need to develop social canons to allow a decent death for children for whom the only possibility is protracted, painful suffering.

I do not mean to imply that one should develop a new basis for civil damages. In the field of medicine, the need is to recognize an ethical category, a concept of wrongful continuance of existence, not a new legal right. The concept of injury for continuance of existence, the proposed analogue of the concept of tort for wrongful life, presupposes that life can be of a negative value such that the medical maxim *primum non nocere* ("first do no harm") would require not sustaining life.[17]

The idea of responsibility for acts that sustain or prolong life is cardinal to the notion that one should not under certain circumstances further prolong the life of a child. Unlike adults, children cannot decide with regard to euthanasia (positive or negative), and if more than a utilitarian justification is sought, it must be sought in a duty not to inflict life on another person in circumstances where that life would be painful and futile. This position must rest on the facts that (1) medicine now can cause the prolongation of the life of seriously deformed children who in the past would have died young and that (2) it is not clear that life so prolonged is a good for the child. Further, the choice is made not on the basis of costs to the parents or to society but on the basis of the child's suffering and compromised existence.

The difficulty lies in determining what makes life not worth living for a child. Answers could never be clear. It seems reasonable, however, that the life of children with diseases that involve pain and no hope of survival should not be prolonged. In the case of Tay-Sachs disease (a disease marked by a progressive increase in spasticity and dementia usually leading to death at age three or four), one can hardly imagine that the terminal stages of spastic reaction to stimuli and great difficulty in swallowing are at all pleasant to the child (even insofar as it can only minimally perceive its circumstances). If such a child develops aspiration pneumonia and is treated, it can reasonably be said that to prolong its life is to inflict suffering. Other diseases give fairly clear portraits of lives not worth living: for example, Lesch-Nyhan disease, which is marked by mental retardation and compulsive self-mutilation.

The issue is more difficult in the case of children with diseases for whom the prospects for normal intelligence and a fair lifestyle do exist, but where these chances are remote and their realization expensive. Children born with meningomyelocele present this dilemma. Imagine, for example, a child that falls within Lorber's fifth category (an IQ of sixty or less, sometimes blind, subject to fits, and always incontinent). Such a child has little prospect of anything approaching a normal life, and there is a good chance of its dying even with treatment.[18] But such judgments are statistical. And if one does not treat such children, some will still survive and, as John Freeman indicates, be worse off if not treated.[19] In such cases one is in a dilemma. If one always treats, one must justify extending the life of those who will ultimately die anyway and in the process subjecting them to the morbidity of multiple surgical procedures. How remote does the prospect of a good life have to be in order not to be worth great pain and expense?[20] It is probably best to decide, in the absence of a positive duty to treat, on the basis of the cost and suffering to parents and society. But, as Freeman argues, the prospect of prolonged or even increased suffering raises the issue of active euthanasia.[21]

If the child is not a person strictly, and if death is inevitable and expediting it would diminish the child's pain prior to death, then it would seem to follow that, all else being equal, a decision for active euthanasia would be permissible, even obligatory.[22] The difficulty lies with "all else being equal," for it is doubtful that active euthanasia could be established as a practice without eroding and endangering children generally, since, as John Lorber has pointed out, children cannot speak in their own behalf.[23] Thus, although there is no argument in principle against the active euthanasia of small children, there could be an argument against such practices based on questions of prudence. To put it another way, even though one might have a duty to hasten the death of a particular child, one's duty to protect children in general could override that first duty. The issue of active euthanasia turns in the end on whether it would have social consequences that refraining would not, on whether (1) it is possible to establish procedural safeguards for limited active euthanasia and (2) whether such practices would have a significant adverse effect on the treatment of small children in general. But since these are procedural issues dependent on sociological facts, they are not open to an answer within the confines of this article. In any event, the concept of the injury of continued existence provides a basis for the justification of the passive euthanasia of small children—a practice already widespread and somewhat established in our society—beyond the mere absence of a positive duty to treat.[24]

Conclusion

Though the lack of certainty concerning questions such as the prognosis of particular patients and the social consequence of active euthanasia of children prevents a clear answer to all the issues raised by the euthanasia of infants, it would seem that this much can be maintained: (1) Since children are not persons strictly but exist in and through their families, parents are the appropriate ones to decide whether or not to treat a deformed child when (a) there is not only little likelihood of full human life but also great likelihood of suffering if the life is prolonged, or (b) when the cost of prolonging life is very great. Such decisions must be made in consort with a physician who can accurately give estimates of cost and prognosis and who will be able to help the parents with the consequences of their decision. (2) It is reasonable to speak of a duty not to treat a small child when such treatment will only prolong a painful life or would in any event lead to a painful death. Though this does not by any means answer all the questions, it does point out an important fact—that medicine's duty is not always to prolong life doggedly but sometimes is quite the contrary.

Notes

1. I am grateful to Laurence B. McCullough and James P. Morris for their critical discussion of this paper. They may be responsible for its virtues, but not for its shortcomings.

2. The concept of extraordinary treatment as it has been developed in Catholic moral theology is useful: treatment is extraordinary and therefore not obligatory if it involves great costs, pain, or inconvenience, and is a grave burden to oneself or others without a reasonable expectation that such treatment would be successful. See Gerald Kelly, S. J., *Medico-Moral Problems* (St. Louis: The Catholic Hospital Association Press, 1958), pp. 128–141. Difficulties are hidden in terms such as "great costs" and "reasonable expectation," as well as in terms such as "successful." Such ambiguity reflects the fact that precise operational definitions are not available. That is, the precise meaning of "great," "reasonable," and "successful" are inextricably bound to particular circumstances, especially particular societies.

3. I will use the term euthanasia in a broad sense to indicate a deliberately chosen course of action or inaction that is known at the time of decision to be such as will expedite death. This use of euthanasia will encompass not only positive or active euthanasia (acting in order to expedite death) and negative or passive euthanasia (refraining from action in order to expedite death), but acting and refraining in the absence of a direct intention that

death occur more quickly (that is, those cases that fall under the concept of double effect). See note 4.

4. But both active and passive euthanasia can be appreciated in terms of the Catholic moral notion of double effect. When the doctrine of double effect is invoked, one is strictly not intending euthanasia, but rather one intends something else. That concept allows actions or omissions that lead to death (1) because it is licit not to prolong life *in extremis* (allowing death is not an intrinsic evil), (2) if death is not actually willed or actively sought (that is, the evil is not directly willed), (3) if that which is willed is a major good (for example, avoiding useless major expenditure of resources or serious pain), and (4) if the good is not achieved by means of the evil (for example, one does not will to save resources or diminish pain *by* the death). With regard to euthanasia the doctrine of double effect means that one need not expend major resources in an endeavor that will not bring health but only prolong dying and that one may use drugs that decrease pain but hasten death. See Richard McCormick, *Ambiguity in Moral Choice* (Milwaukee: Marquette University Press, 1973). I exclude the issue of double effect from my discussion because I am interested in those cases in which the good may follow directly from the evil—the death of the child. In part, though, the second section of this paper is concerned with the concept of proportionate good.

5. Raymond S. Duff and A. G. M. Campbell, "Moral and Ethical Dilemmas in the Special-Care Nursery," *The New England Journal of Medicine*, 289 (Oct. 25, 1973), pp. 890–894.

6. Roger Pell, "The Agonizing Decision of Joanne and Roger Pell," *Good Housekeeping* (January 1972), pp. 76–77, 131–135.

7. This somewhat Kantian argument is obviously made in opposition to Kant's position that suicide involves a default of one's duty to oneself ". . . to preserve his life simply because he is a person and must therefore recognize a duty to himself (and a strict one at that)," as well as a contradictory volition: "that man ought to have the authorization to withdraw himself from all obligation, that is, to be free to act as if no authorization at all were required for this withdrawal, involves a contradiction. To destroy the subject of morality in his own person is tantamount to obliterating from the world . . ." Immanuel Kant, *The Metaphysical Principles of Virtue: Part II of the Metaphysics of Morals*, trans. James Ellington (Indianapolis: Bobbs-Merrill, 1964), p. 83; Akademie Edition, VI, 422–423.

8. Norman L. Cantor, "A Patient's Decision to Decline Life-Saving Medical Treatment: Bodily Integrity Versus the Preservation of Life," *Rutgers Law Review*, 26 (Winter 1972), p. 239.

9. By "young child" I mean either an infant or child so young as not yet to be able to participate, in any sense, in a decision. A precise operational definition of "young child" would clearly be difficult to develop. It is also not clear how one would bring older children into such decisions. See, for example, Milton Viederman, "Saying 'No' to Hemodialysis: Exploring Adaptation," and Daniel Burke, "Saying 'No' to Hemodialysis: An Acceptable Decision," both in *The Hastings Center Report*, 4 (September 1974), pp. 8–10, and John E. Schowalter, Julian B. Ferholt, and Nancy M. Mann, "The Adolescent Patient's Decision To Die," *Pediatrics*, 51 (January 1973), pp. 97–103.

10. An appeal to high costs alone is probably hidden in judgments based on statistics: even though there is a chance for a normal life for certain children with apparently severe cases of meningomyelocele, one is not obliged to treat since that chance is small, and the pursuit of that chance is very expensive. Cases of the costs being low but the expected suffering of the child being high will be discussed under the concept of the injury of continued existence. It should be noted that none of the arguments in this paper bear on cases where neither the cost nor the suffering of the child is considerable. Cases in this last category probably include, for example, children born with mongolism complicated only by duodenal atresia.

11. I have in mind here the issue of physicians, hospital administrators, or others being morally compelled to seek an injunction to force treatment of the child in the absence of parental consent. In these circumstances, the physician, who is usually best acquainted with the facts of the case, is the natural advocate of the child.

12. G. Tedeschi, "On Tort Liability for 'Wrongful Life,'" *Israel Law Review*, 1 (1966), p. 513.

13. Zepeda v. Zepeda: 41 Ill. App. 2d 240, 190 N.E. 2d 849 (1963).

14. Williams v. State of New York: 46 Misc. 2d 824, 260 N.Y.S. 2d 953 (Ct. Cl., 1965).

15. Torts: "Illegitimate Child Denied Recovery Against Father for 'Wrongful Life,'" *Iowa Law Review*, 49 (1969), p. 1009.

16. It is one thing to have a conceptual definition of the injury of continued existence (for example, causing a person to continue to live under circumstances of severe pain and deprivation when there are no alternatives but death) and another to have an operational definition of that concept (that is, deciding what counts as such severe pain and deprivation). This article has focused on the first, not the second, issue.

17. H. Tristram Engelhardt, Jr., "Euthanasia and Children: The Injury of Continued Existence," *The Journal of Pediatrics*, 83 (July 1973), pp. 170–171.

18. John Lorber, "Results of Treatment of Myelomeningocele," *Developmental Medicine and Child Neurology*, 13 (1971), p. 286.

19. John M. Freeman, "The Shortsighted Treatment of Myelomeningocele: A Long-Term Case Report," *Pediatrics*, 53 (March 1974), pp. 311–313.

20. John M. Freeman, "To Treat or Not To Treat," *Practical Management of Meningomyelocele*, ed. John Freeman (Baltimore: University Park Press, 1974), p. 21.

21. John Lorber, "Selective Treatment of Myelomeningocele: To Treat or Not To Treat," *Pediatrics*, 53 (March 1974), pp. 307–308.

22. I am presupposing that no intrinsic moral distinctions exist in cases such as these, between acting and refraining, between omitting care in the hope that death will ensue (that is, rather than the child living to be even more defective) and acting to ensure that death will ensue rather than having the child live under painful and seriously compromised circumstances. For a good discussion of the distinction between acting and refraining, see Jonathan Bennett, "Whatever the Consequences," *Analysis*, 26 (January 1966), pp. 83–102; P. J. Fitzgerald, "Acting and Refraining," *Analysis*, 27 (March 1967), pp. 133–139; Daniel Dinello, "On Killing and Letting Die," *Analysis*, 31 (April 1971), pp. 83–86.

23. Lorber, "Selective Treatment of Myelomeningocele," p. 308.

24. Positive duties involve a greater constraint than negative duties. Hence it is often easier to establish a duty not to do something (not to treat further) than a duty to do something (to actively hasten death). Even allowing a new practice to be permitted (for example, active euthanasia) requires a greater attention to consequences than does establishing the absence of a positive duty. For example, at common law there is no basis for action against a person who watches another drown without giving aid; this reflects the difficulty of establishing a positive duty.

On Deciding the Care of Severely Handicapped or Dying Persons: With Particular Reference to Infants

Raymond S. Duff and A. G. M. Campbell

In this paper we explore conflicts of interest among those who decide care (patient, family, and physician) for persons who are severely handicapped or dying. We also describe the severe restrictions on choices for death placed on decision-makers by the law and advocate some changes.

From observations of the care of sick persons of all ages[1,2] and from reviews of the work of others, we believe that much controversy results from conflicts between two distinct but closely interrelated philosophies of care, one mainly oriented to the disease and the other focused primarily on the needs of the individual patient (the person). The first philosophy implies that life itself is all that matters; that death represents the ultimate in human and medical failure, something to be avoided at all costs. The second philosophy considers that the quality of life should be the primary concern. Usually inseparable, the aims of these philosophies may occasionally diverge sufficiently to cause conflict and distress and create major dilemmas in decision-making.

While most treatment programs are accepted as being both disease-oriented *and* person-oriented, exceptions may be made. If severely compromised living resulting from disease or its treatment is regarded as worse than death, a patient, in particular situations, within certain limits, and with the guidance of his physician and his family, may choose death for his own sake. If because of incompetence he cannot choose, his family and physician may choose for him. In principle, this is a simple philosophy, but conflicts of interest occur and some errors, abuses, and injustices are no doubt inevitable. For these and other reasons—personal, professional, and social—the disease-oriented philosophy may be supported

Reprinted by permission of the authors and publisher from Pediatrics *47, no. 4 (April 1976). Copyright 1976, American Academy of Pediatrics.*

with remarkable tenacity by the *behavior* of persons deciding care. Nevertheless, it is rarely supported fully by the *attitudes* of individuals closely involved because in some situations it is recognized as being inhumane.

~~The disease-oriented philosophy~~ is common in medicine. This is understandable and appropriate because at any one time the majority of persons receiving care probably derive benefit from it. With the use of medical technology, ~~this approach in its purest form supports a total crusade against disease and death.~~ Freireich, a spokesman for research and clinical care of cancer victims, wrote: "In my opinion, death is an insult, the stupidest, ugliest thing that can happen to a human being."[3] This philosophy is simple, clear, and appealing. It demands aggressive policies in patient care, research, and education. It permits physicians and others great freedom to develop and to apply technology for treating "the disease in the body in the bed."[1] Patients and families frequently go along with it because it permits them to put off facing a very painful experience. Hope, or at least an image of hope, can be kept alive and there is no risk of confrontation with church or state about choices for death.[4]

Actions based on the disease-oriented philosophy have brought great benefits to people throughout the world; many diseases have been prevented or cured, and disabilities and suffering have been reduced. We certainly believe that medical technology must continue to advance. However, the chief difficulty with this philosophy is that all treatments must fail eventually and there is no prudent strategy for coping with failure. Physicians who deal with defective infants or old people—the two groups having the highest mortality rates—know that it is commonly pretended that severely compromised living is not a problem, at least not a medical problem. People wish to believe that death is avoidable or can be postponed to some future date and hence ignored. (Those in the "hospice" movement are an exception.[5]) Decisions involving major human implications are often made in an essentially "technical order."[6] Sometimes these decisions are supported by the profession, hospitals, and courts against the wishes of the patient or the patient's family. Then evasions drive people apart; distrust, suspicion, and alienation are common as the life-enhancing benefits of medicine decline and the dehumanizing indignities and economic costs increase. These consequences may be overlooked because decision-makers in acute care hospitals and the courts may be far removed from convalescent homes, nursing homes, and rehabilitation centers where the final and perhaps the best assessments of the quality of care can be made. For little or no gain, patients and families may suffer much, and, as illustrated in the following story, tragedy may be compounded.

Case 1

Baby girl S, the first born to her parents, had a high lumbar meningomyelocele, hydrocephalus, and paralysis and deformities of her legs. Mrs. S, a social worker who was acquainted with the condition from her work, refused to sign the operation permit for back closure. Her husband supported her position, but the physicians and hospital staff obtained a court order for a series of operations. The parents openly expressed their feelings to the staff, and in turn the staff was hostile to them. After surgery, complications were numerous and the child's brain was damaged severely, but Mr. and Mrs. S resolved to do their best for their baby. They took her home hoping that they had been wrong (as they knew they could have been) and that the best choice had been made. As complications arose, they brought the baby into the hospital several times for further treatment. Each time, they felt the hostility of the staff whom they would have liked to avoid but couldn't. When the baby died at 10 months of age, they were questioned by physicians and the police about whether they had deliberately delayed seeking treatment for "heavy breathing" (diagnosed at autopsy as pneumonia) until their baby was near death.

Subsequently, two healthy children were born, but Mrs. S had to work to help pay the large debt incurred in the care of the first baby. She was away from the children much of the time and was always tired when she was at home. Her husband felt neglected, and the children developed behavioral disorders. When one of the children was diagnosed as suffering from maternal deprivation, Mrs. S was hospitalized for treatment of severe depression. She later reported, "It was just more than I could take." She and Mr. S felt that their first baby should have been "helped to die." They considered that much of the suffering of their baby, themselves, and their other children was senseless and destructive.

They doubted that they or their living children would ever fully recover from the court-ordered treatment of their first child.

Sometimes the disease-oriented philosophy of care is a trap. Technical considerations may dominate decision-making and leave aside personal and family notions of morality. Little opportunity is given to consider the issue that the situation for dying or severely handicapped persons of any age can involve evasions of the prognosis until the sick person is dependent, perhaps infantilized, and sometimes made incompetent by the disease, its treatment, or the sedation used to provide "comfort." Then the family and the doctor drift without knowledge of the patient's wishes concerning his terminal care. From the patient's point of view, his capacity to live, *as he defines living*, is what matters; he may consider a sound body without a mind or a sound mind with no control over the body of negative value. The physicians, though, have avoided the appearance of failure and the associated time-consuming, personally taxing tasks of helping the patient and his family cope with the inevitable.

These problems have been presented in the literature with increasing frequency, especially by selected health professionals and others concerned with ethics.[6] But it seems to us that many of these communications have failed to acknowledge some critically important aspects of the task before us. In spite of the difficulties of facing the problems of severely compromised living and of dying, we must do so without the benefit of hindsight from the dead and the dying, especially those who are incompetent from age or infirmity. Neither the dying nor the severely handicapped can organize to right whatever may be wrong in their care. The living cannot reach the dying, the dead cannot reach back to the living, and there are special reasons why the living find it hard to reach each other in these situations. Some persons, in choosing an earlier death for a family member, note the irony that others, adhering to a more comfortable but impractical and perhaps inhumane morality, can organize and use propaganda viciously against them, while guilt and related conditions prevent them from organizing to support what they believe is just.

In addition, we have encountered far more pessimism and cynicism about the human condition among members of the helping professions (law, clergy, and medicine) than in families of sick persons or defective infants. Perhaps the helping professionals have adopted such views as a result of their constant exposure to the abnormal, the troubled, and the incompetent of society, those who make most of the news. If this impression should be supported by further study, one should ask if these professionals with considerable dominance in decision-making are inflicting harm by failing to support wise choices which patients and families prefer. This issue is important not only because of the risk of tyranny, but because in families already under great strain collapse is all too common and is increasing.[7]

While the medical profession finds it pleasant, comfortable, and rewarding to care for persons who benefit from medical technology, medical traditions demand that that minority of persons who are dying or are severely afflicted must not be ignored. However, in some situations, providing help requires the use of a strongly person-oriented rather than a disease-oriented philosophy of care. We believe that "down deep" almost all physicians and those they serve would agree that there are some occasions when death may be a prudent choice and achieving death (in fact, killing) a sorrowful and painful obligation. At the same time they may support the argument put forth by Rachels that there is no moral difference between active and passive euthanasia.[8] Our observations suggest that physicians are reluctant to admit these views. They may be unwilling or sometimes unable to share the agony of making conscious choices for death; yet, in modern medicine where substantial life and death controls exist, isn't this part of their task? They may fear speaking out against the law, especially if in speaking out they are suspected of breaking the law by secret acts. Should physicians concern themselves primarily with taking care of people or with serving vague or even "laggardly" laws?[9] They may believe their primary role as healers is inconsistent with making choices for death, but we have found that at least a substantial minority of persons believe doctors secretly and rightly practice selective euthanasia. These conditions account for much tension and probably explain why physicians seem so ambivalent about Rachels' argument.[10]

In earlier times when fewer technological and institutional factors stood between the physician and those he served, euthanasia probably occurred in the privacy of family life and almost certainly in hospitals.[11] Of course, discussion of this was taboo. Now, most decisions in the care of severely ill or dying persons are made in semi-public institutions where only the most pleasant-appearing moralities can be discussed freely. This influences decisions in care. Given the present state of the law, in the care of any patient there is real danger and fear regarding the possibility of prosecution if several seemingly reasonable choices are made or even considered. Charges of homicide, abuse or neglect of the sick, conspiracy to commit crime, and others outlined by Robertson could be pressed.[12] Knowing their deliberations may be considered both taboo and criminal, physicians do not feel free to listen to or talk with patients or families about some subjects. Yet, if they are to act responsibly, issues must be reviewed for routine decision-making even if they potentially involve acts considered as criminal. Thus, fears of the law and apprehensions about feelings of personal agony[13] deter physicians from joining patients and families in facing problems realistically. As a result patients and families may be left isolated and afraid.

The law has rarely taken into account these and related ironies of modern medicine. This is understandable because most decisions in medicine involve confidentiality and, hence, secrecy. Even in semipublic places like a hospital, detailed deliberations are not open to scrutiny and, hence, the law has had little toward which to react. Yet, we suspect that there are disagreements among physicians, patients, and families, particularly between physicians, and patients and families, based not necessarily on the physicians' real doubt about the wisdom of patient or family preferences but, in part, on the physicians' undisclosed fears of prosecution. In addition to wanting to protect themselves, physicians also naturally desire to prove the worth of their services.

Because of these and other communication failures most of the disagreements among physicians, families, and patients remain latent. Patient and family preferences may be unknown. Physicians are then quite free to be "moral entrepreneurs"[14] and to introduce actions which patients and families might oppose but cannot because of their ignorance. Physicians have been heard to discuss the medical "programming" of patients and families for certain kinds of decisions, often with the best of intentions. In this regard, Waitskin and Stoeckle report that physicians can dominate decision-making through communication so as to control the patient's or family's uncertainty.[15]

In the case of manifest disagreements, the courts might help. Physicians could seek a court review to protect themselves or perhaps to impose treatment on persons they believe can be helped by their therapy. Nevertheless, when disagreements are encountered we have found much reluctance on the part of physicians to seek court reviews. They seem to find the court's adversary approach to problem-solving threatening, and they resist public exposure which could be detrimental to them and to their practices. Most of all, they, along with those they serve, object to the court's record of responding, almost as a reflex, in favor of life without regard to the quality of life for the patient or to the consequences for the family. No doubt, the more comfortable moralities on which present policies are based are convenient for medical technology and fit well with legal and church traditions, but using them may result in the patient being abandoned to a dehumanizing technology or to a cruel disease.

According to this interpretation, if the law were changed to allow choices for death, those cases which were taken to court probably would involve more important issues. Perhaps physicians, patients, and families could then feel free to tell the court what it needs to know in order to act justly or to decide to stay out of an affair which those involved can settle for themselves. What is needed sounds like a *Catch–22* situation: a change in the law (to permit selective euthanasia) is needed to demonstrate that a change in the law is safe and wise. The law is strongly protective of human integrity and life, and this is right. It is also "addicted to principle" and "constantly fears setting bad precedent."[16] Nevertheless, it can also be responsive to a consensus of social interests and expectations if they seem justified. We recognize that an extremely difficult moral dilemma exists but we outline below the reasons why we believe that euthanasia, either passive or active, can be a safe and humane choice in dealing with selected tragedies.

When competent individuals decide their own care and choose death, there is rarely an issue to be decided. That is their business, though of course some would disagree. When minor or incompetent individuals are involved, tradition calls for their families and physicians to decide care. Despite some conflicts of interest we believe they should continue to make the decision. They have the most to lose or gain, and they have the most intimate knowledge of patient preferences or probable preferences and of family realities. Many safeguards against bad choices are in existence already, and, when experience is acquired with such decisions and their consequences, other safeguards will develop.

For example, the bonds of affection within families can be considered such a safeguard. In the case of parents and their infants, our observations are similar to those of Fletcher.[17] It is difficult to say when parents endow a fetus with personhood and cherish him as part of themselves, but they do this almost without exception before the last trimester of pregnancy whether they wanted the baby originally or not. Fetal movements and the changing social relationships prompted by the evident pregnancy create value and an expectation of more to come. All deaths of potentially viable fetuses (those born after 24 to 26 weeks of gestation) that we have encountered have been associated with feelings of acute grief. There has been a death in the family; that child had become part of the parents and siblings and will be mourned for weeks or months and on special occasions, like anniversaries, for years. The loss and the shared grief of family members is never forgotten. The scars of the hurt and the triumph of coping with it nobly will remain throughout the lives of the survivors.

The willingness of individuals to sacrifice for their own intimate relatives is evident.[18] In situations where decisions for death of a loved one brought about by the withdrawal of "heroics" (a case of passive euthanasia), our observations have indicated the nature of the safeguards against unjust killing. The patient's right to life and treatment has been weighed against his right to relief in death; the conflicts among patient, family, and others were discussed; through genetic linkage, the problems for future generations have been considered; and expert estimates of the future of the sick person with and without treatment have been reviewed. Some contend that patients, families, and physicians cannot engage in effective negotiations involving these complicated ques-

tions. Our research and clinical experiences have led us to the opposite view. When patients and families have the opportunity and, if possible, the time to understand the condition, its treatment, and the limitations of outcomes and when professionals are willing to share the responsibility and the agony of deciding care and its consequences, the importance of the person-oriented philosophy becomes evident: the patient may be relieved of suffering from disease or pointless, dehumanizing treatment. At the same time, family members may be provided with an opportunity to adapt to their loss through appropriate grieving. Just as close, early infant-parent contact may enhance the development of healthy relationships for a living child,[19] so similar contacts (offered and encouraged, perhaps, but never forced) may help the grieving relatives of a dying person of any age. While the cast of characters and their respective social relationships are different in cases of dying infants and dying adults, the bonds of affection, the sorrow, and the fears of acting unwisely are ever-present in both situations. Some of this is illustrated in the following story.

Case 2

A premature infant was believed to have a hopeless prognosis. The parents and doctor, with agreement of the medical and nursing staff, decided to stop all heroics. The parents informed their healthy 3-year-old daughter that her brother probably could not live and, on her request, she was brought to see the baby. Later, after contemplating autopsy and plans for disposition of the baby's body (both discussed at their request), the parents were asked which they preferred—to leave, to be beside their baby's incubator, or to have the baby, with all his tubes and apparatus removed, brought to them in a private room. Immediately, they chose the last. In the company of the doctor, they held their infant for 55 minutes while he died. During this time, they wept, talked to their son or about him, found humor in some incongruities, or were silent. The mother cradled the baby to her bosom most of the time while the father stroked his wife and baby. He told us that the scene of mother and dying child was one of sublime beauty despite its occurrence in the midst of tragedy. He later said he believed that the time interval spent in intimacy with their baby was about two hours, not 55 minutes. She told us, "We had to say hello to him before we could say goodbye." They came to think of this experience as a fitting funeral from which they gained greater strength for living. They helped each other. They also helped their daughter over the ensuing weeks as she overcame her abnormal fears of dying and openly dealt with her guilt for feeling that her bad wishes had killed her brother.

While a positive attitude toward the expression of grief is believed to be desirable,[20] this places some special demands on the hospital staff. In using the person-oriented philosophy, patients, families, and physicians will have to give up the myth that the application of technology provides the most promise in dealing with diseases in all situations. If this is done, the profession will lose power over some decisions in patient care and have less liberty to serve technology, but it will have a broader role in caring for people. Patients and families will less often be able to live by false hope. They will have to bear more openly and more responsibly the uncertainties and related burdens of deciding care, especially when technology fails. Then they may gain more control and more strength to face their troubles and find hope in learning of their inner strength. With suitable professional help, we have seen this occur many times.

The medical profession itself provides another safeguard. Physicians generally use accepted guidelines in deciding care, and we believe they will set limits, though not always as some prefer.[21] Moreover, failure troubles them. They accept death with much reluctance. They know that conflicts exist and have to be resolved. While they are aware of the guidelines which various ethical authorities might demand be followed, they know that human variation and uniqueness will require that they ignore some of the most acceptable guidelines in specific situations. We recognize that choices will vary because an experience of caring for a very defective person may be rewarding for one family but destructive for another. Thus, in apparently similar medical situations physicians may advise differently. Also, against family wishes, they may insist on treatment of persons with a fair prognosis or advise against treatment of persons with a hopeless outlook. They may do this to help patients and families select the "least detrimental alternative" (a concept found useful in analyzing a different kind of human tragedy—contested child custody[22]). If physicians, patients,

and families encounter differences which they cannot resolve, the courts should help to decide when death may be chosen, not (as now) that generally death cannot be chosen.

We find there is little reason to have to defend the policy we support against the philosophical "slippery slope" or "wedge" argument, which holds that allowing a choice of death in one situation will lead to widespread use of that choice for minor difficulties or for the convenience of society or of the family. No doubt the danger is great when leaders of governments or the medical profession alone decide,[23] but the decisions we are discussing can be made only by those who care most for the patient and who must bear the consequences. The agony and the suffering which invariably must be endured by those who decide care provide effective safeguards against abuse with rare exception and that exception is easy to detect if choices are made openly, as we advocate. This assumes that altruism in families is strong. We believe it is. Indeed, as suggested by recent observations of sociobiologists, the foundations of altruism may be inborn.[24] This may have been implied by a hospital chaplain who quoted Pascal, "Sometimes the heart has reasons which reason itself cannot understand."

Thus, *we believe that choices for death, whether by active or passive means, should be permitted.* Such choices should be made only after suitable patient, family, and medical consultation. In addition, the decisions and the consequences should be subjected to suitable medical review so that new knowledge and more wisdom about these problems may be acquired. However, since consensus cannot be expected in all situations, the choice made in each case by the patient, the family, and the physician should be honored. Society should intervene only if three conditions occur: first, if harm is being done to someone; second, if a better alternative is available; third, if it can demonstrate the capacity and the will to support those on whom it imposes an unwelcome choice.

It seems evident that suffering patients (when able), sorrowing families, and concerned physicians have always sought the least detrimental alternative while deciding care in the face of tragedy. Sometimes, despite the law, they have chosen an early death by passive or active means as was required in the varied situations. There is a need in our society for a policy of deciding care according to individual situations as *the parties most involved feel* is correct. In view of the complexities of human experience and human tragedy and the difficulties and conflicts in deciding the proper use of medical technology, this approach to the problem of life and death control seems to make sense.

Essentially, decision-making by "muddling through"[25] probably is the best that we can do, but we need freedom to muddle. Eventually, such a policy will probably be supported by the medical profession, just as we think it is supported now by most persons acquainted with human tragedy. If so, it is likely that less energy will have to be used in dealing with the tensions of the dying, the severely handicapped, and their families and more will be devoted to ensure that they live well.

Notes

1. Duff, R. S., Hollingshead, A. B. Sickness and Society. New York, Harper & Row, 1968.

2. Duff, R. S., Campbell, A. G. M. Moral and ethical dilemmas in the special care nursery. N Engl J Med 289:890, 1973.

3. Freireich, quoted in Ross, W. S. The best medical care for the "hopeless" patient. Med Opinion February 1972, pp 51–55.

4. Furlow, T. W., Jr. A matter of life and death. Pharos 36:84, 1973.

5. Dobihal, E. F., Jr. Talk or terminal care? Conn Med 38:364, 1974.

6. Cassell, E. J. Dying in a technological society. In, Facing Death. Hastings Center Studies, Institute of Society, Ethics and the Life Sciences, 1974, vol 2.

7. Bronfenbrenner, U. The origins of alienation. Sci Am 231:53, 1974.

8. Rachels, J. Active and passive euthanasia. N Engl J Med 292:78, 1975.

9. Maguire, D. C. Death by choice. Garden City, New York, Doubleday & Co, 1974, pp 22–54.

10. Letters to the editor. N Engl J Med 292:863–867, 1975.

11. Forrest, D. M. Modern trends in the treatment of spina bifida: Early closure in spina bifida: Results and problems. Proc R Soc Med 60:763, 1967.

12. Robertson, J. A. Involuntary euthanasia of defective newborns: A legal analysis. Stanford Law Rev 27:213, 1975.

13. Artiss, K. L., Levine, A. S. Doctor-patient relationship in severe illness. N Engl J Med 288:1210, 1973.

14. Friedson, E. Profession of Medicine. New York, Dodd, Mead & Co, 1974, p 244.

15. Waitzkin, H., Stoeckle, J. D. The communication of information about illness. Adv Psychosom Med 8:180, 1972.

16. Freund, P. A. Ethical problems in human experimentation. N Engl J Med 273:687, 1965.

17. Fletcher, J. The parent-child bond in the genetic revolution. Theological Stud 33:457, 1972.

18. Hunt, G. M. Implications of the treatment of myelomeningocele for the child and his family. Lancet 2:1308, 1973.

19. Kennell, J. H., Jerauld, R., Wolfe, H. *et al:* Maternal behavior one year after early and extended postpartum contact. Dev Med Child Neurol 16:172, 1974.

20. MaGraw, R. M. Grief: Its clinical importance and its resolution. Mod Med 40:61, 1972.

21. McCormick, R. A. To save or let die. JAMA 229:172, 1974.

22. Goldstein, J., Freud, A., Solnit, A. J. Beyond the Best Interests of the Child. New York, Macmillan Co, 1973.

23. Alexander, L. Medical science under dictatorship. N Engl J Med 241:39, 1949.

24. Wilson, E. Sociobiology. Cambridge, Massachusetts, Belknap Press, 1975.

25. Lindblom, C. E. The science of "muddling through." Pub Admin Rev 19:79, 1959.

Acknowledgment: The suggestions and editorial assistance of Janet Turk are gratefully acknowledged.

Decision Scenario 1

I had been working as a Bioethics Advisor at University Hospital for three months before I was called in to consult on a pediatrics case. Dr. Savano, the attending obstetrician, asked me to meet with him and Dr. Hinds, one of the staff surgeons, to talk with the father of a newborn girl.

I went to the consulting room with Dr. Savano, and he introduced me and Dr. Hinds to Joel Blake. From what Dr. Savano had already told me, I knew that Mr. Blake was in his early twenties and worked as a clerk at a discount store called the Bargain Barn. The baby's mother was Hilda Godgeburn, and she and Mr. Blake were not married.

Mr. Blake was very nervous. He knew that the baby had been born just three hours or so before and that Ms. Godgeburn was in very good condition. But Dr. Savano had not told him anything about the baby.

"I'm sorry to have to tell you this," Dr. Savano said. "But the baby was born with severe defects."

"My God," Blake said. "What's the matter?"

"It's a condition called spina bifida," Dr. Savano said. "There's a hole in the baby's back just below the shoulder blades, and some of the nerves from the spine are protruding through it. The baby will have little or no control over her legs, and she won't be able to control her bladder or bowels." Dr. Savano paused to see if Mr. Blake was understanding him. "The legs and feet are also deformed to some extent because of the defective spinal nerves."

Mr. Blake was shaking his head, paying close attention but hardly able to accept what he was being told.

"There's one more thing," Dr. Savano said. "The spinal defect is making the head fill up with liquid from the spinal canal. That's putting pressure on the brain. We can be sure that the brain is already damaged, but if the pressure continues, the child will die."

"Is there anything that can be done?" Blake asked. "Anything at all?"

Dr. Savano nodded to Dr. Hinds. "We can do a lot," Dr. Hinds said. "We can drain the fluid from the head, repair the opening in the spine, and later we can operate on the feet and legs."

"Then why aren't you doing it?" Mr. Blake asked. "Do I have to agree to it? If I do, then I agree. Please go ahead."

"It's not that simple," Dr. Hinds said. "You see, we can perform surgery, but that won't turn your baby into a normal child. She will always be paralyzed and mentally retarded. To what extent, we can't say now. Her bodily wastes will have to be drained to the outside by the means of artificial devices that we'll have to connect surgically. There will have to be several operations, probably, to get the drain from her head to work properly. A number of operations on her feet will be necessary."

"Oh, God," Mr. Blake said. "Hilda and I can't take it. We don't have enough money for the operations. And even if we did, we would have to spend the rest of our lives taking care of the child."

"The child could be put into a state institution," Dr. Hinds said.

"That's even worse," Mr. Blake said. "Just handing our problem to somebody else. And what kind of life would she have? A pitiful, miserable life."

None of the rest of us said anything. "You said she would die without the operation to drain her head," Mr. Blake said. "How long would that take?"

"A few hours perhaps," Dr. Savano said. "But we can't be sure. It may take several days, and conceivably she might not die at all."

"Oh, God," Mr. Blake said again. "I don't want her to suffer. Can she just be put to sleep painlessly?"

Dr. Savano didn't answer the question. He seemed not even to hear it. "We'll have to talk to Ms. Godgeburn also," he said. "And before you make up your mind for good, I want you to talk with the Bioethics Advisor. You two discuss the matter, and the Advisor will perhaps bring out some things you haven't thought about. Dr. Hinds will leave you both together now. Let me know when you've reached your final decision and we'll talk again."

Assume that you are the bioethics advisor in this case. Would you attempt to persuade Mr. Blake that attempts should be made to save the child's life?

Do you think he is right in asking that the child be painlessly killed? If such killing is not legally permissible, is this relevant to deciding whether the child should be saved if possible? What considerations for and against such an attempt might you mention to help Mr. Blake in reaching a decision?

Are there any arguments in what you have read that seem to you entirely persuasive in such a case?

What factual considerations (if any) do you consider relevant to resolving the moral issues here?

Decision Scenario 2

Brookhaven, as we will call it, is a long-term health care institution in the Washington metropolitan area. Most of Brookhaven's patients are in residence there for only a few months: either they succumb to their ailments and die or they recover sufficiently to return to their homes.

But for some patients death has no immediate likelihood, nor is recovery a possibility. They linger on at Brookhaven, day after day and year after year. Juli Meyers is such a patient, although that is not really her name.

Juli is seventeen and has been in Brookhaven for six years. But before Brookhaven there were other institutions. In fact, Juli has spent most of her life in hospitals and special care facilities. But Juli does not seem to be aware of any of this.

At Brookhaven she spends her days lying in a bed surrounded with barred metal panels. The bars have been padded with foam rubber. Although most of the time Juli is curled tightly in a fetal position, she sometimes flails around wildly and makes guttural sounds. The padding keeps her from injuring herself.

Juli's body is thin and underdeveloped, with sticklike arms and legs. She is blind and deaf and has no control over her bowels and bladder. She is totally dependent on others to clean her and care for her. She can swallow the food put into her mouth, but she cannot feed herself. She makes no response to the people or events around her.

There is no hope that Juli will ever walk or talk, laugh or cry, or even show the slightest sign of intelligence or awareness. She is the victim of one of the forms of Schilder's disease. The nerve fibers that make up her central nervous system have mostly degenerated. The cause of the degeneration is not fully known, nor is it known how to halt the process. The condition is irreversible, and Juli will never be better than she is.

At birth Juli seemed perfectly normal and healthy, but at three months she began to lose her sight and hearing. She made the gurgling noises typical of babies less and less frequently. By the end of her first year, she made no sounds at all and was completely blind and deaf. Also, she was losing control of her muscles, and her head lolled on her shoulders, like a doll with a broken neck.

She became highly subject to infections, and more than once she had pneumonia. Once when she was on the critical list, a specialist suggested to her mother that it would be pointless to continue treating her. Even if she recovered from the pneumonia, she would remain hopelessly impaired. Mrs. Meyers angrily rejected the suggestion and insisted that everything possible be done to save Juli's life.

Although not wealthy, the family bore the high cost of hospitalization and treatments. Mrs. Meyers devoted herself almost totally to caring for Juli at home, and the other four children in the family received little of her attention. Eventually, Mrs. Meyers began to suffer from severe depression, and when Juli was eight and a half, her parents decided she would have to be placed in an institution. Since then, Juli has changed little. No one expects her to change. Her mother visits her three times a month and brings Juli freshly laundered and ironed clothes.

> *Would Robertson's arguments support Mrs. Meyers's decision not to allow Juli to die? How might a utilitarian criticize the decision?*
>
> *Is the decision compatible with the suggestions for arriving at such decisions made by Duff and Campbell?*
>
> *Would treatment for pneumonia in Juli's case be considered "normal medical measures" on the Roman Catholic view?*
>
> *Are there any grounds for supposing that Juli is being made to suffer what Engelhardt calls "the injury of continued existence?"*
>
> *Would your decision have been the same as Mrs. Meyers's?*
>
> *Is it possible to justify using society's limited medical resources to keep Juli alive?*
>
> *Evaluate the following argument. Opponents of abortion oppose spending public funds for abortion on the grounds that they (the opponents) are being forced to support murder, which is a serious moral evil. Keeping Juli alive is a serious moral evil. Therefore, no public funds should be used for this purpose.*

Decision Scenario 3

Susan Roth was looking forward to being a mother. She had quit her secretarial job three months before her baby was due so she could spend the time getting everything ready. Her husband David was equally enthusiastic, and they spent many hours happily speculating about the way things would be when their baby came. It was their first child.

"I hope they don't mix her up with some other baby," Mrs. Roth said to her husband after delivery.

She didn't know yet that there was little chance of confusion. The Roth infant was seriously deformed. Her arms and legs had failed to develop, her skull was misshapen and her face deformed. Her large intestine emptied through her vagina, and she had no muscular control over her bladder.

When she was told, Mrs. Roth said, "We cannot let it live, for her sake and ours." On the day she left the hospital with the child, Mrs. Roth mixed a lethal dose of a tranquilizing drug with the baby's formula and fed it to her. The child died that evening.

Mrs. Roth and her husband were charged with infanticide. During the court proceedings, Mrs. Roth admitted to the killing but said she was satisfied she had done the right thing. "I know I could not let my baby live like that," she said. "If only she had been mentally abnormal, she would not have known her fate. But she had a normal brain. She would have known. Placing her in an institution might have helped me, but it wouldn't have helped her."

The jury, after deliberating for two hours, found Mrs. Roth and her husband guilty of the charge.

Are laws against infanticide unjust?

Can they be supported on utilitarian grounds?

How might they be criticized on Kantian principles? On Rawls's?

Does the fact that the intelligence of the child is normal support the mother's claim that killing was justifiable? Might normal intelligence make the "injury of continued existence" even greater than subnormal intelligence?

Why might Robertson consider the mother's action morally wrong?

Decision Scenario 4

I can't believe God has done this to me, Mike Chovo said to himself. Tears came to his eyes and his nose started running.

His wife Carol handed him a tissue from the box by her bed. "It's all right, Mikey," she said. "We'll make it all right."

Mike wiped his eyes and blew his nose. The yellow tissue struck him as being absurdly cheerful. Given the circumstances, it seemed totally out of place in the hospital room.

"I know," he said. "But it's going to be so hard, so very hard. And it's going to be terrible for Chris and Jan."

"They'll adjust," Carol said. "In some ways it will be good for them to have a brother like Terry. They'll learn somebody doesn't have to be perfect for you to love them."

"Oh, Jesus," Mike said. "Maybe we should have told them not to do anything. He's in such bad shape. The doctors told me they're not sure he has enough of a brain even to learn who we are. I mean, it may be like he's unconscious all of his life."

Mike pulled another tissue out of the box and held it over his eyes. He pressed hard with his fingertips. He wanted Terry to die, but he couldn't tell Carol that. He could barely allow himself to think it. He wished he hadn't given permission for the operation to drain the fluid from Terry's head. But he couldn't oppose Carol at a time like this.

"But we'll love him anyway," Carol said. "We'll take care of him until God calls him away."

"I wonder if we're doing him a favor. I wonder if he's really fit for this world."

"We couldn't just stand by and let him die," Carol said.

"No, I guess we couldn't." Mike hesitated, then went on. "You know, this one operation won't be the end of them. Dr. Flanners told me that it's not unusual to have to operate ten or twelve times in cases like this."

"It's going to be expensive."

"That's right, and I don't know where we're going to get the money."

"We can probably borrow some from my parents. And if we have to, I guess we can get a second mortgage on the house."

"I guess so," Mike admitted.

Carol looked at Mike and smiled at him. After a moment, he smiled back.

Would the line of reasoning taken by Robertson tend to support the decision made by Carol Chovo?

Might the considerations mentioned by Englehardt be used to argue that it would have been better for the Chovos to allow their son to die?

Does the natural law view require treatment in such a case?

On what grounds might Kantian principles be appealed to in order to justify a decision not to treat Terry Chovo?

In what ways, if any, are such considerations as the financial status of the Chovos and the likely influence on the other two children of having a wholly dependent and defective brother relevant to the decision that faced the parents?

Decision Scenario 5

Irene Towers had been a nurse for almost twelve years; for the last three of those years she had worked in the Neonatal Unit of Halifax County Hospital. It was a job she loved. Even when the infants were ill or required special medical or surgical treatment, she found the job of caring for them immensely rewarding. She knew that without her efforts many of the babies would simply die.

Irene Towers was on duty the night that Siamese twins were born to Corrine

Couchers and brought at once to the Neonatal Unit. Even Irene, with all her experience, was distressed to see them. The twin boys were joined at their midsections in a way that made it impossible to separate them surgically. Because of the position of the single liver and the kidneys, not even one twin could be saved at the expense of the life of the other. Moreover, both children were severely deformed, with incompletely developed arms and legs and misshapen heads. As best as the neurologist could determine, both suffered severe brain damage.

The father of the children was Dr. Harold Couchers. Dr. Couchers, a slightly built man in his early thirties, was a specialist in internal medicine with a private practice.

Irene felt sorry for him the night the children were born. When he went into the room with the obstetrician to examine his sons, he had already been told what to expect. He showed no signs of grief as he stood over the slat-sided crib, but the corners of his mouth were drawn tight and his face was almost unnaturally empty of expression. Most strange for a physician, Irene thought, he merely looked at the children and did not touch them. She was sure that in some obscure way he must be blaming himself for what had happened to them.

Later that evening, Irene saw Dr. Couchers sitting in the small conference room at the end of the hall with Dr. Cara Rosen, Corrine Couchers's obstetrician. They were talking earnestly and quietly when Irene passed the open door. Then while she was looking over the assignment sheet at the nursing station, the two of them walked up. Dr. Rosen took a chart from the rack behind the desk and made a notation. After returning the chart, she shook hands with Dr. Couchers and he left.

It was not until the end of her shift that Irene read the chart; Dr. Rosen's note said that the twin boys were to be given neither food nor water. At first, Irene couldn't believe the order. But when she asked her supervisor, she was told that the supervisor had telephoned Dr. Rosen and that the obstetrician had confirmed the order.

Irene said nothing to the supervisor or to anyone else, but she made her own decision. She believed it was wrong to let the children die, particularly in such a horrible way. They deserved every chance to fight for their lives, and she was going to help them the way she had helped hundreds of other babies in the unit.

For the next week and a half, Irene saw to it that the children were given water and fed the standard infant formula. She did it all herself, on her own initiative. Although some of the other nurses on the floor saw what she was doing, none of them said anything to her. One even smiled and nodded to her when she saw Irene feeding the children.

Apparently someone else also disapproved of the order to let the twins die. Thirteen days after their birth, an investigator from the state Family Welfare Agency appeared in the neonatal ward. The rumor was that his visit had been prompted by an anonymous telephone call.

Late in the afternoon of the day of that visit, the deformed twins were made temporary wards of the Agency, and the orders on the chart were changed—the twins were now to be given food and water. On the next day, the county prosecutor's office announced publicly that it would conduct an investigation of the situation and decide whether criminal charges should be brought against Dr. Couchers or members of the hospital staff.

Irene was sure that she had done the right thing. Nevertheless, she was glad to be relieved of the responsibility.

> *Might a utilitarian argument be offered in defense of Dr. Couchers's decision to allow the twins to die?*
>
> *What criticism of such an argument might Robertson offer?*
>
> *Is there a morally relevant distinction between not treating (and allowing to die) and not providing such minimal needs as food and water (and allowing to die)?*
>
> *Following the suggestions of Duff and Campbell, how might a decision about the future of the twins be arrived at?*
>
> *Does Englehardt's line of reasoning support the action taken by Irene Towers?*
>
> *Did Irene Towers exceed the limits of her responsibility or did she act in a morally heroic way?*

3
EUTHANASIA

CASE PRESENTATION
Karen Quinlan

At two in the morning on Tuesday, April 14, 1975, Mrs. Julie Quinlan was awakened by a telephone call. When she hung up she was crying. "Karen is very sick," Mrs. Quinlan said to her husband Joseph. "She's unconscious, and we have to go to Newton Hospital right away."

The Quinlans thought that their twenty-one-year-old adopted daughter might have been in an automobile accident. But the doctor in the intensive care unit told them that wasn't so. Karen was in a critical comatose state of unknown cause and was being given oxygen through a mask taped over her nose and mouth. She had been brought to the hospital by two friends who had been with her at a birthday party. After a few drinks, she had started to pass out, and her friends decided she must be drunk and put her to bed. Then a girl checked on her later in the evening and found that Karen wasn't breathing. Her friends gave her mouth-to-mouth resuscitation and took her to the nearest hospital.

Blood and urine tests showed that Karen had not consumed a dangerous amount of alcohol. They also showed the presence of .6 milligram percent of aspirin and the tranquilizer Valium. Two milligrams would have been toxic and five lethal. Why Karen stopped breathing was mysterious. But it was during that time that part of her brain died from oxygen depletion.

After Karen had been unconscious for about a week, she was moved to St. Clare's Hospital in nearby Denville, where testing and life-support facilities were better. Dr. Robert J. Morse, a neurologist, and Dr. Arshad Javed, a pulmonary internist, became her physicians. Additional tests were made. Extensive brain damage was confirmed, and several possible causes of the coma were ruled out.

During the early days, the Quinlans were hopeful. Karen's eyes opened and closed, and her mother and her nineteen-year-old sister, Mary Ellen, thought that they detected signs that she recognized them. But Karen's condition began

to deteriorate. Her weight gradually dropped from one-hundred twenty pounds to seventy. Her body began to contract into a rigid fetal position, until her five-foot two-inch frame was bent into a shape hardly longer than three feet. She was now breathing mechanically, by means of an MA-1 respirator that pumped air through a tube in her throat.

By early July, Karen's physicians, her mother, sister, and brother had come to believe it was hopeless to expect her ever to regain consciousness. Only her father continued to believe it might be possible. But when he told Dr. Morse about some encouraging sign he had noticed, Dr. Morse said to him, "Even if God did perform a miracle so that Karen would live, her damage is so extensive she would spend the rest of her life in an institution." Mr. Quinlan then realized that Karen would never again be as he remembered her. He now agreed with Karen's sister: "Karen would never want to be kept alive on machines like this. She would hate this."

The Quinlans' parish priest, Father Thomas Trapasso, had also assured them that the moral doctrines of the Roman Catholic Church did not require the continuation of extraordinary measures to support a hopeless life. Before making his decision, Mr. Quinlan asked the priest, "Am I playing God?" Father Thomas said, "God has made the decision that Karen is going to die. You're just agreeing with God's decision, that's all."

On July 31, after Karen had been unconscious for three and a half months, the Quinlans gave Drs. Morse and Jared their permission to take Karen off the respirator. The Quinlans signed a letter authorizing the discontinuance of extraordinary procedures and absolving the hospital from all legal liability. "I think you have come to the right decision," Dr. Morse said to Mr. Quinlan.

But the next morning Dr. Morse called Mr. Quinlan. "I have a moral problem about what we agreed on last night," he said. "I feel I have to consult somebody else and see how he feels about it." The next day, Dr. Morse called again. "I find I will not do it," he said. "And I've informed the administrator at the hospital that I will not do it."

The Quinlans were upset and bewildered by the change in Dr. Morse. Later, they talked with the hospital attorney and were told by him that because Karen was over twenty-one, they were no longer her legal guardians. The Quinlans would have to go to court and be appointed to guardianship. After that, the hospital might or might not remove Karen from the respirator.

Mr. Quinlan consulted attorney Paul Armstrong. Because Karen was an adult without income, Mr. Quinlan explained, Medicare was paying the four-hundred and fifty dollars a day it cost to keep her alive. The Quinlans thus had no financial motive in asking that the respirator be taken away. Mr. Quinlan said that his belief that Karen should be allowed to die rested on his conviction that it was God's will, and it was for this reason that he wanted to be appointed Karen's guardian.

Mr. Armstrong filed a plea with Judge Robert Muir of the New Jersey Superior Court on September 12, 1975. He explicitly requested that Mr. Quinlan be appointed Karen's guardian so that he would have "the express power of authorizing the discontinuance of all extraordinary means of sustaining her life." Later, on October 20, Mr. Armstrong argued the case on three constitutional grounds. First, he claimed that there is an implicit right to privacy guaranteed by the Constitution and that this right permits individuals or others acting for them to terminate the use of extraordinary medical measures, even when death may result. This right holds, Armstrong said, unless there are compelling state interests that set it aside.

Second, Armstrong argued that the First Amendment guarantee of religious freedom extended to the Quinlan case. If the Court did not allow them to act in accordance with the doctrines of their church, their religious liberty would be infringed. Finally, Armstrong appealed to the "cruel and unusual punishment" clause of the Eighth Amendment. He claimed that "for the state to require that Karen Quinlan be kept alive, against her will and the will of her family, after the dignity, beauty, promise and meaning of earthly life have vanished, is cruel and unusual punishment."

Karen's mother, sister, and a friend testified that Karen had often talked about not wanting to be kept alive by machines. An expert witness, a neurologist, testified that Karen was in a "chronic vegetative state" and that it was unlikely that she would ever regain consciousness. Doctors testifying for St. Clare's hospital and Karen's physicians agreed with this. But, they argued, her brain still showed patterns of electrical activity, and she still had a discernible pulse. Thus, she could not be considered dead by legal or medical criteria.

On November 10, Judge Muir ruled against Joseph Quinlan. He praised Mr. Quinlan's character and concern, but he decided that Mr. Quinlan's anguish over his daughter might cloud his judgment about her welfare so he should not be made her guardian. Furthermore, Judge Muir said, because Karen is still medically and legally alive, "the Court should not authorize termination of the respirator. To do so would be homicide and an act of euthanasia."

Mr. Armstrong appealed the decision to the New Jersey Supreme Court. On January 26, 1976, the Court convened to hear arguments, and Mr. Armstrong argued substantially as before. But this time the Court's ruling was favorable. The Court agreed that Mr. Quinlan could assert a right of privacy on Karen's behalf and that whatever he decided for her should be accepted by society. It also set aside any criminal liability for removing the respirator, claiming that if death resulted it would not be homicide and that even if it were homicide, it would not be unlawful. Finally, the Court stated that if Karen's physicians believed that she would never emerge from her coma, they should consult an ethics committee to be established by St. Clare's Hospital. If the committee accepted their prognosis, then the respirator could be removed. If Karen's present physicians were then unwilling to take her off the respirator, Mr. Quinlan was free to find a physician who would.

Six weeks after the court decision, the respirator still had not been turned off. In fact, another machine, one for controlling body temperature, had been added. Mr. Quinlan met with Morse and Jared and demanded that they remove the respirator. They agreed to "wean" Karen from the machine, and soon she was breathing without mechanical assistance. Dr. Morse and St. Clare's Hospital were determined that Karen would not die while under their care. Although she was moved to a private room, it was next door to the intensive care unit. They intended to put her back on the respirator at the first sign of breathing difficulty.

Because Karen was still alive, the Quinlans began a long search for a chronic-care hospital. Twenty or more institutions turned them away, and physicians expressed great reluctance to become involved in the case. Finally, Dr. Joseph Fennelly volunteered to treat Karen, and on June 9, she was moved from St. Clare's to the Morris View Nursing Home.

Now, over seven years since Karen Quinlan lapsed into a coma, she continues to breathe. She receives high-nutrient feedings and regular doses of antibiotics to ward off infections. During some periods she is more active than at others, making reflexive responses to touch and sound.

CASE PRESENTATION
The Death of J. K. Collums

On November 16, 1981, sixty-nine-year-old Woodrow Collums went into the Oak Hills Care Center in the small town of Poteet, Texas to visit his seventy-two-year-old brother J. K. Collums. J. K. was a victim of Alzheimer's disease, a poorly understood illness in which the brain undergoes progressive degeneration. J. K. had already reached the point of being unable to care for any of his bodily needs, and he could no longer speak or respond to others. A nasogastric tube fed him the nutrients needed to keep him alive.

"I just stood there and looked at him a few minutes," Woody Collums said about his brother. "He was beyond saying anything to me. So I left and went back to the car, thinking I'd just go on and let the Lord take care of it. But I got to the car, and this gun was in the car."

Mr. Collums decided to shoot his brother, and took the gun back into the room. But once there, he changed his mind. "So I started to leave, and I looked back at him, and I just couldn't go off and leave him like that. I turned around and shot him five times, just as fast as I could shoot him. He never moved. He was the most peaceful looking guy you've ever seen."

Mr. Collums then checked his brother's pulse to be sure that he was dead. He put the pistol down on a bedside tray, and waited for someone to call the police. While waiting, he said to a staff member, "I've killed horses, cows, and dogs that were suffering. He's suffered long enough."

Mr. Collums freely admitted shooting his brother, but he refused to acknowledge that he had murdered him. "I feel like he's been dead since he's been in this condition." he said.

A Bexar County, Texas grand jury indicted Mr. Collums for the shooting of his brother. But even the county prosecutors regarded the action as a clear case of mercy killing. The two brothers had been very close all their lives, and although J. K. Collums had not signed an actual "living will," which is legal in Texas, he had written a letter to his physician in which he expressed his views about being kept alive by extraordinary means. According to J. K. Collums' wife Helen, he said that "if they couldn't do something to help his brain, to please put him to sleep forever." The letter was written before the disease had progressed to the point that he was no longer able to reason and communicate.

When asked if she blamed her brother-in-law for his actions, Helen Collums said, "Oh, no! God, no, no!" She went on to say, "I thank God Jim's out of his misery. I hate to think it had to be done the way it was done, but I understand it. I couldn't ever have shot him. I could have asked for the life supports to be taken away, because I don't believe in life supports. I just think it's cruelty for someone who's terminally ill, to stuff a tube down his nose from May to November. That's agony and cruelty. People don't know about these things. I just hope it helps somebody else, so they don't have to go through what he went through."

Helen Collums now believes she should not have allowed the stomach tube to be put into place. But once it had been, other members of the family refused to allow it to be removed. They thought removing it would constitute murder. Besides, it was not clear that the nursing home would agree to its removal. Court decisions allow the removal of support systems that are "extraordinary means" of prolonging life when the patient has "clearly and convincingly" rejected the use of such means beforehand. But is a feeding tube "extraordinary?"

Woodrow Collums received much public sympathy, but not everyone approved of his action. Theresa Brock, the administrator of the Oak Hills Care Center, expressed the opposition view. "None of us knows," she said, "and nobody here can tell you, nobody on this earth can tell you, what Jim was able to feel, or perceive, or think or know, and it's not up to any of us to end somebody's life for them."

Everyone agreed that J. K. Collums could still recognize his wife and could still pucker his lips as if to kiss her. He did just that on the day that he died.

In February of 1982, Woodrow Collums pleaded guilty to a charge of murder. He waived a jury trial, and at a punishment hearing he told Judge Tom Rickhoff about what he had done. Mr. Collums said of his brother, "He looked like he was just begging me to get him out of his misery. I regret having to do what I did, but I don't regret doing it. I felt he would have done it himself if he could have."

Mr. Collums's lawyer, Roy Barrera, expressed the hope that the hearing would help people understand the need for euthanasia. "If we can do mercy killings for animals to relieve pain and suffering," he said, "I just can't see where under the proper conditions a human being would be given any less than what we give animals."

Judge Rickhoff was faced with the decision of whether to send Mr. Collums to jail or to put him on probation. On March 4, Judge Rickhoff ruled that Mr. Collums was to be placed on probation for a period of ten years. During that time, he would be required to spend ten hours each week working at homes for the elderly.

Introduction

Death comes to us all. We hope that when it comes it will be swift and allow us to depart without prolonged suffering, our dignity intact. We also hope that it will not force burdens on our family and friends, making them pay both financially and emotionally by our lingering and hopeless condition.

Such considerations give euthanasia a strong appeal. Should we not be able to snip the thread of life when the weight of suffering and hopelessness grows too heavy to bear? The answer to this question is not so easy as it may seem, for hidden within it are a number of complicated moral issues.

Just what is euthanasia? The word comes from the Greek for "good death," and in English it has come to have the meaning "easy death." But this does very little to help us understand the concept. For consider this: if we give ourselves an easy death, are we committing suicide? If we assist someone else to an easy death (with or without that person's permission), are we committing murder? Anyone who opposed killing (either of one's self or of others) on moral grounds might also consider it necessary to object to euthanasia.

It may be, however, that the answer to both of these questions is no. But if it is, then it is necessary to specify the conditions that distinguish euthanasia from both suicide and murder. Only then would it be possible to argue, without contradiction, that euthanasia is morally acceptable but the other two forms of killing are not. (Someone believing that suicide is morally legitimate would not object to euthanasia carried out by the person herself, but he would still have to deal with the problem posed by the euthanasia/murder issue.)

Active and Passive Euthanasia

We have talked of euthanasia as though it involved directly taking the life of a person, either one's own life or the life of another. However, some philosophers distinguish between "active euthanasia" and "passive euthanasia," which in turn rests on a distinction between *killing* and *letting die*. To kill someone (including one's self) is to take a definite action to end his or her life (administering a lethal injection, for example). To allow someone to die, by contrast, is to take no steps to prolong a person's life when those steps seem called for (failing to give an injection of antibiotics, for example). Active euthanasia, then, is direct killing and is an act of commission. Passive euthanasia is an act of omission.

This distinction is used in most contemporary codes of medical ethics (that of the American Medical Association, for example) and is also recognized in the Anglo-American tradition of law. Except in special circumstances, it is illegal to deliberately cause the death of another person. It is not, however, illegal (except in special circumstances) to allow a person to die. Clearly, one might consider active euthanasia morally wrong while recognizing passive euthanasia as morally legitimate.

Some philosophers, however, have argued that the active-passive distinction is morally irrelevant with respect to euthanasia. Both are cases of causing death, and it is the circumstances in which death is caused, not the manner of causing it, that is of moral importance. (This is the claim defended by James Rachels in his essay, "Active and Passive Euthanasia," included in this chapter.) Furthermore, the active-passive distinction is not always clear-cut. If a person dies after special life-sustaining equipment has been withdrawn, is this a case of active or passive euthanasia? Or is it a case of euthanasia at all?

Voluntary and Nonvoluntary Euthanasia

Philosophers and other writers on euthanasia have often thought it important to distinguish between *voluntary* and *nonvoluntary* euthanasia. Voluntary euthanasia includes cases in which a person takes his or her own life, either directly or by refusing treatment. But it also includes cases in which a person deputizes another to act in accordance with his wishes. Thus, a person might instruct her family not to permit the use of artificial support systems, should she become unconscious, suffer from brain damage, and be unable to speak for herself. Or a person might request that he be given a lethal injection, after suffering third-degree burns over most of his body and being told that he has virtually no hope of recovery. That the individual explicitly consents to death is a necessary feature of voluntary euthanasia.

Nonvoluntary (or involuntary) euthanasia includes those cases in which the decision about death is not made by the person who is to die. Here the person gives no specific consent or instructions, and the decision is made by family, friends, or physician. The distinction between voluntary and nonvoluntary euthanasia is not always a clear one. Physicians sometimes assume that people are "asking" to die, even when no explicit request has been made. Also the wishes and attitudes that people express when they are *not* in extreme life-threatening medical situations may be too vague for us to be certain that they would choose death when they are in such a situation. Is "I never want to be hooked up to one of those machines" an adequate indication that the person who says this does not want to be put on a respirator should he meet with an accident and fall into a comatose state?

If the distinctions we have made are considered legitimate and relevant, it is clear that there are six cases in which euthanasia becomes a moral decision:

1. Self-administered euthanasia
   a. active
   b. passive
2. Other-administered euthanasia
   a. active and voluntary
   b. active and nonvoluntary
   c. passive and voluntary
   d. passive and nonvoluntary

Even these possibilities do not exhaust the cases that euthanasia presents us with. For example, notice that the voluntary/nonvoluntary distinction does not appear in connection with self-administered euthanasia in our scheme. It might be argued that it should, for a person's decision to end his life (actively or passively) may well not be a wholly voluntary or free decision. People who are severely depressed by their illness and decide to end their lives, for example, might not be thought of as having made a voluntary choice. Hence, one might approve of self-administered voluntary euthanasia, yet think that the nonvoluntary form should not be permitted. It should not be allowed not because it is necessarily morally wrong, but because it would not be a genuine decision by the person. The person might be thought of as suffering from a psychiatric disability.

Ethical Theories

Roman Catholicism explicitly rejects all forms of euthanasia as against the natural law duty to preserve life. It considers euthanasia as morally identical with either suicide or murder. This position is not as rigid as it may seem, however. As we have already seen in the introductory chapter and in the last chapter, the principle of double effect makes it morally acceptable to give medication for the relief of pain—even if the indirect result of the medication will be to shorten the life of the recipient. The intended result is not the death of the person but the relief of suffering. The difference in intention is thus considered to be a morally significant one. Those not accepting the principle of double effect would be likely to classify the administration of a substance that would relieve pain but would also cause death as a case of euthanasia.

Furthermore, on the Catholic view there is no moral obligation to continue treatment when a person is medically hopeless. It is legitimate to allow people to die as a result of their illness or injury, even though their lives might be lengthened by the use of extraordinary means. Additionally, we may legitimately make the same decisions about ourselves that we make about others who are in no condition to decide. Thus, without intending to kill ourselves, we may choose measures for the relief of pain that may secondarily hasten our end. Or we may refuse extraordinary treatment and let "nature" take its course, let "God's will" determine the outcome. (See the introductory chapter for a fuller discussion of the Roman Catholic position on euthanasia and extraordinary means of sustaining life.)

At first sight, utilitarianism would seem to endorse euthanasia in all of its forms. Whenever suffering is great and the condition of the person is one without legitimate medical hope, then the principle of utility might be invoked to approve putting the person to death. After all, in such a case we seem to be acting to end suffering and to bring about a state of affairs in which happiness exceeds unhappiness. Thus, whether the person concerned is ourself or another, euthanasia would seem to be a morally right action.

A utilitarian might argue in this way, but this is not the only way in which the principle of utility might be applied. It could be argued, for example, that since life is a necessary condition for happiness, it is wrong to destroy that condition because, by doing so, the possibility of all future happiness is lost. Furthermore, a rule utilitarian might well argue that a rule like "The taking of a human life is permissible when suffering is intense and the condition of the person permits no legitimate hope" would be open to abuse. Consequently, in the long run the rule would actually work to increase the amount of unhappiness in the world. Obviously, it is not possible to say there is such a thing as "the" utilitarian view of euthanasia. The principle of utility supplies a guide for an answer, but it is not itself an answer.

Euthanasia presents a considerable difficulty for Kant's ethics. For Kant, an autonomous rational being has a duty to preserve his or her life. Thus, one cannot rightly refuse needed medical care or commit suicide. Yet our status as autonomous rational beings also endows us with an inherent dignity. If that status is destroyed or severely compromised, as it is when people become comatose and unknowing because of illness or injury, then it is not certain that we have a duty to maintain our lives under such conditions. It may be more in keeping with our freedom and dignity for us to instruct others either to put us to death or to take no steps to keep us alive should we ever be in such a state. Voluntary euthanasia may be compatible with (if not required by) Kant's ethics.

By a similar line of reasoning, it may be that nonvoluntary euthanasia might be seen as a duty that we have to others. We might argue that by putting to death a comatose and hopeless person we are recognizing the dignity that person possessed in his or her previous state. Also, as we mentioned in the last chapter, it might also be argued that a human being in a vegetative state is not a person in the relevant moral sense. Thus, our ordinary duty to preserve life does not hold.

The view of the moral legitimacy of euthanasia suggested by Rawls's theory was discussed in the introductory chapter and in the introduction to Chapter 2. Some of the implications for euthanasia that follow from Ross's theory are presented by the Brandt essay included in this chapter, and we will briefly mention some of them below.

The Selections

The six selections that make up this chapter represent the diversity of issues and responses the euthanasia problem evokes. Chief Justice Richard J. Hughes, the author of the unanimous decision on the Quinlan case by the New Jersey Supreme Court, supports the claim that a legally based right of privacy permits a patient to decide to refuse medical treatment. Hughes also claims, more controversially, that this right can be exercised by a parent or guardian when the patient herself is in no position to do so. This means, then, that the patient is dependent upon the "best judgment" of others as to what she would wish. In the opinion of the court, removal of life-sustaining equipment would not be a case of homicide (or any other kind of wrongful killing), even if the patient should die as a result. Thus, the court seems to endorse implicitly the principle of double effect.

J. Gay-Williams's "The Wrongfulness of Euthanasia" presents a statement of the conservative view. Gay-Williams defines "euthanasia" as intentionally taking the life of a person who is believed to be suffering from some illness or injury from which recovery cannot reasonably be expected. Gay-Williams rejects passive euthanasia as a *name* for actions that are usually designated by the phrase but seems to approve of the actions themselves. Gay-Williams argues that euthanasia as intentional killing goes against natural law because it violates the natural inclination to preserve life. Furthermore, both self-interest and possible practical consequences of euthanasia provide reasons for rejecting it.

The traditional view that there is an important moral difference between active and passive euthanasia is one accepted by J. Gay-Williams. Active euthanasia involves killing and passive euthanasia letting die, and this fact has led many physicians and philosophers to reject active euthanasia as morally wrong, even while approving of passive euthanasia. James Rachels's essay challenges both the use and moral significance of the distinction. Since both forms of euthanasia result in the death of a person, Rachels argues that active euthanasia ought to be preferred to passive. It is more humane because it allows suffering to be brought to a speedy end. Furthermore, Rachels claims, the distinction itself can be shown to be morally irrelevant. Is there, he asks, any genuine moral difference between drowning a child and merely watching a child drown and doing nothing to save it?

Finally, Rachels attempts to show that the bare fact that there is a difference between killing and letting die doesn't make active euthanasia wrong. Killing of any kind is right or wrong depending on the intentions and circumstances in which it takes place, and if the intentions and circumstances are of a certain kind, then active euthanasia can be morally right.

For these reasons, Rachels suggests that the approval given to the active-passive euthanasia distinction in the Code of Ethics of the American Medical Association is unwise. He encourages physicians to rely upon the distinction only to the extent that they are forced to do so by law but not to give it any significant moral weight. In particular, they should not make use of it when writing new policies or guidelines.

Philippa Foot, as part of her broader concerns in her essay "Euthanasia," develops a distinction between active and passive euthanasia by using the notion of a "right to life." She argues that Rachels's criticisms of the distinction as morally irrelevant and inhumane in application are unsound, and she offers cases to show the value of making and using the distinction.

The basic issue considered by Foot, however, is this one: "Whether it is ever sufficient justification of the choice of the death of another that death can be counted a benefit rather than harm, and that this is why the choice is made." To put the question more directly (although less accurately), Foot asks if we are ever justified in killing people for their own good. In answering this question, Foot analyzes the notion of "ordinary human life" and considers when someone's life might be regarded as not worth living any longer.

But is it legitimate for us to decide when someone else's life is not worth living any longer? Foot thinks not. Everyone has a right to life (in a sense she specifies), and when rights are involved, it is what a person wants that counts. Thus, even if someone would be better off dead, if he wants to live, then we are not justified in killing him. (Nonvoluntary active euthanasia cannot be supported.) Furthermore, if a person both wants to live and has a right to the services of doctors and others, then nonvoluntary passive euthanasia is not justified either.

In the case of those whose wishes we don't know (for example, those in a comatose state), Foot argues that to take the life of such a person would infringe his right. Thus, she rejects nonvoluntary, active euthanasia in such cases. But, she points out, there may be reason to believe, on the basis of generally shared social attitudes at a certain time, that a comatose person probably would not want to be kept alive artificially. Nonvoluntary passive euthanasia may thus sometimes be acceptable.

It is important to notice that although Foot endorses voluntary euthanasia (active and passive) as morally legitimate, she does not claim that we have a *duty* to kill a person who has decided his or her life is no longer worth living. Such a person may not know his own mind, may be depressed, or may be mistaken about his condition, and we may be in a better position to judge whether life is really worthless to him. Thus, for Foot, explicit consent by the person merely guarantees that we would not be infringing his right to life by following his direction to allow him to die.

All writers on euthanasia must, implicitly or explicitly, deal with the moral principle "It is morally wrong to kill innocent human beings." Richard Brandt points out that this form of the principle is more useful as a principle of determining blame than for guiding us in making decisions. He suggests that a more appropriate principle can be based on Ross's statement that we have a strong prima facie obligation not to kill any human being except in justifiable self-defense—unless we have an even stronger prima facie moral obligation to do something that cannot be done without killing.

Another of Ross's prima facie obligations is that we not cause injury to another person. Brandt points out that this opens the possibility, in connection with the prima facie obligation not to kill, that killing is not always an injury. In general, Brandt suggests, I have not injured a person if I treat him in a way that he would want me to if he were fully rational. Someone in an irreversible coma is "beyond injury," Brandt argues. If he has left instructions that in such cases his life should be ended, then we are under a prima facie obligation to do so. If he has left no such instructions, then we may attempt to determine what his wishes would be from what we know about him as a person. We can also use for evidence what we know to be the *rational* choice in the circumstances. Of course, Brandt says, if a person left instructions that his life is to be maintained, if possible, under any circumstances, then we have a prima facie obligation to respect this preference also.

Like so many issues, euthanasia has traditionally been discussed only in the back rooms of medicine. Often decisions about whether to allow a patient to die are made by physicians acting on their own authority. Such decisions do not represent so much an arrogant claim to godlike wisdom as an acknowledgment of the physician's obligation to do what is best for the patient. Most physicians admit that allowing or helping a patient to die is sometimes the best assistance that can be given. Decisions made in this fashion depend on the beliefs and judgment of particular physicians. Because these may differ from those of the patient concerned, it is quite possible that the physician's decision may differ from the wishes of the patient.

The same is the case with hospital policies regulating the practice of euthanasia. Some hospitals regularly note on the charts of certain patients codes that indicate to the staff that those patients are not to be resuscitated. ("DNR"—Do Not Resuscitate—is one such code.) Such policies make no fine discriminations but are frequently applied merely to anyone who happens to be over a certain age—sixty-five, for example.

But covert decisions and secret policies are becoming practices of the past as euthanasia is discussed more widely and openly. Increasingly, people want to be sure that they have some say in what happens to them should they fall victim to hopeless injury or illness.

One indication of this newly developing interest is the California "Natural Death Act," passed by the California legislature on August 30, 1977. The act permits a competent adult to sign a directive that will authorize physicians to withhold or discontinue "mechanical" or "artificial" life-support equipment if the person is judged to be "terminal" and if "death is imminent."

The strength of the legislation is that it allows a person to express in an explicit manner how he or she wishes to be treated before treatment is needed. In this way, the autonomy of the individual is recognized. Even though unconscious or comatose, a person can continue to exert control over his or her life. This, in turn, means that physicians need not—and should not—be the decisive voice in deciding upon the continuation or use of special medical equipment.

But some critics of the law claim that it does not go far enough in protecting autonomy and making death easier, where this is what is wanted. They point out that the directive specified in the law would have made no difference in the case of Karen Quinlan. She had not been diagnosed as having a "terminal condition" at least two weeks prior to being put on a respirator, yet this is one of the requirements of the act. Consequently, the directive would have been irrelevant to her condition.

Nor, for that matter, would those people be allowed to die who wish to, if their disease or injury does not involve treatment by "artificial" or "mechanical" means. Thus, a person suffering from throat cancer would simply have to bear the pain and wait for a "natural" death.

However, in favor of such directives, it should also be said that had J. K. Collums signed the one that is legal in the state of Texas, he could have avoided being attached to a life-support system.

Whatever may be thought of the merits of the Natural Death Act, that it exists at all is a sure indication that more public attention is being given to euthanasia than ever before. Although the California bill was the first of its kind, at present seven other states have also adopted "right-to-die" legislation.

Another sign of change is the recent concern with the medical circumstances in which people die. The medical ideal of a "hospital death," one in which the patient's temperature, pulse rate, and respiration are brought within normal limits by medication and machinery, is being severely challenged. A new ideal of a natural death seems to be emerging. In this view, the kind of support that a dying patient needs is psychological counseling and contact with family and friends, rather than heroic medical efforts.

An acceptance of death as a normal end of life and the development of new means of caring for the dying may ease the problem of euthanasia. If those who are hopeless and near death are offered an alternative to either euthanasia or an all-out medical effort to preserve their lives, they may choose that alternative. "Death with dignity" need not always mean choosing a lethal injection.

In the Matter of Karen Quinlan, an Alleged Incompetent

The Supreme Court of New Jersey

Background Note. The decision of the court was issued on March 31, 1976. It was delivered by Chief Justice Hughes. The following abridgement omits references and case citations.

Constitutional and Legal Issues

I. The Free Exercise of Religion

Simply stated, the right to religious beliefs is absolute but conduct in pursuance thereof is not wholly immune from governmental restraint. So it is that, for the sake of life, courts sometimes (but not always) order blood transfusions for Jehovah's Witnesses (whose religious beliefs abhor such procedure), forbid exposure to death from handling virulent snakes or ingesting poison (interfering with deeply held religious sentiments in such regard), and protect the public health as in the case of compulsory vaccination (over the strongest of religious objections). . . . The Public interest is thus considered paramount, without essential dissolution of respect for religious beliefs.

We think, without further examples, that, ranged against the State's interest in the preservation of life, the impingement of religious belief, much less religious "neutrality" as here, does not reflect a constitutional question, in the circumstances at least of the case presently before the Court. Moreover, like the trial court, we do not recognize an independent parental right of religious freedom to support the relief requested.

II. Cruel and Unusual Punishment

Similarly inapplicable to the case before us is the Constitution's Eighth Amendment protection against cruel and unusual punishment which, as held by the trial court, is not relevant to situations other than the imposition of penal sanctions. Historic in nature, it stemmed from punitive excesses in the infliction of criminal penalties. We find no precedent in law which would justify its extension to the correction of social injustice or hardship, such as, for instance, in the case of poverty. The latter often condemns the poor and deprived to horrendous living conditions which could certainly be described in the abstract as "cruel and unusual punishment." Yet the constitutional base of protection from "cruel and unusual punishment" is plainly irrelevant to such societal ills which must be remedied, if at all, under other concepts of constitutional and civil right.

So it is in the case of the unfortunate Karen Quinlan. Neither the State, nor the law, but the accident of fate and nature, has inflicted upon her conditions which though in essence cruel and most unusual, yet do not amount to "punishment" in any constitutional sense.

Neither the judgment of the court below, nor the medical decision which confronted it, nor the law and equity perceptions which impelled its action, nor the whole factual base upon which it was predicated, inflicted "cruel and unusual punishment" in the constitutional sense.

III. The Right of Privacy

It is the issue of the constitutional right of privacy that has given us most concern, in the exceptional circumstances of this case. Here a loving parent, *qua* parent and raising the rights of his incompetent and profoundly damaged daughter, probably irreversibly doomed to no more than a biologically vegetative remnant of life, is before the court. He seeks authorization to abandon specialized technological procedures which can only maintain for a time a body having no potential for resumption or continuance of other than a "vegetative" existence.

We have no doubt, in these unhappy circumstances, that if Karen were herself miraculously lucid for an interval (not altering the existing prognosis of the condition to which she would soon return) and perceptive of her irreversible condition, she could effectively decide

From In the Matter of Karen Quinlan, an Alleged Incompetent. *Supreme Court of New Jersey, 70 N.J. 10, 355 A. 2d 647.*

upon discontinuance of the life-support apparatus, even if it meant the prospect of natural death. To this extent we may distinguish [a case] which concerned a severely injured young woman (Delores Heston), whose life depended on surgery and blood transfusion; and who was in such extreme shock that she was unable to express an informed choice (although the Court apparently considered the case as if the patient's own religious decision to resist transfusion were at stake), but most importantly a patient apparently salvable to long life and vibrant health;—a situation not at all like the present case.

We have no hesitancy in deciding, in the instant diametrically opposite case, that no external compelling interest of the State could compel Karen to endure the unendurable, only to vegetate a few measurable months with no realistic possibility of returning to any semblance of cognitive or sapient life. We perceive no thread of logic distinguishing between such a choice on Karen's part and a similar choice which, under the evidence in this case, could be made by a competent patient terminally ill, riddled by cancer and suffering great pain; such a patient would not be resuscitated or put on a respirator in the example described by Dr. Korein, and *a fortiori* would not be kept *against his will* on a respirator.

Although the Constitution does not explicitly mention a right of privacy, Supreme Court decisions have recognized that a right of personal privacy exists and that certain areas of privacy are guaranteed under the Constitution. The Court has interdicted judicial intrusion into many aspects of personal decision, sometimes basing this restraint upon the conception of a limitation of judicial interest and responsibility, such as with regard to contraception and its relationship to family life and decision.

The Court in *Griswold* found the unwritten constitutional right of privacy to exist in the penumbra of specific guarantees of the Bill of Rights "formed by emanations from those guarantees that help give them life and substance." Presumably this right is broad enough to encompass a patient's decision to decline medical treatment under certain circumstances, in much the same way as it is broad enough to encompass a woman's decision to terminate pregnancy under certain conditions.

The claimed interests of the State in this case

are essentially the preservation and sanctity of human life and defense to the right of the physician to administer medical treatment according to his best judgment. In this case the doctors say that removing Karen from the respirator will conflict with their professional judgment. The plaintiff answers that Karen's present treatment serves only a maintenance function; that the respirator cannot cure or improve her condition but at best can only prolong her inevitable slow deterioration and death; and that the interests of the patient, as seen by her surrogate, the guardian, must be evaluated by the court as predominant, even in the face of an option *contra* by the present attending physicians. Plaintiff's distinction is significant. The nature of Karen's care and the realistic chances of her recovery are quite unlike those of the patients discussed in many of the cases where treatments were ordered. In many of those cases the medical procedure required (usually a transfusion) constituted a minimal bodily invasion and the chances of recovery and return to functioning life were very good. We think that the State's interest *contra* weakens and the individual's right to privacy grows as the degree of bodily invasion increases and the prognosis dims. Ultimately there comes a point at which the individual's rights overcome the State interest. It is for that reason that we believe Karen's choice, if she were competent to make it, would be vindicated by the law. Her prognosis is extremely poor,—she will never resume cognitive life. And the bodily invasion is very great,—she requires 24-hour intensive nursing care, antibiotics, and the assistance of a respirator, a catheter and feeding tube.

Our affirmance of Karen's independent right of choice, however, would ordinarily be based upon her competency to assert it. The sad truth, however, is that she is grossly incompetent and we cannot discern her supposed choice based on the testimony of her previous conversation with friends, where such testimony is without sufficient probative weight. Nevertheless we have concluded that Karen's right of privacy may be asserted on her behalf by her guardian under the peculiar circumstances here present.

If a putative decision by Karen to permit this non-cognitive, vegetative existence to terminate by natural forces is regarded as a valuable incident of her right of privacy, as we believe it to be, then it should not be discarded solely on the basis that her condition prevents her conscious exercise of the choice. The only practical way to prevent destruction of the right is to permit the guardian and family of Karen to render their best judgment, subject to the qualifications hereinafter stated, as to whether she would exercise it in these circumstances. If their conclusion is in the affirmative this decision should be accepted by a society the overwhelming majority of whose members would, we think, in similar circumstances, exercise such a choice in the same way for themselves or for those closest to them. It is for this reason that we determine that Karen's right of privacy may be asserted in her behalf, in this respect, by her guardian and family under the particular circumstances presented by this record. [Sections IV (Medical Factors), V (Alleged Criminal Liability), and VI (Guardianship of the Person) omitted.]

Declaratory Relief

We thus arrive at the formulation of the declaratory relief which we have concluded is appropriate to this case. Some time has passed since Karen's physical and mental condition was described to the Court. At that time her continuing deterioration was plainly projected. Since the record has not been expanded we assume that she is now even more fragile and nearer to death than she was then. Since her present treating physicians may give reconsideration to her present posture in the light of this opinion, and since we are transferring to the plaintiff as guardian the choice of the attending physician and therefore other physicians may be in charge of the case who may take a different view from that of the present attending physicians, we herewith declare the following affirmative relief on behalf of the plaintiff. Upon the concurrence of the guardian and family of Karen, should the responsible attending physicians conclude that there is no reasonable possibility of Karen's ever emerging from her present comatose condition to a cognitive, sapient state and that the life-support apparatus now being administered to Karen should be discontinued, they shall consult with the hospital "Ethics Committee" or like body of the institution in which Karen is then hospitalized. If that consultative body agrees that there is no reasonable possibility of Karen's ever emerging from her present comatose condition to a cognitive, sapient state, the present life-support system may be withdrawn and said action shall be without any civil or criminal liability therefor on the part of any participant, whether guardian, physician, hospital or others. We herewith specifically so hold.

The Wrongfulness of Euthanasia

J. Gay-Williams

My impression is that euthanasia—the idea, if not the practice—is slowly gaining acceptance within our society. Cynics might attribute this to an increasing tendency to devalue human life, but I do not believe this is the major factor. The acceptance is much more likely to be the result of unthinking sympathy and benevolence. Well-publicized, tragic stories like that of Karen Quinlan elicit from us deep feelings of compassion. We think to ourselves, "She and her family would be better off if she were dead." It is an easy step from this very human response to the view that if someone (and others) would be better off dead, then it must be all right to kill that person.[1] Although I respect the compassion that leads to this conclusion, I believe the conclusion is wrong. I want to show that euthanasia is wrong. It is inherently wrong, but it is also wrong judged from the standpoints of self-interest and of practical effects.

Before presenting my arguments to support this claim, it would be well to define "euthanasia." An essential aspect of euthanasia is that it involves taking a human life, either one's own or that of another. Also, the person whose life is taken must be someone who is believed to be suffering from some disease or injury from which recovery cannot reasonably be expected. Finally, the action must be deliberate and intentional. Thus, euthanasia is intentionally taking the life of a presumably hopeless person. Whether the life is one's own or that of another, the taking of it is still euthanasia.

It is important to be clear about the deliberate and intentional aspect of the killing. If a hopeless person is given an injection of the wrong drug by mistake and this causes his death, this is wrongful killing but not euthanasia. The killing cannot be the result of accident. Furthermore, if the person is given an injection of a drug that is believed to be necessary to treat his disease or better his condition and the person dies as a result, then this is neither wrongful killing nor euthanasia. The intention was to make the patient well, not kill him. Similarly, when a patient's condition is such that it is not reasonable to hope that any medical procedures or treatments will save his life, a failure to implement the procedures or treatments is not euthanasia. If the person dies, this will be as a result of his injuries or disease and not because of his failure to receive treatment.

The failure to continue treatment after it has been realized that the patient has little chance of benefitting from it has been characterized by some as "passive euthanasia." This phrase is misleading and mistaken.[2] In such cases, the person involved is not killed (the first essential aspect of euthanasia), nor is the death of the person intended by the withholding of additional treatment (the third essential aspect of euthanasia). The aim may be to spare the person additional and unjustifiable pain, to save him from the indignities of hopeless manipulations, and to avoid increasing the financial and emotional burden on his family. When I buy a pencil it is so that I can use it to write, not to contribute to an increase in the gross national product. This may be the unintended consequence of my action, but it is not the aim of my action. So it is with failing to continue the treatment of a dying person. I intend his death no more than I intend to reduce the GNP by not using medical supplies. His is an unintended dying, and so-called "passive euthanasia" is not euthanasia at all.

1. The Argument from Nature

Every human being has a natural inclination to continue living. Our reflexes and responses fit us to fight attackers, flee wild animals, and dodge out of the way of trucks. In our daily lives we exercise the caution and care necessary to protect ourselves. Our bodies are similarly structured for survival right down to the molecular level. When we are cut, our capillaries seal shut, our blood clots, and fibrogen is produced to start the process of healing the wound. When we are invaded by bacteria, antibodies are produced to fight against the alien organisms, and their remains are swept out of the body by special cells designed for clean-up work.

Euthanasia does violence to this natural goal of survival. It is literally acting against nature because all the processes of nature are bent towards the end of bodily survival. Euthanasia defeats these subtle mechanisms in a way that, in a particular case, disease and injury might not.

It is possible, but not necessary, to make an appeal to revealed religion in this connection.[3] Man as trustee of his body acts against God, its rightful possessor, when he takes his own life. He also violates the commandment to hold life sacred and never to take it without just and compelling cause. But since this appeal will persuade only those who are prepared to accept that religion has access to revealed truths, I shall not employ this line of argument.

It is enough, I believe, to recognize that the organization of the human body and our patterns of behavioral responses make the continuation of life a natural goal. By reason alone, then, we can recognize that euthanasia sets us against our own nature.[4] Furthermore, in doing so, euthanasia does violence to our dignity. Our dignity comes from seeking our ends. When one of our goals is survival, and actions are taken that eliminate that goal, then our natural dignity suffers. Unlike animals, we are conscious through reason of our nature and our ends. Euthanasia involves acting as if this dual nature—inclination towards survival and awareness of this as an end—did not exist. Thus, euthanasia denies our basic human character and requires that we regard ourselves or others as something less than fully human.

2. The Argument from Self-Interest

The above arguments are, I believe, sufficient to show that euthanasia is inherently wrong. But there are reasons for considering it wrong when judged by standards other than reason. Because death is final and irreversible, euthanasia contains within it the possibility that we will work against our own interest if we practice it or allow it to be practiced on us.

Contemporary medicine has high standards of excellence and a proven record of accomplishment, but it does not possess perfect and complete knowledge. A mistaken diagnosis is possible, and so is a mistaken prognosis. Consequently, we may believe that we are dying of a disease when, as a matter of fact, we may not be. We may think that we have no hope of recovery when, as a matter of fact, our chances are quite good. In such circumstances, if euthanasia were permitted, we would die needlessly. Death is final and the chance of error too great to approve the practice of euthanasia.

Also, there is always the possibility that an experimental procedure or a hitherto untried technique will pull us through. We should at least keep this option open, but euthanasia closes it off. Furthermore, spontaneous remission does occur in many cases. For no apparent reason, a patient simply recovers when those all around him, including his physicians, expected him to die. Euthanasia would just guarantee their expectations and leave no room for the "miraculous" recoveries that frequently occur.

Finally, knowing that we can take our life at any time (or ask another to take it) might well incline us to give up too easily. The will to live is strong in all of us, but it can be weakened by pain and suffering and feelings of hopelessness. If during a bad time we allow ourselves to be killed, we never have a chance to reconsider. Recovery from a serious illness requires that we fight for it, and anything that weakens our determination by suggesting that there is an easy way out is ultimately against our own interest. Also, we may be inclined towards euthanasia because of our concern for others. If we see our sickness and suffering as an emotional and financial burden on our family, we may feel that to leave our life is to make their lives easier.[5] The very presence of the possibility of euthanasia may keep us from surviving when we might.

3. The Argument from Practical Effects

Doctors and nurses are, for the most part, totally committed to saving lives. A life lost is, for them, almost a personal failure, an insult to their skills and knowledge. Euthanasia as a practice might well alter this. It could have a corrupting influence so that in any case that is severe doctors and nurses might not try hard enough to save the patient. They might decide that the patient would simply be "better off dead" and take the steps necessary to make that come about. This attitude could then carry over to their dealings with patients less seriously ill. The result would be an overall decline in the quality of medical care.

Finally, euthanasia as a policy is a slippery slope. A person apparently hopelessly ill may be allowed to take his own life. Then he may be permitted to deputize others to do it for him should he no longer be able to act. The judgment of others then becomes the ruling factor. Already at this point euthanasia is not personal and voluntary, for others are acting "on behalf of" the patient as they see fit. This may well incline them to act on behalf of other patients who have not authorized them to exercise their judgment. It is only a short step, then, from voluntary euthanasia (self-inflicted or authorized), to directed euthanasia administered to a patient who has given no authorization, to involuntary euthanasia conducted as part of a social policy.[6] Recently many psychiatrists and sociologists have argued that we define as "mental illness" those forms of behavior that we disapprove of.[7] This gives us license then to lock up those who display the behavior. The category of the "hopelessly ill" provides the possibility of even worse abuse. Embedded in a social policy, it would give society or its representatives the authority to eliminate all those who might be considered too "ill" to function normally any longer. The dangers of euthanasia are too great to all to run the risk of approving it in any form. The first slippery step may well lead to a serious and harmful fall.

I hope that I have succeeded in showing why the benevolence that inclines us to give approval

of euthanasia is misplaced. Euthanasia is inherently wrong because it violates the nature and dignity of human beings. But even those who are not convinced by this must be persuaded that the potential personal and social dangers inherent in euthanasia are sufficient to forbid our approving it either as a personal practice or as a public policy.

Suffering is surely a terrible thing, and we have a clear duty to comfort those in need and to ease their suffering when we can. But suffering is also a natural part of life with values for the individual and for others that we should not overlook. We may legitimately seek for others and for ourselves an easeful death, as Arthur Dyck has pointed out.[8] Euthanasia, however, is not just an easeful death. It is a wrongful death. Euthanasia is not just dying. It is killing.

Notes

1. For a sophisticated defense of this position see Philippa Foot, "Euthanasia," *Philosophy and Public Affairs*, vol. 6 (1977), pp. 85–112 [see below, pp. 163–74]. Foot does not endorse the radical conclusion that euthanasia, voluntary and involuntary, is always right.

2. James Rachels rejects the distinction between active and passive euthanasia as morally irrelevant in his "Active and Passive Euthanasia," *New England Journal of Medicine*, vol. 292, pp. 78–80. But see the criticism by Foot, pp. 100–103 [pp. 167–69 below].

3. For a defense of this view see J. V. Sullivan, "The Immorality of Euthanasia," in *Beneficent Euthanasia*, ed. Marvin Kohl (Buffalo, New York: Prometheus Books, 1975), pp. 34–44.

4. This point is made by Ray V. McIntyre in "Voluntary Euthanasia: The Ultimate Perversion," *Medical Counterpoint*, vol. 2, pp. 26–29.

5. See McIntyre, p. 28.

6. See Sullivan, "Immorality of Euthanasia," pp. 34–44, for a fuller argument in support of this view.

7. See, for example, Thomas S. Szasz, *The Myth of Mental Illness*, rev. ed. (New York: Harper & Row, 1974).

8. Arthur Dyck, "Beneficent Euthanasia and Benemortasia," Kohl, op. cit., pp. 117–129.

Active and Passive Euthanasia

James Rachels

The distinction between active and passive euthanasia is thought to be crucial for medical ethics. The idea is that it is permissible, at least in some cases, to withhold treatment and allow a patient to die, but it is never permissible to take any direct action designed to kill the patient. This doctrine seems to be accepted by most doctors, and it is endorsed in a statement adopted by the House of Delegates of the American Medical Association on December 4, 1973:

> The intentional termination of the life of one human being by another—mercy killing—is contrary to that for which the medical profession stands and is contrary to the policy of the American Medical Association.
>
> The cessation of the employment of extraordinary means to prolong the life of the body when there is irrefutable evidence that biological death is imminent is the decision of the patient and/or his immediate family. The advice and judgment of the physician should be freely available to the patient and/or his immediate family.

However, a strong case can be made against this doctrine. In what follows I will set out some of the relevant arguments, and urge doctors to reconsider their views on this matter.

To begin with a familiar type of situation, a patient who is dying of incurable cancer of the throat is in terrible pain, which can no longer be satisfactorily alleviated. He is certain to die within a few days, even if present treatment is continued, but he does not want to go on living for those days since the pain is unbearable. So he asks the doctor for an end to it, and his family joins in the request.

Suppose the doctor agrees to withhold treatment, as the conventional doctrine says he

Reprinted by permission from the New England Journal of Medicine 292, *no. 2 (January 9, 1975): 78–80.*

may. The justification for his doing so is that the patient is in terrible agony, and since he is going to die anyway, it would be wrong to prolong his suffering needlessly. But now notice this. If one simply withholds treatment, it may take the patient longer to die, and so he may suffer more than he would if more direct action were taken and a lethal injection given. This fact provides strong reason for thinking that, once the initial decision not to prolong his agony has been made, active euthanasia is actually preferable to passive euthanasia, rather than the reverse. To say otherwise is to endorse the option that leads to more suffering rather than less, and is contrary to the humanitarian impulse that prompts the decision not to prolong his life in the first place.

Part of my point is that the process of being "allowed to die" can be relatively slow and painful, whereas being given a lethal injection is relatively quick and painless. Let me give a different sort of example. In the United States about one in 600 babies is born with Down's syndrome. Most of these babies are otherwise healthy—that is, with only the usual pediatric care, they will proceed to an otherwise normal infancy. Some, however, are born with congenital defects such as intestinal obstructions that require operations if they are to live. Sometimes, the parents and the doctor will decide not to operate, and let the infant die. Anthony Shaw describes what happens then:

> . . . When surgery is denied [the doctor] must try to keep the infant from suffering while natural forces sap the baby's life away. As a surgeon whose natural inclination is to use the scalpel to fight off death, standing by and watching a salvageable baby die is the most emotionally exhausting experience I know. It is easy at a conference, in a theoretical discussion, to decide that such infants should be allowed to die. It is altogether different to stand by in the nursery and watch as dehydration and infection wither a tiny being over hours and days. This is a terrible ordeal for me and the hospital staff—much more so than for the parents who never set foot in the nursery.[1]

I can understand why some people are opposed to all euthanasia, and insist that such infants must be allowed to live. I think I can also understand why other people favor destroying these babies quickly and painlessly. But why should anyone favor letting "dehydration and infection wither a tiny

being over hours and days"? The doctrine that says that a baby may be allowed to dehydrate and wither, but may not be given an injection that would end its life without suffering, seems so patently cruel as to require no further refutation. The strong language is not intended to offend, but only to put the point in the clearest possible way.

My second argument is that the conventional doctrine leads to decisions concerning life and death made on irrelevant grounds.

Consider again the case of the infants with Down's syndrome who need operations for congenital defects unrelated to the syndrome to live. Sometimes, there is no operation, and the baby dies, but when there is no such defect, the baby lives on. Now, an operation such as that to remove an intestinal obstruction is not prohibitively difficult. The reason why such operations are not performed in these cases is, clearly, that the child has Down's syndrome and the parents and doctor judge that because of that fact it is better for the child to die.

But notice that this situation is absurd, no matter what view one takes of the lives and potentials of such babies. If the life of such an infant is worth preserving, what does it matter if it needs a simple operation? Or, if one thinks it better that such a baby should not live on, what difference does it make that it happens to have an unobstructed intestinal tract? In either case, the matter of life and death is being decided on irrelevant grounds. It is the Down's syndrome, and not the intestines, that is the issue. The matter should be decided, if at all, on that basis, and not be allowed to depend on the essentially irrelevant question of whether the intestinal tract is blocked.

What makes this situation possible, of course, is the idea that when there is an intestinal blockage, one can "let the baby die," but when there is no such defect there is nothing that can be done, for one must not "kill" it. The fact that this idea leads to such results as deciding life or death on irrelevant grounds is another good reason why the doctrine should be rejected.

One reason why so many people think that there is an important moral difference between active and passive euthanasia is that they think killing someone is morally worse than letting someone die. But is it? Is killing, in itself, worse than letting die? To investigate this issue, two cases may be considered that are exactly alike except that one involves killing whereas the other involves letting someone die. Then, it can be asked whether this difference makes any difference to the moral assessments. It is important that the cases be exactly alike, except for this one difference, since otherwise one cannot be confident that it is this difference and not some other that accounts for any variation in the assessments of the two cases. So, let us consider this pair of cases:

In the first, Smith stands to gain a large inheritance if anything should happen to his six-year-old cousin. One evening while the child is taking his bath, Smith sneaks into the bathroom and drowns the child, and then arranges things so that it will look like an accident.

In the second, Jones also stands to gain if anything should happen to his six-year-old cousin. Like Smith, Jones sneaks in planning to drown the child in his bath. However, just as he enters the bathroom Jones sees the child slip and hit his head, and fall face down in the water. Jones is delighted; he stands by, ready to push the child's head back under if it is necessary, but it is not necessary. With only a little thrashing about, the child drowns all by himself, "accidentally," as Jones watches and does nothing.

Now Smith killed the child, whereas Jones "merely" let the child die. That is the only difference between them. Did either man behave better, from a moral point of view? If the difference between killing and letting die were in itself a morally important matter, one should say that Jones's behavior was less reprehensible than Smith's. But does one really want to say that? I think not. In the first place, both men acted from the same motive, personal gain, and both had exactly the same end in view when they acted. It may be inferred from Smith's conduct that he is a bad man, although that judgment may be withdrawn or modified if certain further facts are learned about him—for example, that he is mentally deranged. But would not the very same thing be inferred about Jones from his conduct? And would not the same further considerations also be relevant to any modification of this judgment? Moreover, suppose Jones pleaded, in his own defense, "After all, I didn't do anything except just stand there and watch the child drown. I didn't kill him; I only let him die." Again, if letting die were in itself less bad than killing, this defense should have at least some weight. But it does not. Such a "defense" can only be regarded as a grotesque perversion of moral reasoning. Morally speaking, it is no defense at all.

Now, it may be pointed out, quite properly, that the cases of euthanasia with which doctors are concerned are not like this at all. They do not involve personal gain or the destruction of normal healthy children. Doctors are concerned only with cases in which the patient's life is of no further use to him, or in which the patient's life has become or will soon become a terrible burden. However, the point is the same in these cases: the bare difference between killing and letting die does not, in itself, make a moral difference. If a doctor lets a patient die, for humane reasons, he is in the same moral position as if he had given the patient a lethal injection for humane reasons. If his decision was wrong—if, for example, the patient's illness was in fact curable—the decision would be equally regrettable no matter which method was used to carry it out. And if the doctor's decision was the right one, the method used is not in itself important.

The AMA policy statement isolates the crucial issue very well; the crucial issue is "the intentional termination of the life of one human being by another." But after identifying this issue, and forbidding "mercy killing," the statement goes on to deny that the cessation of treatment is the intentional termination of a life. This is where the mistake comes in, for what is the cessation of treatment, in these circumstances, if it is not "the intentional termination of the life of one human being by another"? Of course it is exactly that, and if it were not, there would be no point to it.

Many people will find this judgment hard to accept. One reason, I think, is that it is very easy to conflate the question of whether killing is, in itself, worse than letting die, with the very different question of whether most actual cases of killing are more reprehensible than most actual cases of letting die. Most actual cases of killing are clearly terrible (think, for example, of all the murders reported in the newspapers), and one hears of such cases every day. On the other hand, one hardly ever hears of a case of letting die, except for the actions of doctors who are motivated by humanitarian reasons. So one learns to think of killing in a much worse light than of letting die. But this does not mean that there is something about killing that makes it in itself worse than letting die, for it is not the bare difference between killing and letting die that makes the difference in these cases. Rather, the other factors—the murderer's motive of personal gain, for example, contrasted with the doctor's humanitarian motivation—account for different reactions to the different cases.

I have argued that killing is not in itself any worse than letting die; if my contention is right, it follows that active euthanasia is not any worse than passive euthanasia. What arguments can be given on the other side? The most common, I believe, is the following:

"The important difference between active and passive euthanasia is that, in passive euthanasia, the doctor does not do anything to bring about the patient's death. The doctor does nothing, and the patient dies of whatever ills already afflict him. In active euthanasia, however, the doctor does something to bring about the patient's death: he kills him. The doctor who gives the patient with cancer a lethal injection has himself caused his patient's death; whereas if he merely ceases treatment, the cancer is the cause of the death."

A number of points need to be made here. The first is that it is not exactly correct to say that in passive euthanasia the doctor does nothing, for he does do one thing that is very important: he lets the patient die. "Letting someone die" is certainly different, in some respects, from other types of action—mainly in that it is a kind of action that one may perform by way of not performing certain other actions. For example, one may let a patient die by way of not giving medication, just as one may insult someone by way of not shaking his hand. But for any purpose of moral assessment, it is a type of action nonetheless. The decision to let a patient die is subject to moral appraisal in the same way that a decision to kill him would be subject to moral appraisal: it may be assessed as wise or unwise, compassionate or sadistic, right or wrong. If a doctor deliberately let a patient die who was suffering from a routinely curable illness, the doctor would certainly be to blame for what he had done, just as he would be to blame if he had needlessly killed the patient. Charges against him would then be appropriate. If so, it would be no defense at all for him to insist that he didn't "do anything." He would have done something very serious indeed, for he let his patient die.

Fixing the cause of death may be very important from a legal point of view, for it may determine whether criminal charges are brought against the doctor. But I do not think that this notion can be used to show a moral difference between active and passive euthanasia. The reason why it is considered bad to be the cause of someone's death is that death is regarded as a great evil—and so it is. However, if it has been decided that euthanasia—even passive euthanasia—is desirable in a given case, it has also been decided that in this instance death is no greater an evil than the patient's continued existence. And if this is true, the usual reason for not wanting to be the cause of someone's death simply does not apply.

Finally, doctors may think that all of this is only of academic interest—the sort of thing that philosophers may worry about but that has no practical bearing on their own work. After all, doctors must be concerned about the legal consequences of what they do, and active euthanasia is clearly forbidden by the law. But even so, doctors should also be concerned with the fact that the law is forcing upon them a moral doctrine that may well be indefensible, and has a considerable effect on their practices. Of course, most doctors are not now in the position of being coerced in this matter, for they do not regard themselves as merely going along with what the law requires. Rather, in statements such as the AMA policy statement that I have quoted, they are endorsing this doctrine as a central point of medical ethics. In that statement, active euthanasia is condemned not merely as illegal but as "contrary to that for which the medical profession stands," whereas passive euthanasia is approved. However, the preceding considerations suggest that there is really no moral difference between the two, considered in themselves (there may be important moral differences in some cases in their *consequences*, but, as I pointed out, these differences may make active euthanasia, and not passive euthanasia, the morally preferable option). So, whereas doctors may have to discriminate between active and passive euthanasia to satisfy the law, they should not do any more than that. In particular, they should not give the distinction any added authority and weight by writing it into official statements of medical ethics.

Note

1.   A. Shaw, "Doctor, Do We Have a Choice?" *The New York Times Magazine,* January 30, 1972, p. 54.

Euthanasia

Philippa Foot

1. Defining "Euthanasia"

The widely used *Shorter Oxford English Dictionary* gives three meanings for the word "euthanasia": the first, "a quiet and easy death"; the second, "the means of procuring this"; and the third, "the action of inducing a quiet and easy death." It is a curious fact that no one of the three gives an adequate definition of the word as it is usually understood. For "euthanasia" means much more than a quiet and easy death, or the means of procuring it, or the action of inducing it. The definition specifies only the manner of the death, and if this were all that was implied a murderer, careful to drug his victim, could claim that his act was an act of euthanasia. We find this ridiculous because we take it for granted that in euthanasia it is death itself, not just the manner of death, that must be kind to the one who dies.

To see how important it is that "euthanasia" should not be used as the dictionary definition allows it to be used, merely to signify that a death was quiet and easy, one has only to remember that Hitler's "euthanasia" program traded on this ambiguity. Under this program, planned before the War but brought into full operation by a decree of 1 September 1939, some 275,000 people were gassed in centers which were to be a model for those in which Jews were later exterminated. Anyone in a state institution could be sent to the gas chambers if it was considered that he could not be "rehabilitated" for useful work. As Dr. Leo Alexander reports, relying on the testimony of a neuropathologist who received 500 brains from one of the killing centers,

> In Germany the exterminations included the mentally defective, psychotics (particularly schizophrenics), epileptics and patients suffering from infirmities of old age and from various organic neurological disorders such as infantile paralysis, Parkinsonism, multiple sclerosis and brain tumors. . . . In truth, all those unable to work and considered nonrehabilitable were killed.[1]

These people were killed because they were "useless" and "a burden on society"; only the manner of their deaths could be thought of as relatively easy and quiet.

Let us insist, then, that when we talk about euthanasia we are talking about a death understood as a good or happy event for the one who dies. This stipulation follows etymology, but is itself not exactly in line with current usage, which would be captured by the condition that the death should *not* be an evil rather than that it *should* be a good. That this is how people talk is shown by the fact that the case of Karen Ann Quinlan and others in a state of permanent coma is often discussed under the heading of "euthanasia." Perhaps it is not too late to object to the use of the word "euthanasia" in this sense. Apart from the break with the Greek origins of the word there are other unfortunate aspects of this extension of the term. For if we say that the death must be supposed to be a good to the subject we can also specify that it shall be for his sake that an act of euthanasia is performed. If we say merely that death shall not be an evil to him, we cannot stipulate that benefiting him shall be the motive where euthanasia is in question. Given the importance of the question, For whose sake are we acting? it is good to have a definition of euthanasia which brings under this heading only cases of opting for death for the sake of the one who dies. Perhaps what is most important is to say either that euthanasia is to be for the good of the subject or at least that death is to be no evil to him, thus refusing to talk Hitler's language. However, in this paper it is the first condition that will be understood, with the additional proviso that by an act of euthanasia we mean one of inducing or otherwise opting for death for the sake of the one who is to die.

A few lesser points need to be cleared up. In the first place it must be said that the word "act" is

Philippa Foot, "Euthanasia," Philosophy & Public Affairs, Vol. 6, no. 2 (Winter 1977). Copyright © 1977 by Philippa Foot. Reprinted by permission. Editor's note: This is a selection from the original, and section headings have been added.

not to be taken to exclude omission; we shall speak of an act of euthanasia when someone is deliberately allowed to die, for his own good, and not only when positive measures are taken to see that he does. The very general idea we want is that of a choice of action or inaction directed at another man's death and causally effective in the sense that, in conjunction with actual circumstances, it is a sufficient condition of death. Of complications such as overdetermination, it will not be necessary to speak.

A second, and definitely minor, point about the definition of an act of euthanasia concerns the question of fact versus belief. It has already been implied that one who performs an act of euthanasia thinks that death will be merciful for the subject since we have said that it is on account of this thought that the act is done. But is it enough that he acts with this thought, or must things actually be as he thinks them to be? If one man kills another, or allows him to die, thinking that he is in the last stages of a terrible disease, though in fact he could have been cured, is this an act of euthanasia or not? Nothing much seems to hang on our decision about this. The same condition has got to enter into the definition whether as an element in reality or only as an element in the agent's belief. And however we define an act of euthanasia culpability or justifiability will be the same: if a man acts through ignorance his ignorance may be culpable or it may not.[2]

2. When Is Life Good?

These are relatively easy problems to solve, but one that is dauntingly difficult has been passed over in this discussion of the definition, and must now be faced. It is easy to say, as if this raised no problems, that an act of euthanasia is by definition one aiming at the *good* of the one whose death is in question, and that it is *for his sake* that his death is desired. But how is this to be explained? Presumably we are thinking of some evil already with him or to come on him if he continues to live, and death is thought of as a release from this evil. But this cannot be enough. Most people's lives contain evils such as grief or pain, but we do not therefore think that death would be a blessing to them. On the contrary life is generally supposed to be a good even for someone who is unusually

unhappy or frustrated. How is it that one can ever wish for death for the sake of the one who is to die? This difficult question is central to the discussion of euthanasia, and we shall literally not know what we are talking about if we ask whether acts of euthanasia defined as we have defined them are ever morally permissible without first understanding better the reason for saying that life is a good, and the possibility that it is not always so.

If a man should save my life he would be my benefactor. In normal circumstances this is plainly true; but does one always benefit another in saving his life? It seems certain that he does not. Suppose, for instance, that a man were being tortured to death and was given a drug that lengthened his sufferings; this would not be a benefit but the reverse. Or suppose that in a ghetto in Nazi Germany a doctor saved the life of someone threatened by disease, but that the man once cured was transported to an extermination camp; the doctor might wish for the sake of the patient that he had died of the disease. Nor would a longer stretch of life always be a benefit to the person who was given it. Comparing Hitler's camps with those of Stalin, Dmitri Panin observes that in the latter the method of extermination was made worse by agonies that could stretch out over months.

> Death from a bullet would have been bliss compared with what many millions had to endure while dying of hunger. The kind of death to which they were condemned has nothing to equal it in treachery and sadism.[3]

These examples show that to save or prolong a man's life is not always to do him a service: it may be better for him if he dies earlier rather than later. It must therefore be agreed that while life is normally a benefit to the one who has it, this is not always so.

The judgment is often fairly easy to make—that life is or is not a good to someone—but the basis for it is very hard to find. When life is said to be a benefit or a good, on what grounds is the assertion made? . . .

Do we think that life can be a good to one who suffers a lot of pain? Clearly we do. What about severely handicapped people; can life be a good to them? Clearly it can be, for even if someone is almost completely paralyzed, perhaps living in an iron lung, perhaps able to move things only by means of a tube held between his lips, we do not rule him out order if he says that some benefactor saved his life. Nor is it different with mental handicap. There are many fairly severely handicapped people—such as those with Down's Syndrome (Mongolism)—for whom a simple affectionate life is possible. What about senility? Does this break the normal connection between life and good? Here we must surely distinguish between forms of senility. Some forms leave a life which we count someone as better off having than not having, so that a doctor who prolonged it would benefit the person concerned. With some kinds of senility this is however no longer true. There are some in geriatric wards who are barely conscious, though they can move a little and swallow food put into their mouths. To prolong such a state, whether in the old or in the very severely mentally handicapped, is not to do them a service or confer a benefit. But of course it need not be the reverse: only if there is suffering would one wish for the sake of the patient that he should die.

It seems, therefore, that merely being alive even without suffering is not a good, and that we must make a distinction similar to that which we made when animals were our topic. [The distinction was between merely being alive and operating normally.] But how is the line to be drawn in the case of men? What is to count as ordinary human life in the relevant sense? If it were only the very senile or very ill who were to be said not to have this life it might seem right to describe it in terms of *operation*. But it will be hard to find the sense in which the men described by Panin were not operating, given that they dragged themselves out to the forest to work. What is it about the life that the prisoners were living that makes us put it on the other side of the dividing line from that of some severely ill or suffering patients, and from most of the physically or mentally handicapped? It is not that they were in captivity, for life in captivity can certainly be a good. Nor is it merely the unusual nature of their life. In some ways the prisoners were living more as other men do than the patient in an iron lung. . . .

The suggested solution to the problem is, then, that there is a certain conceptual connection between *life* and *good* in the case of human beings as in that of animals and even plants. Here, as there, however, it is not the mere state of being alive that can determine, or itself count as, a good,

but rather life coming up to some standard of normality. It was argued that it is as part of ordinary life that the elements of good that a man may have are relevant to the question of whether saving his life counts as benefiting him. Ordinary human lives, even very hard lives, contain a minimum of basic goods, but when these are absent the idea of life is no longer linked to that of good. And since it is in this way that the elements of good contained in a man's life are relevant to the question of whether he is benefited if his life is preserved, there is no reason why it should be the balance of good and evil that counts.

It should be added that evils are relevant in one way when, as in the examples discussed above, they destroy the possibility of ordinary goods, but in a different way when they invade a life from which the goods are already absent for a different reason. So, for instance, the connection between *life* and *good* may be broken because consciousness has sunk to a very low level, as in extreme senility or severe brain damage. In itself this kind of life seems to be neither good nor evil, but if suffering sets in one would hope for a speedy end.

The idea we need seems to be that of life which is ordinary human life in the following respect—that it contains a minimum of basic human goods. What is ordinary in human life—even in very hard lives—is that a man is not driven to work far beyond his capacity; that he has the support of a family or community; that he can more or less satisfy his hunger; that he has hopes for the future; that he can lie down to rest at night. Such things were denied to the men in the Vyatlag camps described by Panin; not even rest at night was allowed them when they were tormented by bed-bugs, by noise and stench, and by routines such as body-searches and bath-parades—arranged for the night time so that work norms would not be reduced. Disease too can so take over a man's life that the normal human goods disappear. When a patient is so overwhelmed by pain or nausea that he cannot eat with pleasure, if he can eat at all, and is out of the reach of even the most loving voice, he no longer has ordinary human life in the sense in which the words are used here. And we may now pick up a thread from an earlier part of the discussion by remarking that crippling depression can destroy the enjoyment of ordinary goods as effectively as external circumstances can remove them.

This, admittedly inadequate, discussion of the sense in which life is normally a good, and of the reasons why it may not be so in some particular case, completes the account of what euthanasia is here taken to be. An act of euthanasia, whether literally act or rather omission, is attributed to an agent who opts for the death of another because in his case life seems to be an evil rather than a good. The question now to be asked is whether acts of euthanasia are ever justifiable. But there are two topics here rather than one. For it is one thing to say that some acts of euthanasia considered only in themselves and their results are morally unobjectionable, and another to say that it would be all right to legalize them. Perhaps the practice of euthanasia would allow too many abuses, and perhaps there would be too many mistakes. Moreover the practice might have very important and highly undesirable side effects, because it is unlikely that we could change our principles about the treatment of the old and the ill without changing fundamental emotional attitudes and social relations. The topics must, therefore, be treated separately. In the next part of the discussion, nothing will be said about the social consequences and possible abuses of the practice of euthanasia, but only about acts of euthanasia considered in themselves.

What we want to know is whether acts of euthanasia, defined as we have defined them, are ever morally permissible. To be more accurate, we want to know whether it is ever sufficient justification of the choice of death for another that death can be counted a benefit rather than harm, and that this is why the choice is made.

3. Justice and Charity

It will be impossible to get a clear view of the area to which this topic belongs without first marking the distinct grounds on which objection may lie when one man opts for the death of another. There are two different virtues whose requirements are, in general, contrary to such actions. An unjustified act of killing, or allowing to die, is contrary to justice or to charity, or to both virtues, and the moral failings are distinct. Justice has to do with what men *owe* each other in the way of noninterference and positive service. When used in this wide sense, which has its history in the doctrine of the cardinal virtues, justice is not especially connected with, for instance, law courts

but with the whole area of rights, and duties corresponding to rights. Thus murder is one form of injustice, dishonesty another, and wrongful failure to keep contracts a third; chicanery in a law court or defrauding someone of his inheritance are simply other cases of injustice. Justice as such is not directly linked to the good of another, and may require that something be rendered to him even where it will do him harm, as Hume pointed out when he remarked that a debt must be paid even to a profligate debauchee who "would rather receive harm than benefit from large possessions."[5] Charity, on the other hand is the virtue which attaches us to the good of others. An act of charity is in question only where something is not demanded by justice, but a lack of charity and of justice can be shown where a man is denied something which he both needs and has a right to; both charity and justice demand that widows and orphans are not defrauded, and the man who cheats them is neither charitable nor just.

It is easy to see that the two grounds of objection to inducing death are distinct. A murder is an act of injustice. A culpable failure to come to the aid of someone whose life is threatened is normally contrary, not to justice, but to charity. But where one man is under contract, explicit or implicit, to come to the aid of another injustice too will be shown. Thus injustice may be involved either in an act or an omission, and the same is true of a lack of charity; charity may demand that someone be aided, but also that an unkind word not be spoken.

The distinction between charity and justice will turn out to be of the first importance when voluntary and nonvoluntary euthanasia are distinguished later on. This is because of the connection between justice and rights, and something should now be said about this. I believe it is true to say that wherever a man acts unjustly he has infringed a right, since justice has to do with whatever a man is owed, and whatever he is owed is his as a matter of right. Something should therefore be said about the different kinds of rights. The distinction commonly made is between having a right in the sense of having a liberty, and having a "claim-right" or "right of recipience."[6] The best way to understand such a distinction seems to be as follows. To say that a man has a right in the sense of a liberty is to say that no one can demand that he do not do the thing which he has a right to do. The fact that he has a right to do it consists in the fact that a certain kind of objection does not lie against his doing it. Thus a man has a right in this sense to walk down a public street or park his car in a public parking space. It does not follow that no one else may prevent him from doing so. If for some reason I want a certain man not to park in a certain place I may lawfully park there myself or get my friends to do so, thus preventing him from doing what he has a right (in the sense of a liberty) to do. It is different, however, with a claim-right. This is the kind of right which I have in addition to a liberty when, for example, I have a private parking space; now others have duties in the way of noninterference, as in this case, or of service, as in the case where my claim-right is to goods or services promised to me. Sometimes one of these rights gives other people the duty of securing to me that to which I have a right, but at other times their duty is merely to refrain from interference. If a fall of snow blocks my private parking space there is normally no obligation for anyone else to clear it away. Claim rights generate duties; sometimes these duties are duties of noninterference; sometimes they are duties of service. If your right gives me the duty not to interfere with you I have "no right" to do it; similarly, if your right gives me the duty to provide something for you I have "no right" to refuse to do it. What *I* lack is the right which is a liberty; I am not "at liberty" to interfere with you or to refuse the service.

4. Right to Life

Where in this picture does the right to life belong? No doubt people have the right to live in the sense of a liberty, but what is important is the cluster of claim-rights brought together under the title of the right to life. The chief of these is, of course, the right to be free from interferences that threaten life. If other people aim their guns at us or try to pour poison into our drink we can, to put it mildly, demand that they desist. And then there are the services we can claim from doctors, health officers, bodyguards, and firemen; the rights that depend on contract or public arrangement. Perhaps there is no particular point in saying that the duties these people owe us belong to the right to life; we might as well say that all the services owed to anyone by tailors, dressmakers, and couturiers belong to a right called the right to be elegant. But contracts such as those understood in

the patient-doctor relationship come in in an important way when we are discussing the rights and wrongs of euthanasia, and are therefore mentioned here. . . .

Let us now ask how the right to life affects the morality of acts of euthanasia. Are such acts sometimes or always ruled out by the right to life? This is certainly a possibility; for although an act of euthanasia is, by our definition, a matter of opting for death for the good of the one who is to die, there is, as we noted earlier, no direct connection between that to which a man has a right and that which is for his good. It is true that men have the right only to the kind of thing that is, in general, a good: we do not think that people have the right to garbage or polluted air. Nevertheless, a man may have the right to something which he himself would be better off without; where rights exist it is a man's will that counts, not his or anyone else's estimate of benefit or harm. So the duties complementary to the right to life—the general duty of noninterference and the duty of service incurred by certain persons—are not affected by the quality of a man's life or by his prospects. Even if it is true that he would be, as we say, "better off dead," so long as he wants to live this does not justify us in killing him and may not justify us in deliberately allowing him to die. All of us have the duty of noninterference, and some of us may have the duty to sustain his life. Suppose, for example, that a retreating army has to leave behind wounded or exhausted soldiers in the wastes of an arid or snowbound land where the only prospect is death by starvation or at the hands of an enemy notoriously cruel. It has often been the practice to accord a merciful bullet to men in such desperate straits. But suppose that one of them demands that he should be left alive? It seems clear that his comrades have no right to kill him, though it is a quite different question as to whether they should give him a life-prolonging drug. The right to life can sometimes give a duty of positive service, but does not do so here. What it does give is the right to be left alone.

5. Active and Passive Euthanasia

Interestingly enough we have arrived by way of a consideration of the right to life at the distinction normally labeled "active" versus "passive" euthanasia, and often thought to be irrelevant to the moral issue.[7] Once it is seen that the right to life is a distinct ground of objection to certain acts of euthanasia, and that this right creates a duty of noninterference more widespread than the duties of care there can be no doubt about the relevance of the distinction between passive and active euthanasia. Where everyone may have the duty to leave someone alone, it may be that no one has the duty to maintain his life, or that only some people do.

Where then do the boundaries of the "active" and "passive" lie? In some ways the words are themselves misleading, because they suggest the difference between act and omission which is not quite what we want. Certainly the act of shooting someone is the kind of thing we were talking about under the heading of "interference," and omitting to give him a drug a case of refusing care. But the act of turning off a respirator should surely be thought of as no different from the decision not to start it; if doctors had decided that a patient should be allowed to die, either course of action might follow, and both should be counted as passive rather than active euthanasia if euthanasia were in question. The point seems to be that interference in a course of treatment is not the same as other interference in a man's life, and particularly if the same body of people are responsible for the treatment and for its discontinuance. In such a case we could speak of the disconnecting of the apparatus as killing the man, or of the hospital as allowing him to die. By and large, it is the act of killing that is ruled out under the heading of noninterference, but not in every case.

Doctors commonly recognize this distinction, and the grounds on which some philosophers have denied it seem untenable. James Rachels, for instance, believes that if the difference between active and passive is relevant anywhere, it should be relevant everywhere, and he has pointed to an example in which it seems to make no difference which is in question. If someone saw a child drowning in a bath it would seem just as bad to let it drown as to push its head under water.[7] If "it makes no difference" means that one act would be as iniquitous as the other this is true. It is not that killing is *worse* than allowing to die, but that the two are contrary to distinct virtues, which gives the possibility that in some circumstances one is impermissible and the other permissible. In the circumstances invented by Rachels, both are

wicked: it is contrary to justice to push the child's head under the water—something one has no right to do. To leave it to drown is not contrary to justice, but it is a particularly glaring example of lack of charity. Here it makes no practical difference because the requirements of justice and charity coincide; but in the case of the retreating army they did not: charity would have required that the wounded soldier be killed had not justice required that he be left alive.[8] In such a case it makes all the difference whether a man opts for the death of another in a positive action, or whether he allows him to die. An analogy with the right to property will make the point clear. If a man owns something he has the right to it even when its possession does him harm, and we have no right to take it from him. But if one day it should blow away, maybe nothing requires us to get it back for him; we could not deprive him of it, but we may allow it to go. This is not to deny that it will often be an unfriendly act or one based on an arrogant judgment when we refuse to do what he wants. Nevertheless, we would be within our rights, and it might be that no moral objection of any kind would lie against our refusal.

It is important to emphasize that a man's rights may stand between us and the action we would dearly like to take for his sake. They may, of course, also prevent action which we would like to take for the sake of others, as when it might be tempting to kill one man to save several. But it is interesting that the limits of allowable interference, however uncertain, seem stricter in the first case than the second. Perhaps there are no cases in which it would be all right to kill a man against his will *for his own sake* unless they could equally well be described as cases of allowing him to die, as in the example of turning off the respirator. However, there are circumstances, even if these are very rare, in which one man's life would justifiably be sacrificed to save others, and "killing" would be the only description of what was being done. For instance, a vehicle which had gone out of control might be steered from a path on which it would kill more than one man to a path on which it would kill one.[9] But it would not be permissible to steer a vehicle towards someone in order to kill him, against his will, for his own good. An analogy with property rights illustrates the point. One may not destroy a man's property against his will on the grounds that he would be better off without it; there are however circumstances in which it could be destroyed for the sake of others. If his house is liable to fall and kill him that is his affair; it might, however, without injustice be destroyed to stop the spread of a fire.

We see then that the distinction between active and passive, important as it is elsewhere, has a special importance in the area of euthanasia. It should also be clear why James Rachels' other argument, that it is often "more humane" to kill than to allow to die, does not show that the distinction between active and passive euthanasia is morally irrelevant. It might be "more humane" in this sense to deprive a man of the property that brings evils on him, or to refuse to pay what is owed to Hume's profligate debauchee; but if we say this we must admit that an act which is "more humane" than its alternative may be morally objectionable because it infringes rights.

6. Right to Service

So far we have said very little about the right to service as opposed to the right to noninterference, though it was agreed that both might be brought under the heading of "the right to life." What about the duty to preserve life that may belong to special classes of persons such as bodyguards, firemen, or doctors? Unlike the general public they are not within their rights if they merely refrain from interfering and do not try to sustain life. The subject's claim-rights are two-fold as far as they are concerned and passive as well as active euthanasia may be ruled out here if it is against his will. This is not to say that he has the right to any and every service needed to save or prolong his life; the rights of other people set limits to what may be demanded, both because they have the right not to be interfered with and because they may have a competing right to services. Furthermore one must inquire just what the contract or implicit agreement amounts to in each case. Firemen and bodyguards presumably have a duty which is simply to preserve life, within the limits of justice to others and of reasonableness to themselves. With doctors it may however be different, since their duty relates not only to preserving life but also to the relief of suffering. It is not clear what a doctor's duties are to his patient if life can be prolonged only at the cost of suffering or suffering relieved only by

measures that shorten life. George Fletcher has argued that what the doctor is under contract to do depends on what is generally done, because this is what a patient will reasonably expect.[10] This seems right. If procedures are part of normal medical practice then it seems that the patient can demand them however much it may be against his interest to do so. Once again it is not a matter of what is "most humane."

That the patient's right to life may set limits to permissible acts of euthanasia seems undeniable. If he does not want to die no one has the right to practice active euthanasia on him, and passive euthanasia may also be ruled out where he has a right to the services of doctors or others.

Perhaps few will deny what has so far been said about the impermissibility of acts of euthanasia, simply because we have so far spoken about the case of one who positively wants to live, and about his rights, whereas those who advocate euthanasia are usually thinking either about those who wish to die or about those whose wishes cannot be ascertained either because they cannot properly be said to have wishes or because, for one reason or another, we are unable to form a reliable estimate of what they are. The question that must now be asked is whether the latter type of case, where euthanasia though not involuntary would again be nonvoluntary, is different from the one discussed so far. Would we have the right to kill someone for his own good so long as we had no idea that he positively wished to live? And what about the life-prolonging duties of doctors in the same circumstances? This is a very difficult problem. On the one hand, it seems ridiculous to suppose that a man's right to life is something which generates duties only where he has signalled that he wants to live; as a borrower does indeed have a duty to return something lent on indefinite loan only if the lender indicates that he wants it back. On the other hand, it might be argued that there is something illogical about the idea that a right has been infringed if someone incapable of saying whether he wants it or not is deprived of something that is doing him harm rather than good. Yet on the analogy of property we would say that a right has been infringed. Only if someone had earlier told us that in such circumstances he would not want to keep the thing could we think that his right had been waived. Perhaps if we could make confident judgments about what anyone in such circumstances would wish, or what he would have wished beforehand had he considered the matter, we could agree to consider the right to life as "dormant," needing to be asserted if the normal duties were to remain. But as things are we cannot make any such assumption; we simply do not know what most people would want, or would have wanted, us to do unless they tell us. This is certainly the case so far as active measures to end life are concerned. Possibly it is different, or will become different, in the matter of being kept alive, so general is the feeling against using sophisticated procedures on moribund patients, and so much is this dreaded by people who are old or terminally ill. Once again the distinction between active and passive euthanasia has come on the scene, but this time because most people's attitudes to the two are so different. It is just possible that we might presume, in the absence of specific evidence, that someone would not wish, beyond a certain point, to be kept alive; it is certainly not possible to assume that he would wish to be killed.

7. Voluntary Euthanasia

In the last paragraph we have begun to broach the topic of voluntary euthanasia, and this we must now discuss. What is to be said about the case in which there is no doubt about someone's wish to die: either he has told us beforehand that he would wish it in circumstances such as he is now in, and has shown no sign of a change of mind, or else he tells us now, being in possession of his faculties and of a steady mind. We should surely say that the objections previously urged against acts of euthanasia, which it must be remembered were all on the ground of rights, had disappeared. It does not seem that one would infringe someone's right to life in killing him with his permission and in fact at his request. Why should someone not be able to waive his right to life, or rather, as would be more likely to happen, to cancel some of the duties of noninterference that this right entails? (He is more likely to say that he should be killed by this man at this time in this manner, than to say that anyone may kill him at any time and in any way.) Similarly someone may give permission for the destruction of his property, and request it. The important thing is that he gives a critical permission, and it seems

that this is enough to cancel the duty normally associated with the right. If someone gives you permission to destroy his property it can no longer be said that you have no right to do so, and I do not see why it should not be the case with taking a man's life. An objection might be made on the ground that only God has the right to take life, but in this paper religious as opposed to moral arguments are being left aside. Religion apart, there seems to be no case to be made out for an infringement of rights if a man who wishes to die is allowed to die or even killed. But of course it does not follow that there is no moral objection to it. Even with property, which is after all a relatively small matter, one might be wrong to destroy what one had the right to destroy. For, apart from its value to other people, it might be valuable to the man who wanted it destroyed, and charity might require us to hold our hand where justice did not.

8. The Morality of Euthanasia

Let us review the conclusion of this part of the argument, which has been about euthanasia and the right to life. It has been argued that from this side come stringent restrictions on the acts of euthanasia that could be morally permissible. Active nonvoluntary euthanasia is ruled out by that part of the right to life which creates the duty of noninterference though passive nonvoluntary euthanasia is not ruled out, except where the right to life-preserving action has been created by some special condition such as a contract between a man and his doctor, and it is not always certain just what such a contract involves. Voluntary euthanasia is another matter: as the preceding paragraph suggested, no right is infringed if a man is allowed to die or even killed at his own request.

Turning now to the other objection that normally holds against inducing the death of another, that it is against charity, or benevolence, we must tell a very different story. Charity is the virtue that gives attachment to the good of others, and because life is normally a good, charity normally demands that it should be saved or prolonged. But as we so defined an act of euthanasia that it seeks a man's death for his own sake—for his good—charity will normally speak in favor of it. This is not, of course, to say that charity can require an act of euthanasia which justice forbids, but if an act of euthanasia is not contrary to justice—that is, it does not infringe rights—charity will rather be in its favor than against.

Once more the distinction between nonvoluntary and voluntary euthanasia must be considered. Could it ever be compatible with charity to seek a man's death although he wanted to live, or at least had not let us know that he wanted to die? It has been argued that in such circumstances active euthanasia would infringe his right to life, but passive euthanasia would not do so, unless he had some special right to life-preserving service from the one who allowed him to die. What would charity dictate? Obviously when a man wants to live there is a presumption that he will be benefited if his life is prolonged, and if it is so the question of euthanasia does not arise. But it is, on the other hand, possible that he wants to live where it would be better for him to die: perhaps he does not realize the desperate situation he is in, or perhaps he is afraid of dying. So, in spite of a very proper resistance to refusing to go along with a man's own wishes in the matter of life and death, someone might justifiably refuse to prolong the life even of someone who asked him to prolong it, as in the case of refusing to give the wounded soldier a drug that would keep him alive to meet a terrible end. And it is even more obvious that charity does not always dictate that life should be prolonged where a man's own wishes, hypothetical or actual, are not known.

So much for the relation of charity to nonvoluntary passive euthanasia, which was not, like nonvoluntary active euthanasia, ruled out by the right to life. Let us now ask what charity has to say about voluntary euthanasia both active and passive. It was suggested in the discussion of justice that if of sound mind and steady desire a man might give others the *right* to allow him to die or even to kill him, where otherwise this would be ruled out. But it was pointed out that this would not settle the question of whether the act was morally permissible, and it is this that we must now consider. Could not charity speak against what justice allowed? Indeed it might do so. For while the fact that a man wants to die suggests that his life is wretched, and while his rejection of life may itself tend to take the good out of the things he might have enjoyed, nevertheless his wish to die might here be opposed for his own sake just as

it might be if suicide were in question. Perhaps there is hope that his mental condition will improve. Perhaps he is mistaken in thinking his disease incurable. Perhaps he wants to die for the sake of someone else on whom he feels he is a burden, and we are not ready to accept this sacrifice whether for ourselves or others. In such cases, and there will surely be many of them, it could not be for his own sake that we kill him or allow him to die, and therefore euthanasia as defined in this paper would not be in question. But this is not to deny that there could be acts of voluntary euthanasia both passive and active against which neither justice nor charity would speak.

We have now considered the morality of euthanasia both voluntary and nonvoluntary, and active and passive. The conclusion has been that nonvoluntary active euthanasia (roughly, killing a man against his will or without his consent) is never justified; that is to say, that a man's being killed for his own good never justifies the act unless he himself has consented to it. A man's rights are infringed by such an action, and it is therefore contrary to justice. However, all the other combinations, nonvoluntary passive euthanasia, voluntary active euthanasia, and voluntary passive euthanasia are sometimes compatible with both justice and charity. But the strong condition carried in the definition of euthanasia adopted in this paper must not be forgotten; an act of euthanasia as here understood is one whose purpose is to benefit the one who dies.

9. Present Practices

In the light of this discussion let us look at our present practices. Are they good or are they bad? And what changes might be made, thinking now not only of the morality of particular acts of euthanasia but also of the indirect effects of instituting different practices, of the abuses to which they might be subject and of the changes that might come about if euthanasia became a recognized part of the social scene.

The first thing to notice is that it is wrong to ask whether we should introduce the practice of euthanasia as if it were not something we already had. In fact we do have it. For instance it is common, where the medical prognosis is very bad, for doctors to recommend against measures to prolong life, and particularly where a process of degeneration producing one medical emergency after another has already set in. If these doctors are not certainly within their legal rights this is something that is apt to come as a surprise to them as to the general public. It is also obvious that euthanasia is often practiced where old people are concerned. If someone very old and soon to die is attacked by a disease that makes his life wretched, doctors do not always come in with life-prolonging drugs. Perhaps poor patients are more fortunate in this respect than rich patients, being more often left to die in peace; but it is in any case a well recognized piece of medical practice, which is a form of euthanasia.

No doubt the case of infants with mental or physical defects will be suggested as another example of the practice of euthanasia as we already have it, since such infants are sometimes deliberately allowed to die. That they are deliberately allowed to die is certain; children with severe spina bifida malformations are not always operated on even where it is thought that without the operation they will die; and even in the case of children with Down's Syndrome who have intestinal obstructions the relatively simple operation that would make it possible to feed them is sometimes not performed.[11] Whether this is euthanasia in our sense or only as the Nazis understood it is another matter. We must ask the crucial question, "Is it for the sake of the child himself that the doctors and parents choose his death?" In some cases the answer may really be yes, and what is more important it may really be true that the kind of life which is a good is not possible or likely for this child, and that there is little but suffering and frustration in store for him.[12] But this must presuppose that the medical prognosis is wretchedly bad, as it may be for some spina bifida children. With children who are born with Down's Syndrome it is, however, quite different. Most of these are able to live on for quite a time in a reasonably contented way, remaining like children all their lives but capable of affectionate relationships and able to play games and perform simple tasks. The fact is, of course, that the doctors who recommend against life-saving procedures for handicapped infants are usually thinking not of them but rather of their parents and of other children in the family or of the "burden on society" if the children survive. So it is not for

their sake but to avoid trouble to others that they are allowed to die. When brought out into the open this seems unacceptable: at least we do not easily accept the principle that adults who need special care should be counted too burdensome to be kept alive. It must in any case be insisted that if children with Down's Syndrome are deliberately allowed to die this is not a matter of euthanasia except in Hitler's sense. And for our children, since we scruple to gas them, not even the manner of their death is "quiet and easy"; when not treated for an intestinal obstruction a baby simply starves to death. Perhaps some will take this as an argument for allowing active euthanasia, in which case they will be in the company of an S.S. man stationed in the Warthgenau who sent Eichmann a memorandum telling him that "Jews in the coming winter could no longer be fed" and submitting for his consideration a proposal as to whether "it would not be the most humane solution to kill those Jews who were incapable of work through some quicker means."[13] If we say we are *unable* to look after children with handicaps we are no more telling the truth than was the S.S. man who said that the Jews could not be fed.

Nevertheless if it is ever right to allow deformed children to die because life will be a misery to them, or not to take measures to prolong for a little the life of a newborn baby whose life cannot extend beyond a few months of intense medical intervention, there is a genuine problem about active as opposed to passive euthanasia. There are well-known cases in which the medical staff has looked on wretchedly while an infant died slowly from starvation and dehydration because they did not feel able to give a lethal injection. According to the principles discussed in the earlier part of this paper they would indeed have had no right to give it, since an infant cannot ask that it should be done. The only possible solution—supposing that voluntary active euthanasia were to be legalized—would be to appoint guardians to act on the infant's behalf. In a different climate of opinion this might not be dangerous, but at present, when people so readily assume that the life of a handicapped baby is of no value, one would be loath to support it.

Finally, on the subject of handicapped children, another word should be said about those with severe mental defects. For them too it might sometimes be right to say that one would wish for death for their sake. But not even severe mental handicap automatically brings a child within the scope even of a possible act of euthanasia. If the level of consciousness is low enough it could not be said that life is a good to them, any more than in the case of those suffering from extreme senility. Nevertheless if they do not suffer it will not be an act of euthanasia by which someone opts for their death. Perhaps charity does not demand that strenuous measures are taken to keep people in this state alive, but euthanasia does not come into the matter, any more than it does when someone is, like Karen Ann Quinlan, in a state of permanent coma. Much could be said about this last case. It might even be suggested that in the case of unconsciousness this "life" is not the life to which "the right to life" refers. But that is not our topic here.

What we must consider, even if only briefly, is the possibility that euthanasia, genuine euthanasia, and not contrary to the requirements of justice or charity, should be legalized over a wider area. Here we are up against the really serious problem of abuse. Many people want, and want very badly, to be rid of their elderly relatives and even of their ailing husbands or wives. Would any safeguards ever be able to stop them describing as euthanasia what was really for their own benefit? And would it be possible to prevent the occurrence of acts which were genuinely acts of euthanasia but morally impermissible because infringing the rights of a patient who wished to live?

Perhaps the furthest we should go is to encourage patients to make their own contracts with a doctor by making it known whether they wish him to prolong their life in case of painful terminal illness or of incapacity. A document such as the Living Will seems eminently sensible, and should surely be allowed to give a doctor following the previously expressed wishes of the patient immunity from legal proceedings by relatives.[14] Legalizing active euthanasia is, however, another matter. Apart from the special repugnance doctors feel towards the idea of a lethal injection, it may be of the very greatest importance to keep a psychological barrier up against killing. Moreover it is active euthanasia which is the most liable to abuse. Hitler would not have been able to kill 275,000 people in his "euthanasia" program if he had had to wait for them to need life-saving treatment. But there are other objections to active euthanasia, even voluntary active euthanasia. In the first place it would be hard to devise procedures that would protect people from being persuaded into giving their consent. And secondly the possibility of active voluntary euthanasia might change the social scene in ways that would be very bad. As things are, people do, by and large, expect to be looked after if they are old or ill. This is one of the good things that we have, but we might lose it, and be much worse off without it. It might come to be expected that someone likely to need a lot of looking after should call for the doctor and demand his own death. Something comparable could be good in an extremely poverty-stricken community where the children genuinely suffered from lack of food; but in rich societies such as ours it would surely be a spiritual disaster. Such possibilities should make us very wary of supporting large measures of euthanasia, even where moral principle applied to the individual act does not rule it out.

Notes

I would like to thank Derek Parfit and the editors of *Philosophy & Public Affairs* for their very helpful comments.

1. Leo Alexander, "Medical Science under Dictatorship," *New England Journal of Medicine*, 14 July 1949, p. 40.

2. For a discussion of culpable and nonculpable ignorance see Thomas Aquinas, *Summa Theologica*, First Part of the Second Part, Question 6, article 8, and Question 19, articles 5 and 6.

3. Dmitri Panin, *The Notebooks of Sologdin* (London, 1976), pp. 66–67.

4. David Hume, *Treatise*, Book III, Part II, Section 1.

5. See, for example D. D. Raphael, "Human Rights Old and New," in D. D. Raphael, ed., *Political Theory and the Rights of Man* (London, 1967), and Joel Feinberg, "The Nature and Value of Rights," *The Journal of Value Inquiry* 4, no. 4 (Winter 1970): 243–257. Reprinted in Samuel Gorovitz, ed., *Moral Problems in Medicine* (Englewood Cliffs, New Jersey, 1976).

6. See, for example, James Rachels, "Active and Passive Euthanasia," *New England Journal of Medicine* 292, no. 2 (9 Jan. 1975): 78–80.

7. Ibid.

8. It is not, however, that justice and charity conflict. A man does not lack charity because he refrains from an act of injustice which would have been for someone's good.

9. For a discussion of such questions, see my article "The Problem of Abortion and the Doctrine of Double Effect," *Oxford Review*, no. 5 (1967); reprinted in Rachels, *Moral Problems*, and Gorovitz, *Moral Problems in Medicine*.

10. *George Fletcher,* "Legal Aspects of the Decision not to Prolong Life," *Journal of the American Medical Association* 203, no. 1 (1 Jan. 1968): 119–122. Reprinted in Gorovitz.

11. I have been told this by a pediatrician in a well-known medical center in the United States. It is confirmed by Anthony M. Shaw and Iris A. Shaw, "Dilemma of Informed Consent in Children," *The New England Journal of Medicine* 289, no. 17 (25 Oct. 1973): 885–890. Reprinted in Gorovitz.

12. It must be remembered, however, that many of the social miseries of spina bifida children could be avoided. Professor R. B. Zachary is surely right to insist on this. See, for example, "Ethical and Social Aspects of Spina Bifida," *The Lancet,* 3 Aug. 1968, pp. 274–276. Reprinted in Gorovitz.

13. Quoted by Hannah Arendt, *Eichmann in Jerusalem* (London 1963), p. 90.

14. Details of this document are to be found in J. A. Behnke and Sissela Bok, eds., *The Dilemmas of Euthanasia* (New York, 1975), and in A. B. Downing, ed., *Euthanasia and the Right to Life: The Case for Voluntary Euthanasia* (London, 1969).

A Moral Principle About Killing

Richard Brandt

One of the Ten Commandments states: "Thou shalt not kill." The commandment does not supply an object for the verb, but the traditional Catholic view has been that the proper object of the verb is "innocent human beings" (except in cases of extreme necessity), where "innocent" is taken to exclude persons convicted of a capital crime or engaged in an unjust assault aimed at killing, such as members of the armed forces of a country prosecuting an unjust war. Thus construed, the prohibition is taken to extend to suicide and abortion. (There is a qualification: that we are not to count cases in which the death is not wanted for itself or intended as a *means* to a goal that is wanted for itself, provided that in either case the aim of the act is the avoidance of some evil greater than the death of the person.) Can this view that all killing of innocent human beings is morally wrong be defended, and if not, what alternative principle can be?

This question is one the ground rules for answering which are far from a matter of agreement. I should myself be content if a principle were identified that could be shown to be one that would be included in any moral system that rational and benevolent persons would support for a society in which they expected to live. Apparently others would not be so content; so in what follows I shall simply aim to make some observations that I hope will identify a principle with which the consciences of intelligent people will be comfortable. I believe the rough principle I will suggest is also one that would belong to the moral system rational and benevolent people would want for their society.

Let us begin by reflecting on what it is to kill. The first thing to notice is that *kill* is a biological term. For example, a weed may be killed by being sprayed with a chemical. The verb *kill* involves essentially the broad notion of death—the change from the state of being biologically alive to the state of being dead. It is beyond my powers to give any general characterization of this transition, and it may be impossible to give one. If there is one, it is one that human beings, flies, and ferns all share; and to kill is in some sense to bring that transition about. The next thing to notice is that at least human beings do not live forever, and hence killing a human being at a given time must be construed as *advancing the date* of its death, or as *shortening its life*. Thus it may be brought about that the termination of the life of a person occurs at the time t instead of at the time $t + k$. Killing is thus shortening the span of organic life of something.

There is a third thing to notice about *kill*. It is a term of causal agency and has roots in the legal tradition. As such, it involves complications. For instance, suppose I push a boulder down a mountainside, aiming it at a person X and it indeed strikes X, and he is dead after impact and not before (and not from a coincidental heart

This article first appeared in the book Beneficent Euthanasia, *edited by Marvin Kohl, published by Prometheus Books, Buffalo, N.Y., 1975, and is reprinted by permission.*

attack); in that case we would say that I killed X. On the other hand, suppose I tell Y that X is in bed with Y's wife, and Y hurries to the scene, discovers them, and shoots X to death; in that case, although the unfolding of events from my action may be as much a matter of causal law as the path of the boulder, we should *not* say that I killed X. Fortunately, for the purpose of principles of the morally right, we can sidestep such complications. For suppose I am choosing whether to do *A* or *B* (where one or the other of these "acts" may be construed as essentially *in*action—for example, *not* doing what I know is the one thing that will *prevent* someone's death); then it is enough if I know, or have reason to think it highly probable, that were I to do *A*, a state of the world including the death of some person or persons would ensue, whereas were I to do *B*, a state of the world of some specified different sort would ensue. If a moral principle will tell me in this case whether I am to do *A* or *B*, that is all I need. It could be that a moral principle would tell me that I am absolutely never to perform any action *A*, such that were I to do it the death of some innocent human being would ensue, provided there is some alternative action I might perform, such that were I to do it no such death would ensue.

It is helpful, I think, to reformulate the traditional Catholic view in a way that preserves the spirit and intent of that view (although some philosophers would disagree with this assessment) and at the same time avoids some conceptions that are both vague and more appropriate to a principle about when a person is morally blameworthy for doing something than to a principle about what a person ought morally to do. The terminology I use goes back, in philosophical literature, to a phrase introduced by W. D. Ross, but the conception is quite familiar. The alternative proposal is that there is a *strong prima facie obligation* not to kill any human being except in justifiable self-defense; in the sense (of prima facie) that it is morally *wrong* to kill any human being except in justifiable self-defense *unless* there is an even stronger prima facie moral obligation to do something that cannot be done without killing. (The term *innocent* can now be omitted, since if a person is not innocent, there may be a stronger moral obligation that can only be discharged by killing him; and this change is to the good since it is not obvious that we have no prima facie obligation to avoid killing people even

if they are not innocent.) This formulation has the result that sometimes, to decide what is morally right, we have to compare the stringencies of conflicting moral obligations—and that is an elusive business; but the other formulation either conceals the same problem by putting it in another place, or else leads to objectionable implications. (Consider one implication of the traditional formulation, for a party of spelunkers in a cave by the oceanside. It is found that a rising tide is bringing water into the cave and all will be drowned unless they escape at once. Unfortunately, the first man to try to squeeze through the exit is fat and gets wedged inextricably in the opening, with his head inside the cave. Somebody in the party has a stick of dynamite. Either they blast the fat man out, killing him, or all of them, including him, will drown. The traditional formulation leads to the conclusion that all must drown.)

Let us then consider the principle: "There is a strong prima facie moral obligation not to kill any human being except in justifiable self-defense." I do not believe we want to accept this principle without further qualification; indeed, its status seems not to be that of a basic principle at all, but derivative from some more-basic principles. W. D. Ross listed what he thought were the main basic prima facie moral obligations; it is noteworthy that he listed a prima facie duty not to *cause injury*, but he did not include an obligation not to kill. Presumably this was no oversight. He might have thought that killing a human being is always an injury, so that the additional listing of an obligation not to kill would be redundant; but he might also have thought that killing is sometimes *not* an injury and that it is prima facie obligatory not to kill only when, and because, so doing would injure a sentient being.

What might be a noninjurious killing? If I come upon a cat that has been mangled but not quite killed by several dogs and is writhing in pain, and I pull myself together and put it out of its misery, I have killed the cat but surely not *injured* it. I do not injure something by relieving its pain. If someone is being tortured and roasted to death and I know he wishes nothing more than a merciful termination of life, I have not injured him if I shoot him; I have done him a favor. In general, it seems I have not injured a person if I treat him in a way in which he would want me to treat him if he were fully rational, or in a way to which he would be indifferent if he were fully rational. (I do not think that terminating the life of a human fetus in the third month is an injury; I admit this view requires discussion.[1])

Consider another type of killing that is not an injury. Consider the case of a human being who has become unconscious and will not, it is known, regain consciousness. He is in a hospital and is being kept alive only through expensive support-ive measures. Is there a strong prima facie moral obligation not to withdraw these measures and not to take positive steps to terminate his life? It seems obvious that if he is on the only kidney machine and its use could *save* the life of another person, who could lead a normal life after temporary use, it would be wrong not to take him off. Is there an obligation to continue, or not to terminate, if there is no countering obligation? I would think not, with an exception to be mentioned; and this coincides with the fact that he is *beyond* injury. There is also not an obligation *not* to preserve his life, say, in order to have his organs available for use when they are needed.

There seems, however, to be another morally relevant consideration in such a case—knowledge of the patient's own wishes when he was con-scious and in possession of his faculties. Suppose he had feared such an eventuality and prepared a sworn statement requesting his doctor to termi-nate his life at once in such circumstances. Now, if it is morally obligatory to some degree to carry out a person's wishes for disposal of his body and pos-sessions after his death, it would seem to be equally morally obligatory to respect his wishes in case he becomes a "vegetable." In the event of the existence of such a document, I would think that if he can no longer be injured we are free to with-draw life-sustaining measures and also to take positive steps to terminate life—and are even morally bound, prima facie, to do so. (If, however, the patient had prepared a document directing that his body be preserved alive as long as possible in such circumstances, then there would be a prima facie obligation *not* to cease life-sustaining measures and not to terminate. It would seem ob-vious, however, that such an obligation would fall far short of giving the patient the right to con-tinued use of a kidney machine when its use by another could save that person's life.) Some per-sons would not hesitate to discontinue life-sustaining procedures in such a situation, but would balk at more positive measures. But the hesitation to use more positive procedures, which veterinarians employ frequently with animals, is surely nothing but squeamishness; if a person is in the state described, there can be no injury to him in positive termination more or less than that in allowing him to wither by withdrawing life-supportive procedures.

If I am right in my analysis of this case, we must phrase our basic principle about killing in such a way as to take into account (1) whether the killing would be an injury and (2) the person's own wishes and directives. And perhaps, more important, any moral principle about killing must be viewed simply as an implicate of more basic principles about these matters.

Let us look for corroboration of this proposal to how we feel about another type of case, one in which termination would be of positive benefit to the agent. Let us suppose that a patient has a terminal illness and is in severe pain, subject only to brief remissions, with no prospect of any event that could make his life good, either in the short or long term. It might seem that here, with the patient in severe pain, at least life-supportive measures should be discontinued, or positive termination adopted. But I do not think we would accept this inference, for in this situation the patient, let us suppose, has his preferences and is able to express them. The patient may have strong religious convictions and prefer to go on living despite the pain; if so, surely there is a prima facie moral obligation not positively to terminate his life. Even if, as seemingly in this case, the situation is one in which it would be *rational* for the agent, from the point of view of his own welfare, to direct the termination of his life,[2] it seems that if he (irrationally) does the opposite, there is a prima facie moral obligation not to terminate and some prima facie obligation to sustain it. Evidently a person's own expressed wishes have moral force. (I believe, however, that we think a person's expressed wishes have *less* moral force when we think the wishes are irrational.)

What is the effect, in this case, if the patient himself expresses a preference for termination and would, if he were given the means, terminate his own existence? Is there a prima facie obligation to sustain his life—and pain—against his will? Surely not. Or is there an obligation *not* to take positive measures to terminate his life im-mediately, thereby saving the patient much discomfort? Again, surely not. What possible reason could be offered to justify the claim that the answer is affirmative, beyond theological ones about God's will and our being bound to stay alive at His pleasure? The only argument I can think of is that there is some consideration of public policy, to the effect that a recognition of such moral permission might lead to abuses or to some other detriment to society in the long run. Such an argument does seem weak.

It might be questioned whether a patient's request should be honored, if made at a time when he is in pain, on the grounds that it is not rational. (The physician may be in a position to see, however, that the patient is quite right about his prospects and that his personal welfare would be maximized by termination.) It might also be questioned whether a patient's formal declaration, written earlier, requesting termination if he were ever in his present circumstances, should be honored, on the grounds that at the earlier time he did not know what it would be like to be in his present situation. It would seem odd, however, if *no* circumstances are identifiable in which a patient's request for termination is deemed to have moral force, when his request *not* to terminate is thought morally weighty in the same circumstances, even when this request is clearly irrational. I think we may ignore such arguments and hold that, in a situation in which it is rational for a person to choose termination of his life, his expressed wish is morally definitive and removes both the obligation to sustain life and the obligation not to terminate.

Indeed, there is a question whether or not in these circumstances a physician has not a moral obligation at least to withdraw life-supporting measures, and perhaps positively to terminate life. At least there seems to be a general moral obligation to render assistance when a person is in need, when it can be given at small cost to oneself, and when it is requested. The obligation is the stronger when one happens to be the only person in a position to receive such a request or to know about the situation. Furthermore, the physician has acquired a special obligation if there has been a long-standing personal relationship with the patient—just as a friend or relative has special obligations. But since we are discussing not the possible obligation to terminate but the obligation *not* to terminate, I shall not pursue this issue.

The patient's own expression of preference or consent, then, seems to be weighty. But suppose he is unable to express his preference; suppose that his terminal disease not only causes him great pain but has attacked his brain in such a way that he is incapable of thought and of rational speech. May the physician, then, after consultation, take matters into his own hands? We often think we know what is best for another, but we think one person should not make decisions for another. Just as we must respect the decision of a person who has decided after careful reflection that he wants to commit suicide, so we must not take the liberty of deciding to bring another's life to a close contrary to his wishes. So what may be done? Must a person suffer simply because he cannot express consent? There is evidence that can be gathered about what conclusions a person would draw if he were in a state to draw and express them. The patient's friends will have some recollection of things he has said in the past, of his values and general ethical views. Just as we can have good reason to think, for example, that he would vote Democratic if voting for president in a certain year, so we can have good reason to think he would take a certain stand about the termination of his own life in various circumstances. We can know of some persons who because of their religious views would want to keep on living until natural processes bring their lives to a close. About others we can know that they decidedly would not take this view. We can also know what would be the *rational* choice for them to make, and our knowledge of this can be *evidence* about what they would request if they were able. There are, of course, practical complications in the mechanics of a review board of some kind making a determination of this sort, but they are hardly insurmountable.

I wish to consider one other type of case, that of a person who, say, has had a stroke and is leading, and for some time can continue to lead, a life that is comfortable but one on a very low level, *and* who has antecedently requested that his life be terminated if he comes, incurably, into such a situation. May he then be terminated? In this case, unlike the others, there are probably ongoing pleasant experiences, perhaps on the level of some animals, that seem to be a good thing. One can hardly say that *injury* is being done such a person by keeping him alive; and one might say that some slight injury is being done him by terminating his existence. There is a real problem here. Can the (slight) goodness of these experiences stand against the weight of an earlier firm declaration requesting that life be terminated in a situation of hopeless senility? There is no *injury* in keeping the person alive despite his request, but there seems something *indecent* about keeping a mind alive after a severe stroke, when we know quite well that, could he have anticipated it, his own action would have been to terminate his life. I think that the person's own request should be honored; it should be if a person's expressed preferences have as much moral weight as I think they should have.

What general conclusions are warranted by the preceding discussion? I shall emphasize two. First, there is a prima facie obligation *not* to terminate a person's existence when this would injure him (except in cases of self-defense or of senility of a person whose known wish is to be terminated in such a condition) *or* if he wishes not to be terminated. Second, there is *not* a prima facie obligation not to terminate when there would be *no* injury, or when there would be a positive benefit (release from pain) in so doing, provided the patient has not declared himself otherwise or there is evidence that his wishes are to that effect. Obviously there are two things that are decisive for the morality of terminating a person's life: whether so doing would be an *injury* and whether it conforms to what is known of his *preferences*.

I remarked at the outset that I would be content with some moral principles if it could be made out that rational persons would want those principles incorporated in the consciences of a group among whom they were to live. It is obvious why rational persons would want these principles. They would want injury avoided both because they would not wish others to injure them and because, if they are benevolent, they would not wish others injured. Moreover, they would want weight given to a person's own known prefer-

ences. Rational people do want the decision about the termination of their lives, where that is possible; for they would be uncomfortable if they thought it possible that others would be free to terminate their lives without consent. The threat of serious illness is bad enough without that prospect. On the other hand, this discomfort would be removed if they knew that termination would not be undertaken on their behalf without their explicit consent, except after a careful inquiry had been made, both into whether termination would constitute an injury and whether they would request termination under the circumstances if they were in a position to do so.

If I am right in all this, then it appears that killing a person is not something that is just prima facie wrong *in itself;* it is wrong roughly only if and because it is an *injury* of someone, or if and because it is contrary to the *known preferences* of someone. It would seem that a principle about the prima facie wrongness of killing is *derivative* from principles about when we are prima facie obligated not to injure and when we are prima facie obligated to respect a person's wishes, at least about what happens to his own body. I do not, however, have any suggestions for a general statement of principles of this latter sort.

Notes

1. See my "The Morality of Abortion" in *The Monist*, 56 (1972), pp. 503–26; and, in revised form, in [*Abortion: Pro and Con*, ed. R. L. Perkins (General Learning Press, 1975)].

2. See my "The Morality and Rationality of Suicide," in James Rachels, ed., *Moral Problems* [Harper & Row, 1975]; and, in revised form, in E. S. Shneidman, ed., *Suicidology: Current Developments* [Grune & Stratton, 1976].

Natural Death Act

The State of California

Legislative Counsel's Digest

AB 3060, Keene. Cessation of medical care for terminal patients.

No existing statute prescribes a procedure whereby a person may provide in advance for the withholding or withdrawal of medical care in the

From California Health and Safety Code, Part I, Division 7, Chapter 3.9, Section 7188. Approved by the Governor on the 30th of September, 1976.

event the person should suffer a terminal illness or mortal injury.

This bill would expressly authorize the withholding or withdrawal of life-sustaining procedures, as defined, from adult patients afflicted with a terminal condition, as defined, where the patient has executed a directive in the form and manner prescribed by the bill. Such a directive would generally be effective for five years from the date of execution unless sooner revoked in a specified manner. This bill would relieve physicians, licensed health professionals acting under the direction of a physician, and health facilities from civil liability, and would relieve physicians and licensed health professionals acting under the direction of a physician from criminal prosecution or charges of unprofessional conduct, for withholding or withdrawing life-sustaining procedures in accordance with the provisions of the bill.

The bill would provide that such a withholding or withdrawal of life-sustaining procedures shall not constitute a suicide nor impair or invalidate life insurance, and the bill would specify that the making of such a directive shall not restrict, inhibit, or impair the sale, procurement, or issuance of life insurance or modify existing life insurance. The bill would provide that health insurance carriers, as prescribed, could not require execution of a directive as a condition for being insured for, or receiving, health care services.

The bill would make it a misdemeanor to willfully conceal, cancel, deface, obliterate, or damage the directive of another without the declarant's consent. Any person, not justified or excused by law, who falsifies or forges the directive of another or willfully conceals or withholds personal knowledge of a prescribed revocation with the intent to cause a withholding or withdrawal of life-sustaining procedures contrary to the wishes of the declarant and thereby causes life-sustaining procedures to be withheld or withdrawn, and death to thereby be hastened, would be subject to prosecution for unlawful homicide. . . .

The people of the State of California do enact as follows:

Chapter 3.9. Natural Death Act

7188. Any adult person may execute a directive directing the withholding or withdrawal of life-sustaining procedures in a terminal condition. The directive shall be signed by the declarant in the presence of two witnesses not related to the declarant by blood or marriage and who would not

be entitled to any portion of the estate of the declarant upon his decease under any will of the declarant or codicil thereto then existing or, at the time of the directive, by operation of law then existing. In addition, a witness to a directive shall not be the attending physician an employee of the attending physician or a health facility in which the declarant is a patient, or any person who has a claim against any portion of the estate of the declarant upon his decease at the time of the execution of the directive. The directive shall be in the following form:

DIRECTIVE TO PHYSICIANS

Directive made this _____ day of _____ (month, year).

I _____, being of sound mind, willfully, and voluntarily make known my desire that my life shall not be artificially prolonged under the circumstances set forth below, do hereby declare:

1. If at any time I should have an incurable injury, disease, or illness certified to be a terminal condition by two physicians, and where the application of life-sustaining procedures would serve only to artificially prolong the moment of my death and where my physician determines that my death is imminent whether or not life-sustaining procedures are utilized, I direct that such procedures be withheld or withdrawn, and that I be permitted to die naturally.

2. In the absence of my ability to give directions regarding the use of such life-sustaining procedures, it is my intention that this directive shall be honored by my family and physician(s) as the final expression of my legal right to refuse medical or surgical treatment and accept the consequences from such refusal.

3. If I have been diagnosed as pregnant and that diagnosis is known to my physician, this directive shall have no force or effect during the course of my pregnancy.

4. I have been diagnosed and notified at least 14 days ago as having a terminal condition by _____ M.D., whose address is _____, and whose telephone number is _____ . I understand that if I have not filled in the physician's name and address, it shall be presumed that I did not have a terminal condition when I made out this directive.

5. This directive shall have no force or effect five years from the date filled in above.

6. I understand the full import of this directive and I am emotionally and mentally competent to make this directive.

Signed _____

City, County, and State of Residence _____

_____

The declarant has been personally known to me and I believe him or her to be of sound mind.

Witness_____

Witness_____

Decision Scenario 1

"Apparently he was inside the tank with an oxygen hose to provide ventilation," Dr. Mangel said. "There was some oil residue on the walls. When Mr. Golenga struck an arc to weld the seam, there was a flash fire."

Mrs. Golenga gripped the hand of her nineteen-year-old son Cervando. Both had been crying, but now listening was so important that they forced back their tears.

"How badly hurt is he?" Mrs. Golenga asked.

"Very badly," Dr. Mangel said. "Most of his body is covered with severe burns, and his lungs are damaged from breathing in the fire and smoke."

"Will he live?" Cervando asked.

"I have to be honest with you and say that I don't think he will," Dr. Mangel said. "We are giving him plasma and saline solutions to rehydrate him and antibiotics to try to stop infections. But he hasn't got much of a chance."

"The pain, what about the pain?" asked Mrs. Golenga.

"There's only so much we can do."

"There's really no hope?" Cervando asked.

"I wouldn't say that," Dr. Mangel said. "There is always hope. But in this case it is very limited. He might die in a few hours or he might die tomorrow or the next day."

"Please," Mrs. Golenga said. "Can you help him die? I know he doesn't want to suffer if he has no real hope. He told me often, 'if something happens to me, don't let them stick me full of needles and keep me alive. Tell them to put me out of my misery.' Can you do that, Doctor?"

"Are you sure that's what he would want?" Dr. Mangel asked.

"My mother is right," Cervando said. "I've heard my father say that many times. He said he never wanted to just lie around and suffer, being a burden to himself and everyone. We want to do as he wanted us to."

"We could stop treating him," Dr. Mangel said. "Then let nature take its course."

"That sounds terrible," Mrs. Golenga said. "To make a man fight for his life when he has no hope and no help. It is cold and cruel."

"I'm sorry," said Dr. Mangel. "It is all that the law permits me to do."

Would Rachels regard this as the kind of case in which active euthanasia would be more humane than passive?

On Foot's analysis, would it be legitimate to conclude that Mr. Golenga's life is not worth living any longer?

According to the conservative view of Gay-Williams, is there anything that might be done to put an end to Mr. Golenga's life that would also be morally acceptable?

Would the line of reasoning taken by Chief Justice Hughes in the Quinlan case make Mrs. Golenga and Cervando the appropriate people to decide whether Mr. Golenga receives additional treatment, is allowed to die, or is killed?

Decision Scenario 2

Mr. Jeffry Box was eighty-one years old when he was brought to Doctor's Hospital. His right side was paralyzed, he spoke in a garbled way, and he had trouble understanding even the simplest matters. His only known relative was a sister four years younger, and she lived half a continent away. When a hospital social worker called to tell her about her brother's condition, she was quite uninterested. "I haven't seen him in fifteen years," she said. "I thought he might already be dead. Just do whatever you think best for him. I'm too old to worry about him."

Neurological tests and x-ray studies showed Mr. Box was suffering from a brain hemorrhage caused by a ruptured blood vessel.

"Can you fix it?" asked Dr. Hollins. She was the resident responsible for Mr. Box's primary care. The man she addressed was Dr. Carl Oceana, the staff's only neurosurgeon.

"Sure," said Dr. Oceana. "I can repair the vessel and clean out the mess. But it won't do much good, you know."

"You mean he'll still be paralyzed?"

"That's right. And he'll still be mentally incoherent. After the operation he'll have to be put in a nursing home or some other chronic-care place, because he won't be able to see to his own needs."

"And if you don't operate?" Dr. Hollins asked.

Dr. Oceana shrugged. "He'll be dead by tomorrow. Maybe sooner, depending on how long it takes for the pressure in his skull to build up."

"What would you do?"

"I know what I would want done to me if I were the patient," said Dr. Oceana. "I'd want people to keep their knives out of my head and let me die a nice, peaceful death."

"But we don't know what he would want," Dr. Hollins said. "He's never been our patient before, and the social worker hasn't been able to find any friends who might tell us what he'd want done."

"Let's just put ourselves in his place," said Dr. Oceana. "Let's do unto others what we would want done unto us."

"That means letting Mr. Box die."

"Exactly."

On what grounds might Brandt approve the view taken by Dr. Oceana?

On what grounds might Gay-Williams object?

Would Foot's principles justify a decision to allow Mr. Box to die?

Would the natural law view make the operation discussed a moral mandate?

Decision Scenario 3

Sigmund Freud, the founder of psychoanalysis, suffered from cancer of the jaw during the last years of his life. At the end, when he had fled to London to escape the Nazis, he was in constant agony. He was operated on and given radium treatments, but the cancer was unstoppable. It destroyed the tissues inside his mouth and, finally, ate through his cheek. The wound gave off a disgusting odor and caused Freud terrible pain.

Ten years before, in Vienna, he had told his personal physician, Dr. Max Schur, "I can stand a great deal of pain and I hate sedatives, but I trust you will not let me suffer unnecessarily." Dr. Schur promised him that he would not. On September 21, 1939 Freud reminded Schur of his promise. "It is only torture now," he told Schur, "and it has no longer any sense."

The next day, Schur injected Freud with a third of a grain of morphine. Freud, who was wholly unaccustomed to sedatives, fell into a deep sleep from which he never recovered. Schur had kept his promise.

Assuming that this is a case of active euthanasia, would Foot regard it as justifiable? Would Rachels, Brandt, or Gay-Williams? Explain the reasoning behind each conclusion.

Decision Scenario 4

When two plainclothes detectives arrived at Virginia Crawford's suburban apartment at 6:30 on a Sunday morning to arrest her for murder, she was not terribly surprised to see them.

She cried when they insisted on putting her in handcuffs before transporting her to the jail in the county court building. Yet she had more or less expected to be arrested eventually.

For almost a month, a police investigation had been conducted at Mercy hospital, where Ms. Crawford worked as a nurse in the intensive care unit. The entire hospital staff knew about the investigation, and Ms. Crawford herself had been questioned on three occasions by officers conducting the inquiry. At the time, her answers had seemed to be satisfactory to the police, and there was no hint that she was under suspicion. Still, she always believed that eventually they would catch up with her.

The investigation centered on the deaths of four elderly patients during the period February 1979 to March 1980. All of the patients were in the intensive care unit at the times of their deaths. Each had been diagnosed as suffering from a terminal illness, and the chart notation on each case indicated that they had all suffered irreversible brain damage and were totally without higher brain functions.

The three women and one man were all unmarried and had no immediate family to take an interest in their welfare. All of them were being kept alive by respirators, and their deaths were caused directly by their respirators being turned off. In each instance of death, Ms. Crawford had been the person in charge of the ICU.

After securing the services of an attorney, Ms. Crawford was released on bail and a time was set for her appearance in court. Through her attorney, Marvin Washington, she made a statement to the media.

"My client has asked me to announce that she fully and freely admits that she was the one who turned off the respirators of the four patients in question at Mercy Hospital. She acted alone and without the knowledge of any other individual. She is prepared to take full responsibility for her actions."

Mr. Washington went on to say that he would request a jury trial for his client. "I am sure," he said, "that no jury will convict Ms. Crawford of murder merely for turning off the life-support systems of people who were already dead."

When asked what he meant by that, Mr. Washington explained. "These patients were no longer people," he said. "Sometime during the course of the treatment, their brains simply stopped functioning in a way that we associate with human life."

Ms. Crawford was present during the reading of her statement, and after a whispered conversation with her attorney, she spoke once for herself. "I consider what I did an act of compassion and humanity," she said. "I consider it altogether moral, and I feel no guilt about it. I did for four people what they would have wanted done, if they had only been in a condition to know."

> *Does the natural law view offer grounds for removing life-support systems for people who are beyond a reasonable hope of recovery? If so, what are they?*
>
> *Would Gay-Williams oppose the actions of Ms. Crawford?*
>
> *According to Brandt, can Ms. Crawford be said to have done anyone an injury?*
>
> *Would Foot regard the actions of Ms. Crawford as defensible?*

Decision Scenario 5

"I'm ready to die now," Zema Radford said to the physician who stood by her hospital bed.

"I don't think you really mean that," Dr. Carl Tang said. "You're very ill, so you aren't really in a position to make a decision like that."

"My mind is quite clear at the moment. I'll admit it isn't always, but now I know what I want. I want you to take away all these nasty tubes and wires."

"We really can't do that, Mrs. Radford. Without them you would die, and none of us wants to be responsible for your death."

Mrs. Radford was eighty-three-years-old, and disease had wasted her body. She lay curled on the narrow bed, her frail left arm outside the sheet so the line from the IV bag would not be obstructed. Thin green wires leading to the machine monitoring her heart rate snaked across a corner of the bed.

"Can't a patient refuse treatment?" she asked Dr. Tang.

"Ordinarily, yes. But usually only ambulatory patients do that. And, of course, we have to be sure the patient is mentally competent."

"I'm really too weak to argue," Mrs. Radford said. "If I had any of my family with me, I would ask them to help me die. I don't, so I have to ask you."

"I'll take it up with your other doctors. I can't promise what we'll do, but we'll discuss it."

According to Foot, does Mrs. Radford have a right to risk dying by demanding that her life-support equipment be removed?

If Dr. Tang believes that removing the equipment will result in the death of Mrs. Radford, would he be right, according to Gay-Williams, in refusing to remove it?

If Dr. Tang holds such a belief, then according to Rachels, would he be equally justified in killing Mrs. Radford as in removing the equipment?

Would the reasoning in the court decision in the Quinlan case tend to support Mrs. Radford's request?

Part II
RIGHTS

4

PATERNALISM, TRUTH TELLING, AND CONFIDENTIALITY

CASE PRESENTATION
Laetrile and Government Regulation

In 1920 Ernst Krebs, a California physician, derived a substance from crushed apricot pits which he hoped could be used to improve the taste of bootleg whiskey. The substance contained traces of poisonous cyanide, which occurs naturally in apricot pits, and was considered too dangerous for human use by Dr. Krebs.

But in 1952 Ernst Krebs, Jr., claimed to have purified the substance, making it safe for human consumption. The substance, now called Laetrile, was put forward by Dr. and Mr. Krebs as an effective cure for cancer. Cancer, Mr. Krebs, claimed, involves certain cells that contain an abnormal amount of a certain enzyme. This enzyme triggers the release of cyanide from Laetrile, and the cyanide destroys tumor cells. Normal cells do not contain the enzyme, Krebs claimed. Rather, they contain another enzyme that neutralizes the cyanide. Consequently, cancerous cells are destroyed while whole, normal cells are protected.

Krebs's theory is considered to be wrong by the scientific community. The enzyme that is supposed to release the cyanide is found in smaller amounts in cancer cells than in normal cells. The enzyme that is supposed to neutralize the cyanide in normal cells is found in an equal amount in cancerous cells. Also, the destructive effects of cyanide are general and not at all limited to cancerous cells.

A number of tests and investigations involving Laetrile have been conducted. In 1953, the California Medical Association Cancer Commission discovered that all but one of forty-four people treated with Laetrile were either dead or still suffered from active cancer. In 1963, the Cancer Advisory Council reported to the California Department of Public Health that Laetrile was of no therapeutic value in diagnosed cases of cancer. The use of it was then made illegal in California. In 1965, Canadian investigators reported that Laetrile was ineffective in cancer therapy.

Between 1957 and 1975, five series of animal tests involving Laetrile were conducted by the National Cancer Institute. No evidence was found to support the claim that Laetrile was an effective therapy in cancer treatment. These results were confirmed by the work at four other research centers.

Between 1972 and 1976, the Memorial Sloan-Kettering Institute investigated the use of Laetrile in the treatment of tumors in mice and rats. About thirty-seven separate experiments were conducted, and one investigator did report that Laetrile might inhibit tumor growth. These findings could not be duplicated by others, and it was claimed that the investigator's techniques were not sufficiently sensitive. The head of the Sloan-Kettering laboratory, Dr. C. Chester Stock, commented on the work done by his group: "Laetrile is not active against cancer. If something is active, we would see it consistently active, which we have not seen with our Laetrile experiments."

Despite the rejection of Laetrile by the medical and scientific community, a great number of people who have sought out Laetrile treatment have testified to its effectiveness. No case has been regarded as scientifically persuasive, however. Some people never had cancer and were, at most, the victims of misdiagnosis. Others wrongly thought themselves cured of cancer. Still others have had their symptoms improve temporarily (something fairly frequent in cancer) and have wrongly attributed the improvement to the use of Laetrile.

Supporters of Laetrile were unsuccessful in their attempts to secure its approval as a legitimate drug by the Food and Drug Administration. To gain approval, Laetrile would have to be shown to be both safe and effective, and no evidence adequate to support the claim of effectiveness could be produced. In 1970 advocates of Laetrile began describing it as a vitamin—"vitamin B-17." Under this description, it was believed that the substance could escape the FDA regulations and be marketed legally to those who wanted it. It was also suggested that cancer is a result of vitamin B-17 deficiency.

No scientific evidence supports this view, however. Laetrile is not a vitamin, and no disease has been discovered that results from a deficiency of it. Laetrile has no nutritional value and plays no role in cellular metabolism, growth, or development.

In 1974 the FDA took legal action against two products, marketed as health foods, that contained a chemical substance identical with Laetrile. The manufacturers were placed under a permanent injunction forbidding the manufacture and sale of the products by a California Federal court in 1975. In 1976, a New Jersey Federal court placed a similar product under an injunction, forbidding its transport across state lines. The California court observed that the chemical substance (Laetrile) in the products it was considering was not a vitamin and that the products were adulterated foods. The New Jersey court held that the sale of the product that it was considering constituted fraud.

Public response to the scientific and legal attitude towards Laetrile has not always been one of acquiescence. A court decision permitting an individual to import Laetrile for personal use was won by Glen Rutherford of Conway

Springs, Kansas in 1971. It was the first of such decisions, and several in various states have since been handed down.

The John Birch Society, a conservative political organization, has also entered the Laetrile controversy. In 1972 one of its members, a California physician named John Richardson, was arrested for dispensing Laetrile. He was convicted, the conviction was overturned, and two retrials both ended with hung juries. A Birch Society ad hoc defense group for Dr. Richardson, headed by Robert Bradford, was turned into the Committee for Freedom of Choice in Cancer Therapy. This group, reportedly composed of twenty-three thousand members, is working for the legalization of Laetrile.

The group argues that the government has no right to interfere with an individual's choice of treatment. This is particularly true, they claim, when the treatment does not produce dangerous side effects. (Laetrile appears to be safe in normal doses. It did cause the death of a ten-month-old child, but this was the result of an accident.)

Pro-Laetrile groups have lobbied strongly for the passage of a "Medical Freedom of Choice" bill, which would set aside the FDA requirement that drugs must be both safe and effective before they can be marketed and require only that they be shown to be safe.

The groups have not succeeded in getting any national legislation passed, but they have been very effective on the state level. Responding to pressure from such pro-Laetrile organizations as the Cancer Control Society and the National Health Federation, the Indiana legislature overrode the governor's veto of a bill to legalize the manufacture and marketing of Laetrile. Similar legislation has also been passed in some twenty-seven states. Laetrile proponents hope to escape the FDA ban on Laetrile by having the substance approved state by state. If no interstate commerce is involved, then the FDA regulations do not apply. Passage of national legislation would make this process unnecessary.

Opponents of the legalization of Laetrile are most concerned about patient-consumer protection. As the FDA *Drug Bulletin* expressed the fear: "No worthless drug is without harm; a patient's choice of Laetrile, to the extent that such choice delays or interferes with swift diagnosis and prompt effective treatment, is potentially fatal."

Laetrile advocates have argued that the substance should at least be available to those who are terminal cases—such people should be allowed to try what they want to try. Opponents, however, argue that use in such cases would give the substance an air of legitimacy. This is the position taken by the American Cancer Society:

> Laetrile supporters would be able to cite the fact that it was given by
> such-and-such a physician, in such-and-such hospital. . . . This immediately
> would give it the status of a viable alternative to proved cancer treatments. And
> the danger is that patients whose cancers are discovered in early stages may
> think that Laetrile is a legitimate therapeutic option.

Consumer Reports sees the pressure groups formed by Laetrile advocates as threatening the effectiveness and integrity of the drug laws:

> Over the past seven decades, Congress has passed increasingly tough drug laws
> to protect consumers from the purveyors of quack remedies. Such laws are now

being jeopardized by the pro-Laetrile forces and by the state legislatures that bow to their demands. In our opinion, approval of Laetrile as an anticancer drug would devastate the carefully structured consumer-protection drug laws enacted in modern times and would open the door to the legitimization of quackery. According to the evidence on hand, Laetrile has no place in the medical marketplace.

In 1979 the National Cancer Institute, responding to immense public pressure, initiated a three-year program of human testing using Laetrile. At a number of medical centers throughout the United States, patients with cancer in advanced stages who could no longer be helped by ordinary therapies and who gave their consent were treated with Laetrile.

It was administered intravenously for twenty-one days, then orally three times a day. Patients were also served the special diet advocated by most Laetrile proponents: fresh fruits and vegetables, whole grains, vitamins, and pancreatic enzymes.

The patient population in the study consisted of 156 people. After a month of the treatment, the cancer had progressed in 50 percent of the patients. After three months, it had progressed in 90 percent. At the end of eight months, only about one-fifth of the original patients were still alive. The figures reflect about the same percentages that would be expected in a group receiving no treatment at all.

Defenders of Laetrile claim that the test results are not valid, because the drug used was not pure Laetrile. A representative of the NCI dismisses the criticism as irrelevant. The drug used in the test was identical in its chemical structure to that derived from "natural" sources.

The Director of the NCI, Vincent DeVita, Jr., summarized the results of the study:

> The findings . . . present public evidence of Laetrile's failure as a cancer treatment. The hollow promise of this drug has led thousands of Americans away from potentially helpful therapy of scientific validity.

The findings of the NCI clinical trials have not changed the views of Laetrile's public defenders. Robert Bradford, head of the Committee for Freedom of Choice in Cancer Therapy, responded to the study in this way: "The whole thing, as far as we are concerned, is a put-up deal to discredit Laetrile."

Thus, despite the position of the FDA, despite the opinion of the scientific and medical community, despite the most recent experimental results, many people continue to look to Laetrile as a source of hope. Laetrile advocates still push for its legalization and its recognition as an alternative therapy.

CASE PRESENTATION
Contraception, Minors, and the Notification Rule

In February of 1982, the federal Department of Health and Human Services issued a regulation to go into effect on April 23. The regulation requires that the parents of minors who receive prescriptions for birth-control drugs or devices from federally funded clinics be sent letters of notification within ten days of the minor's visit.

A minor, for the purpose of the regulation, is any person under the age of eighteen who is not married and is not a member of the armed forces. Notification is not required only when there is reason to believe that the parents might physically harm the minor. Otherwise, the requirement to notify the parents has the force of law.

Since the regulation was first proposed, it has been a source of great controversy. Those who support the regulation claim that because all contraceptives pose a risk to the health of the user, the parents of those minors using them have a right to be informed of the risks. After all, it is the parents who are responsible for the health and well-being of their children, and it is the parents who must be prepared to cope with the potential health problems.

This is fundamentally the position taken by Marjory Mecklenberg, the director of HHS Adolescent Pregnancy Programs and one of the authors of the regulation. "Our minimum responsibility," Ms. Mecklenburg said, "is to protect the health and, in some cases, the life of children receiving prescriptions, who may be at risk of embolism, stroke, and permanent sterility."

> In her view, concern with confidentiality is not adequate to offset the parents' need to know. "We are dealing with children, many of them below 15 years," she said. "We can't allow things to be done to them in the name of confidentiality or privacy by professionals who aren't responsible for them, no matter how well-meaning those professionals may be. They have no ongoing interest in or relation with the child. Although 82 percent of all teenagers on contraceptives are on the pill, half don't return to the clinics for follow-up visits. The real challenge now is to bring the teens and the parents back together again.

Connaught Marshner of the National Pro-Family Coalition praised the bill for helping to restore parental authority and discourage premarital sexual experience. In her view, the regulation would not necessarily lead to more teenager pregnancies. She stated:

> The argument that this will cause an increase in teen-age pregnancy assumes that teenagers can't control their urges and nothing will stop them from having sex. In fact, if children had more discussion with parents, they would hear their parents' point of view, and it would inspire them to control their feelings. I hope that bringing the subject up for discussion will be constructive. We can't avoid having tense discussions, but a tense conversation is better than no conversation at all.

Opponents of the regulation generally agree about the value of promoting parental interest in the sexual activity of their teen-age children. In their opinion, however, the most likely result of enforcing the regulation will be that it will discourage teenagers from seeking contraceptives at all. Many either fear the disapproval of their parents or regard the matter of their own sexuality as a wholly private concern. Although parents need not give their consent in order for contraceptive prescriptions to be obtained, for a large number of teenagers the distinction between consent and notification is virtually nonexistent.

The fear that the use of contraceptives by female teenagers would decrease seems borne out by empirical evidence. In 1980, almost half the initial prescriptions for oral contraceptives among unmarried teenagers were obtained at family planning clinics. A study conducted in 1982, however, showed that 25 percent of the minor patients at such clinics would stop applying for contraceptive prescriptions if their parents were notified.

The almost certain result of such a situation would be a startling increase in the number of teenager pregnancies. This, in turn, would no doubt lead to a substantial increase in the number of abortions among female teenagers.

Furthermore, this part of the population would be put in greater risk of its health for that reason. Among women in their teens, the risks from pregnancy are five times greater than the risk from oral contraceptives. To some extent, then, this offsets the HHS contention that protection of the health of minors is at the basis of the notification requirement.

Some opponents of the regulation also consider it to be discriminatory. For one thing, it affects females, but not males. Male contraceptive devices (condoms) can be bought openly, without the privacy of the buyer being compromised. Female contraceptive devices (such as the IUD) or birth-control pills, by contrast, can be obtained only by prescription. This means that a woman under the age of eighteen who is unmarried and who must rely on a prescription from a federally funded clinic must surrender her privacy under the regulation.

In addition, the regulation applies only to federally funded programs. This means that a minor who can afford her own physician can preserve her privacy. One lacking the financial means to consult a physician privately must pay the price of having her parents informed of her actions, whether or not she consents to it.

Critics also point out that minors who are in the position of having to rely upon federally funded clinics for their contraceptive prescriptions also belong to the group who cannot afford to pay for abortions. Since it is illegal to use federal money to pay for abortions, they must either have unwanted children or try to secure the money for an abortion from private sources. Thus, for this group, the federal government, through its laws and regulations, makes it difficult to obtain both contraceptive prescriptions and abortions.

Critics and defenders of the notification regulation both agree that ultimately its legitimacy will be tested in the courts.

Introduction

Consider the following cases:

1. A state decides to require that all behavioral therapists (that is, all who make use of psychological conditioning techniques to alter behavior patterns) be either licensed psychologists or psychiatrists.

2. A member of the Plymouth Brethren sect is opposed to the "shedding of blood" and refuses to consent to a needed appendectomy, but when his appendix ruptures and he lapses into unconsciousness, the surgical resident operates and saves his life.

3. A physician decides not to tell the parents of an infant who died shortly after

birth that the cause of death was an unpredictable birth defect because he does not wish to influence their desire to have a child.

4.   A janitor employed in an elementary school consults a psychiatrist retained by the school board and tells her that he has on two occasions molested young children; the psychiatrist decides that it is her duty to inform the school board.

There is perhaps no single moral issue that is present in all these cases. Rather, there is a complex of related issues. Each case involves acting on the behalf of someone else—the public, a patient, or a special group. And each action comes into conflict with the desires, rights, or expectations of some person or persons. Even though the issues are related, it is most fruitful to discuss them separately.

Paternalism

Exactly what paternalism is, is itself a matter of dispute. Roughly speaking, we can say that paternalism consists in acting in a way that is believed to protect or advance the interest of a person although acting in this way goes against the person's own immediate desires or limits the person's freedom of choice. (Oversimplifying, paternalism is the view that "Father knows best.") Thus, the first three cases presented above are instances of paternalistic behavior.

It is useful to distinguish what we can call "state paternalism" from "personal paternalism." State paternalism, as the name suggests, is the control exerted by a legislature, agency, or other governmental body over particular kinds of practices or procedures. Such control is typically exercised through laws, licensing requirements, technical specifications, and operational guidelines and regulations. (The first case above is an example of state paternalism.)

By contrast, personal paternalism consists in an individual's deciding, on the basis of his own principles or values, that he knows what is best for another person. The individual then acts in a way that deprives the other person of genuine and effective choice. (Cases two and three are examples of this.) Paternalism is personal when it is not a matter of public or semipublic policy but is a result of private, moral decision making.

State Paternalism in Medical and Health Care

At first sight, state paternalism seems wholly unobjectionable in the medical context. We are all certain to feel more confident in consulting a physician when we know that she or he has had to meet the standards for education, competence, and character set by a state licensing board and medical society. We feel relatively sure that we aren't putting ourselves in the hands of an incompetent quack.

Indeed, that we can feel such assurance can be regarded as one of the marks of the social advancement of medicine. As late as the early twentieth century in the United States, the standards for physicians were low and licensing laws were either nonexistent or poorly enforced. It was possible to qualify as a physician with as little as four months formal schooling and a two-year apprenticeship. Even these requirements were enforced only at prestigious medical schools such as Yale's. Privately owned schools that were run for profit were not overly stringent in their admissions policies or graduation requirements.

In addition, many people practiced a form of medicine not taught in the medical schools. Thompsonists claimed that herbs of the right kind would cure all ailments, and homeopaths believed that minute doses of drugs that would cause disease symptoms in a healthy person would also eliminate those symptoms in a sick person. Hydropaths relied upon externally and internally applied water as the basic treatment modality, and naturopaths emphasized the curative power of proper diet and exercise.

Virtually all of the nonstandard medicine practiced in the nineteenth century we would now regard as quackery. Most of those who practiced it were sincere in their beliefs, but the theories on which their practices were based are ones that we consider to be completely false. Ironically, the irregular practitioners were often more successful than their orthodox counterparts. Whereas standard medicine relied on such "heroic" measures as bleeding and purging, the "quacks" generally stressed minimum intervention and the healing power of nature. Nature quite often turned out to be a better physician than even the best trained physician.

Strict licensing laws and the upgrading of medical schools eventually led to the triumph of a standard medicine based on the theories of the natural sciences. Irregular medicine virtually disappeared from the American scene. Confidence in the scientific basis of medicine was increased with the widespread acceptance of the germ theory of disease, the identification of particular disease-causing bacterial agents, and the development of specific drug therapies that could bring about almost miraculous cures in some diseases. The Pure Food and Drug Laws reflected this confidence, and their enforcement was used as a weapon to protect consumers from practitioners who used therapies that were unproved scientifically. The laws are still used for this purpose.

There is little doubt that rigorous standards and strictly enforced laws have done much to improve medical care in this country. At the very least, they have made it less dangerous to consult a physician. At the same time, however, they have also placed close restrictions on individual freedom of choice. In the nineteenth century, a person could choose among a variety of medical viewpoints. That is no longer so today.

It is no longer the case because we now recognize that some medical viewpoints are wrong and if implemented, may endanger a patient. At the very least, people treated by those who espouse such views run the risk of not getting the best kind of medical care available. Unlike people in the nineteenth century, we are confident that we know (within limits) what kinds of medical therapies are effective and what kinds are useless or harmful. The scientific character of contemporary medicine gives us this confidence.

Secure in these beliefs, our society generally endorses paternalism by the state in the regulation of medical practice. We believe it is important to protect sick people from quacks and charletans, from those who raise false hopes and take advantage of human suffering. We generally accept, then, that the range of choice of health therapy ought to be limited to what we consider to be legitimate and scientific.

This point of view has come under attack in recent years. Most currently, such controversy has centered on the prohibition of the alleged anticancer drug Laetrile by the Food and Drug Administration. (See the Case Presentation for a detailed account of the controversy.) Because of this prohibition, a number of individuals and groups have claimed that they are now unable to choose a therapy that they wish and that this situation is an unwarranted restriction of their rights. It should be enough, they claim, for the government to issue a warning if it thinks one is called for. But after that, everyone should be free to act as he or she chooses.

The debate about Laetrile raises the more general question: To what extent is it legitimate for a government to restrict the actions and choices of its citizens for their own good? It is perhaps not possible to give a wholly satisfactory general answer to this question. No one objects that he is not permitted to drink polluted water from the city water supply or that he is not able to buy candy bars contaminated with insect parts. Yet some do object if they have to drink water that contains fluorides or if they cannot buy candy bars that contain saccharine. But all such limitations result from governmental attempts to protect the health of citizens.

Seeing to the well-being of its citizens certainly has to be recognized as one of the legitimate aims of a government. And such functioning may easily include seeing to their physical health. State paternalism with respect to health seems, in general, to be justifiable. Yet the laws and regulations through which the paternal concern is expressed are certain to come into conflict with the exercise of individual liberties. Perhaps the only way in which conflicts can be resolved is on an issue-by-issue basis. Later, we will discuss some of the limitations that moral theories place on state paternalism.

It is worth noticing that state paternalism in medical and health-care matters may be more pervasive than it seems at first sight. Laws regulating medical practice, the licensing of physicians and medical personnel, regulations governing the licensing and testing of drugs, and guidelines that must be followed in scientific research are some of the more obvious expressions of paternalism. Less obvious is the fact that government research funds can be expended only in prescribed ways and that only certain approved forms of medical care and therapy will be paid for under government-sponsored health programs. For example, it was a political and social triumph for chiropractors and Christian Science Readers when some of their services were included under Medicare coverage. Thus, government money, as well as laws and regulations, can be used in paternalistic ways.

Personal Paternalism in Medical and Health Care

That patients occupy a dependent role with respect to their physicians seems to be true historically, sociologically, and pychologically. The patient is sick, the physician is well. The patient is in need of the knowledge and skills the physician possesses, but the physician does not need those possessed by the patient. The patient seeks out the physician to ask for help, but the physician does not seek out the patient. The patient is a single individual, while the physician represents the institution of medicine with its hospitals, nurses, technicians, consultants, and so on.

In his dependence on the physician, the patient willingly surrenders some of his autonomy. Explicitly or implicitly, he agrees to allow the physician to make certain decisions for him that he would ordinarily make for himself. The physician tells him what to eat and drink and what to avoid, what medicine he should take and when to take it, how much exercise he should get and what kind it should be. The patient consents to run at least part of his life by "doctor's orders" in the hope that he will regain his health or at least improve his condition.

The physician acquires a great amount of power in this relationship. But he also acquires a great responsibility. It has been recognized at least since the time of Hippocrates that the physician has an obligation to act in the best interest of his patient. The patient is willing to transfer part of his autonomy because he is confident that the physician will act in this way.

If this analysis of the present form of the physician-patient relationship is roughly correct, two questions are appropriate.

First, should the relationship be one in which the patient is so dependent on the paternalism of the physician? Perhaps it would be better if patients did not think of themselves as transferring *any* of their autonomy to physicians. Physicians might better be thought of as people offering advice, rather than as ones issuing orders. Thus, patients, free to accept or reject advice, would retain fully their power to govern their own lives. If this is a desirable goal, it is clear that the present nature of the physician-patient relationship needs to be drastically altered.

The problem with this point of view is that the patient is ordinarily not in a position to judge the advice that is offered. The reason for consulting a physician in the first place is to gain the advantage of his knowledge and judgment. Moreover, courses of medical therapy are often complicated ones involving many interdependent steps. A patient could not expect the best treatment if he insisted on accepting some of the steps and rejecting others. As a practical matter, a patient who expects good medical care must pretty much put himself in the hands of his physician.

For this reason, the second question is perhaps based on a more realistic assessment of the nature of medical care: How much autonomy must be given up by the patient? The power of the physician over the patient cannot be absolute. The patient cannot become the slave or creature of the physician—this is not what a patient consents to when he agrees to place himself under the care of a physician. What, then, are the limits of the paternalism that can be legitimately exercised by the physician?

Truth Telling in Medicine

This question arises most forcefully when physicians deceive patients. When, if ever, is it justifiable for a physician to deceive her or his patient?

The paternalistic answer, of course, is that deception by the physician is justified when it is in the best interest of the patient. Suppose, for example, that a transplant surgeon detects signs of tissue rejection in a patient who has just received a donor kidney. The surgeon is virtually certain that within a week the kidney will have to be surgically removed and the patient transferred to dialysis equipment again. Although in no immediate clinical danger, the patient is suffering from postoperative depression. It is altogether possible that if the patient is told at this time that the transplant appears to be a failure, his depression will become more severe. This, in turn, might lead to a worsening of the patient's physical condition, perhaps even to a life-threatening extent.

Eventually the patient will have to be told of the need for another operation. But by the time that need arises, his psychological condition may have improved. Is the surgeon justified in avoiding giving a direct and honest answer to the patient when he asks about his condition? In the surgeon's assessment of the situation, the answer is likely to do the patient harm. His duty as a physician, then, seems to require that he deceive the patient, either by lying to him (an act of commission) or by allowing him to believe (an act of omission) that his condition is satisfactory and the transplant was successful.

Yet doesn't the patient have a right to know the truth from his physician? After all, it is his life that is being threatened. Should he not be told how things stand with him so that he will be in a position to make decisions that affect his own future? Is the surgeon not exceeding the bounds of the powers granted to him by the patient? The patient surely had no intention of completely turning over his autonomy to the surgeon.

This issue is one of "truth telling." Does the physician always owe it to the patient to tell the truth? Some writers (see the selection by Lund in this chapter) make a distinction between lying to the patient and merely being nonresponsive or evasive. But is this really a morally relevant distinction? In either case, the truth is being kept from the patient. Both are instances of medical paternalism.

The use of placebos (from the Latin *placebo* meaning "I shall please") in medical therapy is another issue that raises questions about the legitimate limits of paternalism in medicine. The "placebo effect" is a well-documented psychological phenomenon: even patients who are seriously ill will sometimes show improvement when they are given *any* kind of medication (a sugar pill, for example) or treatment. This can happen even when the medication or treatment is irrelevant to their condition.

The placebo effect can be exploited by physicians for the (apparent) good of their patients. Many patients cannot accept a physician's well-considered judgments. When they come to a physician with a complaint and are told that there is nothing organically wrong with them, that no treatment or medication is called for, they continue to ail. They may then lose confidence in their physician or their inclination to seek medical advice for more serious complaints.

One way to avoid these consequences is for the physician to prescribe a placebo for the patient. Since the patient (we can assume) suffers from no organic disease condition, he is not in need of any genuine medication. And because of the placebo effect, he may actually find himself relieved of the symptoms that caused him to seek medical help. Moreover, the patient feels satisfied that he has been treated, and his confidence in his physician and in medicine in general remains intact.

Since the placebo effect is not at all likely to be produced if the patient knows he is being given an ineffective medication, the physician cannot be candid about the "treatment" prescribed. She must either be silent, say something indefinite like "I think this might help your condition," or lie. Since the placebo effect is more likely to be achieved if the medication is touted as being amazingly effective against complaints like those of the patient, there is a reason for the physician to lie outright. Because the patient may stand to gain a considerable amount of good from placebo therapy, the physician may think of herself as acting in the best interest of her patient.

Despite its apparent advantages, placebo therapy may be open to two ethical criticisms. First, we can ask whether giving placebos is really in the best interest of a patient. It encourages many patients in their belief that drugs can solve their problems. Patients with vague and general complaints may need some kind of psychological counseling, and giving them placebos merely discourages them from coming to grips with their genuine problems. Also, not all placebos are harmless (see the discussion in the introduction to Chapter 5). Some contain active chemicals that produce side effects (something likely to enhance the placebo effect) so the physician who prescribes placebos may be subjecting her patient to some degree of risk.

Second, by deceiving her patient, the physician is depriving him of the chance to make genuine decisions about his own life. Because the person is not genuinely sick, it does not seem legitimate to regard him as having deputized his physician to act in his behalf or as having transferred any of his power or autonomy to the physician. In Kant's terms, the physician is not acknowledging the patient's status as an autonomous rational agent. She is not according him the dignity that he possesses simply by virtue of being human. (A utilitarian who wished to claim that telling the truth to patients is a policy that will produce the best overall benefits could offer essentially the same criticism.)

Deception is not the only issue raised by the general question of the legitimacy of medical paternalism. Another of some importance is difficult to state precisely, but it has to do with the general attitude of physicians towards their patients. Patients often feel that physicians deal with them in a way that is literally paternalistic—that physicians treat them like children.

The physician, like the magician or shaman, is often seen as a figure of power and mystery, one who controls the forces of nature and, by doing so, relieves suffering and restores health. Some physicians like this role and act in accordance with it. They resent having their authority questioned and fail to treat their patients with dignity and respect.

For example, many physicians call their patients by their first names while expecting patients to refer to them as "Dr. X." In our society, women in particular have been most critical of such condescending attitudes displayed by physicians.

More serious is the fact that many physicians do not make a genuine effort to educate patients about the state of their health, the significance of laboratory findings, or the reasons why medication or other therapy is being prescribed. Patients are not only expected to follow orders, but they are expected to do so blindly.

The issue here is not one of informed consent (which we will discuss in detail in the next chapter). For in informed consent, a patient must give permission for a procedure of a special sort to be performed. Here we are talking only about the ordinary medical situation—someone consults a physician because of a shoulder pain or just to get a yearly checkup.

The amount of time that it takes to help a patient understand his medical condition and the reason for the prescribed therapy is, of course, one reason why physicians do not attempt to provide such information. A busy physician in an office practice might see thirty or forty patients a day, and it is difficult to give each of them the necessary amount of attention. Also, patients without a medical background obviously can find it hard to understand medical explanations—particularly in the ways in which they are often given.

The result, for whatever reasons, is a situation in which physicians make decisions about patients without allowing patients to know the basis for them. Explanations are not given, it is sometimes said, because patients "wouldn't understand" or "might draw the wrong conclusions about their illness" or "might worry needlessly." Patients are thus not only *not* provided information, they are discouraged from asking questions or revealing their doubts.

The moral questions here concern the responsibility of the physician. Is it ultimately useful for patients that physicians should play the role of a distant and mysterious figure of power? If so, then it may be that physicians should cultivate the role. Do patients have a right to ask that physicians treat them with the same dignity as physicians treat one another? Should a physician attempt to educate her or his patients about their illnesses? Or is a physician's only real responsibility to provide patients with needed medical treatment?

Furthermore, is it always obvious that the physician knows what will count as the all-around best treatment for a patient? Patients, being human, have values of their own, and they may well not rank their best chance for effective medical treatment above all else. A woman with breast cancer, for example, may wish to avoid having a breast surgically removed (mastectomy) and so prefer another mode of treatment, even though her physician may consider it less effective. Can her physician legitimately withhold from her knowledge of alternate modes of treatment and so allow her no choice? Can he make the decision about treatment himself on the grounds that it is a purely medical matter, one about which the patient has no expert knowledge?

Confidentiality

"Whatever I see or hear, professionally or privately, which ought not be divulged, I will keep secret and tell no one," runs one of the pledges in the Hippocratic Oath.

The tradition of medical practice in the West has taken this injunction very seriously. That it has done so is not entirely due to the high moral character of physicians, for the pledge to secrecy also serves an important practical function. Physicians need to have information of an intimate and highly personal sort in order to make diagnoses and prescribe courses of therapy. If physicians were known to reveal such personal information, then patients would be reluctant to cooperate and the practice of medicine would be adversely affected. Furthermore, because psychological factors play a role in medical therapy, the chances of success in medical treatment are improved when patients can place trust and confidence in their physicians. This aspect of the physician-patient relationship actually forms a part of medical therapy. Of course this is particularly so of the "talking cures" characteristic of some forms of psychiatry.

A number of states recognize the need for "privileged communication" between physician and patient and have laws to protect physicians from being compelled to testify about their patients in court. (These laws present some unexpected difficulties, as H. A. Davidson points out in his essay included in this chapter.) Yet physicians are also members of a society, and the society must attempt to protect the general interest. This sometimes places the physician in the middle of a conflict between the interest of the individual and the interest of society.

For example, physicians are often required by law to act in ways that force them to reveal certain information about their patients. The best instance of this is perhaps the legal obligation to report to health departments the names of those patients who are carriers of such communicable diseases as syphilis and tuberculosis. This permits health authorities to warn those with whom the carriers have come into contact and to guard against the spread of the diseases. Thus, the interest of the society is given precedence over physician-patient confidentiality.

Few people would question society's right to demand that physicians violate a patient's confidence when the issue is that of protecting the health of great numbers of people. More open to question are laws that require physicians to report gunshot wounds or other injuries that might be connected with criminal actions. (In some states, before abortion became legal, physicians were required to report cases of attempted abortion.) Furthermore, physicians as citizens have a legal duty to report any information they may have about a crime unless they are protected by a priviliged-communication law.

Thus, the physician is placed in a position of conflict. If he acts to protect the patient's confidences, then he runs the risk of acting illegally. If he acts in accordance with the law, then he must violate the confidence of his patients. What needs to be decided from a moral point of view is to what extent the laws that place a physician in such a situation are justified.

The physician who is not in private practice but is employed by a government agency or a business organization also encounters similar conflicts. Her obligations run in two directions: to her patients and to her employer. Should a physician who works for a government agency tell her superiors that an employee has confided in her that he is a drug addict? If she does not, the man may be subject to blackmail or bribery. If she does, then she must violate the patient's confidence. Or what if a psychiatrist retained by a company decides that one of the employees is so psychologically disturbed that she cannot function effectively in her job. Should the psychiatrist inform the employer of this, even if it means going against the wishes of the patient? (Consider also the fourth case cited at the beginning of this chapter.)

Even more serious problems arise in psychiatry. Suppose that a patient expresses to his psychiatrist feelings of great anger against someone and even announces that he intends to go out and kill that person. What should the psychiatrist do? Is it his obligation to warn the person being threatened? Should he report the threat to the police? This is fundamentally the issue that was dealt with by the California Supreme Court in the case of *Tarasoff* v. *Regents of the University of California*. (See the selection in this chapter by William J. Curran for a discussion.)

The basic question about confidentiality concerns the extent to which we are willing to go to protect it. It is doubtful that anyone would want to assert that confidentiality should be absolutely guaranteed. But if not, then under what conditions is it better to violate it than to preserve it?

Ethical Theories: Paternalism, Truth Telling, Confidentiality

What we have called state paternalism and personal paternalism are compatible with utilitarian ethical theory. But whether they are justifiable is a matter of controversy. If the principle of utility shows that governmental laws, policies, practices, or regulations increase the general happiness, then they are justified. It can be argued that they are justified even if they restrict the individual's freedom of choice or action because for utilitarianism such freedom has no absolute value. Personal paternalism is justified in a similar way. If a physician believes that she can protect her patient from unnecessary suffering or can relieve his pain by keeping him in ignorance, by lying to him, by giving him placebos or by otherwise deceiving him, then these actions are morally legitimate.

However, John Stuart Mill did not take this view of paternalism. Mill argued that freedom of choice is of such importance that it can be justifiably restricted only when it can be shown that unregulated choice would cause harm to other people. Mill claimed that compelling people to act in certain ways "for their own good" is never legitimate. This position, Mill argued, is one that is justified by the principle of utility. Gerald Dworkin, in the selection included in this chapter, provides an analysis of Mill's position, and there is no need for us to repeat it here. We should note, however, that utilitarianism does not offer a straightforward answer to the question of the legitimacy of paternalism.

What we have said about paternalism also applies more or less to the issue of confidentiality. Generally speaking, if violating confidentiality seems necessary to produce a state of affairs in which happiness is increased, then the violation is justified. This might be the case when, for example, someone's life is in danger or someone is being tried for a serious crime and the testimony of a physician is needed to help establish her innocence. Yet it also might be argued from the point of view of rule utilitarianism that confidentiality is such a basic ingredient in the physician-patient relationship that, in the long run, more good will be produced if confidentiality is never violated.

The Kantian view of paternalism, truth telling, and confidentiality is more clear-cut. Every person is a rational and autonomous agent. As such he or she is entitled to make decisions that affect his or her own life. This means that a person is entitled to receive information relevant to making such decisions and is entitled to the truth, no matter how painful it might be. The use of placebos or any other kind of deception in medicine is morally illegitimate because this would involve denying a person the respect and dignity to which he or she is entitled. The categorical imperative also rules out lying, for the maxim involved in such an action produces a contradiction. (There are special difficulties in applying the categorical imperative that we discussed in the introductory chapter. When these are taken into account, Kant's view is perhaps not quite so straightforward and definite as it first appears.)

It can be argued that Kant's principles also establish that confidentiality should be regarded as absolute. When a person becomes a patient, she does so with the expectation that what she tells her physician will be kept confidential. Thus, in the physician-patient relationship there is an implicit promise. The physician implicitly promises that he will not reveal any information about his patient, either what he has been told or what he has learned for himself. If this analysis is correct, then the physician is under an obligation to preserve confidentiality because keeping promises is an absolute duty. (Here, as in the case of lying, there are difficulties connected with the way in which a maxim is stated. See the introductory chapter for a discussion.)

Ross's principles recognize that everyone has a moral right to be treated as an autonomous agent who is entitled to make decisions affecting his own life. Also, everyone is entitled to know the truth and to be educated in helpful ways. Similarly, if confidentiality is a form of promise keeping, everyone is entitled to expect that it will be kept. Thus, paternalism, lying, and violation of confidence are prima facie morally objectionable. But, of course, it is possible to imagine circumstances in which they would be justified. The right course of action that a physician must follow is one that can be determined only on the basis of the physician's knowledge of the patient, the patient's problem, and the general situation. Thus, Ross's principles rule out paternalism, deception, and violations of confidence as general policies, but they do not make them morally illegitimate in an absolute way.

Rawls's theory of social and political morality is compatible with state paternalism of a restricted kind. No laws, practices, or policies can legitimately violate the rights of individuals. At the same time, however, a society, viewing arrangements from the original position, might decide to institute a set of practices that would promote what they agreed to be their interests. If, for example, health is agreed to be an interest, then they might be willing to grant to the state the power to regulate a large range of matters connected with the promotion of health. Establishing standards for physicians would be an example of such regulation. But they might also go so far as to give the state power to decide (on the advice of experts) what medical treatments are legitimate, what drugs are safe and effective to use, what substances should be controlled or prohibited, and so on. So long as the principles of justice are not violated and so long as the society can be regarded as imposing these regulations on itself for the promotion of its own good, then such paternalistic practices are unobjectionable. With respect to personal paternalism, deception, and confidentiality, Rawls's general theory offers no specific answers. But since Rawls endorses Ross's account of prima facie duties (while rejecting Ross's intuitionism), it seems reasonable to believe that Rawls's view on these matters would be the same as Ross's.

The natural law doctrine of Roman Catholicism suggests that paternalism in both of its forms is legitimate. When the state is organized to bring about such "natural goods" as health, then laws and practices that promote those goods are morally right. Individuals do have a worth in themselves and should be free to direct and organize their own lives. But at the same time, individuals may be ignorant of relevant information, lack the intellectual capacities to determine what is really in their best interest, or be moved by momentary passions and circumstances. For these reasons, the state may act so that people are protected from their own shortcomings, and yet their genuine desires, their "natural ends," are satisfied.

Thus, natural law doctrine concludes that because each individual has an inherent worth, she is entitled to be told the truth in medical situations (and others) and not deceived. But it reasons too that because a physician has superior knowledge, he may often perceive the interest of the patient better than the patient herself. Accordingly, natural law doctrine indicates that although he should avoid lying, a physician is still under an obligation to act for the best interest of his patient. This may mean allowing the patient to believe something that is not so (as in placebo therapy) or withholding information from the patient. In order for this to be morally legitimate, however, the physician's motive must always be that of advancing the welfare of the patient.

In the matter of confidentiality, the natural law doctrine of Roman Catholicism recognizes that the relationship between physician and patient is one of trust, and a physician has a duty not to betray the confidences of her patients. But the relationship is not sacrosanct and the duty is not absolute. When the physician finds herself in a situation in which a greater wrong will be done if she does not reveal a confidence entrusted to her by a patient, then she has a duty to reveal the confidence. If, for example, the physician possesses knowledge that would save someone from death or unmerited suffering, then it is her duty to make this knowledge available, even if by doing so she violates a patient's trust.

We have been able merely to sketch an outline of possible ways in which our ethical theories might deal with the issues involved in paternalism, truth telling, and confidentiality. Some of the views presented are open to challenge, and none of them has been worked out in a completely useful way. That is one of the tasks that remains to be performed.

The Selections

In his essay included in this chapter, Gerald Dworkin attempts to show that even if we place an absolute value on individual choice, then a variety of paternalistic policies can still be justified. In consenting to a system of representative government, we understand that it may act to safeguard our interests in certain ways. But, Dworkin asks, what are the "kinds of conditions which make it plausible to suppose that rational men could reach agreement to limit their liberty even when other men's interests are not affected?"

Dworkin suggests that such conditions are satisfied in cases in which there are "goods" such as health involved—one that everybody needs to pursue other goods. Rational people would agree that attaining such a good should be promoted by the government even when individuals don't recognize it as a good at a particular time. There is a sense, Dworkin argues, in which we are not really imposing such a good on people. What we are really saying is that if everyone knew the facts and assessed them properly, this is what they would choose. Also, we are sometimes influenced by immediate alternatives that look more attractive, or we are careless or depressed and so do not act for what we acknowledge as a good. Thus, we might approve of laws such as ones against cigarette smoking because we know we should not smoke cigarettes.

It is plausible, Dworkin suggests, that rational people would grant to a legislature the right to impose such restrictions on their conduct. But the government has to demonstrate the exact nature of the harmful effects to be avoided. Also, if there is an alternative way of accomplishing the end without restricting liberty, then the society should adopt it.

Perhaps the most common form of paternalism in medicine consists in withholding information from patients. Physician Mack Lipkin, in "On Telling Patients the Truth," provides a defense of the practice. It is usually a practical impossibility to tell patients "the whole truth," he claims. Patients usually simply do not possess enough information about how their bodies work to understand the nature of their disease, and their understanding of the terms used by a physician is likely to be quite different from the meaning intended. Besides, some patients do not wish to be told the truth about their illness. Whether it is a matter of telling the truth or of deceiving patients by giving them placebos, the crucial question, according to Lipkin, is "whether the deception was intended to benefit the patient or the doctor."

Sissela Bok, in "Lies to the Sick and Dying," reviews three arguments that physicians frequently use to justify not telling the truth to their patients. All three are arguments appealed to by Lipkin. However, Bok finds each of them faulty and unpersuasive.

Bok points out that the first of the arguments trades on a confusion between telling "the truth" (that is, everything that is true about a situation) and "truthfulness" (being honest). In effect, the argument asserts that since it is impossible to tell "the truth" to people who are not medical experts, then there is no clear distinction between what is true and what is false. Anything medical said to them is, at best, partially true. When this argument is accepted, Bok claims, the way is open for the physician to decide just how much of "the truth" will be revealed to serve the best interest of the patient.

Are physicians correct in claiming that patients don't want to know the truth? This is an issue that is open to empirical tests. Bok cites studies which show that a large majority of people say they want to be told the truth about themselves, even if they should be diagnosed as having a catastrophic illness.

The last argument examined by Bok holds that information given to a patient might damage the patient (or at least not help the patient), thus proper health care demands that information not be supplied. This argument also has an empirical aspect and is open to challenge on factual grounds. As Bok observes, the harm associated with the disclosure of bad news and risks is probably greatly overestimated. What is more, very real benefits (such as increased cooperation) are never mentioned.

Bok is not willing to go so far as to say that lying to a patient is never justified. She is primarily concerned with showing that withholding the truth is a serious matter that requires justification in each case. Like Ross, she sees telling the truth to be a prima facie obligation that can be set aside only for the sake of some more weighty obligation.

In "Professional Secrecy," Henry A. Davidson presents some of the dilemmas that confidentiality causes for physicians. The physician's obligations to society, her legal situation, her duties to an employer, and her duties to certain third parties can all serve as a source of moral difficulties. Davidson stresses, in particular, the dangers that conflicting obligations pose for the doctor-patient relationship. Unfortunately, although Davidson does much to identify the issues, he offers very little by way of solution. He seems content to rely on "personal judgment, the facing of responsibility, and the path-pointing of the human conscience." Clearly, more than this is needed.

William J. Curran, in the last selection, discusses a case recently decided by the California Supreme Court that has been of particular concern to psychiatrists. The court ruled that therapists at the student health service of the University of California at Berkeley were negligent in their duty to warn a woman named Tarasoff that her life had been threatened by one of their patients. Although the therapists had reported the threat to the police, Ms. Tarasoff was murdered by the patient. The question that Curran addresses is whether or not the therapists had done all they were obligated to do to protect both their patient and the community by reporting the case to the police. But more general issues are also involved here: Does a psychiatrist have a duty to warn at all? Should a patient be told that not everything he tells his psychiatrist will be held in confidence? Is a psychiatrist obliged to seek a court order committing a patient involuntarily to an institution if the patient utters a threat that the psychiatrist judges to be seriously motivated?

Paternalism, truth telling, and confidentiality are bound together in a complicated web of moral issues. We have not identified all of the strands of the web, nor have we traced out their connections with one another. We have, however, mentioned enough difficulties to reveal the seriousness of the issues.

Some of the issues are social ones and require that we decide about the moral legitimacy of certain kinds of laws, practices, and policies. Others are matters of personal morality, ones that concern our obligations to society and to other people. Our ethical theories, we can hope, will provide us with the means of arriving at workable and justifiable resolutions of the issues. But before this point is reached, much intellectual effort and ingenuity will have to be invested.

Paternalism

Gerald Dworkin

Neither one person, nor any number of persons, is warranted in saying to another human creature of ripe years, that he shall not do with his life for his own benefit what he chooses to do with it. *Mill*

I do not want to go along with a volunteer

Reprinted from The Monist *56, no. 1 (January 1972), with the permission of the editor.*

basis. I think a fellow should be compelled to become better and not let him use his discretion whether he wants to get smarter, more healthy or more honest. *General Hershey*

I take as my starting point the "one very simple principle" proclaimed by Mill in *On Liberty* . . . "That principle is, that the sole end for which mankind are warranted, individually or collectively, in interfering with the liberty of action of any of their number, is self-protection. That the only purpose for which power can be rightfully exercised over any member of a civilized community, against his will, is to prevent harm to others. He cannot rightfully be compelled to do or forbear because it will be better for him to do so, because it will make him happier, because, in the opinion of others, to do so would be wise, or even right."[1]

This principle is neither "one" nor "very simple." It is at least two principles; one asserting that self-protection or the prevention of harm to others is sometimes a sufficient warrant and the other claiming that the individual's own good is *never* a sufficient warrant for the exercise of compulsion either by the society as a whole or by its individual members. I assume that no one with the possible exception of extreme pacifists or anarchists questions the correctness of the first half of the principle. This essay is an examination of the negative claim embodied in Mill's principle—the objection to paternalistic interferences with a man's liberty.

I

By paternalism I shall understand roughly the interference with a person's liberty of action justified by reasons referring exclusively to the welfare, good, happiness, needs, interests or values of the person being coerced. One is always well-advised to illustrate one's definitions by examples but it is not easy to find "pure" examples of paternalistic interferences. For almost any piece of legislation is justified by several different kinds of reasons and even if historically a piece of legislation can be shown to have been introduced for purely paternalistic motives, it may be that advocates of the legislation with an anti-paternalistic outlook can find sufficient reasons justifying the legislation without appealing to the reasons which were originally adduced to support it. Thus, for example, it may be that the original legislation requiring motorcyclists to wear safety helmets was

introduced for purely paternalistic reasons. But the Rhode Island Supreme Court recently upheld such legislation on the grounds that it was "not persuaded that the legislature is powerless to prohibit individuals from pursuing a course of conduct which could conceivably result in their becoming public charges," thus clearly introducing reasons of a quite different kind. Now I regard this decision as being based on reasoning of a very dubious nature but it illustrates the kind of problem one has in finding examples. The following is a list of the kinds of interferences I have in mind as being paternalistic.

II

1. Laws requiring motorcyclists to wear safety helmets when operating their machines.

2. Laws forbidding persons from swimming at a public beach when lifeguards are not on duty.

3. Laws making suicide a criminal offense.

4. Laws making it illegal for women and children to work at certain types of jobs.

5. Laws regulating certain kinds of sexual conduct, e.g. homosexuality among consenting adults in private.

6. Laws regulating the use of certain drugs which may have harmful consequences to the user but do not lead to anti-social conduct.

7. Laws requiring a license to engage in certain professions with those not receiving a license subject to fine or jail sentence if they do engage in the practice.

8. Laws compelling people to spend a specified fraction of their income on the purchase of retirement annuities. (Social Security)

9. Laws forbidding various forms of gambling (often justified on the grounds that the poor are more likely to throw away their money on such activities than the rich who can afford to).

10. Laws regulating the maximum rates of interest for loans.

11. Laws against duelling.

In addition to laws which attach criminal or civil penalties to certain kinds of action there are laws, rules, regulations, decrees, which make it

either difficult or impossible for people to carry out their plans and which are also justified on paternalistic grounds. Examples of this are:

1. Laws regulating the types of contracts which will be upheld as valid by the courts, e.g. (an example of Mill's to which I shall return) no man may make a valid contract for perpetual involuntary servitude.

2. Not allowing as a defense to a charge of murder or assault the consent of the victim.

3. Requiring members of certain religious sects to have compulsory blood transfusions. This is made possible by not allowing the patient to have recourse to civil suits for assault and battery and by means of injunctions.

4. Civil commitment procedures when these are specifically justified on the basis of preventing the person being committed from harming himself. (The D.C. Hospitalization of the Mentally Ill Act provides for involuntary hospitalization of a person who "is mentally ill, and because of that illness, is likely to injure *himself* or others if allowed to remain at liberty." The term injure in this context applies to unintentional as well as intentional injuries.)

5. Putting fluorides in the community water supply.

All of my examples are of existing restrictions on the liberty of individuals. Obviously one can think of interferences which have not yet been imposed. Thus one might ban the sale of cigarettes, or require that people wear safety-belts in automobiles (as opposed to merely having them installed) enforcing this by not allowing motorists to sue for injuries even when caused by other drivers if the motorist was not wearing a seat-belt at the time of the accident.

I shall not be concerned with activities which though defended on paternalistic grounds are not interferences with the liberty of persons, e.g. the giving of subsidies in kind rather than in cash on the grounds that the recipients would not spend the money on the goods which they really need, or not including a $1000 deductible provision in a basic protection automobile insurance plan on the ground that the people who would elect it could least afford it. Nor shall I be concerned with measures such as "truth-in-advertising" acts and the

Pure Food and Drug legislation which are often attacked as paternalistic but which should not be considered so. In these cases all that is provided—it is true by the use of compulsion—is information which it is presumed that rational persons are interested in having in order to make wise decisions. There is no interference with the liberty of the consumer unless one wants to stretch a point beyond good sense and say that his liberty to apply for a loan without knowing the true rate of interest is diminished. It is true that sometimes there is sentiment for going further than providing information, for example when laws against usurious interest are passed preventing those who might wish to contract loans at high rates of interest from doing so, and these measures may correctly be considered paternalistic.

III

Bearing these examples in mind let me return to a characterization of paternalism. I said earlier that I meant by the term, roughly, interference with a person's liberty for his own good. But as some of the examples show the class of persons whose good is involved is not always identical with the class of persons whose freedom is restricted. Thus in the case of professional licensing it is the practitioner who is directly interfered with and it is the would-be patient whose interests are presumably being served. Not allowing the consent of the victim to be a defense to certain types of crime primarily affects the would-be aggressor but it is the interests of the willing victim that we are trying to protect. Sometimes a person may fall into both classes as would be the case if we banned the manufacture and sale of cigarettes and a given manufacturer happened to be a smoker as well.

Thus we may first divide paternalistic interferences into "pure" and "impure" cases. In "pure" paternalism the class of persons whose freedom is restricted is identical with the class of persons whose benefit is intended to be promoted by such restrictions. Examples: the making of suicide a crime, requiring passengers in automobiles to wear seat-belts, requiring a Christian Scientist to receive a blood transfusion. In the case of "impure" paternalism in trying to protect the welfare of a class of persons we find that the only way to do so will involve restricting the freedom of other persons besides those who are benefitted.

Now it might be thought that there are no cases of "impure" paternalism since any such case could always be justified on non-paternalistic grounds, i.e. in terms of preventing harms to others. Thus we might ban cigarette manufacturers from continuing to manufacture their product on the grounds that we are preventing them from causing illness to others in the same way that we prevent other manufacturers from releasing pollutants into the atmosphere, thereby causing danger to the members of the community. The difference is, however, that in the former but not the latter case the harm is of such a nature that it could be avoided by those individuals affected if they so chose. The incurring of the harm requires, so to speak, the active co-operation of the victim. It would be mistaken theoretically and hypocritical in practice to assert that our interference in such cases is just like our interference in standard cases of protecting others from harm. At the very least someone interfered with in this way can reply that no one is complaining about his activities. It may be that impure paternalism requires arguments or reasons of a stronger kind in order to be justified since there are persons who are losing a portion of their liberty and they do not even have the solace of having it be done "in their own interest." Of course in some sense, if paternalistic justifications are ever correct then we are protecting others, we are preventing some from injuring others, but it is important to see the differences between this and the standard case.

Paternalism then will always involve limitations on the liberty of some individuals in their own interest but it may also extend to interferences with the liberty of parties whose interests are not in question.

IV

Finally, by way of some more preliminary analysis, I want to distinguish paternalistic interferences with liberty from a related type with which it is often confused. Consider, for example, legislation which forbids employees to work more than, say, 40 hours per week. It is sometimes argued that such legislation is paternalistic for if employees desired such a restriction on their hours of work they could agree among themselves to impose it voluntarily. But because they do not the society imposes its own conception of their

best interests upon them by the use of coercion. Hence this is paternalism.

Now it may be that some legislation of this nature is, in fact, paternalistically motivated. I am not denying that. All I want to point out is that there is another possible way of justifying such measures which is not paternalistic in nature. It is not paternalistic because as Mill puts it in a similar context such measures are "required not to overrule the judgment of individuals respecting their own interest, but to give effect to that judgment: they being unable to give effect to it except by concert, which concert again cannot be effectual unless it receives validity and sanction from the law."[2]

The line of reasoning here is a familiar one first found in Hobbes and developed with great sophistication by contemporary economists in the last decade or so. There are restrictions which are in the interests of a class of persons taken collectively but are such that the immediate interest of each individual is furthered by his violating the rule when others adhere to it. In such cases the individuals involved may need the use of compulsion to give effect to their collective judgment of their own interest by guaranteeing each individual compliance by the others. In these cases compulsion is not used to achieve some benefit which is not recognized to be a benefit by those concerned, but rather because it is the only feasible means of achieving some benefit which *is* recognized as such by all concerned. This way of viewing matters provides us with another characterization of paternalism in general. Paternalism might be thought of as the use of coercion to achieve a good which is not recognized as such by those persons for whom the good is intended. Again while this formulation captures the heart of the matter—it is surely what Mill is objecting to in *On Liberty*—the matter is not always quite like that. For example when we force motorcyclists to wear helmets we are trying to promote a good—the protection of the person from injury—which is surely recognized by most of the individuals concerned. It is not that a cyclist doesn't value his bodily integrity; rather, as a supporter of such legislation would put it, he either places, perhaps irrationally, another value or good (freedom from wearing a helmet) above that of physical well-being or, perhaps, while recognizing the danger in the abstract, he either does not fully appreciate it or he underestimates the likelihood of its occurring. But now we are approaching the question of possible justifications of paternalistic measures and the rest of this essay will be devoted to that question.

V

I shall begin for dialectical purposes by discussing Mill's objections to paternalism and then go on to discuss more positive proposals.

An initial feature that strikes one is the absolute nature of Mill's prohibitions against paternalism. It is so unlike the carefully qualified admonitions of Mill and his fellow Utilitarians on other moral issues. He speaks of self-protection as the *sole* end warranting coercion, of the individual's own goals as *never* being a sufficient warrant. Contrast this with his discussion of the prohibition against lying in *Util[itarianism]*.

> Yet that even this, rule, sacred as it is, admits of possible exception, is acknowledged by all moralists, the chief of which is where the with-holding of some fact . . . would save an individual . . . from great and unmerited evil.[3]

The same tentativeness is present when he deals with justice.

> It is confessedly unjust to break faith with any one: to violate an engagement, either express or implied, or disappoint expectations raised by our own conduct, at least if we have raised these expectations knowingly and voluntarily. Like all the other obligations of justice already spoken of, this one is not regarded as absolute, but as capable of being overruled by a stronger obligation of justice on the other side.[4]

This anomaly calls for some explanation. The structure of Mill's argument is as follows:

1. Since restraint is an evil the burden of proof is on those who propose such restraint.

2. Since the conduct which is being considered is purely self-regarding, the normal appeal to the protection of the interests of others is not available.

3. Therefore we have to consider whether reasons involving reference to the individual's own good, happiness, welfare, or interests are sufficient to overcome the burden of justification.

4. We either cannot advance the interests of the individual by compulsion, or the attempt to do so involves evil which outweighs the good done.

5. Hence the promotion of the individual's own interests does not provide a sufficient warrant for the use of compulsion.

Clearly the operative premise here is 4 and it is bolstered by claims about the status of the individual as judge and appraiser of his welfare, interests, needs, etc.

> With respect to his own feelings and circumstances, the most ordinary man or woman has means of knowledge immeasurably surpassing those that can be possessed by any one else.[5]

> He is the man most interested in his own well-being: the interest which any other person, except in cases of strong personal attachment, can have in it, is trifling, compared to that which he himself has.[6]

These claims are used to support the following generalizations concerning the utility of compulsion for paternalistic purposes.

> The interferences of society to overrule his judgment and purposes in what only regards himself must be grounded on general presumptions; which may be altogether wrong, and even if right, are as likely as not to be misapplied to individual cases.[7]

> But the strongest of all the arguments against the interference of the public with purely personal conduct is that when it does interfere, the odds are that it interferes wrongly and in the wrong place.[8]

> All errors which the individual is likely to commit against advice and warning are far outweighed by the evil of allowing others to constrain him to what they deem his good.[9]

Performing the utilitarian calculation by balancing the advantages and disadvantages we find that:

> Mankind are greater gainers by suffering each other to live as seems good to themselves, than by compelling each other to live as seems good to the rest.[10]

From which follows the operative premise 4.

This classical case of a utilitarian argument with all the premises spelled out is not the only line of reasoning present in Mill's discussion. There are asides, and more than asides, which look quite different and I shall deal with them later. But this is clearly the main channel of Mill's thought and it is one which has been subjected to vigorous attack from the moment it appeared—most often by fellow Utilitarians. The link that they have usually seized on is, as Fitzjames Stephen put it, the absence of proof that the "mass of adults are so well acquainted with their own interests and so much disposed to pursue them that no compulsion or restraint put upon them by any others for the purpose of promoting their interest can really promote them."[11] Even so sympathetic a critic as Hart is forced to the conclusion that:

> In Chapter 5 of his essay Mill carried his protests against paternalism to lengths that may now appear to us as fantastic. . . . No doubt if we no longer sympathise with this criticism this is due, in part, to a general decline in the belief that individuals know their own interest best.[12]

> Mill endows the average individual with "too much of the psychology of a middle-aged man whose desires are relatively fixed, not liable to be artificially stimulated by external influences; who knows what he wants and what gives him satisfaction of happiness; and who pursues these things when he can."[13]

Now it is interesting to note that Mill himself was aware of some of the limitations on the doctrine that the individual is the best judge of his own interests. In his discussion of government intervention in general (even where the intervention does not interfere with liberty but provides alternative institutions to those of the market) after making claims which are parallel to those just discussed, e.g.

> People understand their own business and their own interests better, and care for them more, than the government does, or can be expected to do.[14]

He goes on to an intelligent discussion of the "very large and conspicuous exceptions" to the maxim that:

> Most persons take a juster and more intelligent view of their own interest, and of the means of promoting it than can either be prescribed to them by a general enactment of the legislature, or pointed out in the particular case by a public functionary.[15]

Thus there are things

> of which the utility does not consist in ministering to inclinations, nor in serving the daily uses of life, and the want of which is least felt where the need is greatest. This is peculiarly true of those things which are chiefly useful as tending to raise the character of human beings. The uncultivated cannot be competent judges of cultivation. Those who most need to be made wiser and better, usually desire it least, and, if they desired it, would be incapable of finding the way to it by their own lights.

> . . . . A second exception to the doctrine that individuals are the best judges of their own interest, is when an individual attempts to decide irrevocably now what will be best for his interest at some future and distant time. The presumption in favor of individual judgment is only legitimate, where the judgment is grounded on actual, and especially on present, personal experience; not where it is formed antecedently to experience, and not suffered to be reversed even after experience has condemned it.[16]

The upshot of these exceptions is that Mill does not declare that there should never be government interference with the economy but rather that

> . . . in every instance, the burden of making out a strong case should be thrown not on those who resist but on those who recommend government interference. Letting alone, in short, should be the general practice: every departure from it, unless required by some great good, is a certain evil.[17]

In short, we get a presumption not an absolute prohibition. The question is why doesn't the argument against paternalism go the same way?

I suggest that the answer lies in seeing that in addition to a purely utilitarian argument Mill uses another as well. As a Utilitarian Mill has to show, in Fitzjames Stephen's words, that:

> Self-protection apart, no good object can be attained by any compulsion which is not in itself a greater evil than the absence of the object which the compulsion obtains.[18]

To show this is impossible; one reason being that it isn't true. Preventing a man from selling himself into slavery (a paternalistic measure which Mill himself accepts as legitimate), or from taking heroin, or from driving a car without wearing seatbelts may constitute a lesser evil than allowing him to do any of these things. A consistent Utilitarian can only argue against paternalism on the grounds that it (as a matter of fact) does not maximize the good. It is always a contingent question that may be refuted by the evidence. But there is also a non-contingent argument which runs through *On Liberty*. When Mill states that "there is a part of the life of every person who has come to years of discretion, within which the individuality of that person ought to reign uncontrolled either by any other person or by the public collectively" he is saying something about what it means to be a person, an autonomous agent. It is because coercing a person for his own good denies this status as an independent entity that Mill objects to it so strongly and in such absolute terms. To be able to choose is a good that is independent of the wisdom of what is chosen. A man's "mode of laying out his existence is the best, not because it is the best in itself, but because it is his own mode."[19]

> It is the privilege and proper condition of a human being, arrived at the maturity of his faculties, to use and interpret experience in his own way.[20]

As further evidence of this line of reasoning in Mill consider the one exception to his prohibition against paternalism.

> In this and most civilised countries, for example, an engagement by which a person should sell himself, or allow himself to be sold, as a slave, would be null and void; neither enforced by law nor by opinion. The ground for thus limiting his power of voluntarily disposing of his own lot in life, is apparent, and is very clearly seen in this extreme case. The reason for not interfering, unless for the sake of others, with a person's voluntary acts, is consideration for his liberty. His voluntary choice is evidence that what he so chooses is desirable, or at least endurable, to him, and his good is on the whole best provided for by allowing him to take his own means of pursuing it. But by selling himself for a slave, he abdicates his liberty; he foregoes any future use of it beyond that single act.
>
> He therefore defeats, in his own case, the very purpose which is the justification of allowing him to dispose of himself. He is no longer free; but is thenceforth in a position which has no longer the presumption in its favour, that would be afforded by his voluntarily remaining in it. The principle of freedom cannot require that he should be free not to be free. It is not freedom to be allowed to alienate his freedom.[21]

Now leaving aside the fudging on the meaning of freedom in the last line it is clear that part of this argument is incorrect. While it is true that *future* choices of the slave are not reasons for thinking that what he chooses then is desirable for him, what is at issue is limiting his immediate choice; and since this choice is made freely, the individual may be correct in thinking that his interests are best provided for by entering such a contract. But the main consideration for not allowing such a contract is the need to preserve the liberty of the person to make future choices. This gives us a principle—a very narrow one—by which to justify some paternalistic interferences. Paternalism is justified only to preserve a wider range of freedom for the individual in question. How far this principle could be extended, whether it can justify all the cases in which we are inclined upon reflection to think paternalistic measures justified remains to be discussed. What I have tried to show so far is that there are two strains of argument in Mill—one a straight-forward Utilitarian mode of reasoning and one which relies not on the goods which free choice leads to but on the absolute value of the choice itself. The first cannot establish any absolute prohibition but at most a presumption and indeed a fairly weak one given some fairly plausible assumptions about human psychology; the second while a stronger line of argument seems to me to allow on its own grounds a wider range of paternalism than might be suspected. I turn now to a consideration of these matters.

VI

We might begin looking for principles governing the acceptable use of paternalistic power in cases where it is generally agreed that it is legitimate. Even Mill intends his principles to be applicable only to mature individuals, not those in what he calls "non-age." What is it that justifies us in interfering with children? The fact that they lack some of the emotional and cognitive capacities required in order to make fully rational decisions. It is an empirical question to just what extent children have an adequate conception of their own present and future interests but there is not much doubt that there are many deficiencies. For example it is very difficult for a child to defer gratification for any considerable period of time. Given these deficiencies and given the very real and permanent dangers that may befall the child it becomes not only permissible but even a duty of the parent to restrict the child's freedom in various ways. There is however an important moral limitation on the exercise of such parental power which is provided by the notion of the child eventually coming to see the correctness of his parent's interventions. Parental paternalism may be thought of as a wager by the parent on the child's subsequent recognition of the wisdom of the restrictions. There is an emphasis on what could be called future-oriented consent—on what the child will come to welcome, rather than on what he does welcome.

The essence of this idea has been incorporated by idealist philosophers into various types of "real-will" theory as applied to fully adult persons. Extensions of paternalism are argued for by claiming that in various respects, chronologically mature individuals share the same deficiencies in knowledge, capacity to think rationally, and the ability to carry out decisions that children possess. Hence in interfering with such people we are in effect doing what they would do if they were fully rational. Hence we are not really opposing their will, hence we are not really interfering with their freedom. The dangers of this move have been sufficiently exposed by Berlin in his Two Concepts of Liberty. I see no gain in theoretical clarity nor in practical advantage in trying to pass over the real nature of the interferences with liberty that we impose on others. Still the basic notion of consent is important and seems to me the only acceptable way of trying to delimit an area of justified paternalism.

Let me start by considering a case where the consent is not hypothetical in nature. Under certain conditions it is rational for an individual to agree that others should force him to act in ways in which, at the time of action, the individual may not see as desirable. If, for example, a man knows that he is subject to breaking his resolves when temptation is present, he may ask a friend to refuse to entertain his requests at some later stage.

A classical example is given in the Odyssey when Odysseus commands his men to tie him to the mast and refuse all future orders to be set free, because he knows the power of the Sirens to enchant men with their songs. Here we are on relatively sound ground in later refusing Odysseus' request to be set free. He may even claim to have

changed his mind but since it is just such changes that he wished to guard against we are entitled to ignore them.

A process analogous to this may take place on a social rather than individual basis. An electorate may mandate its representatives to pass legislation which when it comes time to "pay the price" may be unpalatable. I may believe that a tax increase is necessary to halt inflation though I may resent the lower pay check each month. However in both this case and that of Odysseus the measure to be enforced is specifically requested by the party involved and at some point in time there is genuine consent and agreement on the part of those persons whose liberty is infringed. Such is not the case for the paternalistic measures we have been speaking about. What must be involved here is not consent to specific measures but rather consent to a system of government, run by elected representatives, with an understanding that they may act to safeguard our interests in certain limited ways.

I suggest that since we are all aware of our irrational propensities, deficiencies in cognitive and emotional capacities and avoidable and unavoidable ignorance it is rational and prudent for us to in effect take out "social insurance policies." We may argue for and against proposed paternalistic measures in terms of what fully rational individuals would accept as forms of protection. Now, clearly since the initial agreement is not about specific measures we are dealing with a more-or-less blank check and therefore there have to be carefully defined limits. What I am looking for are certain kinds of conditions which make it plausible to suppose that rational men could reach agreement to limit their liberty even when other men's interests are not affected.

Of course as in any kind of agreement schema there are great difficulties in deciding what rational individuals would or would not accept. Particularly in sensitive areas of personal liberty, there is always a danger of the dispute over agreement and rationality being a disguised version of evaluative and normative disagreement.

Let me suggest types of situations in which it seems plausible to suppose that fully rational individuals would agree to having paternalistic restrictions imposed upon them. It is reasonable to suppose that there are "goods" such as health which any person would want to have in order to pursue his own good—no matter how that good is conceived. This is an argument that is used in connection with compulsory education for children but it seems to me that it can be extended to other goods which have this character. Then one could agree that the attainment of such goods should be promoted even when not recognized to be such, at the moment, by the individuals concerned.

An immediate difficulty that arises stems from the fact that men are always faced with competing goods and that there may be reasons why even a value such as health—or indeed life—may be overridden by competing values. Thus the problem with the Christian Scientist and blood transfusions. It may be more important for him to reject "impure substances" than to go on living. The difficult problem that must be faced is whether one can give sense to the notion of a person irrationally attaching weights to competing values.

Consider a person who knows the statistical data on the probability of being injured when not wearing seat belts in an automobile and knows the types and gravity of the various injuries. He also insists that the inconvenience attached to fastening the belt every time he gets in and out of the car outweighs for him the possible risks to himself. I am inclined in this case to think that such a weighing is irrational. Given his life-plans which we are assuming are those of the average person, his interests and commitments already undertaken, I think it is safe to predict that we can find inconsistencies in his calculations at some point. I am assuming that this is not a man who for some conscious or unconscious reasons is trying to injure himself nor is he a man who just likes to "live dangerously." I am assuming that he is like us in all the relevant respects but just puts an enormously high negative value on inconvenience—one which does not seem comprehensible or reasonable.

It is always possible, of course to assimilate this person to creatures like myself. I, also, neglect to fasten my seat belt and I concede such behavior is not rational but not because I weigh the inconvenience differently from those who fasten the belts. It is just that having made (roughly) the same calculation as everybody else I ignore it in my actions. [Note: a much better case of weakness of the will than those usually given in ethics texts.] A plausible explanation for this deplorable habit is that although I know in some intellectual sense what the probabilities and risks are I do not fully appreciate them in an emotionally genuine manner.

We have two distinct types of situation in which a man acts in a non-rational fashion. In one case he attaches incorrect weights to some of his values; in the other he neglects to act in accordance with his actual preferences and desires. Clearly there is a stronger and more persuasive argument for paternalism in the latter situation. Here we are really not—by assumption—imposing a good on another person. But why may we not extend our interference to what we might call evaluative delusions? After all in the case of cognitive delusions we are prepared, often, to act against the expressed will of the person involved. If a man believes that when he jumps out the window he will float upwards—Robert Nozick's example—would not we detain him, forcibly if necessary? The reply will be that this man doesn't wish to be injured and if we could convince him that he is mistaken as to the consequences of his action he would not wish to perform the action. But part of what is involved in claiming that a man who doesn't fasten his seat-belts is attaching an irrational weight to the inconvenience of fastening them is that if he were to be involved in an accident and severely injured he would look back and admit that the inconvenience wasn't as bad as all that. So there is a sense in which if I could convince him of the consequences of his action he also would not wish to continue his present course of action. Now the notion of consequences being used here is covering a lot of ground. In one case it's being used to indicate what will or can happen as a result of a course of action and in the other it's making a prediction about the future evaluation of the consequences—in the first sense—of a course of action. And whatever the difference between facts and values—whether it be hard and fast or soft and slow—we are genuinely more reluctant to consent to interferences where evaluative differences are the issue. Let me now consider another factor which comes into play in some of these situations which may make an important difference in our willingness to consent to paternalistic restrictions.

Some of the decisions we make are of such a character that they produce changes which are in one or another way irreversible. Situations are created in which it is difficult or impossible to return to anything like the initial stage at which the decision was made. In particular some of these changes will make it impossible to continue to make reasoned choices in the future. I am thinking specifically of decisions which involve taking drugs that are physically or psychologically addictive and those which are destructive of one's mental and physical capacities.

I suggest we think of the imposition of paternalistic interferences in situations of this kind as being a kind of insurance policy which we take out against making decisions which are far-reaching, potentially dangerous and irreversible. Each of these factors is important. Clearly there are many decisions we make that are relatively irreversible. In deciding to learn to play chess I could predict in view of my general interest in games that some portion of my free-time was going to be pre-empted and that it would not be easy to give up the game once I acquired a certain competence. But my whole life-style was not going to be jeopardized in an extreme manner. Further it might be argued that even with addictive drugs such as heroin one's normal life plans would not be seriously interfered with if an inexpensive and adequate supply were readily available. So this type of argument might have a much narrower scope than appears to be the case at first.

A second class of cases concerns decisions which are made under extreme psychological and sociological pressures. I am not thinking here of the making of the decision as being something one is pressured into—e.g. a good reason for making duelling illegal is that unless this is done many people might have to manifest their courage and integrity in ways in which they would rather not do so—but rather of decisions such as that to commit suicide which are usually made at a point where the individual is not thinking clearly and calmly about the nature of his decision. In addition, of course, this comes under the previous heading of all-too-irrevocable decision. Now there are practical steps which a society could take if it wanted to decrease the possibility of suicide—for example not paying social security benefits to the survivors or as religious institutions do, not allowing such persons to be buried with the same status as natural deaths. I think we may count these as interferences with the liberty of persons to attempt suicide and the question is whether they are justifiable.

Using my argument schema the question is whether rational individuals would consent to such limitations. I see no reason for them to consent to an absolute prohibition but I do think it is reasonable for them to agree to some kind of enforced waiting period. Since we are all aware of the possibility of temporary states, such as great fear or depression, that are inimical to the making of well-informed and rational decisions, it would be prudent for all of us if there were some kind of institutional arrangement whereby we were restrained from making a decision which is (all too) irreversible. What this would be like in practice is difficult to envisage and it may be that if no practical arrangements were feasible then we would have to conclude that there should be no restriction at all on this kind of action. But we might have a "cooling off" period, in much the same way that we now require couples who file for divorce to go through a waiting period. Or, more far-fetched, we might imagine a Suicide Board composed of a psychologist and another member picked by the applicant. The Board would be required to meet and talk with the person proposing to take his life, though its approval would not be required.

A third class of decisions—these classes are not supposed to be disjoint—involves dangers which are either not sufficiently understood or appreciated correctly by the persons involved. Let me illustrate, using the example of cigarette smoking, a number of possible cases.

1. A man may not know the facts—e.g. smoking between 1 and 2 packs a day shortens life expectancy 6.2 years, the costs and pain of the illness caused by smoking, etc.

2. A man may know the facts, wish to stop smoking, but not have the requisite will-power.

3. A man may know the facts but not have them play the correct role in his calculation because, say, he discounts the danger psychologically because it is remote in time and/or inflates the attractiveness of other consequences of his decision which he regards as beneficial.

In case 1 what is called for is education, the posting of warnings, etc. In case 2 there is no theoretical problem. We are not imposing a good on someone who rejects it. We are simply using coercion to enable people to carry out their own goals. (Note: There obviously is a difficulty in that only a subclass of the individuals affected wish to be prevented from doing what they are doing.) In case 3 there is a sense in which we are imposing a good on someone since given his current appraisal of the facts he doesn't wish to be restricted. But in another sense we are not imposing a good since what is being claimed—and what must be shown or at least argued for—is that an accurate accounting on his part would lead him to reject his current course of action. Now we all know that such cases exist, that we are prone to disregard dangers that are only possibilities, that immediate pleasures are often magnified and distorted.

If in addition the dangers are severe and far-reaching we could agree to allowing the state a certain degree of power to intervene in such situations. The difficulty is in specifying in advance, even vaguely, the class of cases in which intervention will be legitimate.

A related difficulty is that of drawing a line so that it is not the case that all ultra-hazardous activities are ruled out, e.g. mountain-climbing, bull-fighting, sports-car racing, etc. There are some risks—even very great ones—which a person is entitled to take with his life.

A good deal depends on the nature of the deprivation—e.g. does it prevent the person from engaging in the activity completely or merely limit his participation—and how important to the nature of the activity is the absence of restriction when this is weighed against the role that the activity plays in the life of the person. In the case of automobile seat belts, for example, the restriction is trivial in nature, interferes not at all with the use or enjoyment of the activity, and does, I am assuming, considerably reduce a high risk of serious injury. Whereas, for example, making mountain-climbing illegal prevents completely a person engaging in an activity which may play an important role in his life and his conception of the person he is.

In general the easiest cases to handle are those which can be argued about in the terms which Mill thought to be so important—a concern not just for the happiness or welfare, in some broad sense, of the individual but rather a concern for the autonomy and freedom of the person. I suggest that we would be most likely to consent to paternalism in those instances in which it preserves and enhances for the individual his ability to rationally consider and carry out his own decisions.

I have suggested in this essay a number of types of situations in which it seems plausible that rational men would agree to granting the legislative powers of a society the right to impose restrictions on what Mill calls "self-regarding" conduct.

However, rational men knowing something about the resources of ignorance, ill-will and stupidity available to the law-makers of a society—a good case in point is the history of drug legislation in the United States—will be concerned to limit such intervention to a minimum. I suggest in closing two principles designed to achieve this end.

In all cases of paternalistic legislation there must be a heavy and clear burden of proof placed on the authorities to demonstrate the exact nature of the harmful effects (or beneficial consequences) to be avoided (or achieved) and the probability of their occurrence. The burden of proof here is twofold—what lawyers distinguish as the burden of going forward and the burden of persuasion. That the authorities have the burden of going forward means that it is up to them to raise the question and bring forward evidence of the evils to be avoided. Unlike the case of new drugs where the manufacturer must produce some evidence that the drug has been tested and found not harmful, no citizen has to show with respect to self-regarding conduct that it is not harmful or promotes his best interests. In addition the nature and cogency of the evidence for the harmfulness of the course of action must be set at a high level. To paraphrase a formulation of the burden of proof for criminal proceedings—better 10 men ruin themselves than one man be unjustly deprived of liberty.

Finally I suggest a principle of the least restrictive alternative. If there is an alternative way of accomplishing the desired end without restricting liberty then although it may involve great expense, inconvenience, etc. the society must adopt it.

Notes

1. J. S. Mill, *Utilitarianism* and *On Liberty* (Fontana Library Edition, ed. by Mary Warnock, London, 1962), p. 135. All further quotes from Mill are from this edition unless otherwise noted.

2. J. S. Mill, *Principles of Political Economy* (New York: P. F. Collier and Sons, 1900), p. 442.

3. Mill, *Utilitarianism* and *On Liberty*, p. 174.

4. *Ibid.*, p. 299.

5. *Ibid.*, p. 207.

6. *Ibid.*, p. 206.

7. *Ibid.*, p. 207.

8. *Ibid.*, p. 214.

9. *Ibid.*, p. 207.

10. *Ibid.*, p. 138.

11. J. F. Stephen, *Liberty, Equality, Fraternity* (New York: Henry Holt & Co., n.d.), p. 24.

12. H. L. A. Hart, *Law, Liberty and Morality* (Stanford: Stanford University Press, 1963), p. 32.

13. *Ibid.,* p. 33.

14. Mill, *Principles,* II, 448.

15. *Ibid.,* II, 458.

16. *Ibid.,* II, 459.

17. *Ibid.,* II, 451.

18. Stephen, p. 49.

19. Mill, *Utilitarianism* and *On Liberty,* p. 197.

20. *Ibid.,* p. 186

21. *Ibid.,* pp. 235–236.

On Telling Patients the Truth

Mack Lipkin

Should a doctor always tell his patients the truth? In recent years there has been an extraordinary increase in public discussion of the ethical problems involved in this question. But little has been heard from physicians themselves. I believe that gaps in understanding the complex interactions between doctors and patients have led many laymen astray in this debate.

It is easy to make an attractive case for always telling patients the truth. But as L. J. Henderson, the great Harvard physiologist-philosopher of decades ago, commented:

> To speak of telling the truth, the whole truth and nothing but the truth to a patient is absurd. Like absurdity in mathematics, it is absurd simply because it is impossible. . . . The notion that the truth, the whole truth, and nothing but the truth can be conveyed to the patient is a good specimen of that class of fallacies called by Whitehead "the fallacy of misplaced concreteness." It results from neglecting factors that cannot be excluded from the concrete situation and that are of an order of magnitude and relevancy that make it imperative to consider them. Of course, another fallacy is also often involved, the belief that diagnosis and prognosis are more certain than they are. But that is another question.

Words, especially medical terms, inevitably carry different implications for different people. When these words are said in the presence of anxiety-laden illness, there is a strong tendency to hear selectively and with emphases not intended by the doctor. Thus, what the doctor means to convey is obscured.

Indeed, thoughtful physicians know that transmittal of accurate information to patients is often impossible. Patients rarely know how the body functions in health and disease, but instead have inaccurate ideas of what is going on; this hampers the attempts to "tell the truth."

Take cancer, for example. Patients seldom know that while some cancers are rapidly fatal, others never amount to much; some have a cure rate of 99 percent, others less than 1 percent; a cancer may grow rapidly for months and then stop growing for years; may remain localized for years or spread all over the body almost from the beginning; some can be arrested for long periods of time, others not. Thus, one patient thinks of cancer as curable, the next thinks it means certain death.

How many patients understand that "heart trouble" may refer to literally hundreds of different abnormalities ranging in severity from the trivial to the instantly fatal? How many know that the term "arthritis" may refer to dozens of different types of joint involvement? "Arthritis" may raise a vision of the appalling disease that made Aunt Eulalee a helpless invalid until her death years later; the next patient remembers Grandpa grumbling about the damned arthritis as he got up from his chair. Unfortunately but understandably, most people's ideas about the implications of medical terms are based on what they have heard about a few cases.

The news of serious illness drives some patients to irrational and destructive behavior; others handle it sensibly. A distinguished philosopher forestalled my telling him about his cancer by saying, "I want to know the truth. The only thing I couldn't take and wouldn't want to know about is cancer." For two years he had watched his mother die slowly of a painful form of cancer. Several of my physician patients have indicated they would not want to know if they had a fatal illness.

Most patients should be told "the truth" to the extent that they can comprehend it. Indeed, most doctors, like most other people, are uncomfortable with lies. Good physicians, aware that some may be badly damaged by being told more than they want or need to know, can usually ascertain the patient's preferences and needs.

Discussions about lying often center about the use of placebos. In medical usage, a "placebo" is a treatment that has no specific physical or chemical action on the condition being treated, but is given to affect symptoms by a psychologic mechanism, rather than a purely physical one. Ethicists believe that placebos necessarily involve a partial or complete deception by the doctor, since the patient is allowed to believe that the treatment has a specific effect. They seem unaware that placebos, far from being inert (except in the rigid pharmacological sense), are among the most powerful agents known to medicine.

Placebos are a form of suggestion, which is a direct or indirect presentation of an idea, followed by an uncritical, i.e., not thought-out, acceptance. Those who have studied suggestion or looked at medical history know its almost unbelievable potency; it is involved to a greater or lesser extent in the treatment of every conscious patient. It can induce or remove almost any kind of feeling or thought. It can strengthen the weak or paralyze the strong; transform sleeping, feeding, or sexual patterns; remove or induce a vast array of symptoms; mimic or abolish the effect of very powerful

drugs. It can alter the function of most organs. It can cause illness or a great sense of well-being. It can kill. In fact, doctors often add a measure of suggestion when they prescribe even potent medications for those who also need psychologic support. Like all potent agents, its proper use requires judgment based on experience and skill.

Communication between physician and the apprehensive and often confused patient is delicate and uncertain. Honesty should be evaluated not only in terms of a slavish devotion to language often misinterpreted by the patient, but also in terms of intent. *The crucial question is whether the deception was intended to benefit the patient or the doctor.*

Physicians, like most people, hope to see good results and are disappointed when patients do poorly. Their reputations and their livelihood depend on doing effective work; purely selfish reasons would dictate they do their best for their patients. Most important, all good physicians have a deep sense of responsibility toward those who have entrusted their welfare to them.

As I have explained, it is usually a practical impossibility to tell patients "the whole truth." Moreover, often enough, the ethics of the situation, the true moral responsibility, may demand that the naked facts not be revealed. The now popular complaint that doctors are too authoritarian is misguided more often than not. Some patients who insist on exercising their right to know may be doing themselves a disservice.

Judgment is often difficult and uncertain. Simplistic assertions about telling the truth may not be helpful to patients or physicians in times of trouble.

Lies to the Sick and Dying

Sissela Bok

Deception as Therapy

A forty-six-year-old man, coming to a clinic for a routine physical checkup needed for insurance purposes, is diagnosed as having a form of cancer likely to cause him to die within six

months. No known cure exists for it. Chemotherapy may prolong life by a few extra months, but will have side effects the physician does not think warranted in this case. In addition, he believes that such therapy should be reserved for patients with a chance for recovery or remission. The patient has no symptoms giving him any reason to believe that he is not perfectly healthy. He expects to take a short vacation in a week.

For the physician, there are now several choices involving truthfulness. Ought he to tell the patient what he has learned, or conceal it? If asked, should he deny it? If he decides to reveal the diagnosis, should he delay doing so until after the patient returns from his vacation? Finally, even if he does reveal the serious nature of the diagnosis, should he mention the possibility of chemotherapy and his reasons for not recommending it in this case? Or should he encourage every last effort to postpone death?

In this particular case, the physician chose to inform the patient of his diagnosis right away. He did not, however, mention the possibility of chemotherapy. A medical student working under him disagreed; several nurses also thought that the patient should have been informed of this possibility. They tried, unsuccessfully, to persuade the physician that this was the patient's right. When persuasion had failed, the student elected to disobey the doctor by informing the patient of the alternative of chemotherapy. After consultation with family members, the patient chose to ask for the treatment.

Doctors confront such choices often and urgently. What they reveal, hold back, or distort will matter profoundly to their patients. Doctors stress with corresponding vehemence their reasons for the distortion or concealment: not to confuse a sick person needlessly, or cause what may well be unnecessary pain or discomfort, as in the case of the cancer patient; not to leave a patient without hope, as in those many cases where the dying are not told the truth about their condition; or to improve the chances of cure, as where unwarranted optimism is expressed about some form of therapy. Doctors use information as part of the therapeutic regimen; it is given out in amounts, in admixtures, and according to timing believed best for patients. Accuracy, by comparison, matters far less.

Lying to patients has, therefore, seemed an especially excusable act. Some would argue that doctors, and *only* doctors, should be granted the right to manipulate the truth in ways so undesirable for politicians, lawyers, and others.[1] Doctors are trained to help patients; their relationship to patients carries special obligations, and they know much more than laymen about what helps and hinders recovery and survival.

Even the most conscientious doctors, then, who hold themselves at a distance from the quacks and the purveyors of false remedies, hesitate to forswear all lying. Lying is usually wrong, they argue, but less so than allowing the truth to harm patients. B. C. Meyer echoes this very common view:

> [O]urs is a profession which traditionally has been guided by a precept that transcends the virtue of uttering truth for truth's sake, and that is, "so far as possible, do no harm."[2]

Truth, for Meyer, may be important, but not when it endangers the health and well-being of patients. This has seemed self-evident to many physicians in the past—so much so that we find very few mentions of veracity in the codes and oaths and writings by physicians through the centuries. This absence is all the more striking as other principles of ethics have been consistently and movingly expressed in the same documents.

The two fundamental principles of doing good and not doing harm—of beneficence and nonmaleficence—are the most immediately relevant to medical practitioners, and the most frequently stressed. To preserve life and good health, to ward off illness, pain, and death—these are the perennial tasks of medicine and nursing. These principles have found powerful expression at all times in the history of medicine. In the Hippocratic Oath physicians promise to:

> use treatment to help the sick . . . but never with a view to injury and wrong-doing.[3]

And a Hindu oath of initiation says:

> Day and night, however thou mayest be engaged, thou shalt endeavor for the relief of patients with all thy heart and soul. Thou shalt not desert or injure the patient even for the sake of thy living.[4]

But there is no similar stress on veracity. It is absent from virtually all oaths, codes, and prayers. The Hippocratic Oath makes no mention of truthfulness to patients about their condition, prognosis, or treatment. Other early codes and prayers are equally silent on the subject. To be sure, they often refer to the confidentiality with which doctors should treat all that patients tell them; but there is no corresponding reference to honesty toward the patient. One of the few who appealed to such a principle was Amatus Lusitanus, a Jewish physician widely known for his skill, who, persecuted, died of the plague in 1568. He published an oath which reads in part:

> If I lie, may I incur the eternal wrath of God and of His angel Raphael, and may nothing in the medical art succeed for me according to my desires.[5]

Later codes continue to avoid the subject. Not even the Declaration of Geneva, adopted in 1948 by the World Medical Association, makes any reference to it. And the Principles of Medical Ethics of the American Medical Association[6] still leave the matter of informing patients up to the physician.

Given such freedom, a physician can decide to tell as much or as little as he wants the patient to know, so long as he breaks no law. In the case of the man mentioned at the beginning of this chapter, some physicians might feel justified in lying for the good of the patient; others might be truthful. Some may conceal alternatives to the treatment they recommend; others not. In each case, they could appeal to the AMA Principles of Ethics. A great many would choose to be able to lie. They would claim that not only can a lie avoid harm for the patient, but that it is also hard to know whether they have been right in the first place in making their pessimistic diagnosis; a "truthful" statement could therefore turn out to hurt patients unnecessarily. The concern for curing and for supporting those who cannot be cured then runs counter to the desire to be completely open. This concern is especially strong where the prognosis is bleak; even more so when patients are so affected by their illness or their medication that they are more dependent than usual, perhaps more easily depressed or irrational.

Physicians know only too well how uncertain a diagnosis or prognosis can be. They know how hard it is to give meaningful and correct answers regarding health and illness. They also know that disclosing their own uncertainty or fears can reduce those benefits that depend upon faith in recovery. They fear, too, that revealing grave risks, no matter how unlikely it is that these will come about, may exercise the pull of the "self-fulfilling prophecy." They dislike being the bearers of uncertain or bad news as much as anyone else. And

last, but not least, sitting down to discuss an illness truthfully and sensitively may take much-needed time away from other patients.

These reasons help explain why nurses and physicians and relatives of the sick and dying prefer not to be bound by rules that might limit their ability to suppress, delay, or distort information. This is not to say that they necessarily plan to lie much of the time. They merely want to have the freedom to do so when they believe it wise. And the reluctance to see lying prohibited explains, in turn, the failure of the codes and oaths to come to grips with the problems of truth-telling and lying.

But sharp conflicts are now arising. Doctors no longer work alone with patients. They have to consult with others much more than before; if they choose to lie, the choice may not be met with approval by all who take part in the care of the patient. A nurse expresses the difficulty which results as follows:

> From personal experience I would say that the patients who aren't told about their terminal illness have so many verbal and mental questions unanswered that many will begin to realize that their illness is more serious than they're being told. . . .
>
> Nurses care for these patients twenty-four hours a day compared to a doctor's daily brief visit, and it is the nurse many times that the patient will relate to, once his underlying fears become overwhelming. . . . This is difficult for us nurses because being in constant contact with patients we can see the events leading up to this. The patient continually asks you, "Why isn't my pain decreasing?" or "Why isn't the radiation treatment easing the pain?" . . . We cannot legally give these patients an honest answer as a nurse (and I'm sure I wouldn't want to) yet the problem is still not resolved and the circle grows larger and larger with the patient alone in the middle.[7]

The doctor's choice to lie increasingly involves co-workers in acting a part they find neither humane nor wise. The fact that these problems have not been carefully thought through within the medical profession, nor seriously addressed in medical education, merely serves to intensify the conflicts.[8] Different doctors then respond very differently to patients in exactly similar predicaments. The friction is increased by the fact that relatives often disagree even where those giving medical care to a patient are in accord on how to approach the patient. Here again, because physicians have not worked out to common satisfaction the question of whether relatives have the right to make such requests, the problems are allowed to be haphazardly resolved by each physician as he sees fit.

The Patient's Perspective

The turmoil in the medical profession regarding truth-telling is further augmented by the pressures that patients themselves now bring to bear and by empirical data coming to light. Challenges are growing to the three major arguments for lying to patients: that truthfulness is impossible; that patients do not want bad news; and that truthful information harms them.

The first of these arguments . . . confuses "truth" and "truthfulness" so as to clear the way for occasional lying on grounds supported by the second and third arguments. At this point, we can see more clearly that it is a strategic move intended to discourage the question of truthfulness from carrying much weight in the first place, and thus to leave the choice of what to say and how to say it up to the physician. To claim that "since telling the truth is impossible, there can be no sharp distinction between what is true and what is false"[9] is to try to defeat objections to lying before even discussing them. One need only imagine how such an argument would be received, were it made by a car salesman or a real estate dealer, to see how fallacious it is.

In medicine, however, the argument is supported by a subsidiary point: even if people might ordinarily understand what is spoken to them, patients are often not in a position to do so. This is where paternalism enters in. When we buy cars or houses, the paternalist will argue, we need to have all our wits about us; but when we are ill, we cannot always do so. We need help in making choices, even if help can be given only by keeping us in the dark. And the physician is trained and willing to provide such help.

It is certainly true that some patients cannot make the best choices for themselves when weakened by illness or drugs. But most still can. And even those who are incompetent have a right to have someone—their guardian or spouse perhaps—receive the correct information.

The paternalistic assumption of superiority to patients also carries great dangers for physicians themselves—it risks turning to contempt. The following view was recently expressed in a letter to a medical journal:

> As a radiologist who has been sued, I have reflected earnestly on advice to obtain Informed Consent but have decided to "take the risks without informing the patient" and trust to "God, judge, and jury" rather than evade responsibility through a legal gimmick. . . .
>
> [I]n a general radiologic practice many of our patients are uninformable and we would never get through the day if we had to obtain their consent to every potentially harmful study.
>
> . . . We still have patients with language problems, the uneducated and the unintelligent, the stolid and the stunned who cannot form an Informed Opinion to give an Informed Consent; we have the belligerent and the panicky who do not listen or comprehend. And then there are the Medicare patients who comprise 35 percent of general hospital admissions. The bright ones wearily plead to be left alone. . . . As for the apathetic rest, many of them were kindly described by Richard Bright as not being able to comprehend because "their brains are so poorly oxygenated."[10]

The argument which rejects informing patients because adequate truthful information is impossible in itself or because patients are lacking in understanding must itself be rejected when looked at from the point of view of patients. They know that liberties granted to the most conscientious and altruistic doctors will be exercised also in the "Medicaid Mills"; that the choices thus kept from patients will be exercised by not only competent but incompetent physicians; and that even the best doctors can make choices patients would want to make differently for themselves.

The second argument for deceiving patients refers specifically to giving them news of a frightening or depressing kind. It holds that patients do not, in fact, generally want such information. That they prefer not to have to face up to serious illness and death. On the basis of such a belief, most doctors in a number of surveys stated that they do not, as a rule, inform patients that they have an illness such as cancer.

When studies are made of what patients desire to know, on the other hand, a large majority say that they *would* like to be told of such a diagnosis.[11] All these studies need updating and should be done with larger numbers of patients and nonpatients. But they do show that there is generally a dramatic divergence between physicians and patients on the factual question of whether patients want to know what ails them in cases of serious illness such as cancer. In most of the studies, over 80 percent of the persons asked indicated that they would want to be told.

Sometimes this discrepancy is set aside by doctors who want to retain the view that patients do not want unhappy news. In reality, they claim, the fact that patients say they want it has to be discounted. The more someone asks to know, the more he suffers from fear which will lead to the denial of the information even if it is given. Informing patients is, therefore, useless; they resist and deny having been told what they cannot assimilate. According to this view, empirical studies of what patients say they want are worthless since they do not probe deeply enough to uncover this universal resistance to the contemplation of one's own death.

This view is only partially correct. For some patients, denial is indeed well established in medical experience. A number of patients (estimated at between 15 percent and 25 percent) will give evidence of denial of having been told about their illness, even when they repeatedly ask and are repeatedly informed. And nearly everyone experiences a period of denial at some point in the course of approaching death.[12] Elisabeth Kübler-Ross sees denial as resulting often from premature and abrupt information by a stranger who goes through the process quickly to "get it over with." She holds that denial functions as a buffer after unexpected shocking news, permitting individuals to collect themselves and to mobilize other defenses. She describes prolonged denial in one patient as follows:

> She was convinced that the x-rays were "mixed up"; she asked for reassurance that her pathology report could not possibly be back so soon and that another patient's report must have been marked with her name. When none of this could be confirmed, she quickly asked to leave the hospital, looking for another physician in the vain hope "to get a better explanation for my

troubles." This patient went "shopping around" for many doctors, some of whom gave her reassuring answers, others of whom confirmed the previous suspicion. Whether confirmed or not, she reacted in the same manner, she asked for examination and reexamination. . . .[13]

But to say the denial is universal flies in the face of all evidence. And to take any claim to the contrary as "symptomatic" of deeper denial leaves no room for reasoned discourse. There is no way that such universal denial can be proved true or false. To believe in it is a metaphysical belief about man's condition, not a statement about what patients do and do not want. It is true that we can never completely understand the possibility of our own death, any more than being alive in the first place. But people certainly differ in the degree to which they can approach such knowledge, take it into account in their plans, and make their peace with it.

Montaigne claimed that in order to learn both to live and to die, men have to think about death and be prepared to accept it.[14] To stick one's head in the sand, or to be prevented by lies from trying to discern what is to come, hampers freedom—freedom to consider one's life as a whole, with a beginning, a duration, an end. Some may request to be deceived rather than to see their lives as thus finite; others reject the information which would require them to do so; but most say that they want to know. Their concern for knowing about their condition goes far beyond mere curiosity or the wish to make isolated personal choices in the short time left to them; their stance toward the entire life they have lived, and their ability to give it meaning and completion, are at stake.[15] In lying or withholding the facts which permit such discernment, doctors may reflect their own fears (which, according to one study,[16] are much stronger than those of laymen) of facing questions about the meaning of one's life and the inevitability of death.

Beyond the fundamental deprivation that can result from deception, we are also becoming increasingly aware of all that can befall patients in the course of their illness when information is denied or distorted. Lies place them in a position where they no longer participate in choices concerning their own health, including the choice of whether to be a "patient" in the first place. A terminally ill person who is not informed that his illness is incurable and that he is near death cannot make decisions about the end of his life; about whether or not to enter a hospital, or to have surgery; where and with whom to spend his last days; how to put his affairs in order—these most personal choices cannot be made if he is kept in the dark, or given contradictory hints and clues. . . .

The reason why even doctors who recognize a patient's right to have information might still not provide it brings us to the third argument against telling all patients the truth. It holds that the information given might hurt the patient and the concern for the right to such information is therefore a threat to proper health care. A patient, these doctors argue, may wish to commit suicide after being given discouraging news, or suffer a cardiac arrest, or simply cease to struggle, and thus not grasp the small remaining chance for recovery. And even where the outlook for a patient is very good, the disclosure of a minute risk can shock some patients or cause them to reject needed protection such as a vaccination or antibiotics.

The factual basis for this argument has been challenged from two points of view. The damages associated with the disclosure of sad news or risks are rarer than physicians believe; and the *benefits* which result from being informed are more substantial, even measurably so. Pain is tolerated more easily, recovery from surgery is quicker, and cooperation with therapy is greatly improved. The attitude that "what you don't know won't hurt you" is proving unrealistic; it is what patients do not know but vaguely suspect that causes them corrosive worry.

It is certain that no answers to this question of harm from information are the same for all patients. If we look, first, at the fear expressed by physicians that informing patients of even remote or unlikely risks conected with a drug prescription or operation might shock some and make others refuse the treatment that would have been best for them, it appears to be unfounded for the great majority of patients. Studies show that very few patients respond to being told of such risks by withdrawing their consent to the procedure and that those who do withdraw are the very ones who might well have been upset enough to sue the physician had they not been asked to consent beforehand.[17] It is possible that on even rarer occa-

sions especially susceptible persons might manifest physical deterioration from shock; some physicians have even asked whether patients who die after giving informed consent to an operation, but before it actually takes place, somehow expire because of the information given to them.[18] While such questions are unanswerable in any one case, they certainly argue in favor of caution, a real concern for the person to whom one is recounting the risks he or she will face, and sensitivity to all signs of distress.

The situation is quite different when persons who are already ill, perhaps already quite weak and discouraged, are told of a very serious prognosis. Physicians fear that such knowledge may cause the patients to commit suicide, or to be frightened or depressed to the point that their illness takes a downward turn. The fear that great numbers of patients will commit suicide appears to be unfounded.[19] And if some do, is that a response so unreasonable, so much against the patient's best interest that physicians ought to make it a reason for concealment or lies? Many societies have allowed suicide in the past; our own has decriminalized it; and some are coming to make distinctions among the many suicides which ought to be prevented if at all possible, and those which ought to be respected.[20]

Another possibile response to very bleak news is the triggering of physiological mechanisms which allow death to come more quickly—a form of giving up or of preparing for the inevitable, depending on one's outlook. Lewis Thomas, studying responses in humans and animals, holds it not unlikely that:

> . . . there is a pivotal movement at some stage in the body's reaction to injury or disease, maybe in aging as well, when the organism concedes that it is finished and the time for dying is at hand, and at this moment the events that lead to death are launched, as a coordinated mechanism. Fuctions are then shut off, in sequence, irreversibly, and, while this is going on, a neural mechanism, held ready for this occasion, is switched on. . . .[21]

Such a response may be appropriate, in which case it makes the moments of dying as peaceful as those who have died and been resuscitated so often testify. But it may also be brought on inappropriately, when the organism could have lived on, perhaps even induced malevolently, by external acts intended to kill. Thomas speculates that some of the deaths resulting from "hexing" are due to such responses. Levi-Strauss describes deaths from exorcism and the casting of spells in ways which suggest that the same process may then be brought on by the community.[22]

It is not inconceivable that unhappy news abruptly conveyed, or a great shock given to someone unable to tolerate it, could also bring on such a "dying response," quite unintended by the speaker. There is every reason to be cautious and to try to know ahead of time how susceptible a patient might be to the accidental triggering—however rare—of such a response. One has to assume, however, that most of those who have survived long enough to be in a situation where their informed consent is asked have a very robust resistance to such accidental triggering of processes leading to death. . . .

Apart from the possible harm from information, we are coming to learn much more about the benefits it can bring patients. People follow instructions more carefully if they know what their disease is and why they are asked to take medications; any benefits from those procedures are therefore much more likely to come about. Similarly, people recover faster from surgery and tolerate pain with less medication if they understand what ails them and what can be done for them.

Respect and Truthfulness

Taken all together, the three arguments defending lies to patients stand on much shakier ground as a counterweight to the right to be informed than is often thought. The common view that many patients cannot understand, do not want, and may be harmed by, knowledge of their condition, and that lying to them is either morally neutral or even to be recommended, must be set aside. Instead, we have to make a more complex comparison. Over against the right of patients to knowledge concerning themselves, the medical and psychological benefits to them from this knowledge, the unnecessary and sometimes harmful treatment to which they can be subjected if ignorant, and the harm to physicians, their profession, and other patients from deceptive practices, we have to set a severely restricted and narrowed paternalistic view—that *some* patients cannot understand, *some* do not want, and *some* may be harmed by, knowledge of their condition, and that they ought not to have to be treated like everyone else if this is not in their best interest.

Such a view is persuasive. A few patients openly request not to be given bad news. Others give clear signals to that effect, or are demonstrably vulnerable to the shock or anguish such news might call forth. Can one not in such cases infer implied consent to being deceived?

Concealment, evasion, withholding of information may at times be necessary. But if someone contemplates lying to a patient or concealing the truth, the burden of proof must shift. It must rest, here, as with all deception, on those who advocate it in any one instance. They must show why they fear a patient may be harmed or how they know that another cannot cope with the truthful knowledge. A decision to deceive must be seen as a very unusual step, to be talked over with colleagues and others who participate in the care of the patient. Reasons must be set forth and debated, alternatives weighed carefully. At all times, the correct information must go to *someone* closely related to the patient.

The law already permits doctors to withhold information from patients where it would clearly hurt their health. But this privilege has been sharply limited by the courts. Certainly it cannot be interpreted so broadly as to permit a general practice of deceiving patients "for their own good." Nor can it be made to include cases where patients might calmly decide, upon hearing their diagnosis, not to go ahead with the therapy their doctor recommends.[23] Least of all can it justify silence or lies to large numbers of patients merely on grounds that it is not always easy to tell what a patient wants.

For the great majority of patients, on the contrary, the goal must be disclosure, and the atmosphere one of openness. But it would be wrong to assume that patients can therefore be told abruptly about a serious diagnosis—that, so long as openness exists, there are no further requirements of humane concern in such communication. Dr. Cicely Saunders, who runs the well-known St. Christopher's Hospice in England, describes the sensitivity and understanding which are needed:

> Every patient needs an explanation of his illness that will be understandable and

convincing to him if he is to cooperate in his treatment or be relieved of the burden of unknown fears. This is true whether it is a question of giving a diagnosis in a hopeful situation or of confirming a poor prognosis.

The fact that a patient does not ask does not mean that he has no questions. One visit or talk is rarely enough. It is only by waiting and listening that we can gain an idea of what we should be saying. Silences and gaps are often more revealing than words as we try to learn what a patient is facing as he travels along the constantly changing journey of his illness and his thoughts about it.

. . . So much of the communication will be without words or given indirectly. This is true of all real meeting with people but especially true with those who are facing, knowingly or not, difficult or threatening situations. It is also particularly true of the very ill.

The main argument against a policy of deliberate, invariable denial of unpleasant facts is that it makes such communication extremely difficult, if not impossible. Once the possibility of talking frankly with a patient has been admitted, it does not mean that this will always take place, but the whole atmosphere is changed. We are then free to wait quietly for clues from each patient, seeing them as individuals from whom we can expect intelligence, courage, and individual decisions. They will feel secure enough to give us these clues when they wish.[24]

Above all, truthfulness with those who are suffering does not mean that they should be deprived of all hope: hope that there is a chance of recovery, however small; nor of reassurance that they will not be abandoned when they most need help.

Much needs to be done, however, if the deceptive practices are to be eliminated, and if concealment is to be restricted to the few patients who ask for it or those who can be shown to be harmed by openness. The medical profession has to address this problem.

Notes

1. Plato, *The Republic*, 389 b.
2. B. C. Meyer, "Truth and the Physician," *Bulletin of the New York Academy of Medicine* 45 (1969): 59–71.
3. W. H. S. Jones, trans., *Hippocrates*, Loeb Classical Library (Cambridge, Mass.: Harvard University Press, 1923), p. 164.
4. Reprinted in M. B. Etziony. *The Physician's Creed: An Anthology of Medical Prayers. Oaths and Codes of Ethics* (Springfield, Ill.: Charles C. Thomas, 1973), pp. 15–18.
5. See Harry Friedenwald, "The Ethics of the Practice of Medicine from the Jewish Point of View," *Johns Hopkins Hospital Bulletin*, no. 318 (August 1917), pp. 256–61.
6. "Ten Principles of Medical Ethics," *Journal of the American Medical Association* 164 (1957): 1119–20.
7. Mary Barrett, letter, *Boston Globe*, 16 November 1976, p. 1.
8. Though a minority of physicians have struggled to bring them to our attention. See Thomas Percival, *Medical Ethics*, 3d ed. (Oxford: John Henry Parker, 1849), pp. 132–41; Worthington Hooker, *Physician and Patient* (New York: Baker and Scribner, 1849), pp. 357–82; Richard C. Cabot, "Teamwork of Doctor and Patient Through the Annihilation of Lying." in *Social Service and the Art of Healing* (New York: Moffat, Yard & Co., 1909), pp. 116–70; Charles C. Lund, "The Doctor, the Patient, and the Truth," *Annals of Internal Medicine* 24 (1946): 955; Edmund Davies, "The Patient's Right to Know the Truth," *Proceedings of the Royal Society of Medicine* 66 (1973): 533–36.
9. Lawrence Henderson, "Physician and Patient as a Social System," *New England Journal of Medicine* 212 (1955).
10. Nicholas Demy, Letter to the Editor, *Journal of the American Medical Association* 217 (1971): 696–97.
11. For the views of physicians, see Donald Oken, "What to Tell Cancer Patients," *Journal of the American Medical Association* 175 (1961): 1120–28; and tabulations in Robert Veatch, *Death, Dying, and the Biological Revolution* (New Haven and London: Yale University Press, 1976), pp. 229–38. For the view of patients, see Veatch, ibid; Jean Aitken-Swan and E. C. Easson, "Reactions of Cancer Patients on Being Told Their Diagnosis," *British Medical Journal*, 1959, pp. 779–83; Jim McIntosh, "Patients' Awareness and Desire for Information About Diagnosed but Undisclosed Malignant Disease," *The Lancet* 7 (1976): 300–303; William D. Kelly and Stanley R. Friesen, "Do Cancer Patients Want to Be Told?," *Surgery* 27 (1950): 822–26.
12. See Avery Weisman, *On Dying and Denying* (New York: Behavioral Publications, 1972) Elisabeth Kübler-Ross, *On Death and Dying* (New York: The Macmillan Co., 1969); Ernest Becker, *The Denial of*

Death (New York: Free Press, 1973); Philippe Ariès, *Western Attitudes Toward Death*, trans. Patricia M. Ranum (Baltimore and London: Johns Hopkins University Press, 1974); and Sigmund Freud, "Negation," *Collected Papers*, ed. James Strachey (London: Hogarth Press, 1950), 5: 181–85.

13. Kübler-Ross, *On Death and Dying*, p. 34.

14. Michel de Montaigne, *Essays*, bk. I, chap. 20.

15. It is in literature that these questions are most directly raised. Two recent works where they are taken up with striking beauty and simplicity are May Sarton, *As We Are Now* (New York: W. W. Norton & Co., 1973); and Freya Stark, *A Peak in Darien* (London: John Murray, 1976).

16. Herman Feifel *et al.*, "Physicians Consider Death," *Proceedings of the American Psychoanalytical Association*, 1967, pp. 201–2.

17. See Ralph Alfidi, "Informed Consent: A Study of Patient Reaction," *Journal of the American Medical Association* 216 (1971): 1325–29.

18. See Steven R. Kaplan, Richard A. Greenwald, and Arvey I. Rogers, Letter to the Editor, *New England Journal of Medicine* 296 (1977): 1127.

19. Oken, "What to Tell Cancer Patients"; Veatch,

Death, Dying, and the Biological Revolution; Weisman, *On Dying and Denying.*

20. Norman L. Cantor, "A Patient's Decision to Decline Life-Saving Treatment: Bodily Integrity Versus the Preservation of Life," *Rutgers Law Review* 26: 228–64; Danielle Gourevitch, "Suicide Among the Sick in Classical Antiquity," *Bulletin of the History of Medicine* 18 (1969): 501–18; for bibliography, see Bok, "Voluntary Euthanasia."

21. Lewis Thomas, "A Meliorist View of Disease and Dying," *The Journal of Medicine and Philosophy* 1 (1976): 212–21.

22. Claude Lévi-Strauss, *Structural Anthropology* (New York: Basic Books, 1963), p. 167; See also Eric Cassell, "Permission to Die," in John Behnke and Sissela Bok, eds., *The Dilemmas of Euthanasia* (New York: Doubleday, Anchor Press, 1975), pp. 121–31.

23. See Charles Fried, *Medical Experimentation: Personal Integrity and Social Policy* (Amsterdam and Oxford: North Holland Publishing Co., 1974), pp. 20–24.

24. Cicely M. S. Saunders, "Telling Patients," in S. J. Reiser, W. J. Dyck, A. J. Curran, *Ethics in Medicine* (Cambridge, Massachusetts: M.I.T. Press, 1977), pp. 238–40.

Professional Secrecy

Henry A. Davidson

> If it be what should not be noised abroad, I will keep silence thereon.
>
> *Oath of Hippocrates*

Any physician may be impaled on the horns of the dilemma of confidentiality. The motor vehicle department wants to know the medical status of a cardiac patient. If the doctor keeps silent, he may be unleashing a driver who might suffer a fatal heart attack and kill dozens of people. If he discloses the information, he will be releasing data given to him in confidence.

Most people assume that whatever they tell a doctor is confidential and that if the physician ever tells anyone else, something dreadful will happen to the doctor. They base their confidence on privileged communication statutes, on the American Medical Association code of ethics, on the Hippocratic Oath, and on the general laws on libel

and defamation. So far as the last item is concerned—that is, the libel law—there *is* some degree of protection against a doctor who tells the whole staff room how he treated the mayor for gonorrhea or who gossips about how he handled the police chief in delirium tremens.

Question of Welfare of the Community

The law of privileged communication rarely offers any protection. Where such a law exists, it usually applies only to court room testimony, but not to staff room gossip. Nor is the Hippocratic Oath any help. Here the relevant sentence is: ". . . whatsoever I see or hear in my attendance on the sick, which ought not to be noised abroad, I will keep silence thereon." The question here is the meaning of the phrase "which ought not to be noised abroad." The fact that a man has a contagious disease or has had a bullet wound or has a homicidal impulse—should these things be kept secret? The Oath doesn't say. And the American Medical Association code, consisting of general principles, has a king-sized loophole in it. Here it is: "Confidence . . . should never be revealed unless the law requires it or if necessary to protect the welfare of individuals or the community."

Could it be argued that, to "protect the welfare of the community," the doctor must reveal that the driver of a school bus has cataracts, the pilot of a jet plane is an alcoholic, the janitor in the school building a homosexual, the nurse on the surgical floor a drug addict, a policeman is a paranoiac, or that the engineer on the "limited" train is a diabetic or epileptic subject to unpredictable spells of impaired consciousness? The American Medical Association code would seem to permit the physician to reveal these findings to the responsible authorities under the "protection of the community" clause.

However, this is highly controversial. In 1960 a Maryland psychiatrist testified before a congressional committee that one of his patients was a mentally unstable homosexual. The patient, a code clerk in a government agency, had defected to Moscow. The doctor's testimony was aimed at suggesting to the Kremlin that this clerk's account of United States activities was unreliable. While this psychiatrist was harshly criticized by some of his colleagues, others defended him on the grounds that what he said was "to protect the community."

Privileged Communication: Legal Aspects

In 34 of our states, physician-patient communications are privileged; that is, the doctor may not reveal in court what he learned from a patient in the course of professional attendance. (The patient may loosen the physician's tongue if he wants to, by waiving the privilege.) However, in 16 states[1] there are *no* physician-patient privileges, and a doctor must, under penalty of contempt of court, tell the judge and jury what a patient told him in confidence if the physician is asked in open court.

In a state like New York, which has a confidentiality statute, a special problem is produced when a sick or unconscious patient has accidentally disclosed something detrimental. Consider the following:[2]

> A victim of an automobile accident lay severely injured in the emergency room. Dr. X was preparing to administer the Babinski test when out of one sock fell a packet of heroin.
> Dr. X faced this dilemma: How to resolve the conflict between his desire to respect the confidentiality of the physician-patient relationship and his duty to preserve the law? If he failed to report the incident to the police, he might face a charge of concealing a wrongful act. On the other hand, if he permitted the law to take its course, he would risk a lawsuit for violating the physician-patient relationship.

What the doctor actually did was this: He made no objections when a member of the hospital team picked up the packet of heroin and turned it over to a nurse who promptly called the police. The patient was arrested, tried, and convicted.

One (but apparently only one) of the appellate court justices said that "the purpose of physician-patient privilege is denied if professional diagnosis and treatment could be obtained by this badly injured man only under penalty of disclosure of this evidence of crime." However, a majority of the court held that the accidental finding of the heroin did not constitute an illegal search, and that turning over the narcotic to the police was not a disclosure of information "acquired in a professional capacity by a physician from patient." A vigorous dissent by one of the justices of the appeals court stressed that the patient "was helpless from his injuries, and being subjected to prosecution on this criminal charge should not have been exacted of him as an alternative to foregoing the necessary medical and surgical attention."

Most doctors say that they favor privileged-communication laws, but there is something to be said against them. Some years ago a New York doctor sued a patient who refused to pay his bill. In court the patient said that the physician's services weren't worth the fee. To show what they were worth, the doctor wanted to discuss his treatment of the case. But he wasn't allowed to testify. Said the court: "It is against public policy to permit a physician to make such disclosures even in actions to recover for his services."

It cost that doctor time and money to learn that "privileged communications" between physician and patient can be a two-sided coin. Sometimes, he found, the side the doctor turns up is the wrong one.

"But that's an exceptional case," you may argue. "The law of privileged communications saves many a patient from embarrassment." Suppose you've been treating a patient for sciatica over a two-year period. Last month, he slipped and fell while getting out of a taxi. Now, alleging he never had a backache in his life before the accident, he has sued the cab driver for injuries. One sentence from you on the witness stand—"I've treated this man's sciatica for two years"—would prove him a liar. But the law in your state holds that your treatment of his sciatica is "privileged." So you can't say a word about it in court. As a result, the verdict goes to your patient, and the luckless cabbie loses out.

You have saved your patient from much embarrassment. And you have saved the time and money that a court appearance would have cost you. But here's the big question: Having been "privileged" by law to be a silent partner to perjury and injustice, have you saved your self-respect?

The law of privileged communications is designed to prevent a physician from making any court disclosure of what he has learned about a patient as a result of their professional relationship. This isn't a constitutional privilege of either patient or physician; it's a legislative gift from the state. And there is no such law in many states; 16 of them manage to do without it very nicely.

The law and its application differ widely among the states where it may be invoked. In Louisiana, for instance, it's effective in criminal proceedings only. In Kentucky, the privilege is limited to cases involving vital statistics. In West Virginia, it can be invoked only in cases originating in the court of a justice of the peace.

No matter what form it takes, the privileged-communications law has a commendable purpose: to ensure the privacy of the patient. But it works out better in theory than in practice. By ensuring the patient's privacy, it too often permits a dishonest man to lie about his condition or treatment. And it prevents the doctor from refuting that lie with the truth.

To get an idea of the strange way in which the privilege laws can defeat justice, consider the following cases: (1) A California doctor who'd been sued for malpractice offered to show in court that another patient of his had suffered no ill effects from the same treatment the plaintiff had been given. But the court refused to permit such testimony. It would violate the second patient's privilege. (2) When a certain New York surgeon sued to collect for an operation, he got nowhere. The trouble was he couldn't prove his services without revealing key facts about the patient's condition. And such testimony was forbidden. It was "privileged."

Ordinarily, when a patient sues his doctor for malpractice, the privilege is automatically waived in order to let the doctor defend himself. In most instances, the waiver extends to both the defendant physician and any consultants he might have called in on the case. There have been exceptions to this rule, however. Not long ago, for example, an Indiana court refused to allow a consultant to testify in a malpractice case on the ground that his testimony would breach privilege! A patient may say anything he chooses to promote a fraudulent medical claim. Yet the doctor may be forbidden to refute the lies. A legal device to muzzle the truth is known by the name of "privilege."

"Privileged communication" is unknown in Britain. In some respects, it is a peculiarly American modification of the law. The purpose of a trial is to discover truth. Most jurists believe that it is wrong to put hurdles in the road to truth.

The "privilege" was first set up in 1828, in New York State. The original theory was that if a patient was not guaranteed that his communication would be kept confidential, he would stay away from doctors and his health would suffer. This danger is still sometimes cited as a rationale for physician-patient privilege. However, statistics indicate that states like Massachusetts and Maryland which do *not* have the privilege are as healthy as the states which do.

Do such laws prevent shame and embarrassment for the patient? The chief medical causes of shame to the average layman are abortion, drug addiction, mental illness, and venereal disease. But even in "privilege" states, all facts about these are made publicly available by reports or legal document. And it is highly unlikely that minor embarrassments like hemorrhoids or ringworm will be subject to courtroom controversy.

In New York, dentists as well as physicians are privileged. Nurses are privileged in Arkansas. Physicians (unprivileged) must answer court questions in New Jersey, but newspaper reporters (privileged) need not. And in Georgia and Tennessee, where physicians must tell all about their patients in court, psychologists cannot.

An Indiana doctor was once forbidden to testify about the cause of a patient's death, although such testimony was essential in settling a claim. Yet the death certificate, which listed the cause, was a matter of public record. Everyone but the jury was entitled to the facts. In a similar case, a Michigan court ruled that "although the death certificate is admissible, the physician who made it is prohibited from testifying as to the facts therein stated." An Arkansas court once decided that a notary public who had typed and notarized a patient's history for a doctor could talk about it, but the doctor couldn't.

To compound the confusion, courts within the same state have been known to disagree on what's privileged and what is not. Is an x-ray a "communication" from patient to doctor? Yes, says one judge. No, says another; it's an "observation." Does a patient's own testimony regarding his illness or treatment mean he has waived privilege? One judge says yes; another says no. Finally, consider the situation in Ohio. One judge there has ruled that a doctor working in a public hospital may testify about treatment of a hospital patient in spite of the privilege rule. Why?—Because, says the court, the doctor's contractual relationship is with the hospital, not with the patient.

However, in a recent Ohio case, an intern in a public hospital was not allowed to testify even though he had never treated the patient. Why not?—The court ruled that a doctor-patient relationship existed in the hospital.

One of the physician's thorniest problems is the disclosure to an employer of a pejorative diagnosis. In one case,[3] a doctor sent a report to the United States Air Force indicating that a civilian employee (an accountant) was an alcoholic. The employee sued the doctor but the courts dismissed the suit, presumably because they felt that the physician had a duty to disclose, notwithstanding New York's privileged communication law. In commenting on this, Chayet [1] writes:

> This case might have come under the "substantial danger" doctrine if the patient

had been a pilot. But since he was an accountant, I think that the decision was improper. The proper way of handling such a situation would have been for the Air Force to have instructed the accountant to give the doctor permission to release the record. This permission could have been made a requirement for continued employment.

This might be construed as a sort of blackmail or as compelling an employee to testify against himself; although, of course, it would have lifted the onus from the physician.

Sometimes a breach of confidence is construed as a violation of the right of privacy. Legal recoveries under this right are rare but are becoming more common. The United States Supreme Court set aside Connecticut's law banning birth control by married couples as an invasion of such a right.[4] Actionable under this, in some jurisdictions, would be showing photographs (or movies of) a patient's face to illustrate scars or plastic surgery, or to show obstetrical or operative procedures.[5]

Some efforts have been made to protect physician-patient disclosures under a right of privacy theory. Chayet has argued that a therapist is sometimes an extension of an individual. Since an individual cannot be compelled to testify against himself, a therapist who is privy to medical confidences should likewise be forbidden to disclose what was told to him. A man could not be compelled to disclose in court whether he had acquired venereal disease. The doctor who has this knowledge from the patient (either through history or findings) should, by this theory, be barred from telling anyone about it since that would be a breach of privacy. Courts have not tested this theory, however.

In the absence of a privileged communication law, courts may condone breaches of confidence if made without malice and to accomplish a socially desirable end. In one case[6] the court supported a physician who told an insurance company that the cause of a baby's death was congenital heart disease. This invalidated the insurance policy which did not cover congenital disorders. The parents sued the pediatrician because he revealed this information without their consent and against their interests. In its opinion, the court said:

> Ordinarily, a physician receives information relating to a patient's health in a confidential

capacity. He should not divulge this without the patient's consent except where the public interest or the private interest of the public so demands. Disclosure may, under such compelling circumstances, be made to a person who has a legitimate interest in the patient's health. In this case, the public's interest in an honest result assumed dominance over the individual's right of nondisclosure.

Presumably, the court reasoned this way: the baby's death was honestly excluded by the terms of this policy. Hence, truth and justice require that the suit be dismissed and the doctor supported. Commenting on this, Chayet [1] said:

> This case lays down a much lower standard than that which is required by the ethics of the medical profession. The case illustrates that once a disclosure is made, the courts will go far in searching for a principle of "social importance" to rationalize the disclosure. I do not agree with the results in this case. The doctor should *not* have made a voluntary, out-of-court disclosure of this nature. The law should have granted redress.

Physicians employed by state hospitals or other government agencies may be considered officers or agents of the state. When the problem lines up as community safety versus the patient's personal interest, the doctor can console himself with that thought. Even then, however, he has a duty to protect the patient's interest up to the point where the public is genuinely jeopardized. For instance, in one case, a patient in a public mental hospital had told her doctor about a string of infidelities. The state child welfare agency heard rumors of this and tried to examine the hospital record. If the mother were as promiscuous as rumor said, they were going to take the children away from her. The hospital denied access to the records. Here it was possible to keep the patient's confidence without damaging the community.

Role of Physician and Breach of Confidence

The private practitioner is in the most delicate position of all. He is, after all, the patient's personally selected representative. Where the law requires disclosure (as in handling addicts, for instance), the physician's duty is clear: to obey the law. In the more typical case, the practitioner has to decide (1) the likelihood that the patient actually will carry out a threat that may be the product of fantasy only, (2) whether the doctor can persuade the patient to change his plans, (3) whether he can win the patient's agreement to notifying a responsible family member, or (4) whether concern for public safety requires an immediate disclosure. If the doctor keeps it confidential because he assumes that the patient is only playing a game in fantasy, he is taking a risk which he has to calculate himself. But then, medicine is full of risks, and the practitioner unwilling to take them had better move into another profession.

The industrial doctor is in an especially awkward position. He is an agent of both the patient and the employer. If he is to be effective, the patient must trust him. What does the industrial medical officer do when he learns that the executive vice-president is a homosexual or the sales manager is an alcoholic? If he doesn't do something about it, he may be violating a duty to the employer. If he does, he may be breaching a confidence and employees may never again trust him.

In its September, 1966, issue, the journal *Psychiatric Progress* interviewed several leading physicians on this matter and reported the following discussion [2]: "Under what circumstances, if any, is a breach of doctor-patient confidentiality justified? One doctor answered simply: whenever an innocent person might be harmed by keeping the confidence (spreading contagious disease, for example) or whenever the patient might do irreparable harm to himself if the secret were preserved."

Another doctor answered:

> The physician's fundamental purpose is to protect the patient. This includes protecting him from himself. It seems, therefore, that a breach is justified when it clearly benefits the patient. Thus it is incumbent upon us to protect him from becoming a murderer, because his act will not only *result in penalties and punishment to him,* but leads to our second obligation—to protect society when *it* is clearly in danger. When we have a firm feeling that something tragic *will* happen we must act and take whatever course is necessary. But cases differ and you can't make any hard and fast rules. Different physicians will interpret patient material differently.

Another practitioner replied:

> If I were faced with the question, I would search my conscience and do what I thought

was best under the circumstances. In the case of minors (such as some students) a breach of confidence is often permissible because the parents are legally responsible. I always explain to an adolescent that ordinarily I would never tell his parents anything he told me. But when a situation involves the parents I let the patient know that I am going to tell them, even though he may disapprove. I know that the law can demand information, but that doesn't really *justify* releasing it. Sometimes you have to do things for legal reasons that are not justified medically.

The medical director at a large university said:

There are some circumstances that call for a breach of confidence. At our university, we follow the policy of never violating a confidence except under subpoena: and then only after talking it over with the university's legal department. In other situations, one breaches confidentiality only in very unusual circumstances, as with homicide, suicide, or another action which, if not dealt with immediately, might damage the patient or others.

If possible, one also tells the patient what is being done and why. If that isn't practical, he can tell the next of kin or another responsible person. If a confidence has to be violated, the doctor should consult with a well-versed person of integrity. It's better to share responsibility than to respond impulsively to being on the spot.

One of the country's leading forensic psychiatrists asserted that: A physician should report confidential information only if convinced of a real danger that the patient will carry out some dangerous act. Just being a nuisance is not enough. Another practitioner replied:

While circumstances vary, it is *never* justifiable to reveal contents of patients' fantasies or ideas when no valid purpose would be served.

But the doctor is justified in breaching a confidence when there is danger to the community or to the individual. The patient should be informed that the situation requires some other intervention and that information about his condition must be shared with a relative.

If the patient is incapable of making a rational decision about action to be taken, the physician is justified in going ahead, having first informed the patient of what is being

done. At the same time one indicates to the authority, parent, or spouse, one's concern for the patient.

If a patient says he has committed a criminal act, the physician, after all, does not know whether the information is accurate—it might be delusional. False confessions often follow highly publicized murders. If a patient admits to a criminal act, the doctor has to decide if this is simply a fantasy-projection of guilt feelings, and if any good would be done by reporting it. If an innocent person is in prison when a patient confesses the crime, it would certainly be the duty of the doctor to tell the court. But if a patient says he assaulted someone 10 years ago and that no one has been convicted of the offense, there is scarcely any need to report it. Such decisions require a careful weighing of facts and possibilities, but that is the physician's job.

Another doctor said that it depends

. . . upon the nature of the crime. If a patient says he's going to forge a check, it wouldn't disturb me. If he says he is going to commit serious bodily injury, it *would* disturb me; my action would depend on whether I felt he was likely to do it.

There are many women, for instance, who say they fear they might kill their children. Usually you know they won't. But if you give credence to such a statement, the first obligation is to inform the family that this is a serious problem and that they should be the motivating force in whatever is done. If they refuse and you still feel that a real danger is involved, you are obligated to report to the police.

An adult must be responsible for his own behavior, but if he cannot be, the physician has to share the responsibility, for the sake of both the individual and other persons.

In universities, the college or infirmary physician has a special problem. Release of intimate information by college authorities may well destroy the doctor's usefulness in the university. The college doctor generally has to decide to do one of three things: (1) absolutely refuse to release the information; (2) urge the student to see an outside (private) doctor and make only minimum notes in the college infirmary file; or (3) try to persuade the student that it would be best to permit the physician to discuss the matter with the dean, his parents, or a guidance counselor. When the chips are down, the college authorities can probably impound and read any record in their own infirmary.

With respect to private practitioners, the road may also be a rocky one. If we lived in a simple and tidy little world, it would be easy to say that the doctor's lips should be permanently sealed. But there are a dozen situations in which the question cannot be disposed of that readily. First, there is the legal requirement to report gunshot wounds and contagious disease. Furthermore, a doctor must not be an accomplice to a crime even in the negative sense of saying nothing. Then there is the problem of protecting public interest when it means revealing a confidence. If you know that the driver of a school bus is an alcoholic or epileptic, you should report it. Last year 30 people were killed when a bus driver had a heart attack and plunged his bus into the East River in New York City. The driver's physician had known about the bad heart, had cautioned him not to drive, but felt he could not report it to the company since the patient might lose his job. In New Jersey some years ago, six people were killed when a bus driver had a petit mal seizure. The treating doctor knew about the epilepsy, pleaded with the patient to stop driving, but didn't think he ought to report it to the motor vehicle department.

More and more patients' bills are being paid by third parties; for example, insurance companies, Medicare, welfare funds, Veterans Administration, relief administrations, Blue Shield, and many others. Most of these facilities will not pay the doctor unless they know the conditions which were treated. Furthermore, it is often no solution to get the patient's signature on an authorization or permission form, since this signature may be required if the patient is going to collect his benefits. In effect, the patient is told: either you waive the confidential nature of your doctor-patient relationship or you don't get the benefit, i.e., the award, the indemnity, the compensation, or whatever it is. Thus the patient may be blackmailed into waiving a precious right or may even be cajoled into signing a document, the import of which he simply does not understand. And once the seal of confidentiality is broken, the doctor-patient relationship is radically and irrevocably altered.

This is one problem that cannot be programmed into a computer. There is still no substitute for personal judgment, the facing of responsibility, and the path-pointing of the human conscience.

Notes

1. The states without privilege include eight in the Atlantic group (Maine, Massachusetts, Connecticut, Delaware, Rhode Island, New Hampshire, Vermont, and New Jersey) and eight southern states (Alabama, Florida, Georgia, Kentucky, Maryland, South Carolina, Tennessee, and Texas).

2. *State* vs. *Anonymous,* 269 New York State Second 459. Reported also in Physician's *Legal Brief* (Bloomfield, N.J.: Schering Corp., September, 1966).

3. *Clark* vs. *Geraci,* 208 New York State Second 569.

4. *Griswold* vs. *Connecticut,* 381 U.S. 479.

5. *Feeney* vs. *Young,* 181 New York State 481.

6. *Hague* vs. *Williams,* 181 Atlantic Second 345.

References

1. Chayet, N. *Confidentiality in Psychiatry.* Seminar of the University of California's Colloquium on Law and Psychiatry, Los Angeles, Dec. 4, 1965.

2. Discussion. *Psychiatric Progress* 1:2, 1966.

Confidentiality and the Prediction of Dangerousness in Psychiatry: The Tarasoff Case

William J. Curran

The California Supreme Court continues to make financial awards to patients in suits against physicians with seemingly little regard for the effect of these awards and decisions upon the practice of

Reprinted by permission from the New England Journal of Medicine 293 *(August 7, 1975): 285–286.*

medicine and the availability of insurance to cover this largesse of the judiciary, and without regard for the social consequences of this "money-for-everything" attitude.

The particular case, *Tarasoff vs. Regents of the University of California*,[1] has already become infamous among mental-health programs in California and among college and university student medical programs all over the country as it has taken its course through the various levels of trial and appeals courts in the Golden State.

The facts of the situation are undisputed. A student at the University of California's Berkeley campus was in psychotherapy with the student health service on an outpatient basis. He told his therapist, a psychologist, that he wanted to kill an unmarried girl who lived in Berkeley but who was then on a summer trip to Brazil. The psychologist, with the concurrence of another therapist and the assistant director of the Department of Psychiatry, reported the matter orally to the campus police and on their suggestion sent them a letter requesting detention of the student and his commitment for observation to a mental hospital. The campus police picked up the student for questioning but "satisfied" that he was "rational," released him on his "promise to stay away" from Miss Tarasoff. The police reported back to the director of psychiatry, Dr. Powelson. Dr. Powelson asked for the return of the psychologist's letter to the police and directed that all copies of the letter be destroyed. Nothing more was done at the health service about the matter. Two months later, shortly after Miss Tarasoff's return, the student went to her home and killed her.

The parents of Miss Tarasoff brought suit for damages against the University and against the therapists and the campus police, as employees of the University and individually. In suing Dr. Powelson, the plaintiffs sought not only general money damages for negligence in failure to warn the girl and her parents and to confine the student, but exemplary or punitive damages (which could be assessed in huge amounts as multiples of the general damages or in any amount at the determination of the jury) for malicious and oppressive abandonment of a dangerous patient.

The Superior Court dismissed all these grounds for legal action against the defendants. The Supreme Court, in a four-to-two decision, re-

versed the decision and found that on these facts a cause of action was stated for general damages against all the therapists involved in the case and the assistant director and the director of psychiatry and against the University as their employer for breach of the duty to warn Miss Tarasoff. The Court dismissed the claim for exemplary damages against the therapists. It also dismissed the action against the police as protected from a suit by a statutory immunity, as well as the suit against the therapists for failure to confine the student under a commitment order, again because of a statutory immunity. The Court implied that without the immunity, both these actions might have been meritorious.

It seems to me most physicians would throw up their hands in dismay over this result and the massive contradictions in the assessment of who was and who was not legally responsible for this death. If I were to describe in detail the reasoning of the court, the confusion of the medical mind would be compounded a thousand times.

The Court asserted that the *Principles of Medical Ethics of the American Medical Association*, Section 9, did not bar breaching the confidentiality of this patient "in order to protect the welfare of this individual [the patient] or the community." From this premise the Court jumped wholeheartedly to a positive duty to warn Miss Tarasoff. This is not what the *Principles* said. The traditional code of medical ethics allows a physician in his sound discretion to breach the confidentiality, but does not require it. It is almost impossible to draft an ethical principle to force a duty on physicians to breach confidences. Must they always warn of death threats, but have discretion on less dangerous threats? Must they warn if the patient is psychotic, but not if he is less disturbed? Does this case mean that every time a patient makes a threat against an unnamed person, the therapist must take steps to find out who it is and warn him (of anything at all, from vague threats to murder) or suffer money damages in the thousands or tens of thousands if the threat, or an aspect of the threat, is carried out?

This case was greatly confused by the array of immunities from suits created under California law. It can be strongly argued that the thrust of these immunity statutes regarding the duty to warn should also have been applied to the therapists, since the statutes were intended to encourage police and mental-health personnel to re-lease patients and not confine them on the basis of unreliable diagnoses of dangerousness. In the past it was thought that too many mental patients were confined for years and years because of their threats to other people, rarely carried out, and be-cause of the conservatism of mental-health per-sonnel in exercising any doubt about dangerous-ness in favor of confinement as the safest way to prevent harm to third parties.

It seems clear that the therapists here thought that they had done all they could to protect their patient and the community by reporting the case to the police. They had exercised their discretion to warn the community and to breach the confidence of the patient, for his own sake, and that of the unknown girl. They could hardly warn her, since she was not even in the country at the time. Also, the threat to Miss Tarasoff might actually have been vaguely directed. The student could well have turned his anger and violence toward another person or toward himself. The only basic recourse was to recommend temporary observa-tional commitment. The practice was to make this to the campus police. It was the police who acted, and they decided to release the student with a warning and a promise to stay away from the girl. How many thousands of such warnings—and re-leases—do police departments make every year? How many people then proceed to kill? The im-munity statute was established to encourage re-lease in these circumstances. But the statutory armor had a hole in it. The director of psychiatry was found by the Court to have a "duty" to warn the girl, irrespective of the police action. The Court utilized some precedents, none clearly applicable to this case, to justify its decision. It seems, how-ever, that the real rationale was the aggravated nature of the case—a killing—in which the family was left without someone else to sue. The therapists, particularly Dr. Powelson, could have warned the girl if they had wanted to go against the police action and if they had thought the specific threat to Miss Tarasoff so serious as to war-rant that action. The Court did not apply any test to ascertain the custom of psychiatrists and mental-health programs actually in such situa-tions. The Court declared the duty as a matter of law, regardless of the accepted practices of the profession. As in the *Helling* decision[2] discussed in an earlier column,[3] the Court made the physician a guarantor against harm to this party, here not even a patient, on the basis of its own concept of monetary justice.

Notes

1. 529 P. 2d 553
2. *Helling vs. Carey and Laughlin,* 519 P. 2d 981.
3. Curran W. J. Glaucoma and streptococcal. pharyngitis: diagnostic practices and malpractice liability. N Engl J Med 291:508–509, 1974.

Decision Scenario 1

"I find it incredible that you plan on allowing yourself to be treated by a chiro-practor," Martha Redpath said.

"What's the matter with going to a chiropractor?" Roger Smith asked. "I went to an M.D. and that didn't do any good. I haven't felt really good in years, but he told me there wasn't anything wrong with me."

"Chiropractors are frauds," Martha said. "They work on the basis of a false theory because they claim that all illnesses are caused either directly or indirectly by misalignments of the vertebrae. That is just sheer nonsense."

"Maybe so," said Roger. "But why shouldn't I go if it makes me feel better? I think they help a lot of people."

"Maybe they won't do you any harm. But in general they're dangerous. They keep a lot of people from getting competent medical treatment, because the people go see a chiropractor instead of a physician. Also, chiropractors often give a lot of x rays, even though most of them aren't trained to do that, and that means that a great number of people receive massive doses of harmful radiation."

Ralph shook his head. "I don't say that you're wrong. But it seems to me that everybody ought to be free to choose the kind of treatment that he wants to get. If he thinks a chiropractor can do him some good, then he ought to be able to consult one."

"Look," Martha said, "I'm as much in favor of individual freedom as you are. But a lot of people just aren't well-enough informed to make good choices about their own medical care. I think that we should have laws that make chiropractic 'medicine' illegal. We need to protect people from their own ignorance and from those who take advantage of it."

Using the principles argued for by Dworkin, construct an argument in support of Martha's position.

Is regulation of the sort advocated by Martha compatible with Rawls's theory?

Do such regulations or laws violate Kant's notion of the individual as an autonomous rational agent?

Decision Scenario 2

"I really don't understand you," Dr. Lowell said. "You definitely have cancer of the bladder. We may be able to remove it all surgically, but even if we can't, chemotherapy or radiation treatments have a good chance of success."

"I want none of those," Patricia Jensen said. "I believe that a high-fiber diet and pure, filtered water are more likely to help me. I don't want to be cut or poisoned or burned."

"You're crazy," Dr. Lowell said. "That won't do anything."

"I intend to try it. Even if I'm wrong, it's my life."

"I won't let you," said Dr. Lowell. "Anybody who thinks the way you do about cancer is out of touch with reality. That's one of the marks of mental illness. And I intend to have you declared mentally incompetent to make decisions about your own welfare. I shall speak to the psychiatrists on our staff and ask the hospital lawyer to arrange for a sanity hearing."

"That's fascism!"

"Call it anything you like. But my duty as a physician is to give you the best medical care possible. If that means having you declared mentally incompetent, then so be it."

Dr. Lowell picked up the telephone.

State and evaluate the argument Dr. Lowell offers to justify her intended course of action.

On Ross's view, does Lowell have a prima facie duty to take steps necessary to treat Ms. Jensen? If so, are there other duties that might make this one not an actual duty?

Would Zembaty regard this as a case of defensible paternalism?

Decision Scenario 3

"You realize that I talked to him for only fifteen or twenty minutes," said Dr. Susan Beck.

"Yeah, but you psychiatrists are supposed to be able to size up a guy just by listening to how he says hello," Dr. Mark Brunetti said.

"Now that I've talked to him, tell me more about him," Beck said.

"I presume you learned his name is T. D. Chang?"

"That was written down for me."

"Fine," said Brunetti. "He's fifty-two years old, a Professor of Asian History at Southwestern University. He's married, has two children in college, and has a solid scholarly reputation."

"What was his complaint?" asked Beck.

"About a month ago he began to experience difficult and painful urination. His attending physician examined him, found that he had an enlarged prostate, and treated with sulfa. No joy. So the attending physician sent him here. We're doing an x-ray scan and a punch biopsy in the morning."

"And you want me to tell you how I think he'll take it if you tell him you suspect cancer?"

"Right," said Brunetti. "I don't like to scare people unless I have to. My inclination here is just to keep quiet until we know for sure."

"I think he would take it all right. He shows no tendency towards hysteria, and his background reveals him to be a person who functions well under normal conditions of stress."

"Good, then if I have to tell him, I won't worry about it."

"Mark, do you mean you're *not* going to tell him?"

"That's right. Not until I know for sure. It's a kindness to him. What he doesn't know won't hurt him, and there's no reason to cause him unnecessary anxiety."

"I don't think I agree with that decision," Beck said. "I think a man like Mr. Chang has a right to know as much about his condition as you do."

"That's silly," Brunetti said. "He can't possibly know as much as I do, and he wouldn't know what to make of the information even if I gave it to him. He would probably figure he's going to die in the next hour."

"So you aren't going to tell him what you suspect or why you're doing the biopsy?"

"I'm not that cruel, even if I am a surgeon."

Do the arguments presented by Lipkin support Brunetti's view? What are the arguments?

Are there grounds for considering this a case of legitimate paternalism, as Zembaty conceives it?

What might an act or rule utilitarian say about this situation? Would Ross be likely to consider Beck or Brunetti right?

Using Bok's line of reasoning, what criticisms might be made of the position taken by Brunetti?

Decision Scenario 4

In the late summer, Harold Leithold, a thirty-four-year-old systems analyst, learned that Data-Ink, his employer, was willing to promote him if he agreed to move from New Orleans to the Dallas branch by October. Leithold and his wife both decided the move would be to their advantage and set about preparing for it.

Since his middle twenties, Leithold had suffered from asthma and subacute diabetes. He was careful with his health and was concerned to find a physician in Dallas he could have confidence in. In order to avoid the trouble of having his medical records sent to a new physician and to minimize the risk of their being lost or delayed in transit, he decided it would be wiser to take them with him.

"I would like to have a copy of my records so I can just hand them over to my new doctor," Leithold told his physician.

"I'm afraid I can't permit that," Dr. Solinger said. "So far as the laws of this state are concerned, the records belong to me."

"Surely that's a trivial point," Leithold said. "I just want copies of the records, and I'm willing to pay for them. You can keep the originals."

"There's more to it than that," Dr. Solinger said. "If I give you a copy, then you'll be able to read the records. You're likely to get all confused by them. You'll think you're sicker than you are or have some kind of disease you really don't have."

"I don't think that's very likely," Leithold said. "I'm not a physician, but I'm not a complete idiot either."

"I know you aren't. But you won't understand the terms, and you'll misinterpret things. It's not really right for me to let you have them. Because if I do, I might be responsible for causing you harm."

"Will you send them to my doctor in Dallas?" Leithold asked.

"Sure, be glad to."

"But you won't let me have them."

Dr. Solinger shook his head. "I can't do it. It's for your own good."

According to the definition of paternalism endorsed by Zembaty, is Dr. Solinger acting in a paternalistic way? If so, would she believe his action is justifiable?

Would a Kantian be likely to regard the act as moral?

Is it possible to defend Mr. Leithold's right to his records on utilitarian grounds?

Can the arguments presented by Lipkin be used to support Dr. Solinger's action?

Decision Scenario 5

"Sometimes I think that what I really want to do is to kill people and drink their blood."

Dr. Allen Wolfe looked at the young man in the chair across from him. The face was round and soft and innocent looking, like that of a large baby. But the body had the powerful shoulders of a college wrestler. There was no doubt that Hal Crane had the strength to carry out his fantasies.

"Any people in particular?" Dr. Wolfe asked.

"Women. Girls about my age. Maybe their early twenties."

"But no one you're personally acquainted with."

"That's right. Just girls I see walking down the street or getting off a bus. I have a tremendous urge to stick a knife into their stomachs and feel the blood come out on my hands."

"But you've never done anything like that?"

Crane shook his head. "No, but I'm afraid I might."

Dr. Wolfe considered Crane a paranoid schizophrenic with compulsive tendencies, someone who might possibly act out his fantasies. He was a potentially dangerous person.

"Would you be willing to take my advice and put yourself in a hospital under my care for a while?"

"I don't want to do that," Crane said. "I don't want to be locked up like an animal."

"But you don't really want to hurt other people, do you?"

"I guess not," Crane said. "But I haven't done anything yet."

"But you might," Dr. Wolfe said. "I'm afraid you might let yourself go and kill someone."

Crane smiled. "That's just the chance the world will have to take, isn't it? I told you I'm not going to let myself be locked up."

Suppose that you are Dr. Wolfe. To take the legal steps necessary to have Mr. Crane committed against his will requires that you violate confidentiality. What justification might a utilitarian offer for doing this?

Might a Kantian oppose commitment on the grounds that it would violate Crane's dignity as a person?

As a physician, how would you justify acting to protect others while going against the wishes of your patient?

Should a physician be required by law to act to protect the welfare of others?

How does this case compare with the Tarasoff case discussed by Curran? What actions, on Curran's view, should be taken by Dr. Wolfe?

Decision Scenario 6

A few years ago, a new strain of gonorrhea known as P.P.N.G. (penicillinase-producing Neisseria gonorrhoeae) developed in the Philippines and began spreading to port cities throughout the world. The new strain is resistant to treatment by penicillin, because it produces its own penicillin-destroying enzyme. It does, however, respond to treatment by synthetic antibiotics such as spectrinomycin.

In 1982, the New York Department of Health became concerned about the great increase in the number of cases of P.P.N.G. in the area. In an unorthodox move, the department began to send inspectors to known brothels to test and treat prostitutes for the disease.

"So far we've had excellent cooperation—from madams, prostitutes, and pimps," the Health Commissioner reported. In a few months, the inspectors visited some forty brothels and tested more than three hundred prostitutes. About 40 percent of those tested turned out to have the disease.

Like all venereal diseases, P.P.N.G. spreads through a chain of infections. One infected individual passes the disease to one or more others, and so on. In an effort to break the chain, the health department also obtained lists of clients from "call girls." Inspectors then called the men on the list and arranged to test them for the disease.

The incidence of P.P.N.G. in New York City has been about 40,000 cases annually for each of the last five years. The health department is hopeful that their new inspection program will substantially reduce the incidence of the disease.

Can a utilitarian argument be used to justify the health department inspection program?

Does the inspection program violate the individual's right to privacy and autonomy? Might a Kantian object to the program?

Do the principles argued for by Dworkin support or condemn such a program?

Decision Scenario 7

Jane Montrose told herself that it was just one of the things you had to do if you wanted to get promoted. Talking to eleven department heads might be a bore, but so far they had all been quite nice. And it wasn't even a bad idea. If she were going to be working as an Assistant Vice-President, she would have to deal with all of these people frequently. It made sense for them to have an opportunity to say whether they would feel comfortable working with her.

"How did you learn so much about computers?" Art Davis asked her.

It was a question people always asked. For some reason, they invariably seemed surprised to learn that a woman was comfortable dealing with the mysteries of data processing.

"I have a degree in computer science," she said. "Besides, I've been working with computers for about eight years now. You get to know their ways."

Davis nodded and smiled at her. She was somewhat surprised that he would ask such a naive question. As head of personnel, he more than anyone knew about her educational background and her work history. She wondered if he wasn't just stalling, making polite conversation until he could ask what really interested him.

"How are you doing with your psychiatrist?" Davis asked.

Jane was totally surprised by the question. She had assumed that only her closest friends knew she had been going to a psychiatrist.

"Fine," she said. "I mean, I've been able to work through a lot of problems that were bothering me."

She didn't really want to talk to Davis about her feelings of depression and lack of self-worth that had been troubling her for the last few years. None of it was any of his business.

"Do you think you'll be able to handle new responsibilities? This is a pretty important job you're being considered for, you know."

"I can handle them. I've always done very well at whatever job I've worked at."

"I know you have," Davis said. "But when we see that an employee has been going to a psychiatrist . . . well, that makes us wonder if that person is really to be trusted with a lot of responsibility. I'm sure you understand."

"I don't really. I don't see what my personal problems have to do with my work, assuming they don't get in the way of my doing it. And they never have."

Davis smiled at her in a way that made her very angry. It was the kind of tolerant but superior smile adults usually reserve for children who are talking about things they don't understand.

"What I want to know," Jane said, "is how you knew about my seeing a psychiatrist. I thought my medical records were all confidential."

"They are, so far as I know. But you did put in an insurance claim for payment, and I have to sign off on all the claims. When I did that, I saw you were getting psychiatric help."

"Are you going to make that public?"

"Not public," Davis said. "But I do feel obliged to mention it to the Executive Planning Group. If they're thinking about promoting you, then that's something they ought to know. I'm surprised you didn't volunteer the information yourself."

"I didn't think it was relevant," Jane said. "I didn't tell them I also suffer from hemorrhoids."

"Well, we'll let them judge whether it's relevant."

Does Davis have an obligation to inform the Executive Planning Group that Jane Montrose is receiving psychiatric treatment?

In New York, employees of the state government have the right to send medical claims for psychiatric or psychological services directly to the insurance company. Should this be made a legal right for all employees in all states?

The so-called Privacy Protection Act of 1980 permits federal law-enforcement agencies to secure search warrants and gain access to all private records, except those of the media. Should the Act be restricted to exclude medical and mental-health records?

5
MEDICAL EXPERIMENTATION
AND INFORMED CONSENT

CASE PRESENTATION
The Willowbrook Hepatitis Experiments

The Willowbrook State School in Staten Island, New York is an institution devoted to housing and caring for mentally retarded children. In 1956 a research group led by Saul Krugman and Joan P. Giles of The New York University School of Medicine initiated a long-range study of viral hepatitis at Willowbrook. The children confined there were made experimental subjects of the study.

Hepatitis is a disease affecting the liver that is now known to be caused by one of two (possibly more) viruses. Although the viruses are distinct, the results they produce are the same. The liver becomes inflamed and increases in size as the invading viruses replicate themselves. Also part of the tissue of the liver may be destroyed and the liver's normal functions impaired. Often the flow of bile through the ducts is blocked, and bilirubin (the major pigment in bile) is forced into the blood and urine. This produces the symptom of yellowish or jaundiced skin.

The disease is generally relatively mild, although permanent liver damage can be produced by it. The symptoms are ordinarily flulike—mild fever, tiredness, inability to keep food down. The viruses causing the disease are transmitted orally through contact with the feces and bodily secretions of infected people.

Krugman and Giles were interested in determining the natural history of viral hepatitis—the mode of infection and the course of the disease over time. They also wanted to test the effectiveness of gamma globulin as an agent for inoculating against hepatitis. (Gamma globulin is a protein complex extracted from the blood serum that contains antigens, substances that trigger the production of specific antibodies to counter infectious agents.)

Krugman and Giles considered Willowbrook to be a good choice for investigation because viral hepatitis occurred more or less constantly in the institution. In the jargon of medicine, the disease was endemic. That this was so was recognized in 1949, and it continued to be so as the number of children in the school increased to over five thousand in 1960. Krugman and Giles claimed that "under the chronic circumstances of multiple and repeated exposure . . . most newly admitted children became infected within the first six to twelve months of residence in the institution."

Over a fourteen-year period, Krugman and Giles collected over twenty-five thousand serum specimens from more than seven hundred patients. Samples were taken before exposure, during the incubation period of the virus, and for periods after the infection. In an effort to get the kind of precise data they considered most useful, Krugman and Giles decided to deliberately infect some of the incoming children with the strain of the hepatitis virus prevalent at Willowbrook.

They justified their decision in the following way:

> It was inevitable that susceptible children would become infected in the institution. Hepatitis was especially mild in the 3- to 10-year age group at Willowbrook. These studies would be carried out in a special unit with optimum isolation facilities to protect the children from other infectious diseases such as shigellosis [dysentary caused by a bacillus], and parasitic and respiratory infections which are prevalent in the institution.

Most important, Krugman and Giles claimed to see the child's being an experimental subject as in the best medical interest of the child, for not only would the child receive special care, but infection with the milder form of hepatitis would provide protection against the more virulent and damaging forms. As they say: "It should be emphasized that the artificial induction of hepatitis implies a 'therapeutic' effect because of the immunity which is conferred."

Krugman and Giles obtained what they considered to be adequate consent from the parents of the children used as subjects. Where they were unable to obtain consent, they did not include the child in the experiment. In the earlier phases of the study, parents were provided with relevant information either by letter or orally, and written consent was secured from them. In the later phases, a group procedure was used:

> First, a psychiatric social worker discusses the project with the parents during a preliminary interview. Those who are interested are invited to attend a group session at the institution to discuss the project in greater detail. These sessions are conducted by the staff responsible for the program, including the physician, supervising nurses, staff attendants, and psychiatric social workers. . . . Parents in groups of six to eight are given a tour of the facilities. The purposes, potential benefits, and potential hazards of the program are discussed with them, and they are encouraged to ask questions. Thus, all parents can hear the response to questions posed by the more articulate members of the group. After leaving this briefing session parents have an opportunity to talk with their private physicians who may call the unit for more information. Approximately two weeks after each visit, the psychiatric social worker contacts the parents for their decision. If the decision is in the affirmative, the consent is signed but parents are informed that signed consent may be withdrawn any time before the beginning of the

program. It has been clear that the group method has enabled us to obtain more thorough informed consent. Children who are wards of the state or children without parents have never been included in our studies.

Krugman and Giles point out that their studies have been reviewed and approved by the New York State Department of Mental Hygiene, the New York State Department of Mental Health, the Armed Forces Epidemological Board, and the human experimentation committees of the New York University School of Medicine and the Willowbrook School. They also stress that, although they were under no obligation to do so, they chose to meet the World Medical Association's Draft Code on Human Experimentation.

The value of the research conducted by Krugman and Giles has been recognized as significant in furthering a scientific understanding of viral hepatitis and methods for treating it. Yet serious moral doubts have been raised about the nature and conduct of the experiments. In particular, many have questioned the use of retarded children as experimental subjects, some claiming that children should never be experimental subjects in investigations that are not directly therapeutic. Others have raised questions about the ways in which consent was obtained from the parents of the children, suggesting that parents were implicitly blackmailed into giving their consent. The letters to the British medical journal *Lancet* and the selection from Paul Ramsey's *The Patient as Person* presented in this chapter discuss these issues.

Introduction

In 1947, an international tribunal meeting in Nuremberg convicted fifteen German physicians of 'war crimes and crimes against humanity." The physicians were charged with taking part in "medical experiments without subjects' consent." But the language of the charge fails to indicate the cruel and barbaric nature of the experiments. Here are just some of them:

At the Ravensbrueck concentration camp, experiments were conducted to test the effectiveness of the drug sulfanilamide. Cuts were deliberately made on the bodies of people, then the wounds were infected with bacteria. The infection was worsened by forcing wood shavings and ground glass into the cuts. Then sulfanilamide and other drugs were tested for their effectiveness in combating the infection.

At the Dachau concentration camp, healthy inmates were injected with extracts from the mucous glands of mosquitos to produce malaria. Various drugs were then used to determine their relative effectiveness.

At Buchenwald, numerous healthy people were deliberately infected with the spotted-fever virus merely for the purpose of keeping the virus alive. Over 90 percent of those infected died as a result.

Also at Buchenwald, various kinds of poisons were secretly administered to a number of inmates to test their efficacy. Either the inmates died or they were killed at once so that autopsies could be performed. Some experimental subjects were shot with poisoned bullets.

At Dachau, to help the German Air Force, investigations were made into the limits of human endurance and existence at very high altitudes. People were placed in sealed chambers then subjected to very high and very low atmospheric pressures. As the indictment puts it, "Many victims died as a result of these experiments and others suffered grave injury, torture, and ill-treatment."

Seven of the physicians convicted were hanged, and the other eight received long prison terms. From the trial there emerged the Nuremberg Code, a statement of the principles that should be followed in conducting medical research with human subjects. (The principles of the code appear as a selection in this chapter.)

Despite the moral horrors that were revealed at Nuremberg, few people doubt the need for medical experimentation involving human subjects. The extent to which contemporary medicine has become effective in the treatment of disease and illness is due almost entirely to the fact that it has become *scientific* medicine. This means that contemporary medicine must conduct inquiries in which data are gathered to test hypotheses and general theories related to disease processes and their treatment. Investigations involving nonhuman organisms are essential, but ultimate tests of the correctness and effectiveness of medical treatments must involve human beings as research subjects. Human physiology and psychology are sufficiently different to make animal studies alone inadequate.

The German physicians tried at Nuremberg were charged with conducting experiments without the consent of their subjects. The notion that consent must be given before a person becomes an experimental subject is still considered to be the basic requirement that must be met for an experiment to be morally legitimate. Ordinarily, it is not merely consent—saying yes—but *informed consent* that is demanded. The basic idea is simply that a person decides to participate in research after he or she has been provided with background information relevant to making the decision.

This same notion of informed consent is also considered a requirement that has to be satisfied before a person can legitimately be subjected to medical treatment. Thus, people are asked to agree to submit themselves to such ordinary medical procedures as blood transfusion or to other procedures such as surgical operations or radiation therapy.

The underlying idea of informed consent in both research and treatment is that people have a right to control what is done to their bodies. The notion of informed consent is thus a recognition of an individual's autonomy—of the right to make decisions governing one's own life. This right is recognized both in practice and in the laws of our society. (Quite often, malpractice suits turn on the issue of whether a patient's informed consent was valid.)

In the abstract, informed consent seems a clear and straightforward notion. After all, we all have an intuitive grasp of what it is to make a decision after we have been supplied with information. Yet in practice informed consent has proved to be a slippery and troublesome concept. In this introduction, we will attempt to identify some of the moral and practical difficulties that make the concept controversial and hard to apply. Our focus will be on informed consent in the context of human experimentation. But most of the issues that arise here also arise in connection with giving and securing informed consent for the application of medical therapies. (They also arise in special forms in abortion and euthanasia.) In effect, then, we will be considering the entire topic.

Before starting our discussion of informed consent, it will be useful to have some idea of what takes place in a typical medical experiment. Perhaps the most common type of research involves the testing of new drugs. Let us consider, then, a sketch of what is involved in such testing.

Drug Testing

Traditions of medical research and regulations of the United States Food and Drug Administration more or less guarantee that the development of new drugs follows a set procedure. The procedure consists of two major parts: preclinical and clinical testing.

When it is thought likely that a chemical substance might be useful, animal experiments are conducted to determine how toxic it is. These tests are also used to estimate the drug's therapeutic index (the ratio of a dose producing toxic effects to a dose producing desired effects). The effects of the substance on particular organs and tissues, as well as on the whole animal, are studied. Efforts are made to determine the drug's potential side effects and hazards (whether, for example, it is carcinogenic).

Clinical testing of the substance occurs in three phases. In phase one, normal human volunteers are used to determine whether the drug produces any toxic effects. If these results are acceptable, then in phase two the drug is administered to a limited number of patients who might be expected to benefit from it. If the drug produces desirable results and has no serious side effects, then phase three studies are initiated. The drug is administered to a larger number of patients by a larger number of clinical investigators. Such trials usually take place at teaching hospitals or in large public institutions. Successful results achieved in this phase ordinarily lead to the licensing of the drug for general use.

In the clinical part of testing, careful procedures are followed to attempt to exclude bias in the results. Investigators want their tests to be successful and patients want to get well, and either or both of these factors may influence test results. Investigators may perceive a patient as "improved" just because they want or expect him to be. What is more, all medications produce a "placebo effect." That is, when patients are given inactive substances (placebos), they nevertheless often show improvement.

To rule out these kinds of influences, a common procedure followed in drug testing is the "double-blind" test design. In this design, a certain number of patients are given the drug being tested, and the remainder of the test group are given placebos. (In some cases, an established drug may be used instead of or in addition to placebos.) Neither the investigators nor the patients are allowed to know who is receiving the drug and who is not—both are kept "blind." Sometimes a test group is divided so that part receives placebos all of the time, part only some of the time, and part receives genuine medication all of the time.

Often placebos are no more than just sugar pills. Yet, frequently, substances are prepared to produce side effects like those of the drug being tested. If, for example, the drug causes drowsiness, a placebo will be used that produces drowsiness. In this way, investigators will not be able to learn which patients are being given placebos on the basis of irrelevant observations.

The double-blind test design is employed in many kinds of clinical investigation, not just in drug testing. Thus, the testing of new vaccines and therapies often follow the same form. A major variation is the "single-blind" design, in which those who must evaluate the results of some treatment are kept in ignorance of which patients have received it.

The "Informed" Part of Informed Consent

At first sight, consent is no more than agreement. A person consents when he or she says "yes" when asked to be a research subject. But legitimate or valid consent cannot be merely saying yes. If people are to be treated as autonomous agents, they must have the opportunity to *decide* whether they wish to become participants in research. Deciding, whatever else it may be, is a process in which we reason about an issue at hand. We consider such matters as the risks to our participation, its possible advantages to ourselves and others, the risks and advantages of other alternatives that are offered to us, and our own values. In short, valid consent requires that we deliberate before we decide.

But genuine deliberation requires both information and understanding. These two requirements are the source of difficulties and controversies. After all, medical research and treatment are highly technical enterprises. They are based on complicated scientific theories that are expressed in a special vocabulary and involve unfamiliar concepts.

For this reason, some physicians and investigators have argued that it is virtually useless to provide patients with relevant scientific information about research and treatment. Patients without the proper scientific background, they argue, simply don't know what to make of the information. Not only do patients find it puzzling, they find it frightening. Thus, some have suggested, informed consent is at worst a pointless charade and at best a polite fiction. The patient's interest is best served by allowing a physician to make the decision.

This obviously paternalistic point of view (see Chapter 4) implies, in effect, that all patients are incompetent to decide their best interest and that physicians must assume the responsibility of acting for them. An obvious objection to this view is that it assumes that because patients lack a medical background, they cannot be given information in a form they can understand that is at least adequate to allow them to decide how they are to be treated. Thus, it can be argued, proponents of this view confuse the difficulty of communication with the impossibility of communication. It is true that it is often hard to explain technical medical matters to a layperson, but this hardly makes it legitimate to conclude that people should turn over their right to determine what is done to them to physicians. Rather, it imposes on physicians and researchers the obligation to find a way to explain medical matters to their patients.

The information provided to patients must be usable. That is, they must understand enough about the proposed research and treatment in order to deliberate and reach a decision. From the standpoint of the researcher, the problem here is to determine when the patient has an adequate understanding to make informed consent valid. Patients, being people, do not like to appear stupid and say they do not understand an explanation. Also, they may believe they understand an explanation when, as a matter of fact, they do not.

At present, there seems to be no generally accepted solution to the problem of determining when a patient understands the information provided to him or her. It seems reasonable to think that some kind of behavioral criteria—such as answering questions about the research project—would be best. But this is an area that requires empirical investigation.

The "Consent" Part of Informed Consent

We have talked so far as though the issue of gaining the legitimate agreement of someone to be a research subject involved only providing information to an ordinary person in ordinary circumstances and then allowing the person to decide. But the matter is more complicated than this because often either the person or the circumstances possess special features. These features can call into question the very possibility of valid consent.

It is generally agreed that in order to be valid, consent must be voluntary. The person must of his or her "own free will" agree to become a research subject. This means that the person must be capable of acting voluntarily. That is, the person must be *competent*.

This is an obvious and sensible requirement that is accepted by virtually everyone. But the difficulty lies in specifying just what it means to be competent. One answer is that a person is competent if he or she is capable of acting rationally. Since we have some idea of what it is to act rationally, this is a movement in the direction of an answer. The problem with it, however, is that people sometimes decide to act for the sake of moral (or religious) principles in ways that may not seem reasonable. For example, someone may volunteer to be a subject in a potentially hazardous experiment because she believes the experiment holds out the promise of helping countless others. In terms of self-interest alone, such an action would not be reasonable.

At present we do not have adequate criteria that can specify who is competent and who is not. Quite apart from this general theoretical problem is the issue of how children, the mentally retarded, and those suffering from psychiatric illnesses are to be considered with respect to consent. Should no person in any of these groups be considered capable of giving consent? If so, then is it ever legitimate to secure the consent from some third party, from a parent or guardian? One possibility is simply to rule out all research that involves such people as subjects. But this has the undesirable consequence of severely hampering efforts to gain the knowledge that might be of use either to the people themselves or to others with similar medical problems.

The questions we have raised here are still matters very much under dispute. Later we will consider some of the special problems that arise with children and other special groups as research subjects.

The circumstances in which research is done can also call into question the voluntariness of consent. This is particularly so with prisons, nursing homes, and mental hospitals. These are all what the sociologist Erving Goffman calls "total institutions," for within them all aspects of a person's life are connected with the social structure. People have a definite place in the structure and particular social roles. Moreover, there are social forces at work that both pressure and encourage an inmate to do what is expected of him.

We will discuss below some of the special problems that arise in research with prisoners. Here we need only to point out that the matter of gaining voluntary consent from inmates in institutions may not be possible at all. If it is possible, then it is necessary to specify the kinds of safeguards that need to be followed in order to free them from the pressures that result from the very fact that they are inmates. Those who suffer from psychiatric illnesses may be considered just as capable intellectually of giving consent, but here too safeguards to protect them from the pressures of the institution need to be specified.

To avoid a misimpression, it is also worth pointing out that ordinary patients in hospitals may also be subject to pressures that call into question the voluntariness of the consent that they give. Patients are psychologically predisposed to act in ways that please physicians. Not only do physicians possess a social role that makes them figures of authority, but an ill person feels very dependent on those who may possess the power to make him well. Thus, he will be inclined to go along with any suggestion or recommendation made by a physician. The ordinary patient, like the inmate in an institution, needs protection from the social and psychological pressures that are exerted by circumstances. Otherwise, the voluntariness of consent will be compromised, and the patient cannot act as a free and autonomous agent.

Medical Research and Medical Therapy

Medical therapy aims at relieving the suffering of people and restoring them to health. It attempts to cure diseases, correct disorders, and bring about normal bodily functioning. Its focus is on the individual patient, and his or her welfare is its primary concern.

Medical research, by contrast, is a scientific enterprise. Its aim is to acquire a better understanding of the chemical and physiological processes that are involved in human functioning. It is concerned with the effectiveness of therapies in ending disease processes and restoring functioning. But this concern is not for the patient as an individual. Rather, it is directed toward establishing theories. The hope, of course, is that this theoretical understanding can be used as a basis for treating individuals. But helping a particular patient get well is not a goal of medical research.

The related but distinct aims of medical research and medical therapy are a source of conflict in human experimentation. It is not unusual for a physician to be acting both as a researcher and as a therapist. This means that although she must be concerned with the welfare of her patient, her aims must also include acquiring data that are important to her research project. It is possible, then that she may quite unconsciously encourage her patients to volunteer to be research subjects, provide them with inadequate information on which to base their decisions, or minimize the risks they are likely to be subject to.

The patient, for his part, may be reluctant to question his physician to acquire more information or to help him understand his role and risks in research. Also, as mentioned above, the patient may feel pressured into volunteering for research, just because he wants to do what his physician expects of him.

The aims of therapy and the aims of research may also cause moral difficulties for the physician that go beyond the question of consent. This is particularly so in certain kinds of research. Let's look at some of the ethical issues more specifically.

Placebos and Research

As we saw earlier in the description of a typical drug experiment, placebos are considered to be essential in order to determine the true effectiveness of the drug being tested. In practice, this means that during all or some of the time they are being "treated," patients who are also subjects in a research program will not be receiving genuine medication. They are not, then, receiving the best available treatment for their specific condition.

This is one of the risks that a patient needs to know about before consenting to become a research subject. After all, most people become patients in order to be cured, if possible, of their ailments, not to further science or anything of the kind.

The physician-as-therapist will continue to provide medical care to a patient, for under double-blind conditions the physician does not know who is being given placebos and who is not. But the physician-as-researcher will know that a certain number of people will be receiving medication that cannot be expected to help their condition. Thus, the aims of the physician who is also a researcher come into conflict.

This conflict is particularly severe in cases in which it is reasonable to believe (on the basis of animal experimentation, tissue research, and so on) that an effective disease preventative exists, yet to satisfy scientific rigor, tests of its effectiveness involve the giving of placebos. This was the case with the development of a polio vaccine by Thomas Weller, John F. Enders, and Fredrick C. Robbins in 1960. The initial phase of the clinical testing involved injecting thirty thousand children with a substance known to be useless in the prevention of polio—a placebo injection. It was realized, statistically, that some of those children would get the disease and die from it.

Since Weller, Enders, and Robbins believed that they had an effective vaccine, they can hardly be regarded as acting in the best interest of these children. As physicians they were not acting to protect the interest and well-being of the children. They did, of course, succeed in proving the safety and effectiveness of the polio vaccine. The moral question is whether they were justified in failing to provide thirty thousand children with a vaccine they believed to be effective, even though it had not been tested on a wide scale with humans. That is, did they correctly resolve the conflict between their role as researchers and their role as physicians?

Placebos also present physician-researchers with another conflict. As we noticed in the earlier discussion, placebos are not always just "sugar pills." They often contain active ingredients that produce in patients effects that resemble those caused by the medication being tested—nervousness, vomiting, loss of appetite, and so on. This means that a patient receiving a placebo is sometimes not only failing to receive any medication for his illness, but he is also receiving a medication that may do him some harm. Thus, the physician committed to care for the patient and to relieve his suffering is at odds with the researcher who may be harming the patient. Do the aims of scientific research and its potential benefits to others justify treating patients in this fashion? Here is another moral question that the physician must face in particular and we must face in general.

We should not leave the topic of the use of placebos without mentioning that it is possible to make use of an experimental design in research that does not require giving placebos to a control group. An investigator can compare the results of two treatment forms: a standard treatment whose effectiveness is known and a new treatment with a possible but not proven effectiveness. This is not as satisfactory scientifically as the other approach because the researcher must do without a control group that has received no genuine treatment. But it does provide a way out of the dilemma of both providing medical care and conducting research.

Therapeutic and Nontherapeutic Research

We have mentioned the conflict that faces the physician who is also an investigator. But the patient who has to decide whether or not to consent to become a research subject is faced with a similar conflict.

Some research holds out the possibility of a direct and immediate advantage to those patients who agree to become subjects. For example, a new drug may, on the basis of limited trials, promise to be more effective in treating an illness than those drugs in standard use. Or a new surgical procedure may turn out to give better results than one that would ordinarily be used. By agreeing to participate in research involving such a drug or procedure, a patient may then have a chance of gaining something more beneficial than he or she would gain otherwise.

Yet the majority of medical research projects do not offer any direct therapeutic advantages to patients who consent to be subjects. The research may eventually benefit many patients, but seldom does it bring direct therapeutic benefits to research participants. Ordinarily, the most that participants can expect to gain is advantages such as having the attention of physicians who are more familiar with their illness than most physicians and receiving close observation and supervision in a research ward.

These are matters that ought to be presented to the patient as information relevant to the decision the patient must make. The patient must then decide whether he or she is willing to become a subject even if there are no special therapeutic advantages to be gained. It is in making this decision that one's moral beliefs can play a role. Some people volunteer to become research subjects without hope of reward because they believe that their action may eventually be of help to others.

Let us now turn to examining some of the problems posed by medical research in dealing with special groups. We will also consider some of the related issues that are involved in fetal research.

Research Involving Children

One of the most controversial areas of all medical experimentation has been that involving children as research subjects. The Willowbrook project discussed in the Case Presentation of this chapter is just one among many investigations that have drawn severe criticism and, quite often, court action.

The obvious question is: Why should children ever be made research subjects? Children clearly lack the physical, psychological, and intellectual maturity of adults. It does not seem that they are as capable as adults of giving informed consent because they can hardly be expected to grasp the nature of research and the possible risks to themselves. Furthermore, because they have not yet developed their capacities, it seems wrong to subject children to risks that might alter, for the worse, the course of their lives. They are in a position of relative dependency, relying upon adults to provide the conditions for their existence and development. It seems almost a betrayal of trust to allow children to be subjected to treatment that is of potential harm to them.

Such considerations help explain why we generally regard research involving children with deep suspicion. It is easy to imagine children being exploited and their lives heedlessly blighted by callous researchers. Some writers have been sufficiently concerned by the possibility of dangers and abuses that they have advocated an end to all research with children as subjects.

But there is another side to the coin. Biologically, children are not just small adults. Their bodies are developing, growing systems. Not only are there anatomical differences, there are also differences in metabolism and biochemistry. For example, some drugs are absorbed and metabolized more quickly in children than in adults, whereas other drugs continue to be active for a longer time. Often some drugs produce different effects when administered to children. Furthermore, just because the bodies of children are still developing, their nutritional needs are different. Findings based on adult subjects cannot simply be extrapolated to children, any more than results based on animal studies can be extrapolated to human beings.

Also, children are prone to certain kinds of diseases (measles, for example) that are either less common in adults or occur in different forms. It is important to know the kinds of therapies that are most successful in the treatment of children afflicted with them. Finally, even familiar surgical procedures cannot be employed in a straightforward way with children. Their developing organ systems are sufficiently different that special pediatric techniques must often be devised.

For many medical purposes, children must be thought of almost as if they were wholly different organisms. Their special biological features set them apart and mark them as subjects requiring special study. To gain the kind of knowledge and understanding required for effective medical treatment of children, it is often impossible to limit research solely to adults.

Failing to conduct research on children raises its own set of ethical issues. It seems likely that if children are excluded from investigations, then the development of pediatric medicine will be severely hindered. In general, this would mean that children would receive medical therapies that are less effective than might be possible. Also, since it is known that children differ significantly from adults in drug reactions, it seems wrong to subject children to the risks of drugs and drug dosages that have been tested only on adults.

Research involving children also seems necessary to avoid causing long-term harm to numerous people. The use of pure oxygen in the environments of prematurely born babies in the early 1940s resulted in blindness and impaired vision in a great number of cases. It was not until a controlled study was done that such damage was traced to the effects of the oxygen. Had the research not been allowed, the chances are very good that the practice would have continued and thousands more infants would have been blinded.

Yet even if we agree that not all research involving children should be forbidden, we still have to face up to the issues that such research generates. Without attempting to be complete, we can mention the following three issues as among the more prominent.

First, who is to be considered a child? For infants and children in elementary school, this question is not a difficult one. But what about people in their teens? Then the line becomes hard to draw. Indeed, perhaps it is not possible to draw a line at all without being arbitrary. The concern behind the question is with the acquisition of autonomy, of self-direction and responsibility. It is obvious on the basis of ordinary experience that people develop at different rates, and some people at sixteen are more capable of taking charge of their own lives than others are at twenty. Some teenagers are more capable of understanding the nature and hazards of a research project than are many people who are much older.

This suggests that many people who are legally children may be quite capable of giving their informed consent. Of course many others probably are not, so that decisions about capability would have to rest on an assessment of the individual. Where medical procedures that have a purely therapeutic aim are concerned, an individual who is capable of deciding whether it is in his or her best interest should probably be the one to decide. The issue may be somewhat different when the aim is not therapy. In such cases, a better policy might be to set a lower limit on the age at which consent can be given. The problem is, of course, what should that limit be?

Second, can anyone else consent on behalf of a child? Parents or guardians have a duty to act for the sake of the welfare of a child under their care. In effect, they have a duty to substitute their judgment for that of the child. We generally agree to this because most often we consider the judgment of an adult more mature and informed than a child's. And because the responsibility for care rests with the adult, we customarily recognize that the adult has a right to decide. It is almost as though the adult's autonomy is being shared with the child—almost as though the child were an extension of the adult.

Society and its courts have recognized limits on the power of adults to decide for children. When it seems that the adult is acting in an irresponsible or unreasonable manner, then society steps in to act as a protector of the child's right to be cared for. Thus, courts have ordered that life-saving procedures or blood transfusions be performed on children even when their parents or guardians have decided against it.

What sort of limits should govern a parent's or guardian's decision to allow a child to become a research subject? Can one person really give informed consent for another? Is it reasonable to believe that if a parent would allow herself to be the subject of an experiment, then it is also right for her to consent to her child's becoming a subject? Or should something more be required before consent for a child's participation can be considered legitimate?

Third, should children be allowed to be subjects of research that does not offer them a chance of direct therapeutic benefits? Perhaps the "something more" that parents or guardians ought to require before consenting on behalf of a child is the genuine possibility that the research will bring the child direct benefits. This would be in accordance with a parent's duty to seek the welfare of the child. It is also a way of recognizing that the parent's autonomy is not identical with that of the child: one may have the right to take a risk one's self without having the right to impose the risk on someone else.

This seems like a reasonable limitation, and it has been advocated by some writers. (See the Freedman selection in this chapter, for example.) Yet there are difficulties with the position. Some research virtually free from risk (coordination tests, for example) might be stopped because of its lack of a "direct therapeutic value." More important, however, much research promising immense long-term benefits would have to be halted. Research frequently involves the withholding of accepted therapies without any guarantee that what is used in their place will be as effective. Sometimes the withholding of accepted treatment is beneficial. Thus, as it turned out, in the research on the incidence of blindness in premature infants in the 1940s, premature infants who were not kept in a pure oxygen environment were better off than those that received ordinary treatment. But no one could know this in advance and such research as this is, at best, ambiguous as to the promise of direct therapy. Sheer ignorance imposes restrictions. Yet if the experiment had not been done, the standard treatment would have continued with its ordinary course of (statistically) disastrous results.

Here, at least, there was the possibility of better results from the experimental treatment. But in research that involves the substitution of placebos for medications or vaccines known to be effective, it is known in advance that some children will not receive medical care considered to be the best. A child who is a subject in such research is then put in a situation in which he or she is subjected to a definite hazard. The limitation on consent that we are considering would rule out such research. But the consequence of doing this would be to restrict the development of new and potentially more effective medications and treatment techniques. That is, future generations of children would be deprived of at least some possible medical advances.

These, then, are some of the issues that we have to face in arriving at a view of the role of children in research. Perhaps the greatest threat to children, however, has to do with social organization. Children, like prisoners, are often grouped together in institutions (schools, orphanages, detention centers, and so on) and are attractive targets for clinical investigators because they inhabit a limited and relatively controlled environment, can be made to follow orders, and do not ask too many questions that have to be answered. It is a misimpression to see researchers in such situations as "victimizing" children, but at the same time, it is clear that careful controls are needed to see that research involving children is legitimate and carried out in a morally satisfactory way.

Research Involving Prisoners

Prisoners are in some respects social outcasts. They have been found guilty of breaking the laws of society and, as a consequence, are removed from it. Stigmatized and isolated, prisoners in the relatively recent past were sometimes thought of as less than human. It seemed only reasonable that such depraved and corrupt creatures should be used as the subjects of experiments that might bring benefits to the members of the society that they wronged. It seemed not only reasonable but fitting.

Accordingly, in the early part of this century, tropical medicine expert Richard P. Strong obtained permission from the Governor of the Philippines to inoculate a number of condemned criminals with plague bacillus. The prisoners were not asked for their consent, but they were rewarded by being provided with cigarettes and cigars.

Episodes of this sort were relatively common during the late nineteenth and early twentieth centuries. But as theories about the nature of crime and criminals changed, it became standard practice to use only volunteers and to secure the consent of the prisoners themselves. In the 1940s, for example, the University of Chicago infected over four hundred prisoners with malaria in an attempt to discover new drugs to treat and prevent the disease. A committee set up by the Governor of Illinois recommended that potential volunteers be informed of the risks, be permitted to refuse without fear of such reprisals as withdrawing privileges, and be protected from unnecessary suffering. The committee suggested also that volunteering to be a subject in a medical experiment is a form of good conduct that should be taken into account in deciding whether a prisoner should be paroled or have his sentence reduced.

But the committee also called attention to a problem of great moral significance. They pointed out that if a prisoner's motive for volunteering is the wish to contribute to human welfare, then a reduction in his sentence would be a reward. But if his motive is to obtain a reduction in sentence, then the possibility of obtaining one is really a form of duress. In this case, the prisoner cannot be regarded as making a free decision.

The issue of duress or "undue influence" as it is called in law is central to the question of deciding whether, and under what conditions, valid informed consent can be obtained for research involving prisoners. To avoid undue influence, some ethicists have argued that prisoners should never be promised any substantial advantages for volunteering to be research subjects. If they volunteer, they should do so for primarily moral or humane reasons.

Others have claimed that becoming research subjects offers prisoners personal advantages that they should not be denied. For example, participation in a research project frees them from the boredom of prison life, gives them an opportunity to increase their feelings of self-worth, and allows them to exercise their autonomy as moral agents. It has been argued, in fact, that prisoners have a *right* to participate in research if the opportunity is offered to them and they wish to do so. To forbid the use of prisoners as research subjects is thus to deny to them, without adequate grounds, a right that all human beings possess. As a denial of their basic autonomy, of their right to take risks and control their own bodies, *not* allowing them to be subjects might constitute a form of cruel and unusual punishment.

By contrast, it can also be argued that prisoners do not deserve to be allowed to exercise such autonomy. It is reasoned that because they have been sentenced for crimes, they should be deprived of the right to volunteer to be research subjects: that right belongs to free citizens. Being deprived of the right to act autonomously is part of their punishment. This is basically the position taken in 1952 by the House of Delegates of the American Medical Association. The Delegates passed a resolution expressing disapproval of the use as research subjects of people convicted of "murder, rape, arson, kidnapping, treason, and other heinous crimes."

A more worrying consideration is the question of whether prisoners can be sufficiently free of undue influence or duress to make their consent legitimate. As we mentioned earlier, prisons are total institutions, and the very institutional framework puts pressures on people to do what is desired or expected of them. There need not be, then, promises of rewards (such as reduced sentences) or overt threats (such as the withdrawing of ordinary privileges) for coercion to be present. That people may volunteer to relieve boredom is itself an indication that they may be acting under duress. That "good conduct" is a factor in deciding whether to grant parole may function as another source of pressure.

The problem presented by prisoners is fundamentally the same as that presented by inmates in other institutions, such as nursing homes and mental hospitals. In these cases, once it has been determined that potential subjects are mentally competent to give consent, then it must also be decided whether the institutional arrangements allow the consent to be "free and voluntary."

Research Involving the Poor

In the eighteenth century, Princess Caroline of England requested the use of six "charity children" as subjects in the smallpox vaccination experiments she was directing. Then, and until quite recently, charity cases, like prisoners, were regarded by some medical researchers as prime research subjects.

A recent and horrible example of medical research involving the poor is the Tuskegee Syphilis Study that was conducted under the auspices of the U.S. Department of Public Health. From 1932 to 1970, a large but undetermined number of black males suffering from the later stages of syphilis were examined at regular intervals to determine the course their disease was taking. The men in the study were poor and uneducated and believed that they were receiving proper medical care from the state and local public health clinics. As a matter of fact, they were given either no treatment or inadequate treatment, and at least forty of them died as a result of factors connected with their disease. Their consent was never obtained, and the nature of the study, its risks, and the alternatives open to them were never explained. It was known when the study began that those with untreated syphilis have a higher death rate than those whose condition is treated, and although the study was started before the advent of penicillin (which is highly effective against syphilis), other drugs were available but were not used in ways to produce the best results. When penicillin became generally available, it still was not used.

The Tuskegee Study clearly violated the Nuremberg Code, but it was not stopped even after the War Crimes trials. It was reviewed in 1969 by a USPH ad hoc committee and it was decided that the study should be phased out in 1970. The reasons for ending the study were not moral ones. It was simply believed that there was nothing of much scientific value to be gained by continuing the work. In 1973, a USPH Ad Hoc Advisory Panel, which had been established as a result of public and congressional pressure to review the Tuskegee Study, presented its final report. It condemned the study both on moral grounds and because of its lack of worth and rigor.

No one today argues seriously that disadvantaged people ought to be made subjects of research simply as a result of their social or economic status. The "back wards" in hospitals whose poor patients once served as a source of research subjects have mostly disappeared as a result of such programs as Medicare and Medicaid. Each person is now entitled to his or her own physician and is not merely under the care of the state or of a private charity.

Yet many research projects continue to be based in large public or municipal hospitals. And such hospitals have a higher percentage of disadvantaged people as patients than do private institutions. For this reason, such people are still more likely to become research subjects than the educated and wealthy. If society continues to accept this state of affairs, special precautions must be taken to see to it that those who volunteer to become research subjects are genuinely informed and free in their decisions.

Research Involving Fetuses

In 1975 legal charges were brought against several physicians in Boston. They had injected antibiotics into living fetuses that were scheduled to be aborted. The aim of the research was to determine by autopsy, after the death of the fetuses, how much of the drug got into the fetal tissues.

Such information is considered to be of prime importance because it increases our knowledge of how to provide medical treatment for a fetus still developing in its mother's womb. It also helps to determine ways in which drugs taken by a pregnant woman may affect a fetus and so points the way towards improved prenatal care.

Other kinds of research involving the fetus also promise to provide important knowledge. Effective vaccines for preventing viral diseases, techniques for treating children with defective immune-system reactions, and hormonal measurements that indicate the status of the developing fetus are just some of the potential advances that are partially dependent on fetal research.

But a number of moral questions arise in connection with such research. Even assuming that a pregnant woman consents to allow the fetus she is carrying to be injected with drugs prior to abortion, is such research ethical? Does the fact that the fetus is going to be aborted alter in any way the moral situation? For example, prior to abortion should the fetus be treated with the same respect and concern for its well-being as a fetus which is not scheduled for abortion?

After the fetus is aborted, if it is viable—if it can live separated from the mother—then we seem to be under an obligation to protect its life. But what if a prenatal experiment threatens its viability? The expectation in abortion is that the fetus will not be viable, but this is not in fact always the case. Does this mean that it is wrong to do anything before abortion to threaten the life of the fetus or reduce its chance for life, even though we do not expect it to live?

These are very difficult questions to answer without first settling the question of whether the fetus is to be considered a person. (See the discussion of this issue in the introduction and selections in Chapter 1.) If the fetus is a person, then it is entitled to the same moral considerations that we extend to other persons. If we decide to take its life, if abortion is considered to be at least sometimes legitimate, then we must be prepared to offer justification. Similarly, if we are to perform experiments on a fetus, even one expected to die, then we must also be prepared to offer justification. Whether the importance of the research is adequate justification is a matter that currently remains to be settled.

If the fetus is not a person, then the question of fetal experimentation becomes less important morally. Since, however, the fetus may be regarded as a potential person, we may still believe it is necessary to treat it with consideration and respect. The burden of justification may be somewhat less weighty, but it may still be there.

Let us assume that the fetus is aborted and is apparently not viable. Typically, before such a fetus dies, its heart beats and its lungs function. Is it morally permissible to conduct research on the fetus before its death? The knowledge that can be gained, particularly of lung functions, can be used to help save the lives of premature infants, and the fetus is virtually certain of dying, whether or not it is made a subject of research.

After the death of a fetus that is either deliberately or spontaneously aborted, are there any moral restraints on what is done with the remains? It is possible to culture fetal tissues and use them for research purposes. These tissues might, in fact, be commercially grown and distributed by biological supply companies in the way that a variety of animal tissues are now dealt with. Exactly when a fetus can be considered to be dead so that its tissues and organs are available for experimentation, even assuming that one approves of their use in this manner, is itself an unanswered question.

Scientists have been concerned about proposed federal guidelines and state laws regulating fetal research. Most investigators fear that they will be forced to operate under such rigid restrictions that research will be slowed or even prohibited. Nearly everyone agrees, however, that some important moral and social decisions must be made about fetal research.

Fetal research has to be considered a part of human experimentation. Not only are many fetuses born alive even when deliberately aborted, but they all possess certain human characteristics and potentialities. But who shall give approval to what is done with the fetus? Who is responsible for consent?

It seems peculiar to say that a woman who has decided to have an abortion is also the one who should consent to research involving the aborted fetus. It can be argued that in deciding to have an abortion she has renounced all interest and responsibility with respect to the fetus. Yet if the fetus does live, we would consider her, at least in part, legally and morally responsible for seeing to its continued well-being.

But if the woman (or the parents) is the one who must give consent for fetal experimentation, are there limits to what she can consent to on behalf of the fetus? With this question we are back where we began. It is obvious that fetal research raises both moral and social issues. We need to decide, then, what is right as a matter of personal conduct and what is right as a matter of social policy. At the moment, issues in each of these areas remain unsettled.

Summary

There are other areas of human experimentation that present special forms of moral problems. We have not discussed, for example, research involving military personnel, college and university students, or dying patients. Moreover, we mentioned only a few of the special difficulties presented by the mentally retarded, psychiatric patients, and old people confined to institutions.

We have, however, raised such a multiplicity of questions about consent and human experimentation that it is perhaps worthwhile to attempt to restate some of the basic issues in a general form. Three issues are particularly noteworthy:

1. Who is competent to consent? (Are children? Are mental patients? If a person is not competent, who—if anyone—should have the power to consent for him or her?)

2. When is consent voluntary? (Is any institutionalized person in a position to offer free consent? How can even hospitalized patients be made free of pressures to consent?)

3. When is information and understanding adequate for genuine decision making? (Can complicated medical information ever be adequately explained to laypeople? Should we attempt to devise tests for understanding?)

Although we have concentrated on the matter of consent in research, there are other morally relevant matters connected with the character of research that we have not discussed. These often relate to research standards. Among them are the following:

1. Is the research of sufficient scientific and medical worth to justify the human risk involved? Research that involves trivial aims or that is unnecessary (when, for example, it merely serves to confirm what is already well established) cannot be used to justify causing any threat to human well-being.

2. Can the knowledge sought be obtained without human experimentation?

3. Have animal (and other) studies been done to minimize so far as is possible the risk to human subjects? A great deal can be learned about the effects of drugs, for example, by using "animal models," and the knowledge gained can be used to minimize the hazards in human trials.

4. Does the design of the research meet accepted scientific standards? Sloppy research that is scientifically worthless means that people have been subjected to risks for no legitimate purpose.

5. Do the investigators have the proper medical or scientific background in order to conduct the research effectively?

6. Is the research designed to minimize the risks and suffering of the participants? As we noted earlier, it is sometimes possible to test new drugs without using placebos. Thus, people in need of medication are not forced to be without treatment for their condition.

7. Have the aims and the design of the research and the qualifications of the investigators been reviewed by a group or committee competent to judge them? Such "peer review" is intended to assure that only research that is worthwhile and that meets accepted scientific standards is conducted. And although such review groups can fail to do their job properly, as they apparently did in the Tuskegee Syphilis Study, they are still necessary instruments of control.

Most writers on experimentation would agree that these are among the questions that must be answered satisfactorily before research involving human subjects is morally acceptable. Obviously, however, a patient who is asked to give his or her consent is in no position to judge whether the research project meets the standards implied by these questions. For this reason, it is important that there be social policies and practices governing research. Everyone should be confident that a research project is, in general, a legitimate one before having to decide whether to volunteer to become a participant.

Special problems are involved in seeing to it that these questions are properly answered. It is enough for our purposes, however, merely to notice that the character of the research and the manner in which it is to be performed are factors that are relevant to determining the moral legitimacy of experimentation involving human subjects.

Ethical Theories: Medical Research and Informed Consent

We have clearly raised too many issues in too many areas of experimentation to discuss how each of several ethical theories might apply to them all. We must limit ourselves to considering a few suggestions about the general issues of human experimentation and informed consent.

Utilitarianism's principle of utility tells us, in effect, to choose those actions that will produce the greatest amount of benefit. Utilitarianism must approve of human experimentation in general since there are cases in which the sacrifices of a few bring great benefits to many. We might, for example, design our social policies to make it worthwhile for people to volunteer for experiments with the view that if people are paid to take risks and are compensated for their suffering or for any damage done to them during the course of a research project, then the society as a whole might benefit.

The principle of utility also tells us to design experiments to minimize suffering and the chance of harm. Also, it forbids us to do research of an unnecessary or trivial kind—research that is not worth its cost in either human or economic resources.

So far as informed consent is concerned, utilitarianism does not seem to require it. If more social good is to be gained by making people research subjects without securing their agreement, then this is morally legitimate. (It is not, of course, necessarily the best procedure to follow. A system of rewards to induce volunteers might be more likely to lead to an increase in general happiness.) Furthermore, the principle of utility suggests that the best research subjects would be "less valuable" members of the society, such as the mentally retarded, the habitual criminal, or the dying. This, again, is not a necessary consequence of utilitarianism, although it is a possible one. If the recognition of rights and dignity would produce a better society in general, then a utilitarian would also say that they must be taken into account in experimentation with human beings.

For utilitarianism, that individual is competent to give consent who is able to balance benefits and risks and then decide what course of action is best for him or her. Thus, if informed consent is taken to be a requirement supported by the principle of utility, those who are mentally ill or retarded or senile have to be excluded from the class of potential experimental subjects. Furthermore, investigators must provide enough relevant information to allow competent people to make a meaningful decision about what is likely to serve their own interests the most.

For Kant, an individual capable of giving consent is one who is rational and autonomous. Kant's principles would thus also rule out as experimental subjects people who are not able to understand experimental procedures, aims, risks, and benefits. People may volunteer for experiments if they expect them to be of therapeutic benefit to themselves, or they may act out of duty and volunteer, thus discharging their imperfect obligation to advance knowledge or to improve human life.

Yet, for Kant, there are limits to the risks that one should take. We have a duty to preserve our lives, so no one should agree to become a subject in an experiment in which the likelihood of death is great. Additionally, no one should subject himself to research in which there is considerable risk that his capacity for rational thought and autonomy will be destroyed. Indeed, Kant's principles appear to require us to regard as morally illegitimate those experiments that seriously threaten the lives or rationality of their subjects. Not only should we not subject ourselves to them, but we should not subject others to them.

Kant's principles also rule out as potential experimental subjects those who are not in a position to act voluntarily, those who cannot exercise their autonomy. This makes it important to determine, from a Kantian point of view, whether children and institutionalized people (including prisoners) can be regarded as free agents capable of moral choice. Also, as in the case of abortion, the status of the fetus must be determined. If the fetus is not a person, then fetal experimentation presents no particular moral problems. But if the fetus is a person, then we must accord it a moral status and act for its sake and not for the sake of knowledge or for others.

Kant's view of people as autonomous rational beings requires that informed consent be obtained for both medical treatment and research. We cannot be forced to accept treatment for "our own good," nor can we be turned into experimental subjects for "the good of others." We must always be treated as ends and never as means only. To be treated in this way requires that others never deliberately deceive us, no matter how good their intentions. In short, we have a right to be told what we are getting into so that we can decide whether we want to go through with it or not.

Ross's theory imposes on researchers prima facie duties to patients that are similar to Kant's requirements. The nature of people as autonomous moral agents requires that their informed consent be obtained. Researchers ought not deceive their subjects, and experiments should be designed in ways in which suffering and the risk of injury or death are minimized.

These are all prima facie duties, of course, and it is possible to imagine situations in which other duties might take precedence over them. In general, however, Ross, like Kant, tells us that human research cannot be based on what is useful, but it must be based on what is right. Ross's principles, like Kant's, do not tell us, however, how we are to deal with such special problems as research involving children or prisoners.

As we saw in the introductory chapter, the principle of double effect and the principle of totality, which are based on the natural law theory of morality, have specific applications to experimentation. Because we hold our bodies in trust, we are responsible for assessing the degree of risk to which we might be put if we agree to become research subjects. Thus, others have an obligation to supply us with the information that we need in order to make our decision. If we decide to give our consent, it must be given freely and not be the consequence of deception or coercion.

If available evidence shows that a sick person may gain benefits from participating in an experiment, then the experiment is justified. But if the evidence shows that the benefits may be slight or if the chance of serious injury or death is relatively great, then the experiment is not justified. In general, the likelihood of a person's benefitting from an experiment must exceed the danger of the person's suffering greater losses. The four requirements that govern the application of the principle of double effect determine what is and what is not an allowable experiment. (See the introductory chapter for a discussion of these.)

People can volunteer for experiments from which they expect no direct benefits. The good they seek in doing so is not their own good but the good of others. But there are limits to what they can subject themselves to. A dying patient, for example, cannot be made the subject of a useless or trivial experiment. The probable value of the knowledge to be gained must balance the risk and suffering the patient is subjected to, and there must be no likelihood that the experiment will seriously injure or kill the patient.

These same restrictions also apply to experiments involving healthy people. The principle of totality forbids a healthy person to submit to an experiment that involves the probability of serious injury, impaired health, mutilation, or death.

The status of the fetus is clear on the Roman Catholic version of the natural law theory: the fetus is a person. As such, the fetus is entitled to the same dignity and respect we accord to other persons. Experiments that involve doing it injury or lessening its chances of life are morally prohibited. But not all fetal research is ruled out. That which may be of therapeutic benefit or which does not directly threaten the fetus's well-being is allowable. Furthermore, research involving fetal tissue or remains is permissible, if it is done for a serious and valuable purpose.

From Rawls's point of view, the difficulty with utilitarianism with respect to human experimentation is that the principle of utility would permit the exploitation of some groups (the dying, prisoners, the retarded) for the sake of others. By contrast, Rawls's principles of justice would forbid all experiments that involve violating a liberty to which a person is entitled by virtue of being a member of society. As a result, all experiments that make use of coercion or deception are ruled out. And since a person has a right to decide what risks she is willing to subject herself to, voluntary informed consent is required of all subjects. Society might, as in utilitarianism, decide to reward those who volunteer to become research subjects. So long as this is a possibility open to all, it is not objectionable.

It would never be right, according to Rawls, to take advantage of those in the society who are least well off to benefit those who are better off. In general, inequalities must be arranged so that they bring benefits (ideally) to everyone or at least to those who are most disadvantaged. Research involving direct therapeutic benefits is clearly acceptable (assuming that there is informed consent), but research that takes advantage of the sick, the poor, the retarded, or the institutionalized and does not benefit them is clearly unacceptable. The status of the fetus—whether or not it is a person in the moral sense—is an issue that has to be resolved before we know how to apply Rawls's principles to fetal research.

We have been able to provide only the briefest sketch here of some of the ways in which our moral theories might apply to the issues in human experimentation. The remarks are not meant to be anything more than suggestive. Clearly, a satisfactory moral theory of human experimentation requires working out the application of principles to problems in detail, as well as resolving such issues as the status of children and fetuses and whether institutionalized people are capable of acting freely.

The Selections

Louis Lasagna in "Some Ethical Problems in Clinical Investigation" discusses some of the issues that face the physician who is in the role of both therapist and researcher. But perhaps the most important aspect of his article is the review of the arguments against informed consent. Lasagna points out that sometimes researchers themselves do not know the risks that may be involved in research, that there are experiments in which information provided to potential subjects can alter the outcome, and that often patients themselves do not wish to be put into a position in which they must make a decision on the basis of information that they are not really competent to evaluate. Taking a basically utilitarian stance, Lasagna suggests that the "greater interest" of society must sometimes be given precedence over the rights of individuals.

This position is in marked contrast to that taken by Hans Jonas in his essay. Jonas argues that if we justify experiments by considering them a right of society, then we are exposing individuals to dangers for the general good. This, for Jonas, is inherently wrong, and no individual should be forced to surrender himself to a social goal.

Any risk that is taken must be voluntary, but obtaining informed consent, Jonas claims, is not sufficient to justify the experimental use of human beings. Two other conditions must be met: subjects must be recruited from those who are most knowledgeable about the circumstances of research and who are intellectually most capable of grasping its purposes and procedures; furthermore, the experiment must be undertaken for an adequate cause. Jonas cautions us that the progress that may come from research is not necessarily worth our efforts or approval, and he reminds us that there are moral values that we ought not to lose in the pursuit of science.

F. J. Ingelfinger claims in "Informed (But Uneducated) Consent" that efforts to secure informed consent from potential patients or subjects are mostly doomed to failure. "The chances are remote," Ingelfinger says, "that the subject really understands what he has consented to—in the sense that the responsible medical investigator understands the goals, nature, and hazards of his study." Nor can the subject be given information that is in any genuine sense complete. In fact, it might even be unethical to present a person with all the contingencies that may be involved in an experiment.

The current procedure, Ingelfinger asserts, is better than ones followed in the past, for then people were not even told that they were going to be research subjects. But beyond this, the process of obtaining informed consent "is no more than an elaborate ritual that, when the patient is uneducated and uncomprehending, confers no more than the semblance of propriety on human experimentation." The subject's only real protection depends on the person directing the research.

Benjamin Freedman claims that an account of what it is to be "free," "informed," and "competent" will allow us to decide when a person is mature enough to give consent and when prisoners are free to consent to participating in experiments. According to Freedman, there is a "right to consent" that arises from our status as persons. To deny someone a right to consent is to deprive him of personhood and autonomy. Also it is often to deprive him of such advantages as direct therapeutic benefits. For these reasons, we should recognize the possibility that prisoners can give valid consent.

Those who claim that full information can never be given to patients or subjects miss the point, Freedman says. The amount and kind of information is relative to the purpose at hand—namely, to permit the patient to make a meaningful decision. Informed consent, then, is possible. Consent must also be responsible, but the only way to decide this is by considering the character of the patient. Finally, Freedman says, consent must be voluntary, and this condition is met when the "reward" for participating does something more than merely raise a person to the ordinary level of rights and freedoms.

In discussing consent and the incompetent, Freedman rejects as invalid proxy consent for research on children. Children, in his view, have a right to "custody, not liberty." They have a right to be cared for, so consent in adults and proxy consent for children are very different.

"The Willowbrook Letters" by Stephen Goldby, Saul Krugman, M. H.

Pappworth, and Geoffrey Edsall concern the moral legitimacy of the study of viral hepatitis that was conducted at the Willowbrook School by Krugman and his associates. (See the Case Presentation for more detail.) Goldby charges that the study was "quite unjustifiable" because it was morally wrong to infect children when no benefit to them could result. Krugman defends himself by claiming that his results demonstrated a "therapeutic effect" for the children involved, as well as for others. He presents four reasons for holding that the infecting of the children was justified.

Pappworth claims that Krugman's defense is presented only after the fact, whereas an experiment is ethical or not in its inception. Moreover, he asserts, consent was obtained through the use of coercion. Parents who wished to put their children in the institution were told that there was room only in the "hepatitis unit."

In the final letter, Edsall defends the Krugman study. The experiments, he asserts, involved no greater risk to the children involved than they would have run in any case. What is more, the results obtained were of general benefit.

Paul Ramsey, in the selection included here, reviews the justifications offered for the Willowbrook experiments presented by Krugman. Ramsey observes that there is nothing about hepatitis that requires that research be conducted on children, that no justification except the needs of the experiment is given for withholding gamma globulin from the subjects, that nothing is said about attempting to control the low-grade epidemic by other means. Furthermore, Ramsey questions the morality of consent secured from the parents of the children. His basic recommendation is that the use of captive populations of children ought to be made legally impossible.

"Good science is ethical science" is a frequently used catch-phrase in the scientific community. But it is clear from our review of the issues in this section that more than a slogan is required to resolve the many moral problems involved in research involving human subjects. As we mentioned earlier, what is required is a patient and careful application of moral theories to specific kinds of cases. This is now being done by philosophers and others, but much work remains.

Some Ethical Problems in Clinical Investigation

Louis Lasagna

One potentially important source of tension in clinical investigation is the fundamental discrepancy in outlook between the clinical investigator and the physician. The two positions are rarely identical. One reads that medical experimentation takes place continually in every doctor's office and that the therapy of disease is an experimental aspect of medicine, but in point of fact, the practice of medicine and the pursuit of a scientific problem are not equivalent.

The physician is primarily concerned with the patient *qua* patient, with getting him well as quickly as possible and with a minimum of discomfort, inconvenience, risk, and cost to the patient. In the practice of his art the doctor has to use any and every measure he considers justified, and he is concerned with what measure (if any) works, not with what contribution (if any) he makes to the body of scientific data.

For the investigator, the primary emphasis is on the research question. This does not mean that he need be callous or lacking in caution; indeed, patients who are in an experiment are likely to be more carefully observed and cared for than if they were not research subjects. (In fact, carefully designed experiments result more often in improved patient care than in exciting new scientific information.) There are good reasons for the preferred status of patients in an experiment. Physicians in a research ward or research institution have usually had the advantage of intensive training, experience, and the intellectual discipline of an academic atmosphere. Further, the patient is, paradoxically, often better served by the restraint observed in the therapeutic approach of the critical experimentalist. The uncritical use of many therapeutic measures can be less desirable than the wise use of a few well-chosen ones; in medicine two and two sometimes add up to minus four, as the patient finds his medications working at cross purposes and yielding iatrogenic illness to boot. Often in controlled trials, for example, the placebo-treated patients turn out to be the lucky ones, as the new "remedy" proves to be toxic or therapeutically ineffective.

Notwithstanding the admirable qualities of many research-oriented physicians, however, there still remain important differences in orientation between the physician and the investigator which may affect the individual patient to a significant degree and which deserve discussion. Take, for example, the patient with metastatic cancer. Here is a serious disease for which we lack good treatment. There would seem to be no ethical problem in giving a desperately ill patient a new compound which may do some good. Yet the situation is only superficially simple.

The first cancer patients to receive an investigational drug often fail to obtain significant therapeutic benefit, and the dose exploration and tolerability studies involved in such early pharmacologic trials are likely to entail a certain amount of serious risk because of the powerful drugs generally required to treat malignant disease. In such a situation, therefore, the physician might well say "No" to the earliest trial of a new drug in cases where the investigator might say "Yes." If one then moves to a problem such as the treatment of pain or of insomnia, where we have remedies which, while not perfect, are for most purposes excellent and reasonably safe, what is the physician to say? Statistically, there is no doubt that the patient has a better chance of adequate relief if given a standard and accepted drug rather than an untried one, no matter how impressive a case for research can be made from the standpoint of society's long-term needs.

Another difficulty stems from the use of both patients and volunteer subjects in medical research. This practice tends to blur the fundamental distinction between these two kinds of subjects. The volunteer (or the patient who is being studied in a way unrelated to his disease) is truly an experimental subject and usually stands to gain little or nothing medically—at least in the near future—from the experience of being exposed to an investigational compound. He may run considerable risk. It seems to me that such a volunteer must be handled quite differently from the patient who is also contributing to research goals but who may derive considerable benefit in the immediate future. To the degree that this distinction is blurred, ethical difficulties will be compounded.

It may be useful to consider the currently controversial issue of obtaining "informed consent" from subjects participating in drug investigation. The new Food and Drug Administration (FDA) regulations governing experimentation on human subjects make it clear that except in rare instances informed written consent must be obtained from anyone who is being given an investigational drug.[1] The FDA has spelled out in great detail the kinds of information that must be supplied to subjects of such experiments. It is interesting to contrast this approach with the usual practice of medicine, in which drug administration also plays an important role, and where patients almost certainly suffer more harm (some avoidable, much of it not) from the use of old drugs than experimental subjects suffer from the prescribing of new drugs by experienced investigators. In ordinary practice, consent is usually not informed, and it is almost never written, except for surgical procedures.

In favor of obtaining informed consent in clinical investigation is the reasonable (and generally held) belief that a person should know what is being done to him and what the risks of participation in an experiment may be. Of course, there are also important legal implications in procedures which—in the absence of consent—may be construed as civil or criminal assault on a person's body. There is a strong common law tradition in this regard which goes back at least as far as Justice Cardozo. In addition, unless a physician or committee other than the investigator is making the final decisions, the patient's informed consent represents a check on the motives of the investigator, motives which may be generally admirable but specifically undesirable, or at least questionable, for the individual patient.

What are the arguments *against* informed consent? To begin with, there are instances in which it would seem clearly not in the patient's best interest to discuss matters with full candor. A person dying of terminal cancer who has been given the few weakly effective available drugs, and whose condition is deteriorating, may gain little from an excessively detailed and frank discussion of the situation when a new drug is available which might possibly provide some benefit. Investigational drug use in psychiatric patients poses similar psychic hazards, including the special risk, if the use of drugs is made to look too much like an experiment, of permanently damaging or destroying the patient-doctor relationship.

One may also argue that obtaining informed consent involves the assumption that the investigator knows the risks of giving the drug, of withholding it, and the alternative risks from the use of other, older agents that might be used instead. The language of the FDA regulations does, it seems to me, imply all this. In fact, this information is available only in small measure.[2] One also assumes that the investigator is capable of the exposition required to present this information to the patient and that the patient is capable of grasping the information. One would also like to think that the patient is capable of making a decision in keeping with his own best interests after hearing the information, although a competent adult should, I suppose, have the freedom to make the wrong decision in the hospital or doctor's office no less than in the voting booth. All of these considerations are not, to be sure, so much arguments against informed consent as examples of the difference between the wish and the achievement.

Some important arguments against consent revolve around the possibility of impeding scientific progress if such consent is routinely obtained. (One could, for "scientific progress," substitute "providing benefit to others, including future generations.") There are some trials that will be impossible if a truly candid explanation has to be provided. One prominent investigator has evinced his skepticism about convincing people to participate in a trial that will last for years and in which some individuals are given drugs to lower their blood pressure and others receive placebos. Since it is not clear that all patients with hypertension should receive drugs, it would seem unethical *not* to perform the trial, but there is disagreement as to whether it is ethical to inform the patients of the nature of the trial while they are participating in it. With postpartum patients, we found in one experiment that if women were approached while they are actually having pain and asked to sign a consent form to participate in an experiment in which they might also receive inert preparations, some 80 to 85 percent refused to participate. (In work conducted on patients of this sort without written consent over a decade or so, we have never seen any evidence of serious harm or discontent; indeed, it is reasonably certain that these patients have received closer attention and better medical care than they would otherwise have received.) This would result in such an idiosyncratic selection of the population that we refused to conduct the trial, not only because of the time that would be required to complete it but because of the very real possibility that the results in such a minority of the population might not provide legitimate basis for predicting effects in the majority.

There is also the chance—even if patients consent to participate—that one may destroy the validity of a trial by inducing introspection of various kinds, producing a sort of Heisenberg effect. Some patients, when they know they are in a trial, will try to outwit the investigator by guessing which medications they are receiving. Other patients will be troubled by the nontherapeutic aspects of the experience, so that one may have difficulty in relating the responses to the usual clinical situation. Although investigators quite rightly tend to emphasize the difference between clinical practice and rigorous clinical investigation, it is nevertheless true that those studying new drugs experimentally wish very much to collect data applicable to the use of the drugs in patients treated by "ordinary" doctors in "routine" medical practice.

Finally, there are some experiments which lose their entire point if all the cards are laid on the table. Take, for example, the investigation of the impact of a placebo. Although some patients report benefits from placebos even when they are told they are receiving "sugar pills," the full power of suggestibility and the patient-doctor relationship would almost certainly be affected by a discussion of the experiment with the subjects. This would be the medical equivalent of "bugging" a jury room to study the jurors' deliberations and then showing the jury the hidden microphones.[3]

Are there alternatives to "double-blind" placebo trials? (It is assumed that the obtaining of consent will be more feasible if patients do not have to agree to receive placebos.) One possibility, in drug investigation, is to demonstrate differences between a new drug and a standard drug. If the new one is significantly better, there is no problem. But what if it is significantly worse? This could mean that the drug is ineffective or merely that it is a *less* effective one—an important distinction. Another possibility is the use of dose-response relationships. If such relationships can be shown for new and old drugs in the same experiment, potency estimates can be made which are in no way dependent on the use of placebos. This is quite possible in a situation such as alleviation of postoperative pain, where the challenge is severe, the response to powerful analgesics is reasonably predictable, and placebos are thus rarely needed or used. In postpartum pain, however, dose-response relationships are rather difficult to elaborate, and the same may be true in studies of hypnotic drugs. This phenomenon has important implications for the admission of new drugs to the marketplace. If placebo studies are abandoned, will the FDA accept clinical comparisons where no dose-response relationships are evident? Not to do so may keep an effective drug off the market, but accepting at face value experiments where no difference is demonstrated between doses or drugs will surely result in the occasional admission of ineffective agents to the market.

Is some less formidable and stylized consent approach acceptable? It is apparently not, in regard to investigational drugs, unless one is willing to flaunt the FDA regulations. On the other hand, it may be possible to modify these regulations so as to make the consent provisions more flexible. If one eliminates the *written* aspects of the present informed consent regulations and substitutes verbal discussion (perhaps even placed on tape for the record) it may be possible to avoid some of the threats to experimentation discussed above while at the same time insuring that a certain amount of discussion with the patient has occurred.[4] I believe that the degree of candor utilized in obtaining consent should be related not only to the specific psychological and clinical problems but also to the expected risks of the experiment.

There is also the possibility of monitoring experimentation by use of peer committees or lay-scientific review boards which go over protocols, checking them carefully for flaws of various kinds, including ethical ones. No investigator should be engaged in research that he would be ashamed to have judged by his scientific colleagues or by a responsible group of laymen and scientists. There is at least theoretical advantage to sharing problems of conscience and morality with individuals not directly involved in the research, and of course ample precedent exists in society for delegation of important decision-making powers to others, although I doubt the legal acceptability of such review as an *alternative* to informed patient consent. It should be remembered, however, that a peer review mechanism may safeguard a subject more efficiently than informed consent; some people will agree to undergo risks that an expert committee would veto on their behalf.

It has been suggested that one way of discouraging unethical research is for editors to prevent the publication of data obtained in unsavory experiments by refusing to accept such manuscripts. Although this is an attractive notion at first glance, one wonders whether in fact important data unethically obtained could or should really be buried in this way. If an unscrupulous investigator were to discover a cure for cancer, would it be ethical to keep this knowledge from being used by others for the benefit of cancer patients, in compulsive adherence to "principle"? Although it is often affirmed that the ends do not justify the means, our society often functions as if they do.

One way of improving the present situation would be to acquaint the public, the regulatory agencies, the governmental granting agencies, and hospital committees with the needs and problems of experimentation. The present FDA regulations on informed consent, for example, quite clearly are the result of a particular climate of opinion. The law is susceptible to change. I heard one distinguished Baltimore judge say recently that the purpose of the law is to harmonize progress with stability. Years ago a property owner possessed the land underneath his feet as far as it went and all of the air directly above his property. With the coming of the airplane, this concept has changed. Similarly, educational facilities once considered "separate but equal" are no longer considered "equal." The law reflects the needs and desires of society as society sees these needs and desires, and it is entirely consistent with history to expect an appropriate legal response from society if it becomes educated to the needs of science and the social benefits of research.[5]

One wonders how many of medicine's greatest advances might have been delayed or prevented by the rigid application of some currently proposed principles to research at large. Even physicians were in a sense intellectually and emotionally unprepared for the earliest triumphs of cardiac surgery. What, then, would have been the layman's reaction to a full exposition of the problems involved in the original Blalock-Taussig shunts? And what of cardiac catheterization? The benefits of this technique have, quite appropriately, won Nobel Prizes for three of the physicians who pioneered in its use, but is it difficult to imagine lay journalists dubbing the early experimentation of these men barbaric and Nazi-like? ("and then, dear readers, these monsters have the temerity to thrust a tube down the length of one's arm into the very chambers of the human heart! The mind of anyone not completely brutalized by prolonged immersion in the bloody charnel houses of Science boggles at the thought.") I doubt, on the other hand, that the public would back—provided they had the facts—legislation like that originally proposed by Senator Thaler in New York State, which would have prohibited pediatric research *of all kinds* in the absence of court orders. Others have already pointed out that such legislation would have rendered impossible the development of the poliomyelitis and other vaccines.

If society is to be educated, there are many items that might be put on the agenda for discussion. The desire to involve the patient in the decision-making process in regard to details of medical care implies that there should be fuller

and franker discussion about the use of everything from drugs to surgical techniques. Whether the public wants this is a matter for debate; I personally doubt it. In my own experience as a physician and investigator, not only are patients usually incapable of making the decisions in question (which is not surprising) but they are usually not desirous of making such decisions. In considerable anxiety a lay friend once called me to say that his physician had disclosed to him the controversy over the long-term use of anticoagulants in the management of patients who had recovered from a cardiac infarct. My friend protested that he was in no position to judge whether his wife should receive anticoagulants and that he really would have preferred his physician to make this judgment. In many complex decision-making situations in medicine, the patient is really more in the position of being on an airplane that has defective landing gear, is running out of gas, and whose pilot has to make some sort of landing in one of several alternate places than in the position of a passenger who is asked whether he wishes to board a plane whose pilot indicates that he is about to fly for the first time with his eyes closed and "no hands."

How much should be told to a patient by a surgeon who is requesting permission to perform an established operation, but one he personally is attempting for the first time? How much should be told to a patient about the hazards of a debilitating series of diagnostic abdominal X-rays, which may subject him to days of restricted food and fluid intake, as well as repeated cathartics? How much should be told to individuals exposed to radiation of any kind, for diagnosis or therapy, in view of the evidence in both insects and mammals that *no* amount of radiation is innocent in regard to genetic damage?

There are many other points that require consideration. What special safeguards are required for the study of prisoners? Of children? Of the psychiatrically ill? Of the mentally retarded? Of the dying patient? If an experimental live virus vaccine is to be given to subjects, should consent also be obtained from neighbors or schoolmates who may pick up the virus from the volunteers and come down with the disease? Should the patients in the adjoining beds be asked for permission when a new antibiotic is given to a patient, in view of the ability of antibiotics to disturb the ecology of the normal bacteria resident in the body and cause the development of resistant strains which can then spread to these patients?

Should individuals be recompensed for damage suffered in the course of research, without any attempt to establish blame? The patient or volunteer who is injured by an experimental drug and loses his earning power thereby is entitled to compensation. The children of a patient who dies as the result of unanticipated mischief from a new diagnostic technique under investigation perhaps ought to expect financial remuneration. This implies not that the investigator must shoulder this burden alone but that the burden must be borne somehow. Who, then, shall pay the bill? In seeking an answer to this question, we should perhaps ask, "Who reaps the benefits of research?" While it is true that the investigator will gain when research is successful, and that with new drugs the pharmaceutical industry will profit, in the final analysis the beneficiary is really society as a whole. It would therefore seem incumbent on society to seek means of walking safely the narrow ledge between the twin abysses of hampered research and uncompensated patient injury. Scientists must not be reckless in their research; neither can they operate in an atmosphere of perpetual fear of disabling economic loss (or destroyed reputations) if unavoidable harm is the result of a well-planned experiment. Patients must not seek court settlements capriciously; neither must they silently suffer pain, injury, or death in the course of research. The problem is both subtle and complex and deserves an honest and equitable solution.

What should be society's attitude toward harm to the individual in return for benefits to the population as a whole? Mass chest X-ray surveys to detect treatable tuberculosis or other pulmonary diseases may cause leukemia in a few. Is the benefit worth the risk? Who shall decide? What means should be taken to safeguard the rights and health of individuals approached to participate in such a survey? Should a simple majority decide whether an entire community's water supply should be fluoridated? We have become reconciled to the ability of a governmental agency to expropriate our land or homes in order to build a new school or a new bridge, but it is not traditional to force anyone to participate in research. Yet society frequently tramples on the rights of individuals in the "greater interest." One can object, but can we deny the existence of the phenomenon? Should

we have different guidelines for individual sacrifice when health or life is at stake, rather than property?

Finally, a word about the effective implantation of an ethical conscience in the minds of physicians and clinical investigators. The doctor becomes increasingly accustomed to a life which does not allow for leisurely contemplation. He is by trade a nonagnostic. Even when he makes a decision not to treat, for example, he is not suspending judgment but expressing the belief that "no treatment" is better than treatment. He must continually choose between remedies even when he has poor basis for making a choice. The doctor is likely to be propelled increasingly in the direction of quick decisions which at times resemble reflex responses. In this pragmatic, frenetic existence he may quickly absorb the moral atmosphere around him without questioning it. It is my conviction, therefore, that ethical problems must be integrated into the doctor's life at the earliest possible moment. I do not believe that it will be effective to bring up such matters relatively late in the medical career, although the doctor will certainly require constant reinforcement throughout his professional life. The medical student must be made, from the beginning, to consider the ethical aspects of medicine, in regard to *both* practice and research. Many a liver biopsy or laboratory test is now performed in the name of science, with little benefit to the patient. A medical student made emotionally immune to the casual performance of risky procedures by the tacit acceptance of such procedures by his mentors is unlikely to be excessively concerned as a physician or investigator with the subtleties of ethical and moral issues. Some way must be found to incorporate these matters so firmly into his moral fabric that he cannot avoid the ethical implications of his acts. I submit that the successful development of such an ethical conscience, combined with professional skill, will protect the patient or experimental subject much more effectively than any laws or regulations.

I have previously said that for the ethical, experienced investigator no laws are needed and for the unscrupulous incompetent no laws will help, except to allow the injured subjects to obtain compensation or to punish the offending scientists. Between these extremes there still remain many investigators who will unquestionably be constrained in some way by legislation. But it is unlikely that subjects will be *optimally* protected from harm without additional safeguards imposed by the scientific community itself. These safeguards will range all the way from exercise of wisdom and judgment to the invoking of statistical monitoring techniques to halt experiments that were ethical at the outset but cannot ethically be continued.

Some are fond of quoting Claude Bernard when he said, in *An Introduction to the Study of Experimental Medicine*, "The principle of medical and surgical morality, therefore, consists in never performing on man an experiment which might be harmful to him in any extent, even though the result might be highly advantageous to science, i.e., to the health of others."[6] This statement is irrelevant to much of clinical investigation, where patients usually are involved in procedures that may be of considerable benefit to them, although they necessarily involve some risk (like almost everything else in the world). One might point out that Claude Bernard also said, "So, among the experiments that may be tried on man, those that can only harm are forbidden, those that are innocent are permissible, and those that may do good are obligatory."[7] The investigator is responsible not only to the patients currently under his care but also to the many that will never be seen by him. Is this responsibility to mankind less noble than that of the physician concerned with the care of the individual patient?

Bernard's statement is—like my own remarks—full of ambivalence. As J. Bronowski has put it, one of society's major tasks is to reconcile the welfare of man with the welfare of men.[8] In clinical investigation, as in other societal activities, the good of the individual and the good of society are often not identical and sometimes mutually exclusive. I believe it is inevitable that the many will continue to benefit on occasion from the contributions—sometimes involuntary—of the few. The problem is to know when to say "Halt!" There are some societal "gains" that may only be available at an excessively high price. We cannot afford to have the cancer of moral decay that comes from frequent and flagrant disregard of human rights gnawing away at the body of science. We should, therefore, in a very real sense welcome the present and continuing debate on ethics in clinical investigation. That harm has come

from exaggerated stories is unquestioned, as is the possibility that additional harm to patients may occur, but I believe that in the long run both the public and science will benefit from a searching analysis of the roots of our ethical conduct.

Notes

1. While the FDA rules apply only to investigational drugs, the issue of consent is relevant to all clinical investigation because of both legal implications and current National Institutes of Health policies on human experimentation which affect the conduct of grantees.

2. It is surrealistic to read, in an editorial in a leading American medical journal, the statement: "How much more important it is to have informed consent, when the potential risk is unknown!"

3. Dinnerstein et al., in an interesting paper, have reviewed some of the literature on the differential effects of drugs in different experimental settings. Their desire to study the effects of drugs "in a completely concealed form, with the subject not even knowing when he has been drugged" and under situations with different "cover stories" would be out of the question if rigid application of this principle of "total disclosure" were made. Albert J. Dinnerstein, Milton Lowenthal, and Bernard Blitz, "The Interaction of Drugs with Placebos in the Control of Pain and Anxiety," *Perspectives in Biology and Medicine*, 10 (1966), 103–117.

4. It is important to remember that there is no *necessary* relation between a consent procedure that satisfies the law and one that safeguards the patient.

5. John Dewey once warned that part of the public protest against experimentation is related to old misunderstandings and dreads about science. He was talking about animal experimentation, but it may be useful to remember his warning to be "on the alert against every revival of the spirit of animosity to discovery and to the application of the fruits of discovery." One does not need to accuse everyone who is concerned about the ethics of clinical investigation of being antiscientific to believe that at least some of the hue and cry can be traced to antiscientism.

6. Claude Bernard, *An Introduction to the Study of Experimental Medicine* (New York: Dover Publications, 1957), p. 101.

7. Ibid., p. 102.

8. J. Bronowski, *Science and Human Values* (London: Hutchinson & Co., 1961), p. 78.

Philosophical Reflections on Experimenting with Human Subjects

Hans Jonas

Experimenting with human subjects is going on in many fields of scientific and technological progress. It is designed to replace the overall instruction by natural, occasional experience with the selective information from artificial, systematic experiment which physical science has found so effective in dealing with inanimate nature. Of the new experimentation with man, medical is surely the most legitimate; psychological, the most dubious; biological (still to come), the most dangerous. I have chosen here to deal with the first only, where the case *for* it is strongest and the task of adjudicating conflicting claims hardest. . . .

The Peculiarity of Human Experimentation

Experimentation was originally sanctioned by natural science. There it is performed on inanimate objects, and this raises no moral problems. But as soon as animate, feeling beings become the subjects of experiment, as they do in the life sciences and especially in medical research, this innocence of the search for knowledge is lost and questions of conscience arise. The depth to which moral and religious sensibilities can become aroused over these questions is shown by the vivisection issue. Human experimentation must sharpen the issue as it involves ultimate questions of personal dignity and sacrosanctity. One profound difference between the human experiment and the physical (besides that between animate and inanimate, feeling and unfeeling nature) is this: The physical experiment employs small-scale, artificially devised substitutes for that about which knowledge is to be obtained, and the experimenter extrapolates from these models and simulated conditions to nature at large. Something deputizes for the "real thing"—balls rolling down an in-

clined plane for sun and planets, electric discharges from a condenser for real lightning, and so on. For the most part, no such substitution is possible in the biological sphere. We must operate on the original itself, the real thing in the fullest sense, and perhaps affect it irreversibly. No simulacrum can take its place. Especially in the human sphere, experimentation loses entirely the advantage of the clear division between vicarious model and true object. Up to a point, animals may fulfill the proxy role of the classical physical experiment. But in the end man himself must furnish knowledge about himself, and the comfortable separation of noncommital experiment and definitive action vanishes. An experiment in education affects the lives of its subjects, perhaps a whole generation of schoolchildren. Human experimentation for whatever purpose is always *also* a responsible, nonexperimental, definitive dealing with the subject himself. And not even the noblest purpose abrogates the obligations this involves.

This is the root of the problem with which we are faced: Can both that purpose and this obligation be satisfied? If not, what would be a just compromise? Which side should give way to the other? The question is inherently philosophical as it concerns not merely pragmatic difficulties and their arbitration, but a genuine conflict of values involving principles of a high order. May I put conflict in these terms. On principle, it is felt, human beings *ought* not to be dealt with in that way (the "guinea pig" protest); on the other hand, such dealings are increasingly urged on us by considerations, in turn appealing to principle, that claim to override those objections. Such a claim must be carefully assessed, especially when it is swept along by a mighty tide. Putting the matter thus, we have already made one important assumption rooted in our "Western" cultural

Reprinted by permission of Daedalus, *Journal of the American Academy of Arts and Sciences, Spring 1969, Boston, Mass. This essay is included, on pp. 105–131, in a 1980 reedition of Jonas's* Philosophical Essays: From Current Creed to Technological Man, *published by the University of Chicago Press.*

tradition: The prohibitive rule is, to that way of thinking, the primary and axiomatic one; the permissive counter-rule, as qualifying the first, is secondary and stands in need of justification. We must justify the infringement of a primary inviolability, which needs no justification itself; and the justification of its infringement must be by values and needs of a dignity commensurate with those to be sacrificed.

Health as a Public Good

The cause invoked [for medical experimentation] is health and, in its more critical aspect, life itself—clearly superlative goods that the physician serves directly by curing and the researcher indirectly by the knowledge gained through his experiments. There is no question about the good served or about the evil fought—disease and premature death. But a good to whom and an evil to whom? Here the issue tends to become somewhat clouded. In the attempt to give experimentation the proper dignity (on the problematic view that a value becomes greater by being "social" instead of merely individual), the health in question or the disease in question is somehow predicated on the social whole, as if it were society that, in the persons of its members enjoyed the one and suffered the other. For the purposes of our problem, public interest can then be pitted against private interest, the common good against the individual good. Indeed, I have found health called a national resource, which of course it is, but surely not in the first place.

In trying to resolve some of the complexities and ambiguities lurking in these conceptualizations, I have pondered a particular statement, made in the form of a question, which I found in the *Proceedings* of the earlier *Daedalus* conference: "Can society afford to discard the tissues and organs of the hopelessly unconscious patient when they could be used to restore the otherwise hopelessly ill, but still salvageable individual?" And somewhat later: "A strong case can be made that society can ill afford to discard the tissues and organs of the hopelessly unconscious patient; they are greatly needed for study and experimental trial to help those who can be salvaged."[1] I hasten to add that any suspicion of callousness that the "commodity" language of these statements may suggest is immediately dispelled by the name of the speaker, Dr. Henry K. Beecher, for whose

humanity and moral sensibility there can be nothing but admiration. But the use, in all innocence, of this language gives food for thought. Let me, for a moment, take the question literally. "Discarding" implies proprietary rights—nobody can discard what does not belong to him in the first place. Does society then own my body? "Salvaging" implies the same and, moreover, a use-value to the owner. Is the life-extension of certain individuals then a public interest? "Affording" implies a critically vital level of such an interest—that is, of the loss or gain involved. And "society" itself—what is it? When does a need, an aim, an obligation become social? Let us reflect on some of these terms.

What Society Can Afford

"Can Society afford . . .?" Afford what? To let people die intact, thereby withholding something from other people who desperately need it, who in consequence will have to die too? These other, unfortunate people indeed cannot afford not to have a kidney, heart, or other organ of the dying patient, on which they depend for an extension of their lease on life; but does that give them a right to it? And does it oblige society to procure it for them? What is it that *society* can or cannot afford—leaving aside for the moment the question of what it has a *right* to? It surely can afford to lose members through death; more than that, it is built on the balance of death and birth decreed by the order of life. This is too general, of course, for our question, but perhaps it is well to remember. The specific question seems to be whether society can afford to let some people die whose death might be deferred by particular means if these were authorized by society. Again, if it is merely a question of what society can or cannot afford, rather than of what it ought or ought not to do, the answer must be: Of course, it can. If cancer, heart disease, and other organic, noncontagious ills, especially those tending to strike the old more than the young, continue to exact their toll at the normal rate of incidence (including the toll of private anguish and misery), society can go on flourishing in every way.

Here, by contrast, are some examples of what, in sober truth, society cannot afford. It cannot afford to let an epidemic rage unchecked; a persistent excess of deaths over births, but neither—we must add—too great an excess of births over deaths; too low an average life expectancy even if demographically balanced by fertility, but neither too great a longevity with the necessitated correlative dearth of youth in the social body; a debilitating state of general heath; and things of this kind. These are plain cases where the whole condition of society is critically affected, and the public interest can make its imperative claims. The Black Death of the Middle Ages was a *public* calamity of the acute kind; the life-sapping ravages of endemic malaria or sleeping sickness in certain areas are a public calamity of the chronic kind. Such situations a society as a whole can truly not "afford," and they may call for extraordinary remedies, including, perhaps, the invasion of private sacrosanctities.

This is not entirely a matter of numbers and numerical ratios. Society, in a subtler sense, cannot "afford" a single miscarriage of justice, a single inequity in the dispensation of its laws, the violation of the rights of even the tiniest minority, because these undermine the moral basis on which society's existence rests. Nor can it, for a similar reason, afford the absence or atrophy in its midst of compassion and of the effort to alleviate suffering—be it widespread or rare—one form of which is the effort to conquer disease of any kind, whether "socially" significant (by reasons of number) or not. And in short, society cannot afford the absence among its members of *virtue*, with its readiness for sacrifice beyond defined duty. Since its presence—that is to say, that of personal idealism—is a matter of grace and not of decree, we have the paradox that society depends for its existence on intangibles of nothing less than a religious order, for which it can hope, but which it cannot enforce. All the more must it protect this most precious capital from abuse.

For what objectives connected with the medico-biological sphere should this reserve be drawn upon—for example, in the form of accepting, soliciting, perhaps even imposing the submission of human subjects to experimentation? We postulate that this must be not just a worthy cause, as any promotion of the health of anybody doubtlessly is, but a cause qualifying for transcendent social sanction. Here one thinks first of those cases critically affecting the whole condition, present and future, of the community we have illustrated. Something equivalent to what in the political sphere is called "clear and present danger" may be invoked and a state of emergency proclaimed, thereby suspending certain otherwise inviolable prohibitions and taboos. We may observe that averting a disaster always carries greater weight than promoting a good. Extraordinary danger excuses extraordinary means. This covers human experimentation, which we would like to count, as far as possible, among the extraordinary rather than the ordinary means of serving the common good under public auspices. Naturally, since foresight and responsibility for the future are of the essence of institutional society, averting disaster extends into long-term prevention, although the lesser urgency will warrant less sweeping licenses.

Society and the Cause of Progress

Much weaker is the case where it is a matter not of saving but of improving society. Much of medical research falls into this category. As stated before, a permanent death rate from heart failure or cancer does not threaten society. So long as certain statistical ratios are maintained, the incidence of disease and of disease-induced mortality is not (in the strict sense) a "social" misfortune. I hasten to add that it is not therefore less of a human misfortune, and the call for relief issuing with silent eloquence from each victim and all potential victims is of no lesser dignity. But it is misleading to equate the fundamentally human response to it with what is owed to society: it is owed by man to man—and it is thereby owed by society to the individuals as soon as the adequate ministering to these concerns outgrows (as it progressively does) the scope of private spontaneity and is made a public mandate. It is thus that society assumes responsibility for medical care, research, old age, and innumerable other things not originally of the public realm (in the original "social contract"), and they become duties toward "society" (rather than directly toward one's fellow man) by the fact that they are socially operated.

Indeed, we expect from organized society no longer mere protection against harm and the securing of the conditions of our preservation, but active and constant improvement in all the domains of life: the waging of the battle against nature, the enhancement of the human estate—in short, the promotion of progress. This is an expansive goal, one far surpassing the disaster norm of our previous reflections. It lacks the urgency of the latter, but has the nobility of the free, forward thrust. It surely is worth sacrifices. It is not at all a question of what society can afford, but of what it is committed to, beyond all necessity, by our mandate. Its trusteeship has become an established, ongoing, institutionalized business of the body politic. As eager beneficiaries of its gains, we now owe to "society," as its chief agent, our individual contributions toward its *continued pursuit*. I emphasize "continued pursuit." Maintaining the existing level requires no more than the orthodox means of taxation and enforcement of professional standards that raise no problems. The more optional goal of pushing forward is also more exacting. We have this syndrome: Progress is by our choosing an acknowledged interest of society, in which we have a stake in various degrees; science is a necessary instrument of progress; research is a necessary instrument of science; and in medical science experimentation on human subjects is a necessary instrument of research. Therefore, human experimentation has come to be a societal interest.

The destination of research is essentially melioristic. It does not serve the preservation of the existing good from which I profit myself and to which I am obligated. Unless the present state is intolerable, the melioristic goal is in a sense gratuitous, and this not only from the vantage point of the present. Our descendants have a right to be left an unplundered planet; they do not have a right to new miracle cures. We have sinned against them, if by our doing we have destroyed their inheritance—which we are doing at full blast; we have not sinned against them if by the time they come around arthritis has not yet been conquered (unless by sheer neglect). And generally, in the matter of progress, as humanity had no claim on a Newton, a Michelangelo, or a St. Francis to appear, and no right to the blessings of their unscheduled deeds, so progress, with all our methodical labor for it, cannot be budgeted in advance and its fruits received as a due. Its coming-about at all and its turning out for good (of which we can never be sure) must rather be regarded as something akin to grace.

The Melioristic Goal, Medical Research, and Individual Duty

Nowhere is the melioristic goal more inherent than in medicine. To the physician, it is not gratuitous. He is committed to curing and thus to improving the power to cure. Gratuitous we called it (outside disaster conditions) as a *social* goal, but noble at the same time. Both the nobility and the gratuitousness must influence the manner in which self-sacrifice for it is elicited, and even its free offer accepted. Freedom is certainly the first condition to be observed here. The surrender of one's body to medical experimentation is entirely outside the enforceable "social contract."

Or can it be construed to fall within its terms—namely, as repayment for benefits from past experimentation that I have enjoyed myself? But I am indebted for these benefits not to society, but to the past "martyrs," to whom society is indebted itself, and society has no right to call in my personal debt by way of adding new to its own. Moreover, gratitude is not an enforceable social obligation; it anyway does not mean that I must emulate the deed. Most of all, if it was wrong to exact such sacrifice in the first place, it does not become right to exact it again with the plea of the profit it has brought me. If, however, it was not exacted, but entirely free, as it ought to have been, then it should remain so, and its precedence must not be used as a social pressure on others for doing the same under the sign of duty.

• • •

The "Conscription" of Consent

The mere issuing of the appeal, the calling for volunteers, with the moral and social pressures it inevitably generates, amounts even under the most meticulous rules of consent to a sort of *conscripting*. And some soliciting is necessarily involved. . . . And this is why "consent," surely a nonnegotiable minimum requirement, is not the full answer to the problem. Granting then that soliciting and therefore some degree of conscripting are part of the situation, who may conscript and who may be conscripted? Or less harshly expressed: Who should issue appeals and to whom?

The naturally qualified issuer of the appeal is the research scientist himself, collectively the main carrier of the impulse and the only one with the technical competence to judge. But his being very much an interested party (with vested interests, indeed, not purely in the public good, but in the scientific enterprise as such, in "his" project, and even in his career) makes him also suspect. The ineradicable dialectic of this situation—a delicate incompatibility problem—calls for particular controls by the research community and by public authority that we need not discuss. They can mitigate, but not eliminate the problem. We have to live with the ambiguity, the treacherous impurity of everything human.

Self-Recruitment of the Community

To whom should the appeal be addressed? The natural issuer of the call is also the first natural addressee: the physician-researcher himself and the scientific confraternity at large. With such a coincidence—indeed, the noble tradition with which the whole business of human experimentation started—almost all of the associated legal, ethical, and metaphysical problems vanish. If it is full, autonomous identification of the subject with the purpose that is required for the dignifying of his serving as a subject—here it is; if strongest motivation—here it is; if fullest understanding—here it is; if freest decision—here it is; if greatest integration with the person's total, chosen pursuit—here it is. With the fact of self-solicitation the issue of consent in all its insoluble equivocality is bypassed per se. Not even the condition that the particular purpose be truly important and the project reasonably promising, which must hold in any solicitation of others, need be satisfied here. By himself, the scientist is free to obey his obsession, to play his hunch, to wager on chance, to follow the lure of ambition. It is all part of the "divine madness" that somehow animates the ceaseless pressing against frontiers. For the rest of society, which has a deep-seated disposition to look with reverence and awe upon the guardians of the mysteries of life, the profession assumes with this proof of its devotion the role of a self-chosen, consecrated fraternity, not unlike the monastic orders of the past, and this would come nearest to the actual, religious origins of the art of healing.

• • •

"Identification" as the Principle of Recruitment in General

If the properties we adduced as the particular qualifications of the members of the scientific fraternity itself are taken as general criteria of selection, then one should look for additional subjects where a maximum of identification, understanding, and spontaneity can be expected—that is, among the most highly motivated, the most highly educated, and the least "captive" members of the community. From this naturally scarce resource, a descending order of permissibility leads to greater abundance and ease of supply, whose use should become proportionately more hesitant as the exculpating criteria are relaxed. An inversion of normal "market" behavior is demanded here —namely, to accept the lowest quotation last (and excused only by the greatest pressure of need); to pay the highest price first.

The ruling principle in our considerations is that the "wrong" of reification can only be made "right" by such authentic identification with the cause that it is the subject's as well as the researcher's cause—whereby his role in its service is not just permitted by him, but *willed*. That sovereign will of his which embraces the end as his own restores his personhood to the otherwise depersonalizing context. To be valid it must be autonomous and informed. The latter condition can, outside the research community, only be fulfilled by degrees; but the higher the degree of understanding regarding the purpose and the technique, the more valid becomes the endorsement of the will. A margin of mere trust inevitably remains. Ultimately, the appeal for volunteers should seek this free and generous endorsement, the appropriation of the research purpose into the person's own scheme of ends. Thus, the appeal is in truth addressed to the one, mysterious, and sacred source of any such generosity of the will—"devotion," whose forms and objects of commitment are various and may invest different motivations in different individuals. The following, for instance, may be responsive to the "call" we are discussing: compassion with human suffering, zeal for humanity, reverence for the Golden Rule, enthusiasm for progress, homage to the cause of knowledge, even longing for sacrificial justification (do not call that "masochism," please). On all these, I say, it is defensible and right to draw when the research objective is worthy enough; and it is a prime duty of the research community (especially in view of what we called the "margin of trust") to see that this sacred source is never abused for frivolous ends. For a less than adequate cause, not even the freest, unsolicited offer should be accepted.

The Rule of the "Descending Order" and its Counterutility Sense

We have laid down what must seem to be a forbidding rule to the number-hungry research industry. Having faith in the transcendent potential of man, I do not fear that the "source" will ever fail a society that does not destroy it—and only such a one is worthy of the blessings of progress. But "elitistic" the rule is (as is the enterprise of progress itself), and elites are by nature small. The combined attribute of motivation and information, plus the absence of external pressures, tends to be socially so circumscribed that strict adherence to the rule might numerically starve the research process. This is why I spoke of a descending order of permissibility, which is itself permissive, but where the realization that it is a *descending* order is not without pragmatic import. Departing from the august norm, the appeal must needs shift from idealism to docility, from high-mindedness to compliance, from judgment to trust. Consent spreads over the whole spectrum. I will not go into the casuistics of this penumbral area. I merely indicate the principle of the order of preference: The poorer in knowledge, motivation, and freedom of decision (and that, alas, means the more readily available in terms of numbers and possible manipulation), the more sparingly and indeed reluctantly should the reservoir be used, and the more compelling must therefore become the countervailing justification.

Let us note that this is the opposite of a social utility standard, the reverse of the order by "availability and expendability": The most valuable and scarcest, the least expendable elements of the social organism, are to be the first candidates for risk and sacrifice. It is the standard of *noblesse oblige;* and with all its counterutility and seeming "wastefulness," we feel a rightness about it and perhaps even a higher "utility," for the soul of the community lives by this spirit.[2] It is also the opposite of what the day-to-day interests of research clamor for, and for the scientific community to honor it will mean that it will have to fight a strong temptation to go by routine to the readiest sources of supply—the suggestible, the ignorant, the dependent, the "captive" in various senses.[3] I do not believe that heightened resistance here must cripple research, which cannot be permitted; but it

may indeed slow it down by the smaller numbers fed into experimentation in consequence. This price—a possibly slower rate of progress—may have to be paid for the preservation of the most precious capital of higher communal life.

Experimentation on Patients

So far we have been speaking on the tacit assumption that the subjects of experimentation are recruited from among the healthy. To the question "Who is conscriptable?" the spontaneous answer is: Least and last of all the sick—the most available of all as they are under treatment and observation anyway. That the afflicted should not be called upon to bear additional burden and risk, that they are society's special trust and the physician's trust in particular—these are elementary responses of our moral sense. Yet the very destination of medical research, the conquest of disease, requires at the crucial stage trial and verification on precisely the sufferers from the disease, and their total exemption would defeat the purpose itself. In acknowledging this inescapable necessity, we enter the most sensitive area of the whole complex, the one most keenly felt and most searchingly discussed by the practitioners themselves. No wonder, it touches the heart of the doctor-patient relation, putting its most solemn obligations to the test. There is nothing new in what I have to say about the ethics of the doctor-patient relation, but for the purpose of confronting it with the issue of experimentation some of the oldest verities must be recalled.

The Fundamental Privilege of the Sick

In the course of treatment, the physician is obligated to the patient and to no one else. He is not the agent of society, nor of the interests of medical science, nor of the patient's family, nor of his cosufferers, nor of future sufferers from the same disease. The patient alone counts when he is under the physician's care. By the simple law of bilateral contract (analogous, for example, to the relation of lawyer to client and its "conflict of interest" rule), the physician is bound not to let any other interest interfere with that of the patient in being cured. But manifestly more sublime norms than contractual ones are involved. We may speak of a sacred trust; strictly by its terms, the doctor is, as it were, alone with his patient and God.

There is one normal exception to this—that is, to the doctor's not being the agent of society vis-à-vis the patient, but the trustee of his interests alone: the quarantining of the contagious sick. This is plainly not for the patient's interest, but for that of others threatened by him. (In vaccination, we have a combination of both: protection of the individual and others.) But preventing the patient from causing harm to others is not the same as exploiting him for the advantage of others. And there is, of course, the abnormal exception of collective catastrophe, the analogue to a state of war. The physician who desperately battles a raging epidemic is under a unique dispensation that suspends in a nonspecifiable way some of the structures of normal practice, including possibly those against experimental liberties with his patients. No rules can be devised for the waiving of rules in extremities. And as with the famous shipwreck examples of ethical theory, the less said about it the better. But what is allowable there and may later be passed over in forgiving silence cannot serve as a precedent. We are concerned with non-extreme, non-emergency conditions where the voice of principle can be heard and claims can be adjudicated free from duress. We have conceded that there are such claims, and that if there is to be medical advance at all, not even the superlative privilege of the suffering and the sick can be kept wholly intact from the intrusion of its needs. About this least palatable, most disquieting part of our subject, I have to offer only groping, inconclusive remarks.

The Principle of "Identification" applied to Patients

On the whole, the same principles would seem to hold here as are found to hold with "normal subjects": motivation, identification, understanding on the part of the subject. But it is clear that these conditions are peculiarly difficult to satisfy with regard to a patient. His physical state, psychic preoccupation, dependent relation to the doctor, the submissive attitude induced by treatment—everything connected with his condition and situation makes the sick person inherently less of a sovereign person than the healthy one. Spontaneity of self-offering was almost to be ruled out; consent is marred by lower resistance or cap-

tive circumstance, and so on. In fact, all the factors that make the patient, as a category, particularly accessible and welcome for experimentation at the same time compromise the quality of the responding affirmation that must morally redeem the making use of them. This, in addition to the primacy of the physician's duty, puts a heightened onus on the physician-researcher to limit his undue power to the most important and defensible research objectives and, of course, to keep persuasion at a minimum.

Still, with all the disabilities noted, there is scope among patients for observing the rule of the "descending order of permissibility" that we have laid down for normal subjects, in vexing inversion of the utility order of quantitative abundance and qualitative "expendability." By the principle of this order, those patients who most identify with and are cognizant of the cause of research—members of the medical profession (who after all are sometimes patients themselves)—come first; the highly motivated and educated, also least dependent, among the lay patients come next; and so on down the line. An added consideration here is seriousness of condition, which again operates in inverse proportion. Here the profession must fight the tempting sophistry that the hopeless case is expendable (because in prospect already expended) and therefore especially usable; and generally the attitude that the poorer the chances of the patient, the more justifiable his recruitment for experimentation (other than for his own benefit). The opposite is true.

Nondisclosure as a Borderline Case

Then there is the case where ignorance of the subject, sometimes even of the experimenter, is of the essence of the experiment (the "double blind"-control group-placebo syndrome). It is said to be a necessary element of the scientific process. Whatever may be said about its ethics in regard to normal subjects, especially volunteers, it is an outright betrayal of trust in regard to the patient who believes that he is receiving treatment. Only supreme importance of the objective can exonerate it, without making it less of a transgression. The patient is definitely wronged even when not harmed. And ethics apart, the practice of such deception holds the danger of undermining the faith in the *bona fides* of treatment, the beneficial intent of the physician—the very basis of the doctor-patient relationship. In every respect it follows that concealed experiment on patients—that is, experiment under the guise of treatment—should be the rarest exception, at best, if it cannot be wholly avoided.

This has still the merit of a borderline problem. The same is not true of the other case of necessary ignorance of the subject—that of the unconscious patient. Drafting him for nontherapeutic experiments is simply and unqualifiedly impermissible; progress or not, he must never be used, on the inflexible principle that utter helplessness demands utter protection.

When preparing this paper, I filled pages with a casuistics of this harrowing field, but then scrapped most of it, realizing my dilettante status. The shadings are endless, and only the physician-researcher can discern them properly as the cases arise. Into his lap the decision is thrown. The philosophical rule, once it has admitted into itself the idea of a sliding scale, cannot really specify its own application. It can only impress on the practitioner a general maxim or attitude for the exercise of his judgment and conscience in the concrete occasions of his work. In our case, I am afraid, it means making life more difficult for him.

It will also be noted that, somewhat at variance with the emphasis in the literature, I have not dwelt on the element of "risk" and very little on that of "consent." Discussion of the first is beyond the layman's competence; the emphasis on the second has been lessened because of its equivocal character. It is a truism to say that one should strive to minimize the risk and to maximize the consent. The more demanding concept of "identification," which I have used, includes "consent" in its maximal or authentic form, and the assumption of risk is its privilege.

No Experiments on Patients Unrelated to Their Own Disease

Although my ponderings have, on the whole, yielded points of view rather than definite prescriptions, premises rather than conclusions, they have led me to a few unequivocal yeses and nos. The first is the emphatic rule that patients should be experimented upon, if at all, *only* with reference to *their disease*. Never should there be added to the gratuitousness of the experiment as such the gra-

tuitousness of service to an unrelated cause. This follows simply from what we have found to be the *only* excuse for infracting the special exemption of the sick at all—namely, that the scientific war on disease cannot accomplish its goal without drawing the sufferers from disease into the investigative process. If under this excuse they become subjects of experiment, they do so *because*, and only because, of *their* disease.

This is the fundamental and self-sufficient consideration. That the patient cannot possibly benefit from the unrelated experiment therapeutically, while he might from experiment related to his condition, is also true, but lies beyond the problem area of pure experiment. I am in any case discussing nontherapeutic experimentation only, where *ex hypothesi* the patient does not benefit. Experiment as part of therapy—that is, directed toward helping the subject himself—is a different matter altogether and raises its own problems but hardly philosophical ones. As long as a doctor can say, even if only in his own thought: "There is no known cure for your condition (or: You have responded to none); but there is promise in a new treatment still under investigation, not quite tested yet as to effectiveness and safety; you will be taking a chance, but all things considered, I judge it in your best interest to let me try it on you"—as long as he can speak thus, he speaks as the patient's physician and may err, but does not transform the patient into a subject of experimentation. Introduction of an untried therapy into the treatment where the tried ones have failed is not "experimentation on the patient."

Generally, and almost needless to say, with all the rules of the book, there is something "experimental" (because tentative) about every individual treatment, beginning with the diagnosis itself; and he would be a poor doctor who would not learn from every case for the benefit of future cases, and a poor member of the profession who would not make any new insights gained from his treatments available to the profession at large. Thus, knowledge may be advanced in the treatment of any patient, and the interest of the medical art and all sufferers from the same affliction as well as the patient himself may be served if something happens to be learned from his case. But his gain to knowledge and future therapy is incidental to the *bona fide* service to the present patient. He has the right to expect that the doctor does nothing to him just in order to learn.

In that case, the doctor's imaginary speech would run, for instance, like this: "There is nothing more I can do for you. But you can do something for me. Speaking no longer as your physician but on behalf of medical science, we could learn a great deal about future cases of this kind if you would permit me to perform certain experiments on you. It is understood that you yourself would not benefit from any knowledge we might gain; but future patients would." This statement would express the purely experimental situation, assumedly here with the subject's concurrence and with all cards on the table. In Alexander Bickel's words: "It is a different situation when the doctor is no longer trying to make [the patient] well, but is trying to find out how to make others well in the future."[4]

But even in the second case, that of the nontherapeutic experiment where the patient does not benefit, at least the patient's own disease is enlisted in the cause of fighting that disease, even if only in others. It is yet another thing to say or think: "Since you are here—in the hospital with its facilities—anyway, under our care and observation anyway, away from your job (or, perhaps, doomed) anyway, we wish to profit from your being available for some other research of great interest we are presently engaged in." From the standpoint of merely medical ethics, which has only to consider risk, consent, and the worth of the objective, there may be no cardinal difference between this case and the last one. I hope that the medical reader will not think I am making too fine a point when I say that from the standpoint of the subject and his dignity there is a cardinal difference that crosses the line between the permissible and the impermissible, and this by the same principle of "Identification" I have been invoking all along. Whatever the rights and wrongs of any experimentation on any patient—in the one case, at least that residue of identification is left him that it is his own affliction by which he can contribute to the conquest of that affliction, his own kind of suffering which he helps to alleviate in others; and so in a sense it is his own cause. It is totally indefensible to rob the unfortunate of this intimacy with the purpose and make his misfortune a convenience for the furtherance of alien concerns.

Conclusion

. . . I wish only to say in conclusion that if some of the practical implications of my reasonings are felt to work out toward a slower rate of progress, this should not cause too great dismay. Let us not forget that progress is an optional goal, not an unconditional commitment, and that its tempo in particular, compulsive as it may become, has nothing sacred about it. Let us also remember that a slower progress in the conquest of disease would not threaten society, grievous as it is to those who have to deplore that their particular disease be not yet conquered, but that society would indeed be threatened by the erosion of those moral values whose loss, possibly caused by too ruthless a pursuit of scientific progress, would make its most dazzling triumphs not worth having. Let us finally remember that it cannot be the aim of progress to abolish the lot of mortality. Of some ill or other, each of us will die. Our mortal condition is upon us with its harshness but also its wisdom—because without it there would not be the eternally renewed promise of the freshness, immediacy, and eagerness of youth; nor would there be for any of us the incentive to number our days and make them count. With all our striving to wrest from our mortality what we can, we should bear its burden with patience and dignity.

Notes

1. *Proceedings of the Conference on the Ethical Aspects of Experimentation on Human Subjects,* November 3–4, 1967 (Boston, Massachusetts; hereafter called *Proceedings*), pp. 50–51.

2. Socially, everyone is expendable relatively—that is, in different degrees; religiously, no one is expendable absolutely: The "image of God" is in all. If it can be enhanced, then it is not by anyone being expended, but by someone expending himself.

3. This refers to captives of circumstance, not of justice. Prison inmates are, with respect to our problem, in a special class. If we hold to some idea of guilt, and to the supposition that our judicial system is not entirely at fault, they may be held to stand in a special debt to society, and their offer to serve—from whatever motive—may be accepted with a minimum of qualms as a means of reparation.

4. *Proceedings*, p. 33.

Informed (but Uneducated) Consent

F. J. Ingelfinger

The trouble with informed consent is that it is not educated consent. Let us assume that the experimental subject, whether a patient, a volunteer, or otherwise enlisted, is exposed to a completely honest array of factual detail. He is told of the medical uncertainty that exists and that must be resolved by research endeavors, of the time and discomfort involved, and of the tiny percentage risk of some serious consequences of the test procedure. He is also reassured of his rights and given a formal, quasi-legal statement to read. No exculpatory language is used. With his written signature, the subject then caps the transaction, and whether he sees himself as a heroic martyr for the sake of mankind, or as a reluctant guinea pig dragooned for the benefit of science, or whether, perhaps, he is merely bewildered, he obviously has given his "informed consent." Because established routines have been scrupulously observed, the doctor, the lawyer, and the ethicist are content.

But the chances are remote that the subject really understands what he has consented to—in the sense that the responsible medical investigator understands the goals, nature, and hazards of his study. How can the layman comprehend the importance of his perhaps not receiving, as determined by luck of the draw, the highly touted new treatment that his roommate will get? How can he appreciate the sensation of living for days with a multi-lumen intestinal tube passing through his mouth and pharynx? How can he interpret the information that an intravascular catheter and radiopaque dye injection have an 0.01 per cent probability of leading to a dangerous thrombosis or cardiac arrhythmia? It is moreover quite unlikely that any patient-subject can see himself accurately within the broad context of the situation, to weigh the inconveniences and hazards that he will have to undergo against the improvements that the research project may bring to the management of his disease in general and to his own

case in particular. The difficulty that the public has in understanding information that is both medical and stressful is exemplified by [a report that] only half the families given genetic counseling grasped its impact.[1]

Nor can the information given to the experimental subject be in any sense totally complete. It would be impractical and probably unethical for the investigator to present the nearly endless list of all possible contingencies; in fact, he may not himself be aware of every untoward thing that might happen. Extensive detail, moreover, usually enhances the subject's confusion. Epstein and Lasagna showed that comprehension of medical information given to untutored subjects is inversely correlated with the elaborateness of the material presented.[2] The inconsiderate investigator, indeed, conceivably could exploit his authority and knowledge and extract "informed consent" by overwhelming the candidate-subject with information.

Ideally, the subject should give his consent freely, under no duress whatsoever. The facts are that some element of coercion is instrumental in any investigator-subject transaction. Volunteers for experiments will usually be influenced by hopes of obtaining better grades, earlier parole, more substantial egos, or just mundane cash. These pressures, however, are but fractional shadows of those enclosing the patient-subject. Incapacitated and hospitalized because of illness, frightened by strange and impersonal routines, and fearful for his health and perhaps life, he is far from exercising a free power of choice when the person to whom he anchors all his hopes asks, "Say, you wouldn't mind, would you, if you joined some of the other patients on this floor and helped us to carry out some very important research we are doing?" When "informed consent" is obtained, it is not the student, the destitute bum, or the prisoner to whom, by virtue of his condition, the thumb screws of coercion are most

Reprinted by permission from the New England Journal of Medicine 287, 9 (August 31, 1972): 465–466.
Editor's Note: The notes in this essay have been renumbered.

relentlessly applied; it is the most used and useful of all experimental subjects, the patient with disease.

When a man or woman agrees to act as an experimental subject, therefore, his or her consent is marked by neither adequate understanding nor total freedom of choice. The conditions of the agreement are a far cry from those visualized as ideal. Jonas would have the subject identify with the investigative endeavor so that he and the researcher would be seeking a common cause: "Ultimately, the appeal for volunteers should seek . . . free and generous endorsement, the appropriation of the research purpose into the person's [i.e., the subject's] own scheme of ends."[3] For Ramsey, "informed consent" should represent a "covenantal bond between consenting man and consenting man [that] makes them . . . joint adventurers in medical care and progress."[4] Clearly, to achieve motivations and attitudes of this lofty type, an educated and understanding, rather than merely informed, consent is necessary.

Although it is unlikely that the goals of Jonas and of Ramsey will ever be achieved, and that human research subjects will spontaneously volunteer rather than be "conscripted,"[3] efforts to promote educated consent are in order. In view of the current emphasis on involving "the community" in such activities as regional planning, operation of clinics, and assignment of priorities, the general public and its political leaders are showing an increased awareness and understanding of medical affairs. But the orientation of this public interest in medicine is chiefly socioeconomic. Little has been done to give the public a basic understanding of medical research and its requirements not only for the people's money but also for their participation. The public, to be sure, is being subjected to a bombardment of sensation-mongering news stories and books that feature "breakthroughs," or that reveal real or alleged exploitations—horror stories of Nazi-type experimentation on abused human minds and bodies. Muckraking is essential to expose malpractices, but unless accompanied by efforts to promote a broader appreciation of medical research and its methods, it merely compounds the difficulties for both the investigator and the subject when "informed consent" is solicited.

The procedure currently approved in the United States for enlisting human experimental subjects has one great virtue: patient-subjects are put on notice that their management is in part at least an experiment. The deceptions of the past are no longer tolerated. Beyond this accomplishment, however, the process of obtaining "informed consent," with all its regulations and conditions, is no more than an elaborate ritual, a device that, when the subject is uneducated and uncomprehending, confers no more than the semblance of propriety on human experimentation. The subject's only real protection, the public as well as the medical profession must recognize, depends on the conscience and compassion of the investigator and his peers.

Notes

1. [Leonard, Claire O., et al. Genetic counseling: a consumer's view. N Engl J Med 287:433–449, 1972.]
2. Epstein, L. C., Lasagna, L. Obtaining informed consent: form or substance. Arch Intern Med 123:682–688, 1969.
3. Jonas, H. Philosophical reflections on experimenting with human subjects. Daedalus 98:219–247, Spring, 1969.
4. Ramsey, P. The ethics of a cottage industry in an age of community and research medicine. N Engl J Med 284:700–706, 1971.

A Moral Theory of Consent

Benjamin Freedman

Most medical codes of ethics, and most physicians, agree that the physician ought to obtain the "free and informed consent" of his subject or patient before attempting any serious medical procedures, experimental or therapeutic in nature. They agree, moreover, that a proxy consent ought to be

Reprinted by permission of the author and publisher from the Hastings Center Report, *5 (August 1975).*
©*Institute of Society, Ethics and Life Sciences, 360 Broadway, Hastings-on-Hudson, New York.*

obtained on behalf of the incompetent subject. And informed consent is seen as not merely a legal requirement, and not merely a formality: it is a substantial requirement of morality.

Acceptance of this doctrine, however, requires the solution of a number of problems. How much information need be imparted? At what age is a person mature enough to consent on his own behalf? Can prisoners give a "free and informed consent" to be experimented upon? Lurking behind these and similar questions there are more fundamental difficulties. What are the functions of consent for the competent and the incompetent? What is the sense in which the patient/subject must be "free," "informed," and "competent?" It is by way of an approach to these latter questions that I shall attempt to respond to the more specific questions.[1]

I. Consent and the Competent

The negative aspects of the doctrine of informed consent have ordinarily been the focus of attention; difficulties in obtaining the informed consent of the subject/patient render the ethics of experimentation and therapeutic measures questionable. Our common view of informed consent is that, when at all relevant, it represents a minimum condition which ethics imposes upon the physician. It is seen as a necessary condition for medical manipulation, but hardly as a sufficient condition.

The reasons why this is so—why it is not sufficient that an experimenter, for instance, have received informed consent from his subject before proceeding—are quite obvious. The scarcity of medical resources (which includes a scarcity of qualified physician-investigators) forbids us from wasting time upon poorly-designed experiments, or upon experiments which merely replicate well-established conclusions. There seems to be, as well, a limit to the dangers which we (ordinarily) allow subjects to face. We do not, as a matter of policy, think it wise to allow would-be suicides to accomplish their end with the aid of a scientific investigator. Many other reasons could be given for the proposition that a person does not have a right to be experimented upon, even when he has given valid consent to the procedure.

The Right to Consent

But there does seem to exist a positive right of informed consent, which exists in both therapeutic and experimental settings. A person who has the capacity to give valid consent, and who has in fact consented to the procedure in question, has a right to have that fact recognized by us. We all have a duty to recognize a valid consent when confronted with it.

From whence derives this right? It arises from the right which each of us possesses to be treated as a person, and in the duty which all of us have, to have respect for persons, to treat a person as such, and not as an object. For this entails that our capacities for personhood ought to be recognized by all—these capacities including the capacity for rational decision, and for action consequent upon rational decision. Perhaps the worst which we may do to a man is to deny him his humanity, for example, by classifying him as mentally incompetent when he is, in fact, sane. It is a terrible thing to be hated or persecuted; it is far worse to be ignored, to be notified that you "don't count."

If an individual is capable of and has given valid consent, I would argue that he has a right, as against the world but more particularly as against his physician, to have it recognized that valid consent has been given. (The same applies, of course, with still greater force, with regard to *refusals* to consent to medical procedures.) The limited force of this claim must be emphasized: it does not entail a right to be treated, or to be experimented upon. It is a most innocuous right, one which most of us would have little hesitation about granting.

It is, therefore, curious that the literature on informed consent has failed to recognize this right—has, in fact, tacitly denied this right, at least as regards experimentation. In writings on informed consent it seems to have been assumed that if, under certain conditions, it is *doubtful* that vaild consent to an experiment has been granted, it is best to "play it safe" ethically. In cases of doubt, we prefer not to take chances: in this case, we will not take a chance upon violating the canons of ethics by experimenting without being certain that the subject has validly consented to the experiment. Since we do not at present know whether a prisoner can give a valid consent, let us not take chances: we call for a moratorium on prison experimentation. Since we do not know at what age a person has the capacity to give a valid consent, we avoid the problem by setting the age of majority at a point where it is beyond doubt that maturity has been attained. If we must err, we shall ensure that we err in being overly ethical.

The establishment of the innocuous right to have valid consent recognized as such eliminates this expedient. Other writers have conceptualized the conflict as one between a right and, at best, a mere liberty. From the patient's point of view, he has a right to have his health protected by the physician, and a mere liberty to be experimented upon. From the physician-investigator's point of view, he has a duty to protect the subject's health, and a mere liberty to experiment upon the subject (contingent, of course, upon obtaining the subject's consent). A recognition of the claims of personhood and autonomy, however, reveals this to be a conflict between rights and duties. The physician-investigator has a duty to recognize consent when validly offered. When the consent is of doubtful validity, therefore, the physician experiences a conflict between two duties. He will not be ethically well-protected by choosing not to experiment, for there exists the possibility—which, as cases are multiplied, becomes a probability—that he is violating a duty in so choosing. Problems in informed consent present us with a dilemma. It is no longer the case that the burden of proof devolves upon the would-be experimenter. The would-be abstainer-from-experiments may have to prove his case as well.

These considerations give us a new point of departure in investigating problems of informed consent. They show us that there is no "fail-safe" procedure which we can fall back upon in cases of doubt. Rather, what is required is an exhaustive examination of each case and issue, to see whether or not a valid consent has in fact been obtained.

When we fail to recognize a valid consent, of course, more is involved than a denial of personhood. Other benefits may be denied as well. Dr. Vernon Mark, for example, maintains that psychosurgery should not be done on prisoners with epilepsy because of the problem in obtaining a voluntary consent from prisoners.[2] But a resolution of this problem has not been shown to be impossible. Surely, the proper thing to do here would be to see whether prisoners can or cannot give valid consent to such a procedure. To remain satisfied with doubts, to fail to investigate this question, complex though it be, results in a denial of medical treatment for the prisoner, as well as representing a negation of the prisoner's human capacities. In depriving prisoners of the opportunity to serve as subjects in medical experiments, there are losses other than those of human re-

spect.[3] Not the least of these is the loss of an opportunity to be of altruistic service to mankind.[4] Even a child feels at times a need to be useful; in promoting a moratorium on prison experimentation we deny prisoners the satisfaction of this psychic need. We should not need a reminder from John Stuart Mill that there are "higher" as well as "lower" pleasures and needs.

The right to have valid consent recognized as such does not indicate that we must experiment on prisoners. What it does indicate is that we have a moral responsibility to investigate in detail the question of whether prisoners can, under certain conditions, validly consent to experimentation. It also requires that we not prevent a researcher from experimenting on the basis of over-scrupulousness. If prisoners *can* give valid consent, we wrong not only the researcher but the prisoner as well by forbidding prison experimentation.

The Requirement of Information

The most common locution for the requirement which I am discussing is "informed consent"—we require "informed consent" to protect a doctor from legal liability resultant from his therapeutic endeavors, or to ensure the "ethicacy" of an experiment. But I believe "informed consent" to be a serious misnomer for what we do, in fact, want medical practice to conform to.

No lengthy rehearsal of the absurdities consequent upon taking the term "informed consent" at face value is necessary. The claim has been made, and repeated with approval, that "fully informed consent" is a goal which we can never achieve, but toward which we must strive. In order to ensure that fully informed consent has been given, it has seriously been suggested that only medical students or graduate students in the life sciences ought to be accepted as subjects for experimentation. *Reductio ad absurdum* examples of "fully informed consent" have been elaborated, in forms which list all the minutiae of the proposed medical procedure, together with all of its conceivable sequelae. With such a view of "informed consent" and its requirements, it is not surprising to find doctors who claim that since they cannot fully inform patients, they will tell them nothing, but instead will personally assume the responsibility for assuring the subject's safety.

In truth, a *reductio ad absurdum* of this view of "informed consent" need not be constructed; it serves as its own *reductio ad absurdum*. For there is no end to "fully informing" patients. When the doctor wishes to insert a catheter, must he commend to the subject's attention a textbook of anatomy? Although this, of course, would not suffice: he must ensure that the patient understand the text as well. Must he tell the patient the story of Dr. X, that bogey of first-year medical students, who, in a state of inebriation, inserted ("by mistake") his pen-refill instead of the catheter? With, of course, the assurance that *this* physician never gets drunk ("Well, rarely, anyway"). Must the patient be informed of the chemical formula of the catheter? Its melting point?

The basic mistake which is committed by those who harp upon the difficulties in obtaining informed consent (and by critics of the doctrine) is in believing that we can talk about information in the abstract, without reference to any human purpose. It is very likely impossible to talk about "information" in this way; but impossible or not, when we do in fact talk about, or request, information, we do not mean "information in the abstract." If I ask someone to "tell me about those clouds" he will, ordinarily, know what I mean; and he will answer me, in the spirit in which he was asked, by virtue of his professional expertise as an artist, meteorologist, astronomer, soothsayer, or what-have-you. The meteorologist will not object that he cannot tell you the optical refraction index of the clouds, and therefore that he cannot "fully answer" your question. He knows that you are asking him with a given end in mind, and that much information about the cloud is irrelevant *relative to that purpose*.

That this "abstract information" requirement is not in question in obtaining valid consent is hardly an original point, but it is worth repeating. One of the leading court opinions on human experimentation puts it like this: ". . . the patient's interest in information does not extend to a lengthy polysyllabic discourse on all possible complications. A mini-course in medical science is not required. . . ."[5]

The proper question to ask, then, is not "What information must be given?" That would be premature: we must first know for what purpose information is needed. *Why* must the patient be informed? Put that way, the answer is immediately forthcoming. The patient must be informed so that he will know what he is getting into, what he may expect from the procedure, what his likely alternatives are—in short, what the procedure (and forbearance from it) will mean, so that a responsible decision on the matter may be made. This is the legal stance, as well as, I think, a "common sensical" stance; as Alexander Capron writes, the information component in valid consent derives in law from the recognition that information is "necessary to make meaningful the power to decide."[6] The proper test of whether a given piece of information needs to be given is, then, whether the physician, knowing what he does about the patient/subject, feels that that patient/subject would want to know this before making up his mind. Outré, improbable consequences would not ordinarily, therefore, be relevant information. Exceptionally, they will be: for example, when there is a small risk of impotence consequent upon the procedure which the physician proposes to perform upon a man with a great stake in his sexual prowess. This is only sensible.

Our main conclusion, then, is that valid consent entails only the imparting of that information which the patient/subject requires in order to make a responsible decision. This entails, I think, the possibility of a valid yet ignorant consent.

Consider, first, the therapeutic context. It is, I believe, not unusual for a patient to give his doctor *carte blanche* to perform any medical procedure which the physician deems proper in order to effect a cure. He is telling the doctor to act as his agent in choosing which procedure to follow. This decision is neither unwise nor (in any serious sense) an abdication of responsibility and an unwarranted burden upon the physician. We each of us choose to delegate our power of choice in this way in dealing with our auto mechanic or stockbroker.

It may be harder to accept an ignorant consent as valid in the purely experimental context. I think, however, that much of this difficulty is due to our paucity of imagination, our failure to imagine circumstances in which a person might choose to proceed in this way. We might approach such a case, for example, by imagining a Quaker who chooses to serve society by acting as a research subject, but who has a morbid fear of knives and pointed instruments. The Quaker might say to the physician-investigator that he wants to serve science but is afraid that his phobia would overcome his better judgment. He might consequently request that any experiment which would involve use of scalpels, hypodermic needles, and such, be performed without informing him: while, say, he is asleep or unconscious. He might further ask the doctor not to proceed should the experiment involve considerable risk. In such a case, or one similar, we would find an instance of a valid yet ignorant consent to experimentation.

The ostensible differences between the therapeutic and experimental contexts may be resolved into two components: in the therapeutic context it is supposed that the physician knows what the sequelae to treatment will be, which information, by definition, is not available in the experimental situation; and in the therapeutic context the doctor may be said to be seeking his patient's good, in contrast to the experimental context where some other good is being sought. On the basis of these differences it may be claimed that a valid yet ignorant consent is enough permission for therapy, but not for experimentation.

Closer examination, however, reveals that these differences do not necessarily obtain. First, because I believe it would be granted that a valid yet ignorant consent can be given in the "therapeutic-experimental" situation, where a new drug or procedure is being attempted to aid the patient (in the absence of any traditional available therapy). In the therapeutic-experimental situation, as in the purely experimental situation, the sequelae are not known (although of course in both cases some definite result is expected or anticipated). If a valid yet ignorant consent is acceptable in the one, therefore, it must be acceptable in the other.

Secondly, because it is patently not the case that we can expect there to be no good accruing to the subject of an experiment by reason of his participation. There are, commonly, financial and other "tangible" benefits forthcoming (laboratory training, and so on). And it must once again be said that the pleasures of altruism are not negligible. The proposed differences between experimentation and therapy do not stand up, and so we must say that if a valid yet ignorant consent is acceptable in the one it must be acceptable in the other. It must be remembered that this statement only concerns itself with one part of the consent doctrine, which is, itself, only one of the requirements which the ethical experiment must satisfy.

To mention—without claiming totally to resolve—two problems which may be raised at this point: First, it is said that a doctor often does not know what will happen as a consequence of a recommended procedure, and so cannot tell the patient what the patient wants to know. The obvious response to this seems to be right: the physician should, in that case, tell the patient/subject that he does not know what will happen (which does not exclude an explanation of what the doctor expects to happen, and on what he bases this expectation).

Second, it will be objected that the adoption of a requirement such as I propose would forbid the use of placebos and blind experiments. I am not sure that this is so; sometimes it must be the case that the subjects in an experiment may be asked (without introducing artifacts into the results) to consent to an experiment knowing that some will, and some will not, be receiving placebos. Another alternative would be to inform the subjects that the experiment may or may not involve some subjects receiving placebos.[7] I am aware, however, that these remarks are less than adequate responses to these problems.

Our conclusion, then, is that the informing of the patient/subject is not a fundamental requirement of valid consent. It is, rather, derivative from the requirement that the consent be the expression of a responsible choice. The two requirements which I do see as fundamental in this doctrine are that the choice be responsible and that it be voluntary.

The Requirement of Responsibility

What is meant by saying that the choice must be "responsible"? Does this entail that the physician may at any time override a patient's judgment on the basis that, in the physician's view, the patient has not chosen responsibly? Surely not; to adopt such a criterion would defeat the purpose embodied in the doctrine of consent. It would mean that a person's exercise of autonomy is always subject to review.

Still, some such requirement would appear to be necessary. A small child can certainly make choices.[8] Small children can also be intelligent enough to understand the necessary information. Yet surely we would not want to say that a small child can give valid consent to a serious medical procedure.[9] The reason for this is that the child cannot choose *responsibly*.

We are faced with a dilemma. On the one hand, it appears that we must require that the choice be responsible. To require only that the choice be free would yield counter-intuitive results. On the other hand, if we do require that the choice made be a responsible one, we seem to presuppose some body which shall judge the reasonableness of choices; this represents a paternalism which is antithetical to the doctrine of consent. An elderly patient chooses to forgo further life-saving measures. How are we to judge whether or not this choice is a responsible one?

The path between the horns of this dilemma involves saying that the "responsibility" which we require is to be predicated not on the nature of the particular choice, but on the nature of the patient/subject. What we need to know is whether *he* is a responsible man ("in general," so to speak), not whether the choice which has been made is responsible. In this way, we avoid the danger of upholding as "responsible" only those choices which we ourselves feel are good choices. We can and do admit into the community of responsible persons individuals who make choices with which we do not agree.

In this sense, responsibility is a dispositional characteristic. To say that someone is a responsible individual means that he makes choices, typically, on the basis of reasons, arguments, or beliefs—and that he remains open to the claims of reason, so that further rational argument might lead him to change his mind. It is to say that a person is capable of making and carrying through a life-plan—that he is prepared to act on the basis of his choices. It is to say that a person is capable of living with his life-plan; he can live with the consequences of his choices, he *takes responsibility* for his choices.[10] Of course, none of these are absolutes: all responsible people are at times pigheaded, at times short-sighted, at times flighty. That is to say, all responsible men at times act irresponsibly. Should the lack of responsibility persist, of course, to an extreme degree, we may say that the person has left the community of responsible folk.

Voluntarism and Reward

The other requirement of valid consent is that it be given voluntarily. The choice which the consent expresses must be freely made.

We all know some conditions which, if satisfied, make us say that a consent has been given involuntarily. The case which immediately springs to mind occurs when an individual succumbs under a threat: we call this duress or coercion. But the threat need not be overt; and perhaps there need not be a threat at all to render consent involuntary.

Hence, the major problem currently engendered by the requirement of voluntariness. It is typified by the prisoner who "volunteers" for an experiment in the hope or expectation of a reward: significantly higher wages, an opportunity for job training, better health care while involved in the experiment, a favorable report to his parole board. Is the consent which the prisoner offers a voluntary consent? The problem may be stated more generally thus: At what point does reward render consent involuntary?

The problem of reward is particularly difficult, since it involves questions of degree. Is a prisoner's consent involuntary if the reward for his participation in the experiment is a three-month reduction of sentence? Is it relevant here that the prisoner is serving a twenty-year sentence, rather than a one-to-five-year sentence? Does a possible increase in wages from twenty-five cents per hour to one dollar per hour constitute duress? Should we consider the percentage increase, or the increase in absolute value, or the increase in actual value which the seventy-five cent disparity represents in the prison environment?

To some, of course, questions like these have little meaning. They have little meaning to those who are indifferent to the demands of justice and autonomy which the consent doctrine represents, to those who are willing to buy guinea pigs, rather than to reward human beings. And they have little meaning for those who are convinced that prisoners are inherently unfree, and who thus would call for a total cessation of prison experimentation. Each of these positions denies, in an *a priori* fashion, freedom to prisoners; each must be rejected. A recognition of the fact that decisions about consent may be over- as well as under-protective forces us to deal with this sort of question, complex though it may be.

As is so often the case, posing the question in a different way may facilitate response. We have been considering the question of how much reward nullifies the validity of consent, how much reward renders the subject unfree. But is it in fact the case that *reward* is the disruptive factor here?

This problem may be clarified by the following examples. Imagine an upper-middle-class individual, who can provide for his family all of their needs and most of the amenities of civilized life. Let us say that this person is offered one hundred dollars to cross the street—if you like, make it one thousand or ten thousand dollars? He chooses to cross the street. Is his choice *involuntary*? Despite the substantial reward, I think most of us would agree that the consent was freely offered (and would that we should have such problems!).

Consider a person who deeply wants to be an astronaut. He is told that as part of the program he must participate in experiments to determine resistance to high-G conditions. Is his consent to this invalid, involuntary? I think not. We would say, this is part of his job; he should have expected it; and if he can't stand the heat, he should get out of the kitchen. In this vein, consider Evel Knievel, a financially prosperous man, who is offered millions of dollars to perform daredevil stunts. His choice may be bizarre, even crazy: but has his reward rendered it unfree?

Finally, consider a man who is informed by his doctor that he will most likely die unless he has open-heart surgery. His "reward" for consenting is his life; the penalty for not consenting is death. Does this mean this man cannot give the doctor valid consent—morally valid consent—to proceed?

There are two distinctions which, I think, go a long way towards dispelling these problems. First, I think it must be granted that natural contingencies ("acts of God," things which come to pass naturally, those contingencies which we cannot hold anyone responsible for) do not render a person unfree, nor do they render unfree the choices which a person makes in light of those contingencies.[11]

That natural contingencies do not render a man unfree is a point which is apt to be forgotten in the present context. I am not—in the morally relevant sense—lacking in freedom because I cannot, unaided, fly through the air, or live on grass. Nor am I unfree because my heart is about to give out. Nor am I unfree when, recognizing that my heart may give out, I choose to undergo surgery. I may, of course, be so crazed by knowing that I am near death's door that I am in a state of general impotence, and hence must have the choice made for me; but general incompetence is not in question here. The distinction between choices forced by man, and choices forced by nature, is, then, of importance.

The second distinction is between those pressures which are, and those which are not, in Daube's words, "consonant with the dignity and responsibility of free life."[12] I would explain this as follows: there are certain basic freedoms and rights which we possess which *entitle* us (morally) to certain things (or states of affairs). We would all, no doubt, draw up different lists of these rights and freedoms; but included in them would be safety of person, freedom of conscience and religion, a right to a certain level of education, and, for some of us, a right to some level of health care. When the "reward" is such as only to give us the necessary conditions of these rights and freedoms—when all that the reward does is to bring us up to a level of living to which we are entitled, and of which we have been deprived by man—then the "reward," I think, constitutes duress. A reward which accrues to one who has achieved this level, or who can easily achieve it (other than by taking the reward-option), and which hence serves only to grant us "luxury" items, does not constitute duress, and hence does not render choice unfree, no matter how great this reward may be.

The rewards above the moral subsistence level are true rewards. In contrast, we may say (with some touch of metaphor) that the "rewards" which only bring us up to the level to which we were in any event entitled are properly viewed as functioning as *threats:* "Do this, or stay where you are:"—when you should not have been "where you are" in the first place.

The astronaut, Evel Knievel, and the upper-middle-class street-crosser are being granted "luxury" items, and hence are capable of giving free consent. But consider a man who will not be admitted to the hospital for treatment unless he agrees to be a subject in an experiment (unrelated to his treatment). Those who feel, as I do, that we are, here and now, morally entitled to medical treatment would agree, I trust, that this illegitimate option coerces the man into agreeing. Or consider a man who has religious scruples against donating blood, who takes his daughter to a hospital for treatment. He is told that the doctors will not treat her unless the family donates a certain amount of blood. His freedom has been nullified: his "consent" to donating blood is morally invalid. Similarly, the college student whose grade is contingent upon his participation in the instructor's psychological experiments is not validly consenting to serve. He is entitled to have his grade based upon his classroom work.

It yet remains to apply this distinction to our

original problem, prison experimentation. The application will not be attempted here, for we would first need to be clear in our minds what rights and freedoms a prisoner is entitled to. I would not hesitate to say, though, that when a situation is created whereby a prisoner can only receive decent health care by participating in an experiment, he is being coerced into that experiment. I would have little hesitation in claiming that if subjecting himself to experimentation is the only way in which a prisoner could learn a trade which may be used "outside," then that prisoner is being coerced, his consent is not free. When we take into account the condition of our society, these would seem to be reasonable entitlements for the prisoner. Other rewards—for example, higher pay—may or may not constitute rewards above the moral subsistence level; if they are, then consent in light of these rewards could be freely offered. Perhaps too much has been said already; judgments like these must be made in an individualized fashion, one which is sensitive to the realities of prison life.

II. Consent and the Incompetent

In this section will be discussed, first, the question of how the age of majority and minority with reference to valid consent ought to be set; and secondly, the problems associated with the concept of proxy consent.

The Age of Consent

It has been argued that the requirements for obtaining valid consent are that the patient/subject must have consented freely and that he must be a responsible individual. The requirement of voluntariness does not raise any novel problems when applied to minors. Rather, what we usually have in mind when restricting the power of the minor to consent is that he is not, in the sense required, a responsible individual.

I have claimed that to be a responsible individual one must be capable of rationally adopting, following through, and accepting the consequences of a life-plan. The age, therefore, at which society indicates a presumption that individuals can satisfy these conditions can be said to be the age at which society ought to grant the right to give valid consent to serious medical procedures. The examples which spring to mind are the age of conscription and the age of marriageability. At these ages society has indicated that one is capable of acting, in a complex society, as an individual.

This is not an argument like that which says "If you are old enough to fight, then you are old enough to vote." The requirements necessary for being a soldier may be wholly unrelated to the requirements necessary before the franchise may be properly exercised. In contrast, the responsibility which we assume to be possessed by those capable of soldiering and contracting marriage is the same responsibility which is required to make consent valid: the ability to work through and with a life-plan.

The first thing which needs to be said, then, is that the age of consent should be lowered from 21 to 18 in those jurisdictions which have not yet done so. This should not entail merely that an 18-year-old may consent in the absence of parental disapproval; it should be a full power to consent, irrespective of what others might say.

But the setting of an age of consent indicates only a presumption and nothing more. The fact that someone has passed the age of consent is not conclusive proof that he is responsible (in the sense required); the fact that someone is below the age of consent is not conclusive proof of irresponsibility. The presumption may be defeated in either direction.

It is clear, for example, that an adult is not, *ipso facto*, responsible. The adult may be insane.

It is equally clear that a minor need not be irresponsible. People mature at different rates. If evidence of responsibility may be supplied on behalf of one below the age of consent, the presumption of irresponsibility should be defeated. The sort of evidence which would be necessary is that which indicates that the person can work through a life-plan. It may be said that this notion is being approached by the law in the special provisions sometimes made for the "emancipated minor." Marriage or economic self-sufficiency are among the common requirements for being considered an emancipated minor. One of the special prerogatives of the emancipated minor is that he may consent on his own behalf to medical care. I would argue that this should be extended to cover participation in experimentation as well.

Proxy Consent

Proxy consent is consent given on behalf of an individual who is himself incapable of granting consent. The major category of those who require proxy consent are minors, but proxy consent may need to be obtained for the insane or the unconscious as well. My comments will nevertheless be restricted to the case of minors, leaving the other cases to be dealt with by implication. In minors, proxy consent is ordinarily granted by the child's parent or guardian; exceptionally, it may be given by another close relative or by an individual appointed by the court for the specific purpose of granting consent to some procedure.

I have argued that the function of informed consent is to respect the autonomy and dignity of the individual. This cannot be the function of proxy consent. The minor patient/subject cannot fully express autonomy and dignity through choices. It may be said that the function of proxy consent is to protect the right of the parents to raise their child as they see fit, to do with the child as they like. But the child is not the property of the parents; parents do not have an absolute right of disposal over the child. In law we recognize constraints upon the parental power, and common morality affirms the justice in this. What then is the function of proxy consent?

I think it would be best to turn this question on its head. By virtue of what right which the child possesses do we require the granting of proxy consent before a medical procedure may be initiated? What *could* be the source of such an obligation? We ordinarily recognize that there is only one fundamental right possessed by minors, a right to be protected and aided in development. " . . . A child, unlike an adult, has a right 'not to liberty but to custody.' "[13] All other rights which a child possesses, all other duties which we have towards children, are derivative from this single right, and are void when inconsistent with it. Broadly speaking, in consequence of this right, we must do what we may to promote the welfare of the child; we must abstain from doing what will injure the child, physically or otherwise; and, as far as this right goes, we are at liberty to deal with the child in ways which neither help nor hurt.

That proxy consent is ordinarily to be obtained from the parent or guardian of the child is understandable. We feel that the parent has the best interests of the child at heart, and knows how best to seek the child's welfare. It also follows from this right, however, that, when the parent does not have the best interests of the child in mind, the power of proxy consent should be transferred to another. It is on such a basis that society feels justified in removing a child from his parent's custody, and in appointing another to act *in parens patriae*. If this system is to be effective, society must, by and large, act on the basis of shared common views about what the welfare of the child consists of. We cannot allow anything which a parent considers to be a benefit to the child—being boiled in oil to save his eternal soul—to count as action in the child's best interests. This does not preclude a certain amount of leeway in a liberal society as to permitted views of welfare: if most feel that it is better, when the money is available, to send the child to a private school, we yet will not fault an affluent parent who decides to send his child to a public school.

The consequences of these propositions for cases when proxy consent is being sought for the purpose of giving therapy to a child accord well with the way the law handles this subject. The problem situation which arises concerns parents who, because of religious scruples, refuse to consent to needed medical treatment for their child. Jehovah's Witnesses, for example, who believe that blood transfusions are forbidden by the law of God, will not consent on behalf of their child to blood transfusions. Society feels that the benefit of the child is to be found in allowing the procedure. Because of this, the hospital will often turn to a judge, who appoints someone to act *in parens patriae* for the purpose of consenting to the specific procedure. I suggest that if it were clearly the view of society that it is to the mongoloid infant's benefit to survive, should a parent refuse to consent to a life-saving procedure for that infant, a similar course would be followed: the consent of a court-appointed guardian would be substituted.

Proxy consent to experimentation on children is a more complicated matter. In law, there are two kinds of intervention in the person of another which are actionable in the absence of consent: those interventions where harm does, and where harm does not, result. The latter are termed "wrongful" or "harmful touchings" (though no harm has occurred). In other words, the mere *doing* of something to a person without his consent is, in itself, an actionable wrong.

We may say that, corresponding to this division, there are two sorts of experiments: those which do, and those which do not, injure the subject appreciably. Beecher has noted, for example, that "Many thousands of psychomotor tests and sociological studies have been carried out in children during the child's development and have revealed much information of value. . . . Sound nutritional studies without risk have been carried out. So have certain blood studies."[14] It must be added that many studies of value cannot, due to metabolic and other differences, be carried out in adults with results which will be valid for children.

It is clear, on the basis of the principle of benefit, that proxy consent to dangerous or harmful experiments on children cannot be valid. What about those experiments which carry no appreciable risk—the "wrongful touchings" sort? In an adult, it would seem, the right to autonomy, the right "to be let alone," is sufficient basis for the action of wrongful touching. But the child does not have a right to autonomy, except insofar as some measure of autonomy is necessary to promote the child's development and well-being.

Harmless experiments on children, therefore, which satisfy the other canons of medical ethics—good design, well-trained experimenters, and so forth—could be performed. Parents would not be derelict in their duty should they consent, on behalf of their child, to experiments of this sort. Participation in these experiments does not infringe the child's right to welfare, unless they would result in a *harmful* (and not just any) restriction of autonomy.

As I see it, the fundamental problem with those who would forbid *all* experimentation upon children[15] is that they confuse consent in adults with proxy consent for children. These two are fundamentally different requirements. Children are not small adults; our relations with children must not be made to approach as nearly as possible to our relations with adults. There are things which you ought to grant to children which need not be granted to adults: if a child is thirsty you provide him with drink. And there are things which may licitly be done to children which could not be done with adults: if my parents annoy me I may not send them to their room. A child is (morally) a different sort of thing than is an adult; we must adjust our relations with them according to their claims upon us.

Conclusion

This paper represents an attempt to formulate what I call a "moral theory" of the requirement of consent to serious medical procedures. The method used involves an interplay between cases and principles, such that each influences the other. Well-established moral intuitions about cases suggested some principles and called for the rejection of others. These principles in turn, once established, enabled the clarification of a proper approach to other, borderline cases.

Under the influence of situation ethics, much of the work on medical ethics has stressed the respects in which cases differ. This has resulted in the development of an *ad hoc* literature on cases which pose difficulty for the doctrine of informed consent. As the cases accumulated, the doctrine began to seem more and more amorphous.

In contrast, this paper has sought to unify the doctrine of consent. Principles which are developed through considering the problems raised by prison experimentation in turn suggested solutions to other situations; rather than stressing the differences between the experimental and the therapeutic contexts, their similarities were emphasized. There is, I think, a need for such efforts at unification, as there is a need for a literature which is committed to the unique aspects of different cases.

Notes

The research for this paper was begun during an internship at the Institute of Society, Ethics and the Life Sciences in the month of June, 1973. I gratefully acknowledge the help of Drs. Daniel Callahan, Marc Lappé, Peter Steinfels, and Robert Veatch, of the Institute, who helped make my internship profitable and enjoyable. My wife Barbara read the manuscript and suggested a number of needed changes.

1. For examples of a similar method applied to different problems, see Thomas I. Emerson, *Toward A General Theory of the First Amendment* (New York: Vintage Books, 1967).

2. "Brain Surgery in Aggressive Epileptics," in *Hastings Center Report*, February 1973.[Reprinted below, pp. xxx–xxx.]

3. See the insert to Alexander M. Capron's call for a moratorium on prison experimentation, "Medical Research in Prisons," *Hastings Center Report*, June 1973. The insert is a report from the New York *Times*, April 15, 1973, and reads in part: "Ninety-six of the 175 inmates at Lancaster County prison have written to a newspaper here protesting a recent decision by the state to halt all medical experiments on state prisoners. In their letter to the *Lancaster New Era*, they urged that state to allow the research

[which] did not harm them and enabled them to pay off their fines and court costs."

4. See Henry K. Beecher, *Research and the Individual: Human Studies* (Boston: Little, Brown, 1970), p. 56. Professor Beecher notes a study of prison inmates, who, for participation in an experiment involving malaria, received pay but no reduction of sentence. Half of the volunteers cited "altruism" rather than money as their motive for volunteering. Those inmates who did not volunteer "expressed or implied respect for those who did volunteer."

5. *Cobbs* v. *Grant*, 502 P. 2d 1, 11.

6. Alexander M. Capron, "Legal Rights and Moral Rights," in Hilton, *et al.*, eds., *Ethical Issues in Human Genetics* (Plenum Press, 1973), 228.

7. If this sort of explanation were given as a matter of course in *all* experiments, this might still further reduce the problem of artifacts. The remarks, it should be noted, are directed towards medical experiments. By and large, they are inapplicable to, say, experiments in social psychology.

8. The counter-suggestion may be made that children cannot *really* make choices. This would, I think, put too great a weight upon the requirement of voluntarism. We would be recruiting the concepts

of choice and volition to do a job which they have not been designed for.

9. I am speaking of course in the moral, not the legal, context. It may be that in an emergency a child may, in the absence of his parents, give legally valid consent.

10. This gives us the link between "responsible" in the dispositional sense explained here, and "responsible" in the blame-sense of the word ("I'll hold you responsible for that.").

11. The *caveat* must be added: natural contingencies do not have, as their *sole* result, the rendering of a person unfree, in the sense which vitiates consent: a man's brain tumor can make the man an idiot, schizophrenia can make a man insane, but these do not so much affect a person's volition as they do disturb his entire psychic structure.

12. David Daube, quoted in Beecher, p. 146.

13. *In re Gault*, 387 U.S. 1 (1967).

14. Beecher, p. 67.

15. See, for example, Paul Ramsey, "Consent as a Canon of Loyalty With Special Reference to Children in Medical Investigations," in *The Patient as Person* (New Haven: Yale University Press, 1970).

The Willowbrook Letters: Criticism and Defense

SIR.—You have referred to the work of Krugman and his colleagues at the Willowbrook State School in three editorials. In the first article the work was cited as a notable study of hepatitis and a model for this type of investigation. No comment was made on the rightness of attempting to infect mentally retarded children with hepatitis for experimental purposes, in an institution where the disease was already endemic.

The second editorial again did not remark on the ethics of the study, but the third sounded a note of doubt as to the justification for extending these experiments. The reason given was that some children might have been made more susceptible to serious hepatitis as the result of the administration of previously heated icterogenic material.

I believe that not only this last experiment, but the whole of Krugman's study, is quite unjustifiable, whatever the aims, and however academi-

cally or therapeutically important are the results. I am amazed that the work was published and that it has been actively supported editorially by the *Journal of the American Medical Association* and by Ingelfinger in the 1967–68 *Year Book of Medicine*. To my knowledge only the *British Journal of Hospital Medicine* has clearly stated the ethical position on these experiments and shown that it was indefensible to give potentially dangerous infected material to children, particularly those who were mentally retarded, with or without parental consent, when no benefit to the child could conceivably result.

Krugman and Giles have continued to publish the results of their study, and in a recent paper go to some length to describe their method of obtaining parental consent and list a number of influential medical boards and committees that have approved the study. They point out again that, in their opinion, their work conforms to the World

Reprinted by permission of the authors and publisher from The Lancet, *April 10, May 8, June 5, and July 10, 1971.*

Medical Association Draft Code of Ethics on Human Experimentation. They also say that hepatitis is still highly endemic in the school.

This attempted defence is irrelevant to the central issue. Is it right to perform an experiment on a normal or mentally retarded child when no benefit can result to that individual? I think that the answer is no, and that the question of parental consent is irrelevant. In my view the studies of Krugman serve only to show that there is a serious loophole in the Draft Code, which under General Principles and Definitions puts the onus of consent for experimentation on children on the parent or guardian. It is this section that is quoted by Krugman. I would class his work as "experiments conducted solely for the acquisition of knowledge," under which heading the code states that "persons retained in mental hospital or hospitals for mental defectives should not be used for human experiment." Krugman may believe that his experiments were for the benefit of his patients, meaning the individual patients used in the study. If this is his belief he has a difficult case to defend. The duty of a pediatrician in a situation such as exists at Willowbrook State School is to attempt to improve that situation, not to turn it to his advantage for experimental purposes, however lofty the aims.

Every new reference to the work of Krugman and Giles adds to its apparent ethical respectability, and in my view such references should stop, or at least be heavily qualified. The editorial attitude of *The Lancet* to the work should be reviewed and openly stated. The issue is too important to be ignored.

If Krugman and Giles are keen to continue their experiments I suggest that they invite the parents of the children involved to participate. I wonder what the response would be.

Stephen Goldby

SIR.—Dr. Stephen Goldby's critical comments about our Willowbrook studies and our motives for conducting them were published without extending us the courtesy of replying in the same issue of *The Lancet*. Your acceptance of his criticisms without benefit of our response implies a blackout of all comment related to our studies. This decision is unfortunate because our recent studies on active and passive immunisation for the prevention of viral hepatitis, type B, have clearly demonstrated a "therapeutic effect" for the children involved. These studies have provided us with the first indication and hope that it may be possible to control hepatitis in this institution. If this aim can be achieved, it will benefit not only the children, but also their families and the employees who care for them in the school. It is unnecessary to point out the additional benefit to the world-wide populations which have been plagued by an insoluble hepatitis problem for many generations.

Dr. Joan Giles and I have been actively engaged in studies aimed to solve two infectious-disease problems in the Willowbrook State School—measles and viral hepatitis. These studies were investigated in this institution because they represented major health problems for the 5000 or more mentally retarded children who were residents. Uninformed critics have assumed or implied that we came to Willowbrook to "conduct experiments on mentally retarded children."

The results of our Willowbrook studies with the experimental live attenuated measles vaccine developed by Enders and his colleagues are well documented in the medical literature. As early as 1960 we demonstrated the protective effect of this vaccine during the course of an epidemic. Prior to licensure of the vaccine in 1963 epidemics occurred at two-year intervals in this institution. During the 1960 epidemic there were more than 600 cases of measles and 60 deaths. In the wake of our ongoing measles vaccine programme, measles has been eradicated as a disease in the Willowbrook State School. We have not had a single case of measles since 1963. In this regard the children at the Willowbrook State School have been more fortunate than unimmunised children in Oxford, England, other areas in Great Britain, as well as certain groups of children in the United States and other parts of the world.

The background of our hepatitis studies at Willowbrook has been described in detail in various publications. Viral hepatitis is so prevalent that newly admitted susceptible children become infected within 6 to 12 months after entry in the institution. These children are a source of infection for the personnel who care for them and for their families if they visit with them. We were convinced that the solution of the hepatitis problem in this institution was dependent on the acquisition of new knowledge leading to the development of an effective immunising agent. The achievements with smallpox, diphtheria, poliomyelitis, and more recently measles represent dramatic illustrations of this approach.

It is well known that viral hepatitis in children is milder and more benign than the same disease in adults. Experience has revealed that hepatitis in institutionalised, mentally retarded children is also mild, in contrast with measles, which is a more severe disease when it occurs in institutional epidemics involving the mentally retarded. Our proposal to expose a small number of newly admitted children to the Willowbrook strains of hepatitis virus was justified in our opinion for the following reasons: (1) they were bound to be exposed to the same strains under the natural conditions existing in the institution; (2) they would be admitted to a special, well-equipped, and well-staffed unit where they would be isolated from exposure to other infectious diseases which were prevalent in the institution—namely, shigellosis, parasitic infections, and respiratory infections—thus, their exposure in the hepatitis unit would be associated with less risk than the type of institutional exposure where multiple infections could occur; (3) they were likely to have a subclinical infection followed by immunity to the particular hepatitis virus; and (4) only children with parents who gave informed consent would be included.

The statement by Dr. Goldby accusing us of conducting experiments exclusively for the acquisition of knowledge with no benefit for the children cannot be supported by the true facts.

Saul Krugman

SIR.—The experiments at Willowbrook raise two important issues: What constitutes valid consent, and do ends justify means? English law definitely forbids experimentation on children, even if both parents consent, unless done specifically in the interests of each individual child. Perhaps in the U.S.A the law is not so clear-cut. According to Beecher, the parents of the children at Willowbrook were informed that, because of overcrowding, the institution was to be closed; but only a week or two later they were told that there would be vacancies in the "hepatitis unit" for children whose parents allowed them to form part of the hepatitis research study. Such consent, ethically if not legally, is invalid because of its element of coercion, some parents being desperately anxious

to institutionalise their mentally defective children. Moreover, obtaining consent after talking to parents in groups, as described by Krugman, is extremely unsatisfactory because even a single enthusiast can sway the diffident who do not wish to appear churlish in front of their fellow citizens.

Do ends justify the means? Krugman maintains that any newly admitted children would inevitably have contracted infective hepatitis, which was rife in the hospital. But this ignores the statement by the head of the State Department of Mental Hygiene that, during the major part of the 15 years these experiments have been conducted, a gamma-globulin inoculation programme had already resulted in over an 80 percent reduction of that disease in that hospital. Krugman and Pasamanick claim that subsequent therapeutic effects justify these experiments. This attitude is frequently adopted by experimenters and enthusiastic medical writers who wish us to forget completely how results are obtained but instead enjoy any benefits that may accrue. Immunisation was not the purpose of these Willowbrook experiments but merely a by-product that incidentally proved beneficial to the victims. Any experiment is ethical or not at its inception, and does not become so because it achieved some measure of success in extending the frontiers of medicine. I particularly object strongly to the views of Willey, " . . . risk being assumed by the subjects of the experimentation balanced against the potential benefit to the subjects *and* [Willey's italics] to society in general." I believe that experimental physicians never have the right to select martyrs for society. Every human being has the right to be treated with decency, and that right must always supersede every consideration of what may benefit mankind, what may advance medical science, what may contribute to public welfare. No doctor is ever justified in placing society or science first and his obligation to patients second. Any claim to act for the good of society should be regarded with distaste because it may be merely a highflown expression to cloak outrageous acts.

M. H. Pappworth

SIR.—I am astonished at the unquestioning way in which *The Lancet* has accepted the intemperate position taken by Dr. Stephen Goldby concerning the experimental studies of Krugman and Giles on hepatitis at the Willowbrook State School. These investigators have repeatedly explained—for over a decade—that natural hepatitis infection occurs sooner or later in virtually 100% of the patients admitted to Willowbrook, and that it is better for the patient to have a known, timed, controlled infection than an untimed, uncontrolled one. Moreover, the wisdom and human justification of these studies have been repeatedly and carefully examined and verified by a number of very distinguished, able individuals who are respected leaders in the making of such decisions.

The real issue is: Is it not proper and ethical to carry out experiments in children, which would apparently incur no greater risk than the children were likely to run by nature, in which the children generally receive better medical care when artificially infected than if they had been naturally infected, and in which the parents as well as the physician feel that a significant contribution to the future well-being of similar children is likely to result from the studies? It is true, to be sure, that the W.M.A. code says, "Children in institutions and not under the care of relatives should not be the subjects of human experiments." But this unqualified *obiter dictum* may represent merely the well-known inability of committees to think a problem through. However, it has been thought through by Sir Austin Bradford Hill, who has pointed out the unfortunate effects for these very children that would have resulted, were such a code to have been applied over the years.

Geoffrey Edsall

Judgment on Willowbrook

Paul Ramsey

In 1958 and 1959 the *New England Journal of Medicine* reported a series of experiments performed upon patients and new admittees to the Willowbrook State School, a home for retarded children in Staten Island, New York.[1] These experiments were described as "an attempt to control the high prevalence of infectious hepatitis in an institution for mentally defective patients." The experiments were said to be justified because, under conditions of an existing controlled outbreak of hepatitis in the institution, "knowledge obtained from a series of suitable studies could well lead to its control." In actuality, the experiments were designed to duplicate and confirm the efficacy of gamma globulin in immunization against hepatitis, to develop and improve or improve upon that inoculum, and to learn more about infectious hepatitis in general.

The experiments were justified—doubtless, after a great deal of soul searching—for the following reasons: there was a smoldering epidemic throughout the institution and "it was apparent that most of the patients at Willowbrook were naturally exposed to hepatitis virus"; infectious hepatitis is a much milder disease in children; the strain at Willowbrook was especially mild; only the strain or strains of the virus already disseminated at Willowbrook were used; and only those small and incompetent patients whose parents gave consent were used.

The patient population at Willowbrook was 4478, growing at a rate of one patient a day over a three-year span, or from 10 to 15 new admissions per week. In the first trial the existing population was divided into two groups: one group served as uninoculated controls, and the other group was inoculated with 0.01 ml. of gamma globulin per pound of body weight. Then for a second trial new admittees and those left uninoculated before were again divided: one group served as uninoculated controls and the other was inoculated with 0.06 ml. of gamma globulin per pound of body weight. This proved that Stokes et al. had correctly demonstrated that the larger amount would give significant immunity for up to seven or eight months.[2]

Serious ethical questions may be raised about the trials so far described. No mention is made of any attempt to enlist the adult personnel of the institution, numbering nearly 1,000 including

Reprinted by permission of Yale University Press from The Patient as Person *by Paul Ramsey, copyright ©
1970 by Yale University. Editor's Note: The footnotes in this article have been renumbered.*

nearly 600 attendants on ward duty, and new additions to the staff, in these studies whose excusing reason was that almost everyone was "naturally" exposed to the Willowbrook virus. Nothing requires that major research into the natural history of hepatitis be first undertaken in children. Experiments have been carried out in the military and with prisoners as subjects. There have been fatalities from the experiments; but surely in all these cases the consent of the volunteers was as valid or better than the proxy consent of these children's "representatives." There would have been no question of the understanding consent that might have been given by the adult personnel at Willowbrook, if significant benefits were expected from studying that virus.

Second, nothing is said that would warrant withholding an inoculation of some degree of known efficacy from part of the population, or for withholding in the first trial less than the full amount of gamma globulin that had served to immunize in previous tests, except the need to test, confirm, and improve the inoculum. That, of course, was a desirable goal; but it does not seem possible to warrant withholding gamma globulin for the reason that is often said to justify controlled trials, namely, that one procedure is *as likely* to succeed as the other.

Third, nothing is said about attempts to control or defeat the low-grade epidemic at Willowbrook by more ordinary, if more costly and less experimental, procedures. Nor is anything said about admitting no more patients until this goal had been accomplished. This was not a massive urban hospital whose teeming population would have to be turned out into the streets, with resulting dangers to themselves and to public health, in order to sanitize the place. Instead, between 200 and 250 patients were housed in each of 18 buildings over approximately 400 acres in a semirural setting of fields, woods, and well-kept, spacious lawns. Clearly it would have been possible to secure other accommodation for new admissions away from the infection, while eradicating the infection at Willowbrook building by building. This might have cost money, and it would certainly have required astute detective work to discover the source of the infection. The doctors determined that the new patients likely were not carrying the infection upon admission, and that it did not arise from the procedures and routine inocula-

tions given them at the time of admission. Why not go further in the search for the source of the epidemic? If this had been an orphanage for normal children or a floor of private patients, instead of a school for mentally defective children, one wonders whether the doctors would so readily have accepted the hepatitis as a "natural" occurrence and even as an opportunity for study.

The next step was to attempt to induce "passive-active immunity" by feeding the virus to patients already protected by gamma globulin. In this attempt to improve the inoculum, permission was obtained from the parents of children from 5 to 10 years of age newly admitted to Willowbrook, who were then isolated from contact with the rest of the institution. All were inoculated with gamma globulin and then divided into two groups: one served as controls while the other group of new patients were fed the Willowbrook virus, obtained from feces, in doses having 50 percent infectivity, i.e., in concentrations estimated to produce hepatitis with jaundice in half the subjects tested. Then twice the 50 percent infectivity was tried. This proved, among other things, that hepatitis has an "alimentary-tract phase" in which it can be transmitted from one person to another while still "inapparent" in the first person. This, doubtless, is exceedingly important information in learning how to control epidemics of infectious hepatitis. The second of the two articles mentioned above describes studies of the incubation period of the virus and of whether pooled serum remained infectious when aged and frozen. Still the small, mentally defective patients who were deliberately fed infectious hepatitis are described as having suffered mildly in most cases: "The liver became enlarged in the majority, occasionally a week or two before the onset of jaundice. Vomiting and anorexia usually lasted only a few days. Most of the children gained weight during the course of hepatitis."

That mild description of what happened to the children who were fed hepatitis (and who continued to be introduced into the unaltered environment of Willowbrook) is itself alarming, since it is now definitely known that cirrhosis of the liver results from infectious hepatitis more frequently than from excessive consumption of alcohol! Now, or in 1958 and 1959, no one knows what may be other serious consequences of contracting infectious hepatitis. Understanding human volunteers were then and are now needed in the study of this disease, although a South American monkey has now successfully been given a form of hepatitis, and can henceforth serve as our ally in its conquest. But not children who cannot consent knowingly. If Peace Corps workers are regularly given gamma globulin before going abroad as a guard against their contracting hepatitis, and are inoculated at intervals thereafter, it seems that this is the least we should do for mentally defective children before they "go abroad" to Willowbrook or other institutions set up for their care.

Discussions pro and con of the Willowbrook experiments that have come to my attention serve only to reinforce the ethical objections that can be raised against what was done simply from a careful analysis of the original articles reporting the research design and findings. In an address at the 1968 Ross Conference on Pediatric Research, Dr. Saul Krugman raised the question, Should vaccine trials be carried out in adult volunteers before subjecting children to similar tests?[3] He answered this question in the negative. The reason adduced was simply that "a vaccine virus trial may be a more hazardous procedure for adults than for children." Medical researchers, of course, are required to minimize the hazards, but not by moving from consenting to unconsenting subjects. This apology clearly shows that adults and children have become interchangeable in face of the overriding importance of obtaining the research goal. This means that the special moral claims of children for care and protection are forgotten, and especially the claims of children who are most weak and vulnerable. (Krugman's reference to the measles vaccine trials is not to the point.)

The *Medical Tribune* explains that the 16-bed isolation unit set up at Willowbrook served "to protect the study subjects from Willowbrook's other endemic diseases—such as shigellosis, measles, rubella and respiratory and parasitic infections—while exposing them to hepatitis."[4] This presumably compensated for the infection they were given. It is not convincingly shown that the children could by no means, however costly, have been protected from the epidemic of hepatitis. The statement that Willowbrook "had endemic infectious hepatitis and a sufficiently open population so that the disease could never be quieted by exhausting the supply of susceptibles" is at best enigmatic.

Oddly, physicians defending the propriety of the Willowbrook hepatitis project soon begin talking like poorly instructed "natural lawyers"! Dr. Louis Lasagna and Dr. Geoffrey Edsall, for example, find these experiments unobjectionable—both, for the reason stated by Edsall: "the children would apparently incur no greater risk than they were likely to run by nature." In any case, Edsall's examples of parents consenting with a son 17 years of age for him to go to war, and society's agreements with minors that they can drive cars and hurt themselves were entirely beside the point. Dr. David D. Rutstein adheres to a stricter standard in regard to research on infectious hepatitis: "It is not ethical to use human subjects for the growth of a virus for any purpose."[5]

The latter sweeping verdict may depend on knowledge of the effects of viruses on chromasomal difficulties, mongolism, etc., that was not available to the Willowbrook group when their researches were begun thirteen years ago. If so, this is a telling point against appeal to "no discernible risks" as the sole standard applicable to the use of children in medical experimentation. That would lend support to the proposition that we always know that there are unknown and undiscerned risks in the case of an invasion of the fortress of the body—which then can be consented to by an adult in behalf of a child only if it is in the child's behalf medically.

When asked what she told the parents of the subject-children at Willowbrook, Dr. Joan Giles replied, "I explain that there is no vaccine against infectious hepatitis. . . . I also tell them that we can modify the disease with gamma globulin but we can't provide lasting immunity without letting them get the disease."[6] Obviously vaccines giving "lasting immunity" are not the only kinds of vaccine to be used in caring for patients.

Doubtless the studies at Willowbrook resulted in improvement in the vaccine, to the benefit of present and future patients. In September 1966, "a routine program of GG [gamma globulin] administration to every new patient at Willowbrook" was begun. This cut the incidence of icteric hepatitis 80 to 85 percent. Then follows a significant statement in the *Medical Tribune* article: "A similar reduction in the icteric form of the disease has been accomplished among the employees, who began getting routine GG earlier in the study."[7] Not only did the research team (so far as these reports show) fail to consider and adopt the alternative that new admittees to the staff be asked to become volunteers for an investigation that might improve the vaccine against the strain of infectious hepatitis to which they as well as the children were exposed. Instead, the staff was routinely protected earlier than the inmates were! And, as we have seen, there was evidence from the beginning that gamma globulin provided at least some protection. A "modification" of the disease was still an inoculum, even if this provided no lasting immunization and had to be repeated. It is axiomatic to medical ethics that a known remedy or protection—even if not perfect or even if the best exact administration of it has not been proved—should not be withheld from individual patients. It seems to a layman that from the beginning various trials at immunization of all new admittees might have been made, and controlled observation made of their different degrees of effectiveness against "nature" at Willowbrook. This would doubtless have been a longer way round, namely, the "anecdotal" method of investigative treatment that comes off second best in comparison with controlled trials. Yet this seems to be the alternative dictated by our received medical ethics, and the only one expressive of minimal care of the primary patients themselves.

Finally, except for one episode, the obtaining of parental consent (on the premise that this is ethically valid) seems to have been very well handled. Wards of the state were not used, though by law the administrator at Willowbrook could have signed consent for them. Only new admittees whose parents were available were entered by proxy consent into the project. Explanation was made to groups of these parents, and they were given time to think about it and consult with their own family physicians. Then late in 1964 Willowbrook was closed to all new admissions because of overcrowding. What then happened can most impartially be described in the words of an article defending the Willowbrook project on medical and ethical grounds:

> Parents who applied for their children to get in were sent a form letter over Dr. Hammond's signature saying that there was no space for new admissions and that their name was being put on a waiting list.
>
> But the hepatitis program, occupying its own space in the institution, continued to admit new patients as each new study group began. "Where do you find new admissions except by canvassing the people who have applied for admission?" Dr. Hammond asked.
>
> So a new batch of form letters went out, saying that there were a few vacancies in the hepatitis research unit if the parents cared to consider volunteering their child for that. In some instances the second form letter apparently was received as closely as a week after the first letter arrived.[8]

Granting—as I do not—the validity of parental consent to research upon children not in their behalf medically, what sort of consent was that? Surely, the duress upon these parents with children so defective as to require institutionalization was far greater than the duress on prisoners given tobacco or paid or promised parole for their cooperation! I grant that the timing of these events was inadvertent. Since, however, ethics is a matter of criticizing institutions and not only of exculpating or making culprits of individual men, the inadvertence does not matter. This is the strongest possible argument for saying that even if parents have the right to consent to submit the children who are directly and continuously in their care to nonbeneficial medical experimentation, this should not be the rule of practice governing institutions set up for their care.

Such use of captive populations of children for purely experimental purposes ought to be made legally impossible. My view is that this should be stopped by legal acknowledgement of the moral invalidity of parental or legal proxy consent for the child to procedures having no relation to a child's own diagnosis or treatment. If this is not done, canons of loyalty require that the rule of practice (by law, or otherwise) be that children in institutions and not directly under the care of parents or relatives should *never* be used in medical investigations having present pain or discomfort and unknown present and future risks to them, and promising future possible benefits only for others.

Notes

1. Robert Ward, Saul Krugman, Joan P. Giles, A. Milton Jacobs, and Oscar Bodansky, "Infectious Hepatitis: Studies of Its Natural History and Prevention," *New England Journal of Medicine* 258, no. 9 (February 27, 1958): 407–16; Saul Krugman,

Robert Ward, Joan P. Giles, Oscar Bodansky, and A. Milton Jacobs, "Infectious Hepatitis: Detection of the Virus during the Incubation Period and in Clinically Inapparent Infection," *New England Journal of Medicine* 261, no. 15 (October 8, 1959): 729–34. The following account and unannotated quotations are taken from these articles.

2.   J. Stokes, Jr., et al., "Infectious Hepatitis: Length of Protection by Immune Serum Globulin (Gamma Globulin) during Epidemics," *Journal of the American Medical Association* 147 (1951): 714–19. Since the half-life of gamma globulin is three weeks, no one knows exactly why it immunizes for so long a period. The "highly significant protection against hepatitis obtained by the use of gamma globulin," however, had been confirmed as early as 1945 (see Edward B. Grossman, Sloan G. Stewart, and Joseph Stokes, "Post-Transfusion Hepatitis in Battle Casualties," *Journal of the American Medical Association* 129, no. 15 [December 8, 1945]: 991–94). The inoculation *withheld* in the Willowbrook experiments had, therefore, proved valuable.

3.   Saul Krugman, "Reflections on Pediatric Clinical Investigations," in *Problems of Drug Evaluation in Infants and Children*, Report of the Fifty-eighth Ross Conference on Pediatric Research, Dorado Beach, Puerto Rico, May 5–7, 1968 (Columbus: Ross Laboratories), pp. 41–42.

4.   "Studies with Children Backed on Medical, Ethical Grounds," *Medical Tribune and Medical News* 8, no. 19 (February 20, 1967): 1, 23.

5.   *Daedalus*, Spring 1969, pp. 471–72, 529. See also pp. 458, 470–72. Since it is the proper business of an ethicist to uphold the proposition that only retrogression in civility can result from bad moral reasoning and the use of inept examples, however innocent, it is fair to point out the startling comparison between Edsall's "argument" and the statement of Dr. Karl Brandt, plenipotentiary in charge of all medical activities in the Nazi Reich: "Do you think that one can obtain any worth-while, fundamental results without a definite toll of lives? The same goes for technological development. You cannot build a great bridge, a gigantic building—you cannot establish a speed record without deaths!" (quoted by Leo Alexander, "War Crimes: Their Social-Psychological Aspects," *American Journal of Psychiatry* 105, no. 3 [September 1948]: 172). Casualties to progress, or injuries accepted in setting speed limits, are morally quite different from death or maiming or even only risks, or unknown risks, directly and deliberately imposed upon an unconsenting human being.

6.   *Medical Tribune*, February 20, 1967, p. 23.

7.   *Medical Tribune*, February 20, 1967, p. 23.

8.   *Medical Tribune*, February 20, 1967, p. 23.

Principles of the Nuremberg Code

1. The voluntary consent of the human subject is absolutely essential.

2. The experiment should be such as to yield fruitful results for the good of society, unprocurable by other methods or means of study, and not random and unnecessary in nature.

3. The experiment should be so designed and based on the results of animal experimentation and a knowledge of the natural history of the disease or other problem under study that the anticipated results will justify the performance of the experiment.

4. The experiment should be so conducted as to avoid all unnecessary physical and mental suffering and injury.

5. No experiment should be conducted where there is an a priori reason to believe that death or disabling injury will occur; except, perhaps, in those experiments where the experimental physicians also serve as subjects.

6. The degree of risk to be taken should never exceed that determined by the humanitarian importance of the problem to be solved by the experiment.

7. Proper preparations should be made and adequate facilities provided to protect the experimental subject against even remote possibilities of injury, disability, or death.

8. The experiment should be conducted only by scientifically qualified persons. The highest de-

From Trials of War Criminals before the Nuremberg Military Tribunals under Control Council Law No. 10, *vol. 2, pp. 181–182. Washington, D.C.: United States Government Printing Office, 1949.*

gree of skill and care should be required through all stages of the experiment of those who conduct or engage in the experiment.

9. During the course of the experiment the human subject should be at liberty to bring the experiment to an end if he has reached the physical or mental state where continuation of the experiment seems to him to be impossible.

10. During the course of the experiment the scientist in charge must be prepared to terminate the experiment at any stage, if he has probable cause to believe, in the exercise of good faith, superior skill and careful judgment required of him that a continuation of the experiment is likely to result in injury, disability, or death to the experimental subject.

Principles of the Declaration of Helsinki

World Medical Association

I. Basic Principles

1. Biomedical research involving human subjects must conform to generally accepted scientific principles and should be based on adequately performed laboratory and animal experimentation and on a thorough knowledge of the scientific literature.

2. The design and performance of each experimental procedure involving human subjects should be clearly formulated in an experimental protocol which should be transmitted to a specially appointed independent committee for consideration, comment, and guidance.

3. Biomedical research involving human subjects should be conducted only by scientifically qualified persons and under the supervision of a clinically competent medical person. The responsibility for the human subject must always rest with a medically qualified person and never rest on the subject of research, even though the subject has given his or her consent.

4. Biomedical research involving human subjects cannot legitimately be carried out unless the importance of the objective is in proportion to the inherent risk to the subject.

5. Every biomedical research project involving human subjects should be preceded by careful assessment of predictable risks in comparison with foreseeable benefits to the subject or to others. Concern for the interests of the subject must always prevail over the interests of science and society.

6. The right of the research subject to safeguard his or her integrity must always be respected. Every precaution should be taken to respect the privacy of the subject and to minimize the impact of the study on the subject's physical and mental integrity and on the personality of the subject.

7. Doctors should abstain from engaging in research projects involving human subjects unless they are satisfied that the hazards involved are believed to be predictable. Doctors should cease any investigation if the hazards are found to outweigh the potential benefits.

8. In publication of the results of his or her research, the doctor is obliged to preserve the accuracy of the results. Reports of experimentation not in accordance with the principles laid down in this Declaration should not be accepted for publication.

9. In any research on human beings, each potential subject must be adequately informed of the aims, methods, anticipated benefits and potential hazards of the study and the discomfort it may entail. He or she should be informed that he or she is at liberty to abstain from participation in the study and that he or she is free to withdraw his or her consent to participation at any time. The doctor should then obtain the subject's freely given informed consent, preferably in writing.

10. When obtaining informed consent for the research project the doctor should be particularly cautious if the subject is in a dependent rela-

Adopted by the 18th World Medical Assembly, Helsinki, Finland, 1964, and revised by the 29th World Medical Assembly, Tokyo, Japan, October 1975. Reprinted with permission of the World Medical Association, Inc. from the "Declaration of Helsinki," revised edition.

tionship to him or her or may consent under duress. In that case the informed consent should be obtained by a doctor who is not engaged in the investigation and who is completely independent of this official relationship.

11. In case of legal incompetence, informed consent should be obtained from the legal guardian in accordance with national legislation. Where physical or mental incapacity makes it impossible to obtain informed consent, or when the subject is a minor, permission from the responsible relative replaces that of the subject in accordance with national legislation.

12. The research protocol should always contain a statement of the ethical consideration involved and should indicate that the principles enunciated in the present Declaration are complied with.

II. Medical Research combined with Professional Care (Clinical Research)

1. In the treatment of the sick person, the doctor must be free to use a new diagnostic and therapeutic measure, if in his or her judgment it offers hope of saving life, reestablishing health or alleviating suffering.

2. The potential benefits, hazards and discomfort of a new method should be weighed against the advantages of the best current diagnostic and therapeutic methods.

3. In any medical study, every patient—including those of a control group, if any—should be assured of the best proven diagnostic and therapeutic method.

4. The refusal of the patient to participate in a study must never interfere with the doctor-patient relationship.

5. If the doctor considers it essential not to obtain informed consent, the specific reasons for this proposal should be stated in the experimental protocol for transmission to the independent committee (I, 2).

6. The doctor can combine medical research with professional care, the objective being the acquisition of new medical knowledge, only to the extent that medical research is justified by its potential diagnostic or therapeutic value for the patient.

III. Non-therapeutic Biomedical Research involving Human Subjects (Non-clinical Biomedical Research)

1. In any purely scientific application of medical research carried out on a human being, it is the duty of the doctor to remain the protector of the life and health of that person on whom biomedical research is being carried out.

2. The subjects should be volunteers—either healthy persons or patients for whom the experimental design is not related to the patient's illness.

3. The investigator or the investigating team should discontinue the research if in his/her or their judgment it may, if continued, be harmful to the individual.

4. In research on man, the interest of science and society should never take precedence over considerations related to the well-being of the subject.

Decision Scenario 1

You are an agent of the Ethics Committee of the National Association of Physicians. You have been sent to Laural, Mississippi, to look into the experimental work of Dr. Joseph Camwell at the Laural State Hospital.

"Our basic concern," Dr. Camwell tells you, "was to test the effectiveness of a hormone-based substance in controlling conception by the regulation of ovulation."

"A birth control pill."

"Exactly," says Dr. Camwell. "We ran a double-blind test with HB-4, the test substance, and a sucrose-based compound flavored and shaped to be phenomenologically indistinguishable from the tablets of HB-4."

"So that neither the experimenter nor the subjects knew who was getting HB-4 and who was getting the sugar pills. But who were your test subjects?"

"Patients who presented themselves at our state-sponsored outpatient clinic and requested contraceptive medication formed our candidate population. We drew from them subjects with a good medical history, and no present major illnesses, who seemed reliable enough to take their medications on schedule."

"What were the racial percentages?"

"We didn't consider that to be a relevant factor in the experiment. It just happened that about 90 percent of our subjects were black, although race was not a criterion for selection."

"Did you secure from these women their informed consent to be subjects in this experiment?"

"Of course," Dr. Camwell says. "I personally explained to each of them that they were going to participate in an experiment but that it wouldn't hurt them any. I told them they would be given birth control pills that we were testing for effectiveness. 'You might get pregnant while you're taking these pills,' I said."

"But you didn't tell them that at least half of them would be receiving sugar pills that would do absolutely nothing to prevent pregnancy?"

"I think that I warned them sufficiently," says Dr. Camwell. "I told them they might get pregnant. None of these women is able to understand medical sophistications. If I tried to tell them about the experiment, they wouldn't understand me. They knew they might get pregnant, and I figured that was enough."

"Did they all agree to participate?"

"Every last person we approached agreed to participate," Dr. Camwell says. "People always want to help out doctors, and they'll do it if you just put it to them in the right way. I never have any trouble getting subjects for my work."

Would you recommend to the ethics committee that Dr. Camwell's consent procedures be condemned? If so, on what grounds?

Camwell apparently endorses Ingelfinger's view that informed consent is impossible. Evaluate this claim.

What sort of information would have to be provided to the potential subjects to satisy the principles of informed consent argued for by Freedman?

Decision Scenario 2

"In effect," said Dr. Sanchez, "the drug is a powerful tranquilizer. We are not sure how it works, but we know that it has a great calming effect on people diagnosed as schizophrenics. It's much like thorazine, which you may have heard of."

"Does it have any side effects?" Monica Jones asked.

"If taken over a period of a couple of weeks, it produces a palsied condition—muscular tremors, difficulty in walking and in controlling the face muscles, and so on. These don't seem to be permanent."

"That's in schizophrenics," Monica said.

"That's right. We don't know the likely effects in other people. Perhaps you will notice no change whatsoever, and perhaps you will never develop the muscular tremors. But perhaps you'll develop them sooner or more severely. That's part of what we need to find out."

"I'm not in danger of death, then?"

"Not to any great extent. That is, all medication has associated with it some risk. But we don't believe the risk here to be great. There is some possibility of long-term nerve or brain damage. We simply don't know the risks here."

"And you need so-called normal people like me to act as subjects so that you can compare the effects of the drug on us with its effects on schizophrenics?"

"Exactly right," said Dr. Sanchez. "But I should tell you that you may not get the drug. None of us involved in the experiment as patients or experimenters will know who is getting the tranquilizer and who is getting a placebo."

"So maybe I'm not running any risk at all," said Monica.

"Maybe not. But your participation is still important. This drug may do much to relieve the symptoms of a great number of schizophrenics."

"Now if I understand correctly," said Monica Jones, "I will be paid for my participation."

"That's right. You will be paid a flat fee for participation—half at the beginning of the study and the rest at the end. I want you to be clear on one thing, however. You must waive your right to claim compensation due to any injury or ill-effects you may suffer as a result of the medication."

"I understand that. I've got to take a risk. I'm not too happy about that, but I can't get a job and I need the money so I can go back to school next semester."

"Fine," said Dr. Sanchez. "I have the consent forms right here."

Is risking one's health for financial gain compatible with Rawls's principles of justice?

Do Kant's principles allow one to take such a risk?

Does the natural law doctrine of Catholicism?

Would the view of human experimentation advocated by Jonas regard such an experiment as legitimate? Would the view of Lasagna? Would Freedman's theory allow such a financial transaction?

Do you think it is possible for Sanchez to give Jones good reasons for participating that do not involve some form of pressure or duress?

Decision Scenario 3

The drug DES—diethylstilbestrol—was once believed to be effective in preventing miscarriages. But in 1971 sufficient evidence was available to establish a link between DES and vaginal cancer and cervical cell abnormalities in the daughters of women given the drug. About one million women were given DES in the first trimester of pregnancy, and over 120 daughters of these women have been shown to have cancer. Sons, apparently, do not develop cancer, but the group shows a higher than average proportion of genital abnormalities and sterility.

In late 1951 and early 1952, women receiving prenatal care at the University of Chicago's Lying-In Hospital were given unmarked tablets of DES as part of a study conducted by Dr. William Dieckmann. One of those receiving the tablets was Ms. Patsy T. Mink, who later became an Assistant Secretary of State.

"I remember quite clearly the doctor giving me those pills and telling me they were vitamins," Ms. Mink says.

Ms. Mink's daughter Gwendolyn was born in the hospital in 1952. Ms. Mink was not notified that she had been given DES until twenty-four years later. She rushed her daughter to a medical examination, and it was discovered that Gwendolyn had abnormal cell changes in the cervix—a condition known as adenosis and thought to be a precursor of cancer.

Ms. Mink is outraged by the experiment in which she was an unwitting subject. She feels that she was not given the drug for a legitimate medical reason and that she was deceived by her doctor. "There's no way we could know," she says. "If they had given me a choice, if they had said, 'We think you are a risk case and this drug may help you, that's different,' that's the choice we should have been presented with. But I wasn't a risk case, and I wasn't told anything."

Is Ms. Mink's moral outrage justified?

Did those who gave her DES act immorally? After all, at the time she was given the drug there was no reason to believe that it might have harmful effects.

If Ms. Mink's informed consent had been obtained, the outcome would have been exactly the same because she could not have been warned of dangers that no one knew existed. Doesn't this show that the whole notion of informed consent is pointless and that one simply must trust in the integrity and best judgment of a physician, as Ingelfinger suggests?

Decision Scenario 4

"You realize," Dr. Thorne said, "that you may not be in the group that receives medication? You may be in the placebo group for at least part of the time."

"Right," Ms. Ross said. "You're just going to give me some medicine."

"And do you understand the aims of the experiment?"

"You want to help me get better," Ms. Ross suggested hesitantly.

"We hope you get better, of course. But that's not what we're trying to accomplish here. We're trying to find out if this particular medication will help other people in your condition if we can treat them earlier than we were able to treat you."

"You want to help people," Ms. Ross said.

"That's right. Now, do you understand that we may not be helping you in this experiment?"

"But you're going to try?"

"Not exactly. I mean, we aren't going to try to harm you. But we aren't necessarily going to be giving you the preferred treatment for your complaint either. Do you know the difference between research and therapy?"

"Research is when you're trying to find something out. You're searching around."

"That's right. And we're asking you to be part of a research effort. As I told you, there are some risks. Besides the possibility of not getting treatment that you need, the drug may produce some limited hepatic portal damage. We're not sure how much."

"I think I understand," Ms. Ross said.

"I hope so," said Dr. Thorne. "Now I understand that you are freely volunteering to participate in this research."

"Yes, sir. Mrs. Woolerd, she told me if I volunteered I'd get a letter put in my file and I could get early release."

"Mrs. Woolerd told you the Review Board would take your volunteering into account when they considered whether you should be put on work-release."

"Yes, sir. And I'm awfully anxious to get out of here. I've got two children staying with my aunt, and I need to get out of this place quick as I can."

"I understand. We can't promise you release, of course. But your participation will look good on your record. Now I have some papers here I want you to sign."

Discuss some of the difficulties involved in explaining research procedures to nonexperts and determining whether they are aware of the nature and risks of their participation.

What reasons are there for believing that Ms. Ross does not understand what she is volunteering for?

Also discuss the problems involved in securing free and voluntary consent from a person involuntarily confined to an institution (a prisoner, for example).

Is there a reason to believe that Ms. Ross is not giving free consent?

What conditions does Freedman require satisfied before a prisoner's consent can be regarded as legitimate?

Decision Scenario 5

The ad in the newspapers was simple and uninformative:

Subjects (male and female) wanted to
participate in scientific study. Must be 21 or
over. $2.00 per hour.

Karen Barty wrote down the address. She could use the money, and in 1962 $2.00 an hour wasn't bad pay for what was sure to be very little work. Besides, the hours were probably flexible, and she could fit the time into her class schedule.

Next Tuesday morning at ten o'clock, Karen and nine other people reported to room 711 of the Basic Sciences Building in the Western Medical Center. A man who introduced himself as Dr. Carlo Raphael explained what would be required of them as research subjects.

"First of all, you must all sign consent forms," he said. "These state that you are voluntary participants in this study and that for your assistance you will receive a financial reward. If you are not willing to sign the forms, then we cannot accept you as a subject."

He interrupted himself to pass out badly mimeographed sheets of paper that had "Voluntary Consent of Research Subjects" printed at the top. Karen signed hers at once, without bothering to read it. The others in her group, she noticed, did the same thing.

"Very good," Dr. Raphael said, after collecting the forms. "We are going to ask that you provide us with the answers to a series of questions. Some of you may think of these as 'tests,' but I want to assure you that they are not tests in the way you ordinarily think of them. You can neither pass or fail. Just give us your immediate and truthful responses."

With the help of two assistants, Dr. Raphael distributed test booklets with coded answer sheets tucked inside. Everyone was then supplied with a black IBM pencil with soft, black lead.

Karen listened, half bored, as Dr. Raphael explained how the answer sheets were to be filled in. She had heard the same kind of explanation a dozen times before, but she guessed that the same thing always had to be said as part of the test procedure. Despite herself, she felt a twinge of anxiety. It was all well and good to say these weren't tests they were taking, but they were enough like every other test she had taken to make her adrenalin flow.

At noon, they handed in their test booklets and took a break for lunch. When they reported back, it was to another room in the same building. It was not a classroom this time, but a lounge. Steel-framed chairs and sofas covered in grey and orange plastic were set about the room, and the floor was covered with beige carpet, its industrial finish looking flat and somewhat dirty.

A long table at the front was draped with white crepe paper, and pitchers of water surrounded by glasses were set at one end. At the opposite end, a red cafeteria tray with small paper cups was watched over by a woman Karen hadn't seen before.

The cups looked like the sort that are usually filled with nuts or hard candies. When Karen got close enough, she saw that each cup contained only what looked like a single cube of sugar.

That's what it tasted like when Karen got hers. Dr. Raphael lined up the ten subjects, and as each one reached the table, the woman handed over one of the cups.

"Let the cube dissolve in your mouth," Dr. Raphael told them. "Then have some water, if you like, but don't eat or drink anything else. Then you may just sit around in this room and talk to each other."

It was pretty disgusting, just eating plain sugar. But within twenty minutes,

Karen knew that it wasn't just plain sugar. She was sitting on one of the sofas talking to another woman about an English group called the Beatles. The woman had never heard of them, and Karen spelled the name for her.

But as she started to spell it, she suddenly found it very hard to concentrate. She knew where she was and what she was doing, but the woman in front of her began to look strange. She seemed to be surrounded by a halo of brightly colored light. The features of her face lost their outlines and became twisted and distorted.

In a few minutes, Karen gave up trying to talk. Somewhere at the back of her mind, she felt fear and confusion. But what was happening to her wasn't unpleasant. It was interesting, really, and she surrendered herself to the fantastic images that seemed to take over her mind without her being able to control them.

Somewhere in that time, Karen fell asleep or at least she thought she did. She vaguely remembered one of Dr. Raphael's assistants holding her by the arm and leading her back to the classroom. She tried to talk to him, but she wasn't sure what she said. When she was handed another test booklet, she was surprised to find how easy it was to fill out the answer sheet. This time there was no anxiety at all.

By five o'clock that afternoon, Karen was herself again. It was not until seventeen years later that she realized she had been an unwitting participant in a research project sponsored by the army to determine the psychological effects of LSD.

> *What kind of information would Karen Barty have had to be given to satisfy Freedman's principles of informed consent?*
>
> *On what grounds would Jonas disapprove of the way in which Karen was employed as a subject?*
>
> *This was clearly a case of nontherapeutic research. Can a case be made for it on utilitarian grounds?*
>
> *Does Karen have any grounds for claiming compensation if in years after the research she suffers from effects that may reasonably be attributed to her participation as a subject?*
>
> *Suppose that Dr. Raphael had fully informed the group about the nature and aims of the research and warned them about potential dangers. Given that very little was known in 1962 about the possible effects of LSD, would any person be justified in risking life or health by participating in the experiment?*

Decision Scenario 6

"That is truly absurd," Dr. Kuhmwar Raita said. "The mother wanted to get rid of the fetus. That's why she elected to have the abortion in the first place. The fetus has no status. It's just a lump of tissue."

Dr. Alan Smith shook his head in disagreement. "It is not, Kuhmwar. That's just the point. The fetus is not viable, but it's out of the uterus and alive at this very instant."

"Well, it will be dead in a short while, then it will be of no use to me. If I'm going to find out anything about cerebral glucose uptake, I've got to have a functioning system."

"But we can't just kill this child."

"The child, as you call it, is as good as dead. And if we can ever gain an understanding of the fundamental processes involved here, we may actually be able to save the lives of countless babies."

"I can't believe you would resort to such a crude argument."

"Call it whatever you want to, but I think it's right."

Is it possible to construct a utilitarian argument to support the position taken by Dr. Raita?

In what way is the status of the fetus relevant to this issue of fetal experimentation?

Are the issues of fetal experimentation exactly analogous to the arguments about abortion? Or are they more closely analogous to the arguments about human experimentation?

What view might a Kantian take on this question?

Decision Scenario 7

In April of 1979, a suit was filed in Illinois by the Cook County Public Guardian against the Illinois Department of Mental Health. The suit alleged that during the 1950s and 1960s between twenty-five and one hundred patients underwent "unauthorized and secret" surgery at a state mental health center.

The suit charged that the patients, without their consent, were subjected to experimental surgery to remove their adrenal glands. A memo from a psychiatrist was cited that described the health center as "virtually a human dog lab."

A spokesman for the mental health department publicly denied the charges in the suit. He claimed that an internal investigation showed that consent from the patients had been obtained and each had been informed of the possible risks and of the short- and long-term effects.

Moreover, the surgery was said to have a therapeutic aim, as well as an experimental one. A theory at the time suggested that the removal of the adrenal gland might correct a hormonal imbalance that some research psychiatrists believed to be a cause of schizophrenia. Furthermore, it was claimed that only four schizophrenic patients were involved.

As a matter of fact, the surgery did not lead to improvement in any of the patients, and the theory which suggested that it might is no longer held. Those who had their adrenal glands removed required injections of cortisone for the rest of their lives to compensate for the loss of natural secretions from the gland.

Suppose that the charge made by the Public Guardian is correct. What utilitarian argument might be offered to support the use of mental patients as subjects in the experimental sugery?

Clearly the only proper candidates for an experimental procedure aimed at treating schizophrenia are people who are schizophrenics. Is it reasonable to believe that people who suffer from a psychosis are capable of giving informed consent?

On Freedman's view, would proxy consent obtained for such people be legitimate?

Is it possible to argue on Kantian grounds that patients diagnosed as psychotic ought to be allowed to consent to any procedure that may help their condition? If not, why not?

How relevant to the moral issue of consent is the nonmoral question of the degree of confirmation of a theory which is the basis of an experimental procedure with a therapeutic aim?

Part III
CONTROLS

6
BEHAVIOR CONTROL AND PSYCHOSURGERY

CASE PRESENTATION
The Agents

She woke up feeling terrible. Her muscles ached and she was sure the Agents had been injecting her with gold again. That was why her body felt so heavy. She could see the gold in the veins in her wrists, and she knew it was also circulating through her brain. The gold made it very hard to think.

Her mother had gotten gold injections once, she remembered. It was for arthritis, her mother told her. Nancy had believed that then, but now she knew that it was really the Agents who had done it. Now they wanted to control her the way they controlled her mother.

It was only half an hour before her first class at ten o'clock, and she knew she would have to hurry. It took almost twenty minutes to walk from the dorm to Hamilton, and the Agents hated it when she was late. They would criticize her and tell her how worthless she was and how disappointed her parents would be if they knew what she had done.

Her suitemates were already gone, so she had the kitchen to herself as she boiled water for instant coffee. She took the coffee to the table in the hall and sat down to look over her Contemporary Civilization assignment. She hadn't read the Aquinas selection yet so she skimmed it quickly.

She found it very hard to concentrate. Then the Agents began to talk to her. They were starting to do that more often. This time the voice came from Susan's stereo. It was the Agent Nancy called Ostra. She wasn't sure that was his name, but she thought he had told her that once.

"You really need more sex," Ostra said. "Why don't you let Bill Hanley do it to you. He's really good-looking and has a nice body. Wouldn't that feel really good?"

She kept her eyes on her CC book and tried not to listen. The Agents talked about sex so much it was incredible. She hardly thought about it at all herself. And she barely knew Bill Hanley. He was in her biology class, and once he had asked to see her notes for a day he had cut. That was the only conversation they had ever had.

In the last couple of weeks, though, the Agents were always bringing up Bill Hanley. Sometimes they said things that were so explicit and so gross she could hardly stand to hear them. They embarrassed her and made her feel frightened. Now when she went to biology class she couldn't even make herself look at Bill Hanley.

The coffee tasted strange. It had a metallic flavor. It was probably the gold, she thought. The Agents were filling her up with gold. That way they could control her better. Already, they were making her think about sex all the time. Once, in a bar near campus, they made her proposition someone she had just met. She didn't go through with it, but next time she might not be able to resist. The Agents were a lot more powerful than she.

She got up and put on her coat, but she wasn't going to go to class. It was pointless. In the last month, she had attended only about half the time. At first, her suitemates had been worried about her, but after a couple of weeks they all left her alone. They had their own lives to live. Susan and Bonnie, in particular, had been hurt by the way she started staying away from them. They told her how much she had changed and how much they missed the fun they all had together. Sometimes it made her feel sad when she thought about it, but she no longer thought about it much. It was just too hard to be with people.

She opened the window and leaned out to look down at the street. It was noisy and busy. A panel truck was parked by the coffee shop on the corner, and cars were jammed up waiting for the light to change. It was only the middle of October, but the wind blowing up from the river was cold. Fifteen stories up, things seemed unreal.

When Susan found her, she was crouched on the window sill. The toes of her jogging shoes extended over the edge, and her arms were wrapped around her bent legs.

Susan told Bonnie later, "I don't know whether she was going to jump or not. But even if she wasn't, it wouldn't have taken much to make her fall."

The incident was upsetting to Susan. She was particularly bothered by the fact that Nancy seemed so cut off from the world around her. "She was like a zombie," Susan said. "I don't think she even recognized me."

Nancy made no protest when Susan insisted that she accompany her to the Student Health Service. Susan sat with her until one of the physicians on duty was available to see her. Susan insisted on telling the physician how she had discovered Nancy and why she had brought her to the Health Service.

After Susan left, Nancy answered Dr. Branson's questions. But when he asked her to sign the voluntary commitment form, which would allow the hospital to confine her for a maximum of fourteen days, she refused.

"I'm sorry you won't sign," Dr. Branson told her. "From what you've said and from what your friend told me, I think you might try to harm yourself. Do you think that's possible?"

"I don't know," Nancy said. "I suppose so."

"Under the law, in such a case, I have the power to keep you here for twenty-four hours. After that, there has to be a court hearing, even if your parents consent to your being hospitalized."

"You're going to call my parents?"

"I have to do that. You're still a legal minor. But no matter what they say, I have to hospitalize you."

"Then there's nothing I can do about it?"

"I hope we can help you and that you won't have to be here long."

Dr. Branson entered a diagnosis of "schizophrenia—paranoid type" on Nancy's chart. He admitted her to the closed ward of the hospital in which the Student Health Service was located and made arrangements for her to be seen by a staff psychiatrist that afternoon. The psychiatrist prescribed an antipsychotic medication and prepared a report to be submitted by the hospital's legal department at a court hearing. The hearing never took place, however. The next day, after talking with her parents on the telephone, Nancy signed a voluntary commitment form.

Nancy remained hospitalized for six weeks. After her release, she dropped her courses and moved back to her family home. Her parents arranged for her to continue to see a psychiatrist on a weekly basis, and she continued a program of drug treatment and psychotherapy. The following academic year, she signed up for three classes at a college near her home. She no longer received messages from the Agents, but her psychiatrist warned her that she must not be surprised if they appeared again. With help she could look forward to a relatively normal life.

CASE PRESENTATION
The Detroit Psychosurgery Case

Lafayette Clinic is a research facility in Detroit that is part of the Michigan Department of Mental Health. In 1972, the director of the clinic was Dr. J. S. Gottlieb, a psychiatrist, and its chief of neurology was Dr. Ernst Rodin. Both Rodin and Gottlieb had read the book *Violence and the Brain*, by V. H. Mark and F. R. Ervin, shortly after its publication in 1970. They discussed the work and agreed that some of the techniques it described might be useful in treating patients suffering from uncontrollable sexual and aggressive impulses.

Rodin wrote a description of a research project they might conduct: "Proposal for the Study of the Treatment of Uncontrollable Aggression at Lafayette Clinic." The research was to involve a comparative study of the value of surgical versus drug treatment of aggressive patients. The surgical part of the project proposed implanting depth-electrodes in the brains of twelve subjects to study their brain activity and to attempt to locate areas of electrical abnormality. If such an area was found and if, by brain stimulation, it could be linked to aggressive behavior, then stereotactic surgery would be performed. (Stereotactic surgery involves locating relatively precise areas by using careful measurements.) The target areas would then be either resectioned (cut out) or destroyed by electrocoagulation. The ultimate aim of the project was said to be to restore patients to a "useful life" in the community.

The proposal, which requested $164,000, was submitted to the State Department of Mental Health. It was approved and included in the Department's legislative budget request. Although the state legislature held two hearings, no questions were raised about the Rodin proposal. The money was made available in July, 1972.

Even before the allocation of funds, a search was being conducted for suitable subjects. The candidates were those confined in state institutions under the Michigan "Criminal Sexual Psychopath" law. These were people charged with serious sex crimes who were not prosecuted but confined involuntarily for an indeterminate period of time until considered sufficiently "cured" for release.

One such person, identified for the record only as John Doe, was approached by Dr. E. G. Yudashkin, the Director of Ionia State Hospital where Doe was confined. Yudashkin described the project to Doe and told him he would probably be released within six months or a year whether or not he participated. But he also pointed out that successful treatment in the research project would lead to an even speedier release.

Doe was not interested in the drug part of the research program but thought he might volunteer for the surgical part. Yudashkin and two staff physicians explained to him on three occasions what this might involve. But the knowledge of the physicians on this topic was not extensive, and Doe later testified that they gave him a misleadingly simple account. But at the time, Doe decided to consent to becoming a subject, and Rodin was informed of this.

Rodin had decided that it was necessary to broaden the population of candidates from which subjects were to be selected. He had gone to Boston and talked with Vernon Mark about the project, and Mark had been critical of the ethical aspects. Rodin wrote in a memo to Gottlieb:

> When I informed Dr. Mark of our project, namely doing amygdalotomies on patients who do not have epilepsy, he became extremely concerned and stated we had no ethical right in so doing. . . . I then retorted that he was misleading us with his previously cited book and he had no right at all from a scientific point of view to state that in the human, aggression is accompanied by seizure discharges in the amygdala, because he is dealing only with patients who have susceptible brains, namely, temporal lobe epilepsy. . . .
>
> He stated categorically that as far as present evidence is concerned, one has no right to make lesions in a "healthy brain" when the individual suffers from rage attacks only.

Rodin discussed this matter with colleagues, and they decided not to do surgery on patients without verifiable organic brain dysfunctions. They expanded the population to be considered to include retarded, epileptic, and self-mutilating patients.

Lafayette Clinic's Human and Animal Experimentation Committee reviewed the project description and procedures and a draft of the informed-consent form. The committee, charged with protecting the rights and welfare of experimental subjects, raised no questions about the moral issues in the project. They approved it in October of 1972.

The project, as approved, required establishing two review committees to supervise patient selection and to protect patients from unethical practices. The three-member Medical Review Committee was to consider the medical condition and history of potential subjects recommended by Rodin. They were to eliminate patients unsuitable from a medical standpoint. After screening, a three-member Human Rights Review Committee was to determine for each patient whether informed consent was adequate and whether any rights were being infringed. After approval by both committees, a patient would then be given a consent form and a detailed explanation of the procedure to be performed on him. Then he and his family would have a week to consider whether they wished to sign the consent form.

None of this procedure was followed in the case of John Doe. Rodin met with John Doe on October 27. They discussed Doe's medical history for an hour, and at the end Doe indicated that he still wanted to participate in the project as a subject. Rodin read him the consent form, which read in part:

> Since conventional treatment efforts over a period of several years have not enabled me to control my outbursts of rage and anti-social behavior, I submit an application to be a subject in a research project which may offer me a form of effective therapy. This therapy is based upon the idea that episodes of anti-social rage and sexuality might be triggered by a disturbance in certain portions of my brain. I understand that in order to be certain that a significant brain disturbance exists, which might relate to my anti-social behavior, an initial operation will have to be performed. This procedure consists of placing fine wires into my brain, which will record the electrical activity from those structures which play a part in anger and sexuality. These electrical waves can then be studied to determine the presence of an abnormality.
>
> In addition electrical stimulation with weak currents passed through these wires will be done in order to find out if one or several points in the brain can trigger my episodes of violence or unlawful sexuality. In other words this stimulation may cause me to want to commit an aggressive or sexual act, but every effort will be made to have a sufficient number of people present to control me. If the brain disturbance is limited to a small area, I understand that the investigators will destroy this part of my brain with an electrical current. If the abnormality comes from a larger part of my brain, I agree that it should be surgically removed, if the doctors determine that it can be done so, without risk of side effects. Should the electrical activity from the parts of my brain into which the wires have been placed reveal that there is no significant abnormality, the wires will simply be withdrawn.

Rodin talked about the meanings of the terms in the form and explained the risks of the surgical procedures.

Later, John Doe was allowed to call his parents. The only explanation they received before signing the consent form was from him. Doe believed that he was agreeing only to implanting depth-electrodes and not to stereotactic surgery. He thought that additional consent would be required for surgery. He and his parents signed the form.

Eventually, after the signing, both committees were given materials relating to John Doe. The members of the committees were all picked by Rodin. The medical committee never met, but each member considered the materials submitted to them by Rodin. The Human Rights Committee also examined the materials individually. Thus, neither committee ever met to discuss Doe's case, nor did any member of either committee talk with Doe.

John Doe was the only patient located to participate in the entire research program. Yet by the end of December, all the committee reviews were completed, and plans were made to implant the electrodes in John Doe's brain in early January.

Before this could happen, the process was brought to a halt. A psychiatric resident at Lafayette Clinic was bothered by the secret way in which the project was being run. He expressed these concerns to Gabe Kaimowitz, an attorney for the Michigan Medical Committee for Human Rights. In early January, Kaimowitz filed a petition and complaint with the Wayne County Circuit Court that asked that the state Department of Mental Health be required to "show cause . . . why they should not be enjoined from performing psychosurgery or using chemotherapy on persons involuntarily confined in the state hospital system in order to study 'uncontrollable aggression' or for any other similar purpose." Kaimowitz also asked that a writ of habeas corpus be issued to release John Doe and others from state hospitals because they were not receiving treatment.

Soon afterwards, the Department of Mental Health decided to cancel funding for the Rodin project. But the court decided that the legal issues were not moot and that the case should be heard. On March 23, the court also decided that the Criminal Sexual Psychopath law, under which John Doe had been committed, was unconstitutional. The court ordered him released, and John Doe was freed from Ionia State Hospital after eighteen years of confinement.

The court then heard arguments on the major legal and moral issues of the complaint. For the first time, a court was being asked to give an opinion on the legitimacy of psychosurgery and other experimental treatment methods involving people involuntarily confined to institutions.

On July 10, 1973, the court ruled that an involuntarily detained adult in a facility of the State Department of Mental Health cannot give legally adequate consent to "an innovative or experimental surgical procedure on the brain." The court was careful to point out that its ruling was based upon the state of knowledge about psychosurgery at the time of the decision. Furthermore, the court emphasized that an involuntary mental patient can give adequate consent to accepted neurological procedures. In the court's view, then, the type of neurosurgery proposed for Doe was not of the character to which he could give proper consent.

Introduction

In Cordova, Spain, in 1964, José M. R. Delgado climbed into a bullring before an audience of hundreds and waved a red cape at a large bull. The bull charged toward him. Then Delgado pressed a button on a tiny transmitter hidden in his right hand, and the bull immediately stopped in place. Delgado pushed another button, and the bull walked quietly away.

The bull was quite ordinary, except for the fact that Delgado had earlier implanted electrodes at precise locations in its brain and had attached to its skull a miniature radio receiver that he had invented known as a stimoceiver. There are no technological reasons standing in the way of controlling human behavior in a similar way.

Electrical Stimulation of Behavior (ESB), as Delgado's techniques are called, is just one of the forms of altering or controlling behavior that have been developed or have come into relatively widespread use in the last few decades. So far ESB has been employed with human subjects only to treat certain kinds of epilepsy, but other of its possibilities have been discussed. Additional forms of control or modification are currently part of accepted medical practice. All forms raise serious moral and social issues.

The basic question is an obvious one: Is it ever morally legitimate to control or alter human behavior by the deliberate use of technology? But before exploring some of the aspects of this question, it will be useful if we first consider a few of the details of what we can call behavior alteration technology. Although most of the readings in this chapter will focus on the technique that has been most controversial (psychosurgery), all the techniques present similar moral issues.

Behavior Alteration Technologies

Electrical Stimulation of the Brain

Michael Crichton's novel *The Terminal Man* presents as its central character a man named Harry Benson. Benson is a victim of temporal lobe epilepsy. Associated with this brain dysfunction that produces epileptic seizures are episodes during which Benson becomes uncontrollably violent. With his permission and to bring his behavior under control, electrodes are implanted in his brain and connected to a stimoceiver. The stimoceiver sends reports of brain-wave activity to a computer. When characteristic brain-wave patterns indicate the onset of a violent episode, the computer transmits a message that activates the stimoceiver to stimulate the brain with electricity, and the violent episodes are aborted. Unfortunately for Benson, however, the equipment does not work as expected, and therein lies the story of the novel.

Human beings have never been hooked up to a computer as Benson was. But people with psychomotor (or temporal lobe) epilepsy have been treated by ESB. Furthermore, Delgado has succeeded in activating a stimoceiver by a computer assigned to monitor the brain patterns of a chimpanzee and to stimulate the brain when the pattern showed that the animal was on the verge of acting aggressively. In essence, then, the situation depicted in Crichton's novel is already a technological reality.

In his work with animals, Delgado has shown that ESB can be used to make an animal open or shut its eyes, fall asleep, wake up, become sexually aroused, turn its head, sneeze, yawn, or perform various other behaviors. ESB can be used with humans to evoke a sensation, stimulate memory, delay heartbeat, or make a finger move. Probably only a lack of experimental work with people stands in the way of using the technique to manipulate human behavior in the way that animal behavior can be manipulated. The principles appear to be the same, and in Delgado's opinion, only human physiology sets limits to what can be done with ESB to control behavior.

Delgado is just one of the researchers working in the area of monitoring physiological activity and developing technology to modify it through direct intervention. So far techniques are still experimental and have been used on a limited scale for therapeutic ends. Yet broader uses are already being discussed. Two criminologists in an article entitled "The Use of Electronics in the Observation and Control of Human Behavior and Its Possible Use in Rehabilitation and Control" discuss the introduction of such techniques into the criminal justice system:

> In the very near future, a computer technology will make possible alternatives to imprisonment. The development of systems for telemetering information from sensors implanted in or on the body will soon make possible the observation and control of human behavior without actual physical contact. Through such telemetric devices, it will be possible to maintain twenty-four-hour-a-day surveillance over the subject and to intervene electronically or physically to influence and control selected behavior. It will thus be possible to exercise control over human behavior and from a distance without physical contact. The possible implications for criminology and corrections of such telemetric systems are tremendously significant.

It is easy to imagine ESB and similar techniques applied even more broadly than this.

Behavior Modification

Anthony Burgess's novel *A Clockwork Orange* and Stanley Kubrick's film of the same title focus on the life of a young thug named Alex. Alex and his gang live for violence in their society of the near future. They deal out savage beatings and commit a particularly vicious rape. Then Alex is captured by the authorities and subjected to the "Ludovico Technique." Tied to a chair, his eyes forced open by clamps, and injected with a nausea-producing drug, Alex is forced to watch films that show in explicit detail violent murders, muggings, and sexual assaults—acts just like those he has been guilty of. After two weeks, the thought of violence or sex makes Alex become literally sick. Radically altered as a person, sanitized and made safe, he is returned to society.

The novel and the film are science fiction—there is no Ludovico Technique. Now consider this case. A homosexual male in his late twenties is seated in a chair before a screen. A picture of a nude man is flashed on the screen, and a split second later, the man in the chair receives a brief but painful electric shock through the electrodes taped to his arm. A slide of a nude female then appears, and the man receives no shock. The process is repeated several times during a number of sessions.

The man's behavior is being reconditioned by means of a process known as aversion therapy. Similar arrangements are used to help people overcome problems with drinking, smoking, and drug addiction, as well as to treat those who suffer from certain kinds of obsessive-compulsive neuroses.

Aversion therapy is just one form of behavior modification that is based on the theory of operant conditioning that was pioneered by the psychologist B. F. Skinner. Operant conditioning consists in the application of negative or positive reinforcements—punishments or rewards—in such a way that the probability of particular behavioral responses is increased or decreased. The electric shock (negative reinforcer) administered to the homosexual man when he sees pictures of nude males should, in principle, lead towards an extinction of his sexual responses to men. Positive reinforcements can be used in a similar way to increase the probability of some desired response. Thus, praising a student who speaks up in class will increase the probability that she will speak up next time.

Planned programs of reinforcement can be used to shape, maintain, and strengthen the likelihood of any form of behavioral response. Skinner and others have argued that all of our behavior is the result of conditioning factors. Consequently, whether or not we want to condition behavior is not the real question. The issue is whether we want to do it in a conscious, deliberate, and more effective way. In his book *Beyond Freedom and Dignity* and in other works, Skinner has argued that we should restructure society so that the kinds of behavior that contribute to its survival are systematically reinforced and those that do not are extinguished by reconditioning.

As with the other behavior alteration technologies, operant conditioning raises moral and social problems at two levels. Those at the first level concern its therapeutic uses in individual cases, while those at the second concern the legitimacy of extending the techniques so as to make them instruments of social control.

Chemotechnology

Every society in history has succeeded in discovering naturally occurring substances that have psychotropic effects—ones that alter behavior, moods, or thinking. In the last thirty or so years the search for more effective and more specific psychotropic agents has intensified. Although natural substances and traditional agents are still being tested, most work has shifted towards the chemical synthesis of new compounds.

In part this work has been pushed forward by the relatively recent success in treating various kinds of mood and thought disorders by chemotherapy. In 1949, it was shown that lithium hydroxide could be used to control the swings in mood and the hyperactivity typical of manic-depressive illness. In 1952, while attempting to develop a drug for controlling high blood pressure, Swiss chemists synthesized the compound reserpine. Reserpine did lower blood pressure, but it also turned out to have powerful tranquilizing effects. Nathan Kline, an American psychiatrist, learned about these effects and recalled reading that twenty years earlier two Indian physicians had reported using an extract from the snake-root plant called Rauwolfia to treat insanity and lower blood pressure. Because reserpine was the active chemical isolated from Rauwolfia, Kline decided to evaluate the use of reserpine in the treatment of schizophrenia.

The results were immediately successful. The disordered thought, rage, and social withdrawal associated with schizophrenia were virtually eliminated. Hyperactive patients became quiet, and those depressed were made alert and cheerful. Reserpine and another compound discovered somewhat earlier, chloropromazine, became the first effective antischizophrenic agents. In 1955, when the antischizophrenic drugs first came into wide use, the population of U.S. mental hospitals was 560,000. By 1971, it was 330,000, despite the fact that the number of admissions doubled. Other factors were also responsible for the decline, but the antischizophrenic agents were the main cause.

It was also in the 1950s that two important groups of mood-elevating drugs were isolated and tested. (These were the monamine oxidase inhibitors and the tricyclic antidepressants.) Before their discovery, the medical treatment of depression involved the use of stimulants like amphetamines for altering slow body movements and barbiturates for calming agitation. However, these often worsened agitation and psychoses and had only short-term effects. The new drugs (such as Tofranil, the trade name of imipramine) are more effective as antidepressant agents, although they have some serious side effects.

None of these psychotropic substances is now used for any purpose other than therapy. Yet the potential for wider use is a real one. For what we consider to be legitimate health reasons, a great number of communities presently add fluoride compounds to their water supply. The addition of mild tranquilizers to lower the level of hostility and to reduce the instances of violent and aggressive behavior might well be thought by some to be equally justifiable on the grounds of health. Therapy, of course, presents its own problems, which we will discuss later.

Psychotherapy

There are a variety of psychotherapies, each with its own theory and its own way of dealing with people. It is open to question whether psychotherapy should be included in a list of behavior-altering technologies because fundamentally, its method consists only in talking to people. Yet the aim of all forms of psychotherapy is behavioral change. Its goal is to eliminate such symptoms as depression and anxiety and to restore people to normal effective functioning.

Unlike other methods of behavior change that we have considered, psychotherapy requires the voluntary participation of the individual in the process. It also involves a relatively long-term face-to-face relationship with a therapist. For these reasons, psychotherapeutic techniques cannot easily be made the instrument of wide-spread social control.

This is not to say, however, that the techniques cannot be used to instill social values in individuals. With respect to the patient, the therapist is in a powerful position. It is the therapist who is in authority, who defines normal and effective functioning, and who works to get the patient to meet those criteria in his or her own life. The therapist as an agent of the state or of the society is frequently able to shape the behavior of a person to conform to approved patterns.

Psychosurgery

Psychosurgery is the surgical removal or destruction of brain tissue for the purpose of altering behavior, moods, or mental states. With respect to the previous three behavior alteration technologies we have discussed, the number of patients treated by psychosurgery is comparatively low. Yet psychosurgery has generated an immense amount of controversy and raised a number of issues about consent, control, racism, and research. For this reason, we will give more attention to psychosurgery than we have to the other techniques.

It is only relatively recently that the moral and medical legitimacy of psychosurgery has been called into question. For over twenty-five years, it was accepted as a matter of course as just one medical treatment option among others. Psychosurgery was introduced in the 1930s when the Portuguese neurosurgeon Egas Moniz developed the technique known as lobotomy (or sometimes, leukotomy). In this procedure, the white nerve fibers connecting the frontal and prefrontal lobes of the brain are severed. Moniz advocated lobotomy as a therapeutic measure in the treatment of the mentally ill, and for his work he was awarded the Nobel Prize in 1949.

Lobotomies became relatively popular operations in the United States, and perhaps as many as fifty thousand of them were performed. The surgical procedure is a simple one, and many were done by psychiatrists rather than surgeons. The procedure was used in the treatment of a wide variety of diagnosed mental illnesses—severe depression, schizophrenia, manic-depressive syndrome, and a number of less defined complaints.

The therapeutic effectiveness of lobotomies has always been a matter of dispute. Undeniably, however, the procedure did frequently produce unfortunate side effects. Those lobotomized often showed a deadening of emotional responsiveness, a loss of ambition, and a tendency to avoid difficulties of any kind. They have been described as "zombies" and "vegetables." Many of these people are still alive today, living in prisons, mental hospitals, and with their families.

Few lobotomies are performed nowadays, although they are by no means an illegal surgical procedure. They declined in popularity towards the end of the 1950s. The decline was not due to any demonstration of their ineffectiveness in the treatment of mental illness nor to the often shocking results. Rather, it resulted from the introduction of new antischizophrenic and antidepressant drugs (see above). These drugs can alter the symptoms of schizophrenia and relieve depression in ways demonstrably more effective than lobotomy. What is more, unlike lobotomy, they produce no irreversible effects.

Yet there remain many behaviorial and mental conditions considered abnormal that cannot be successfully treated by chemotherapy. Some of these conditions have encouraged the development of new forms of psychosurgery. Furthermore, increased knowledge of the brain, acquired in part from studies involving lobotomy, and advances in biomedical technology now provide the basis for more precise psychosurgical procedures.

The new procedures generally involve altering the brain's limbic system— that part associated with emotional responsiveness and self-awareness. The alterations are made by relying on information gained from stereotactic techniques. These techniques involve using three-dimensional geometrical coordinates, external reference points on the skull, and special x-ray procedures to make a map of the brain's structures. Such a map can then be used in connection with micromanipulators to guide probes or electrodes to exact positions within the brain. (This technique is also used in ESB.) The electrodes then record electrical activity within the brain. Also, they can be used to stimulate the brain to determine neural and motor responses. Areas of the brain that show what is considered to be abnormal patterns of electrical activity, such as those of temporal lobe epilepsy, can be marked on the stereotactic map. If a decision is made to destroy some of the brain tissue, then a relatively strong current can be used to heat the tip of an electrode. Small parts of the brain can be destroyed with accuracy and with little damage to surrounding tissue. Stereotactic surgical procedures are markedly different from those of lobotomy, in which a flat, dull knife is used to destroy a relatively large quantity of brain tissue. Described below are three of the more common or controversial psychosurgical operations.

Cingulotractomy.   The gyri cinguli are convolutions of the brain—one on each hemisphere—that are located directly above the band of fibers that connects the hemispheres (the corpus callosum). In this procedure, an incision is made in the part of the gyrus cingulate that extends to the thalamus—a part of the brain connected by fibers to the sensory areas in the cortex. (In a similar procedure, cingulotomy, the gyrus cingulate is removed from one or both sides.) The procedure is used to treat depression—anxiety states, obsessional neuroses that have not responded to other treatments, and various "neuropsychiatric illnesses." It is perhaps the most frequently performed psychosurgical procedure.

Thalamotomy.   In this procedure, parts of the thalamus are surgically destroyed. Although now most often performed for the treatment of intractable pain, it is employed by the neurosurgeon A. J. Andy of the University of Mississippi in the cases of people he describes as exhibiting "hyper-responsive syndrome," a condition supposedly characterized by violence and unmanageability.

Amygdalotomy.   The amygdaloid body is an almond-shaped mass of gray matter in the limbic structure of the brain. In this procedure, parts of it are destroyed in a carefully controlled fashion. The procedure was originally developed to control temporal lobe epilepsy accompanied by violence. Some have now advocated that its use be extended to people with brain damage who show patterns of uncontrollable rage but have no medical signs of epilepsy.

The main focus of the public controversy over neurosurgery has revolved around its use in the treatment of violent behavior associated with epilepsy. Epilepsy is not a disease, but it is regarded as a symptom of brain dysfunction. Abnormal electrical discharges in the temporal lobe and unusual brain-wave patterns are cited to support this claim. Some epileptics, although certainly not all, occasionally give way to rage and violent actions that they apparently have no control over and later have no memory of. William Sweet and Vernon Mark of the Harvard Medical School and Frank Ervin of UCLA have argued (with others) that both epileptic seizures and uncontrollable violence result from stimulation of the limbic structures that control aggression and emotion. This has led them to advocate neurosurgery (particularly amygdalotomy) as the preferred treatment in such cases.

Mark and Ervin argued this view in their book *Violence and the Brain* (1970) and discussed cases of what they considered to be successful treatment. They also recommended the systematic study of violence in order to determine its physical and social causes, to develop tests to determine dispositions to violence, to assess the effectiveness of treatment methods, and to establish community facilities to help violent persons.

The concern with violence displayed by Mark and Ervin has been seen by some as being primarily a political response to the urban and campus riots of the 1960s and as an attempt to avoid confronting the social issues that caused them—poverty, unemployment, racial discrimination, the Vietnam war, and unsatisfactory conditions in higher education. Thus, Mark and Ervin have sometimes been accused of doing no more than medicalizing social problems.

Opponents of psychosurgery often cite in support of this charge a letter by Sweet, Mark, and Ervin that was published in the *Journal of the American Medical Association* in 1967. The letter admitted that social factors were undoubtedly in a large measure responsible for the civil disturbances then taking place. But the authors also suggested that brain disease, producing "behavioral abnormalities (such as poor impulse control, assaultiveness, and psychoses)," might be an unnoticed cause.

In 1976 the U.S. Congress directed the federal National Commission for the Protection of Human Subjects of Behavioral and Biomedical Research to investigate the practice of psychosurgery. The Commission's final report was submitted to the Secretary of Health, Education, and Welfare in March of 1977. It characterized psychosurgery as an experimental procedure, but claimed that the evidence showed that it could have therapeutic effects in some instances. For this reason, the Commission held that the fact that a person is a mental patient, a child, or a prisoner should not, in itself, rule out that person from receiving psychosurgical treatment. The Commission was concerned, however, that safeguards should be introduced to protect people of both ordinary and special status.

The Commission's major recommendations were: (1) psychosurgery should be performed only at institutions with HEW-approved review boards charged with determining that the surgeon is competent to perform the procedure, that the procedure is appropriate therapy for the patient, and that the patient has given informed consent; (2) psychosurgery on children and involuntarily confined persons should be performed only after informed consent by the patient (by parents or guardians in the case of the underage or incompetent) and only after a court review; (3) HEW should maintain a national information center to assess the safety and value of psychosurgery; (4) institutions not complying with HEW guidelines should be denied any federal funding.

The Commission's recommendations were a disappointment to many, and the report has been challenged on several grounds. For one thing, nearly all psychosurgery currently performed is in private institutions that do not receive federal funds and are not bound by federal regulations. Also, the evidence that the Commission relied on to reach its conclusion that psychosurgery is a relatively safe and effective therapeutic procedure has been challenged as inadequate. The evidence consists of a pilot study of only sixty-one cases. More than half were said to have improved significantly from the surgery. But critics point out that no long-range studies were conducted. What is more, the group included fifteen patients who were operated on to relieve emotional reactions to pain, and such patients may not be representative of the typical psychosurgery patient. Also, the study did not base its statistics on the number of operations (some patients had two or three) but on the number of people. Such considerations lead George J. Annas to suggest that when these factors are taken into account, the success rate for psychosurgery is under 30 percent, which is lower than the placebo success rate in surgery of all kinds.

Some critics see the review boards demanded by the Commission as producing more harm than good. They tend to make psychosurgery appear to be an ordinary and legitimate therapy, and by doing so the review boards and the guidelines may actually encourage the spread of psychosurgery. As Berkeley psychiatrist Lee Coleman expresses the point, the Commission guidelines "label the practice as essentially a therapeutic procedure and declare that review boards would be sufficient to prevent abuse of individuals. There is absolutely no reason to believe it is therapeutic. It is experimental, and in fact it's one of the sloppiest forms of experimentation going on at this time."

Because of the current state of knowledge of the brain, others tend to believe that psychosurgery is no more than a morally illegitimate form of human experimentation. John Seeley, professor of psychiatry at Drew Medical School stresses this aspect: "We don't know that much about the brain to make that kind of surgery safe, and we don't know that much about any particular person. It's morally abhorrent to take that kind of risk without having done the underlying scientific work on animals first, and that's a good decade or more away."

At present there are about three thousand neurosurgeons in the United States. Virtually all of their work is totally unrelated to psychosurgery. Yet there are probably around five hundred psychosurgical procedures performed every year. This relatively small number does not, however, alter the seriousness of the moral questions that psychosurgery raises. In the spring of 1977, Secretary of Health, Education, and Welfare Joseph Califano declared a moratorium on the use of federal funds for psychosurgery. This may quiet the public controversy, while leaving the moral and social issues unresolved.

Issues in Psychosurgery and Behavior Control

The five types of behavior alteration technologies that we have discussed have all been advanced by their developers as real or potentially significant contributions to the relief of human suffering. That is, their advocates have promoted them as therapies for the treatment of disease.

At first view this seems a relatively unproblematical claim that presents no special issues. All we need to do is to rely upon the usual sort of scientific evidence to test the effectiveness of the methods. The moral issues seem to be no different from those that are involved in any other sort of therapy or experimentation involving human subjects.

Yet there is a special problem with behavior alteration technologies. With few exceptions (such as epilepsy), the conditions that they are intended to treat are behavioral or mental disorders. This immediately raises the question of whether it is possible to characterize behavioral or mental "dysfunctions" in a way that is as independent of general social attitudes about what constitutes proper behavior or ways of thinking as is the category of physical disease. It has been suggested by a number of psychiatrists, psychologists, and sociologists that the patterns of behavior or thinking that we call mental illness are just ones that we, as a society, disapprove of. By transforming such patterns into diseases or symptoms of diseases, then we make it legitimate to apply medical measures as "therapies" that "cure" people of them.

If this point of view is correct, then the various forms of behavior alteration technologies may be seen as instruments of implicit social coercion. They are more insidious than overt coercion because the individual, believing himself to be suffering from a genuine disease, may give free and voluntary consent to the treatment that is offered to him. This point of view calls into question all forms of behavior alteration that are based on the notion that the "patients" involved suffer from some kind of disease or dysfunction, because this notion implies an inherent denial of the autonomy of the individual in choosing what sort of life to live. Also, it involves a basic dishonesty, a fraud perpetrated on the "patient."

The question whether "abnormal" ways of behaving and thinking constitute diseases is more of an epistemological or conceptual question than it is a moral one. But it is one whose answer has moral consequences. If general social values are being forced on patients, then we need to ask whether this is a morally legitimate practice. Someone might argue that it is because of the beneficial consequences it has for the society as a whole. By contrast, one might seek to show that the practice does violate personal autonomy and worth and so is a morally objectionable practice. Of course it is not at all clear that there are not genuine diseases constituted or indicated by thought and behavior patterns, and this is the matter that must first be settled.

For our purposes, let us beg this question and assume that there are mental illnesses or diseases. At the beginning, we suggested that the basic moral question is simply, "Is it ever morally legitimate to alter human behavior by the deliberate use of technology?" This question cannot be fruitfully discussed unless we also distinguish the kinds of aims and contexts in which behavior alteration might take place. We need to distinguish, first of all, alteration that is carried out for the purpose of therapy from that which aims at control. In therapy, we expect actions to be taken for the good of the individual concerned; to restore the person to health or normal functioning is the object of treatment. Whereas in control, it is someone else's good or the good of the society that is the aim. That is, the person (or persons) benefiting is someone other than the one whose behavior is being altered. (These aims are not absolutely distinct, of course. Society also benefits from having people in it restored to health, even though the immediate object of treatment is not to benefit society.)

It is also useful to distinguish between treatment that is conducted with the permission of the individual and that which is involuntary. Prima facie there is a difference between an individual who seeks to have his behavior modified and one who is made a patient because of a decision by someone else (court, prison authority, or psychiatrist).

We might say that it is morally permissible to alter the behavior of an individual when it is done for therapeutic purposes and the individual gives his or her informed consent. This seems a reasonable principle, but there are several

Difficulties

difficulties with its application. First is the problem of making the therapy/control distinction in some situations. Prisons and mental institutions, in particular, tend to favor measures that have therapeutic value but also permit control. Sometimes it is debatable which aim is being pursued.

Second, informed consent presents unique problems because of the nature of and need for the therapy. There are reasons to believe that institutions such as prisons and mental hospitals are inherently coercive environments because in a variety of ways the social structure encourages acting in accordance with the wishes of those in authority. Furthermore, inmates in such institutions are under considerable social pressure to modify their behavior—that is why they are there in the first place. Accordingly, it is at least an open question whether informed consent can ever be freely given by such people. Also, so far as mental patients are concerned, the nature of mental illness and our general ignorance about it raise the question whether informed consent is ever meaningful in the case of such persons. For example, is a schizophrenic, who suffers from thought disorders, genuinely capable of making a rational decision about his own welfare?

The approval or giving of consent by a court, board, or guardian in the case of those who might be considered "incompetent" because of their institutionalization, illness, or age is a possible alternative. Yet this has the consequence of placing in the hands of others the ultimate responsibility for the well-being of an individual. In the case of psychosurgery, in particular, this means that others and not the individual involved decide on a procedure that may alter the basic personality of the individual in an irreversible fashion.

Not all behavior alteration techniques are equivalent in the kinds of changes they effect. One might well endorse certain limited kinds of behavior modification or psychotherapy, conditional upon an individual's informed consent, while ruling out forms such as psychosurgery. Permanently altering the emotional responses and thought processes of a person by direct intervention is a very serious undertaking. There is good reason to question whether it should be permitted at all, even for therapeutic reasons.

Another aspect of the consent problem concerns the right of an individual to demand a therapy that he believes will be beneficial to him. Recently, Edmund Kemper, convicted of mass murder and confined to the Correctional Medical Facility in Vacaville, California, requested a court appearance, during which he asserted that he wanted to submit himself to psychosurgery but was kept from doing so by the restrictive laws of California. Kemper is certainly entitled to medical care, but should he be allowed to choose psychosurgery? If psychosurgery is not a genuine therapeutic aid, as its critics have claimed, then claims such as Kemper's have no more moral standing than a request for bodily mutilation. Here, again, an issue that is not in itself a moral one has serious moral implications.

Such an issue can be resolved only by additional scientific investigation. This, in turn, raises a question about the social regulation of research. As we have seen, the critics of psychosurgery claim that its results do not show it to be an effective therapy. Its supporters admit that it is still at an experimental stage.

~~and this is one of the reasons they offer to urge its continued practice.~~ But is it morally defensible to recommend to patients an irreversible procedure that is of questionable therapeutic value? Yet should society seek to regulate or eliminate a medical procedure that is regarded by a number of respected professionals to be of value? If society takes such a step, is this not interfering with the free practice of medical research and treatment?

Similar questions can be raised about research involving the electrical stimulation of the brain. It might be argued that the results of the research would be so threatening to the social structure that work in the area should be halted for the good of all. (For a fuller discussion of similar issues, see the introduction to Chapter 7.)

Ethical Theories: Behavior Control and Psychosurgery

The moral principles of Kant, Ross, Rawls, and Roman Catholicism would all seem to rule out psychosurgery that threatens to destroy or alter substantially the ability of an individual to function as an effective agent. Such a change would mean the destruction of individual autonomy and dignity. Yet two considerations cast doubt on this easy answer. First, those who are candidates for psychosurgery are already considered to be people who are not autonomous agents. They are kept from acting, for example, by severe depression or, as in temporal lobe epilepsy, they are compelled to action by forces over which they have no control. Second, the aim of the surgery is to restore patients to normal functioning, even though this may not always be the outcome. One might argue, then, that at least in some cases psychosurgery holds out the only genuine hope that some individuals have of *becoming* autonomous agents. Such considerations suggest, contrary to what some critics have argued, that psychosurgery itself is not a morally illegitimate procedure. The same arguments that support it can also be used to support chemotherapy, behavior modification, and psychotherapy. Of course, one might object in each of these cases that the techniques are so unreliable as therapies that, no matter what their aim, an individual is more likely to sacrifice autonomy than to gain it. It is for this reason that the empirical question of effectiveness is of such importance in each case.

For utilitarianism, effectiveness is the basic question. If any or all of the putative therapies hold out a genuine hope of increasing the happiness of those receiving them, then each is at least prima facie desirable. Indeed, it could be argued that a wholesale program of therapy should be instituted if that seemed likely to increase the overall happiness and well-being of the society.

ESB, psychotherapy, and behavior modification present special issues. We mentioned them earlier in passing, and they are too complicated for us to discuss here. ESB, since it presents the possibility of direct control of behavior, could, when used in that way, destroy autonomy and make human beings into automata. No moral theory that we have discussed would countenance this. Psychotherapy might well involve encouraging individuals to accept the values of their society. To the extent that it does this in a way that involves the long-term and willing participation of the individual, a way that recognizes the individual's capacity for self-determination and decision making, then it is not morally objectionable. Behavior modification presents a somewhat different case, for there the individual is subjected to manipulation. She is not brought to accept a point of view as the result of rational consideration and persuasion. Yet if the manipulation is with the approval of the individual and is directed towards an end chosen by the individual, then none of the theories we have considered would regard the process as inherently objectionable. The main moral issue in all cases of behavior alteration technologies is that of securing the informed consent of the individual, an issue that we discussed earlier (see Chapter 5).

The Selections

The essay by psychiatrist Thomas Szasz raises the conceptual issue that is fundamental to all moral questions about behavior control: *Is there such a thing as mental illness?*

Szasz argues that what we call "mental illness" is no more than a misleading metaphor. (The mind is no more ill than a sick joke is sick.) The concept of illness implies deviation from a norm or standard. For physical illness, the norm is physiological; but for mental illness, Szasz claims, the norm is socially determined. The social norm is then taken as having the same status as the physiological norm, and in effect, nonconformists become the mentally ill. The result is both a denial of individual autonomy and a failure to deal with the genuine issues at the root of human conflict.

The real problems that we should be dealing with, Szasz argues, are the "problems of living" that people face in society. Once we abandon the "myth of mental illness," we can focus our attention on the genuine ethical and social issues.

More than anyone else, Szasz has forcefully and repeatedly called attention to the contemporary inclination to "medicalize" moral and social problems. As we discussed earlier, when certain patterns of acting, thinking, or talking are identified as "symptoms" of disease, then the way is open to employ medical "therapies" to eliminate them. But if those patterns are no more than deviations from social norms, therapy is simply being employed to force conformity and deny autonomy.

In "Autonomy and Behavior Control," Gerald Dworkin explicitly addresses the issue of the impact that various forms of behavior control have on autonomy. Dworkin analyzes autonomy as consisting of a combination of authenticity and independence. Authenticity (the "true self") may lead us to act to change ourselves or to accept ourselves as we are, but it must be combined with (at least) procedural independence. For Dworkin, procedural independence is lacking when a person's motivations to change or stay the same have been influenced by deception or manipulation.

Employing this analysis of autonomy, Dworkin presents seven guidelines for preferring some means of influencing behavior over others. Specifically, those means are preferred which possess the following features: preserve dignity, rationality, and self-identity; avoid deception; are not physically intrusive, employ enough time to permit the individual to change his mind, and work through cognitive and affective structures so the person is not just a passive subject.

Seymour L. Halleck, in the next selection, directs attention to the problem of consent in connection with behavior change technologies. He distinguishes three kinds of treatment situations—where the patient does not verbally consent, where the treatment is administered under duress, and where the patient consents to or requests treatment. Halleck then specifies the three conditions he believes must be met before treatment is forced on a patient. Not only must the treatment be considered likely to benefit the patient and the patient judged incompetent to evaluate his own interest, but a review board should be established to make the final decision.

Halleck points out that the "voluntary" consent of the patient also presents problems when the patient is confined in an institution. To attempt to overcome the implied coercion in such a situation, Halleck recommends that four basic rules be followed. Finally, Halleck calls attention to what he calls the "insidious aspect" of behavior control in the case of voluntary patients. This aspect is that patients will often seek therapy that will end their present sufferings while it worsens their long-term chances of improvement. This places an obligation on the psychiatrist to encourage patients to become aware of how their symptoms are an effort to influence their environment and how the alleviation of them might change the patient's relationship with the environment. Only then, Halleck suggests, should the psychiatrist agree to short-term therapies such as drugs or behavior modification.

Our last focus in this chapter is psychosurgery. The Case Presentation describes the background of the first court hearing and decision made concerning psychosurgery. The judges of the Michigan Circuit Court held that an involuntarily confined person cannot give adequate consent for psychosurgery.

As mentioned in the case presentation, Vernon Mark considered the intended surgery in the Michigan case morally unjustified. In the selection presented here, however, he argues that it is possible to answer all objections to some forms of psychosurgery in a medically and morally satisfactory way. He argues that medical procedures should be used in treating behavior disorders only when the behavior is due to a brain abnormality. Further, he claims that there is only one sort of behavior for which psychosurgery is proper treatment—personal, violent behavior produced by brain disease or injury. Finally, he discusses the moral problems that are presented by diagnosis that involves social factors and the problems of obtaining proper consent to treatment by psychosurgery.

In the final selection, Stephan L. Chorover examines the empirical evidence which Mark and Ervin offered to show the success they achieved in their two best-known cases. Chorover finds the evidence to be deficient and unpersuasive. He recommends that steps be taken both to control the present practice of psychosurgery and to promote research in developing an understanding of the connection between brain function and behavior. Such an understanding, Chorover suggests, would serve as a defense against the sort of simplistic views that currently form the theoretical basis of psychosurgery.

Like Szasz and others, Chorover is also concerned about the possibility of attempting to solve social problems by defining them as medical. When the causes of deviance are social, then the "psychotechnological treatment of deviants should be regarded as a perversion of medicine and a distinct threat to individual liberty."

The Myth of Mental Illness

Thomas S. Szasz

My aim in this essay is to raise the question "Is there such a thing as mental illness?" and to argue that there is not. Since the notion of mental illness is extremely widely used nowadays, inquiry into the ways in which this term is employed would seem to be especially indicated. Mental illness, of course, is not literally a "thing"—or physical object—and hence it can "exist" only in the same sort of way in which other theoretical concepts exist. Yet, familiar theories are in the habit of posing, sooner of later—at least to those who come to believe in them—as "objective truths" (or "facts"). During certain historical periods, explanatory conceptions such as deities, witches, and microorganisms appeared not only as theories but as self-evident *causes* of a vast number of events. I submit that today mental illness is widely regarded in a somewhat similar fashion, that is, as the cause of innumerable diverse happenings, As an antidote to the complacent use of the notion of mental illness—whether as a self-evident phenomenon, theory, or cause—let us ask this question: What is meant when it is asserted that someone is mentally ill?

In what follows I shall describe briefly the main uses to which the concept of mental illness has been put. I shall argue that this notion has outlived whatever usefulness it might have had and that it now functions merely as a convenient myth.

Mental Illness as a Sign of Brain Disease

The notion of mental illness derives its main support from such phenomena as syphilis of the brain or delirious conditions—intoxications, for instance—in which persons are known to manifest various peculiarities or disorders of thinking and behavior. Correctly speaking, however, these are diseases of the brain, not of the mind. According to one school of thought, *all* so-called mental illness is of this type. The assumption is made that some neurological defect, perhaps a very subtle one, will ultimately be found for all the disorders of thinking and behavior. Many contemporary psychiatrists, physicians, and other scientists hold this view. This position implies that people *cannot* have troubles—expressed in what are *now called* "mental illnesses"—because of differences in personal needs, opinions, social aspiration, values, and so on. *All problems in living* are attributed to physicochemical processes which in due time will be discovered by medical research.

"Mental illnesses" are thus regarded as basically no different than all other diseases (that is, of the body). The only difference, in this view, between mental and bodily diseases is that the former, affecting the brain, manifest themselves by means of mental symptoms, whereas the latter, affecting other organ systems (for example, the skin, liver, etc.), manifest themselves by means of symptoms referable to those parts of the body. This view rests on and expresses what are, in my opinion, two fundamental errors.

In the first place, what central nervous system symptoms would correspond to a skin eruption or a fracture? It would *not* be some emotion or complex bit of behavior. Rather, it would be blindness or a paralysis of some part of the body. The crux of the matter is that a disease of the brain, analogous to a disease of the skin or bone, is a neurological

Reprinted from The American Psychologist, *15, no. 2 (February 1960), pp. 113–18. Copyright 1960 by the American Psychological Association. Reprinted by permission of the publisher and by the author.*

defect, and not a problem in living. For example, a *defect* in a person's visual field may be satisfactorily explained by correlating it with certain definite lesions in the nervous system. On the other hand, a persons *belief*—whether this be a belief in Christianity, in Communism, or in the idea that his internal organs are "rotting" and that his body is, in fact, already "dead"—cannot be explained by a defect or disease of the nervous system. Explanations of this sort of occurrence—assuming that one is interested in the belief itself and does not regard it simply as a "symptom'" or expression of something else that is *more interesting*—must be sought along different lines.

The second error in regarding complex psychosocial behavior, consisting of communication about ourselves and the world about us, as mere symptoms of neurological functioning is *epistemological*. In other words, it is an error pertaining not to any mistakes in observation or reasoning, as such, but rather to the way in which we organize and express our knowledge. In the present case, the error lies in making a symmetrical dualism between mental and physical (or bodily) symptoms, a dualism which is merely a habit of speech and to which no known observation can be found to correspond. Let us see if this is so. In medical practice, when we speak of physical disturbances, we mean either signs (for example, a fever) or symptoms (for example, pain). We speak of mental symptoms, on the other hand, when we refer to a patient's *communication about himself, others, and the world about him.* He might state that he is Napoleon or that he is being persecuted by the Communists. These would be considered mental symptoms *only* if the observer believed that the patient was *not* Napoleon or that he was *not* being persecuted by the Communists. This makes it apparent that the statement that "X is a mental symptom" involves rendering a judgment. The judgment entails, moreover, a covert comparison or matching of the patient's ideas, concepts, or beliefs with those of the observer and the society in which they live. The notion of mental symptom is therefore inextricably tied to the *social* (including *ethical*) *context* in which it is made in much the same way as the notion of bodily symptom is tied to an *anatomical* and *genetic context* (Szasz, 1957a, 1957b).

To sum up what has been said thus far: I have tried to show that for those who regard mental symptoms as signs of brain disease, the concept of mental illness is unnecessary and misleading. For what they mean is that people so labeled suffer from diseases of the brain; and, if that is what they mean, it would seem better for the sake of clarity to say that and not something else.

Mental Illness as a Name for Problems in Living

The term "mental illness" is widely used to describe something which is very different than a disease of the brain. Many people today take it for granted that living is an arduous process. Its hardship for modern man, moreover, derives not so much from a struggle for biological survival as from the stresses and strains inherent in the social intercourse of complex human personalities. In this context, the notion of mental illness is used to identify or describe some feature of an individual's so-called personality. Mental illness—as a deformity of the personality, so to speak—is then regarded as the *cause* of the human disharmony. It is implicit in this view that social intercourse between people is regarded as something *inherently harmonious*, its disturbance being due solely to the presence of "mental illness" in many people. This is obviously fallacious reasoning, for it makes the abstraction "mental illness" into a *cause*, even though this abstraction was created in the first place to serve only as a shorthand expression for certain types of human behavior. It now becomes necessary to ask: "What kinds of behavior are regarded as indicative of mental illness, and by whom?"

The concept of illness, whether bodily or mental, implies *deviation from some clearly defined norm*. In the case of physical illness, the norm is the structural and functional integrity of the human body. Thus, although the desirability of physical health, as such, is an ethical value, what health *is* can be stated in anatomical and physiological terms. What is the norm deviation from which is regarded as mental illness? This question cannot be easily answered. But whatever this norm might be, we can be certain of only one thing: namely, that it is a norm that must be stated in terms of *psychosocial, ethical,* and *legal* concepts. For example, notions such as "excessive repression" or "acting out an unconscious impulse" illustrate the use of psychological concepts for judging (so-called) mental health and illness. The idea that chronic hostility, vengefulness, or divorce are indicative of mental illness would be illustrations of the use of ethical norms (that is, the desirability of love, kindness, and a stable marriage relationship). Finally, the widespread psychiatric opinion that only a mentally ill person would commit homicide illustates the use of a legal concept as a norm of mental health. The norm from which deviation is measured whenever one speaks of a mental illness is a *psychosocial and ethical one*. Yet, the remedy is sought in terms of *medical* measures which—it is hoped and assumed—are free from wide differences of ethical value. The definition of the disorder and the terms in which its remedy are sought are therefore at serious odds with one another. The practical significance of this covert conflict between the alleged nature of the defect and the remedy can hardly be exaggerated.

Having identified the norms used to measure deviations in cases of mental illness, we will now turn to the question: "Who defines the norms and hence the deviation?" Two basic answers may be offered: (a) It may be the person himself (that is, the patient) who decides that he deviates from a norm. For example, an artist may believe that he suffers from a work inhibition; and he may implement this conclusion by seeking help *for* himself from a psychotherapist. (b) It may be someone other than the patient who decides that the latter is deviant (for example, relatives, physicians, legal authorities, society generally, etc.). In such a case a psychiatrist may be hired by others to do something *to* the patient in order to correct the deviation.

These considerations underscore the importance of asking the question "Whose agent is the psychiatrist?" and of giving a candid answer to it (Szasz, 1956, 1958). The psychiatrist (psychologist or nonmedical psychotherapist), it now develops, may be the agent of the patient, of the relatives, of the school, of the military services, of a business organization, of a court of law, and so forth. In speaking of the psychiatrist as the agent of these persons or organizations, it is not implied that his values concerning norms, or his ideas and aims concerning the proper nature of remedial action, need to coincide exactly with those of his employer. For example, a patient in individual psychotherapy may believe that his salvation lies in a new marriage; his psychotherapist need not share this hypothesis. As the patient's agent, however, he must abstain from bringing social or

legal force to bear on the patient which would prevent him from putting his beliefs into action. If his *contract* is with the patient, the psychiatrist (psychotherapist) may disagree with him or stop his treatment; but he cannot engage others to obstruct the patient's aspirations. Similarly, if a psychiatrist is engaged by a court to determine the sanity of a criminal, he need not fully share the legal authorities' values and intentions in regard to the criminal and the means available for dealing with him. But the psychiatrist is expressly barred from stating, for example, that it is not the criminal who is "insane" but the men who wrote the law on the basis of which the very actions that are being judged are regarded as "criminal." Such an opinion could be voiced, of course, but not in a courtroom, and not by a psychiatrist who makes it his practice to assist the court in performing its daily work.

To recapitulate: In actual contemporary social usage, the finding of a mental illness is made by establishing a deviance in behavior from certain psychosocial, ethical, or legal norms. The judgment may be made, as in medicine, by the patient, the physician (psychiatrist), or others. Remedial action, finally, tends to be sought in a therapeutic—or covertly medical—framework, thus creating a situation in which *psychosocial*, *ethical*, and/or *legal deviation* are claimed to be correctible by (so-called) *medical action*. Since medical action is designed to correct only medical deviation, it seems logically absurd to expect that it will help solve problems whose very existence had been defined and established on nonmedical grounds. I think that these considerations may be fruitfully applied to the present use of tranquilizers and, more generally, to what might be expected of drugs of whatever type in regard to the amelioration or solution of problems in human living.

The Role of Ethics in Psychiatry

Anything that people *do*—in contrast to things that *happen* to them (Peters, 1958)—takes place in a context of value. In this broad sense, no human activity is devoid of ethical implications. When the values underlying certain activities are widely shared, those who participate in their pursuit may lose sight of them altogether. The discipline of medicine, both as a pure science (for example, research) and as a technology (for example, therapy), contains many ethical considerations and judgments. Unfortunately, these are often denied, minimized, or merely kept out of focus; for the ideal of the medical profession as well as of the people whom it serves seems to be having a system of medicine (allegedly) free of ethical value. This sentimental notion is expressed by such things as the doctor's willingness to treat and help patients irrespective of their religious or political beliefs, whether they are rich or poor, etc. While there may be some grounds for this belief—albeit it is a view that is not impressively true even in these regards—the fact remains that ethical considerations encompass a vast range of human affairs. By making the practice of medicine neutral in regard to some specific issues of value need not, and cannot, mean that it can be kept free from all such values. The practice of medicine is intimately tied to ethics; and the first thing that we must do, it seems to me, is to try to make this clear and explicit. I shall let this matter rest here, for it does not concern us specifically in this essay. Lest there by any vagueness, however, about how or where ethics and medicine meet, let me remind the reader of such issues as birth control, abortion, suicide, and euthanasia as only a few of the major areas of current ethicomedical controversy.

Psychiatry, I submit, is very much more intimately tied to problems of ethics than is medicine. I use the word "psychiatry" here to refer to that contemporary discipline which is concerned with *problems in living* (and not with diseases of the brain, which are problems for neurology). Problems in human relations can be analyzed, interpreted, and given meaning only within given social and ethical contexts. Accordingly, it *does* make a difference—arguments to the contrary notwithstanding—what the psychiatrist's socioethical orientations happen to be; for these will influence his ideas on what is wrong with the patient, what deserves comment or interpretation, in what possible directions change might be desirable, and so forth. Even in medicine proper, these factors play a role, as for instance, in the divergent orientations which physicians, depending on their religious affiliations, have toward such things as birth control and therapeutic abortion. Can anyone really believe that a psychotherapist's ideas concerning religious belief, slavery, or other similar issues play no role in his practical work? If they do make a difference, what are we to infer from it?

Does it not seem reasonable that we ought to have different psychiatric therapies—each expressly recognized for the ethical positions which they embody—for, say, Catholics and Jews, religious persons and agnostics, democrats and communists, white supremacists and Negroes, and so on? Indeed, if we look at how psychiatry is actually practiced today (especially in the United States), we find that people do seek psychiatric help in accordance with their social status and ethical beliefs (Hollingshead & Redlich, 1958). This should really not surprise us more than being told that practicing Catholics rarely frequent birth control clinics.

The foregoing position which holds that contemporary psychotherapists deal with problems in living, rather than with mental illnesses and their cures, stands in opposition to a currently prevalent claim, according to which mental illness is just as "real" and "objective" as bodily illness. This is a confusing claim since it is never known exactly what is meant by such words as "real" and "objective." I suspect, however, that what is intended by the proponents of this view is to create the idea in the popular mind that mental illness is some sort of disease entity, like an infection or a malignancy. If this were true, one could *catch* or *get* a "mental illness," one might *have* or *harbor* it, one might *transmit* it to others, and finally one could get *rid* of it. In my opinion, there is not a shred of evidence to support this idea. To the contrary, all the evidence is the other way and supports the view that what people now call mental illnesses are for the most part *communications* expressing unacceptable ideas, often framed, moreover, in an unusual idiom. The scope of this essay allows me to do no more than mention this alternative theoretical approach to this problem (Szasz, 1957c).

This is not the place to consider in detail the similarities and differences between bodily and mental illnesses. It shall suffice for us here to emphasize only one important difference between them: namely, that whereas bodily disease refers to public, physicochemical occurrences, the notion of mental illness is used to codify relatively more private, sociopsychological happenings of which the observer (diagnostician) forms a part. In other words, the psychiatrist does not stand *apart* from what he observes, but is, in Harry Stack Sullivan's apt words, a "participant observer." This means that he is *committed* to some picture of what he considers reality—and to what he thinks society considers reality—and he observes and judges the patient's behavior in the light of these considerations. This touches on our earlier observation that the notion of mental symptom itself implies a comparison between observer and observed, psychiatrist and patient. This is so obvious that I may be charged with belaboring trivialities. Let me therefore say once more that my aim in presenting this argument was expressly to criticize and counter a prevailing contemporary tendency to deny the moral aspects of psychiatry (and psychotherapy) and to substitute for them allegedly valuefree medical considerations. Psychotherapy, for example, is being widely practiced as though it entailed nothing other than restoring the patient from a state of mental sickness to one of mental health. While it is generally accepted that mental illness has something to do with man's social (or interpersonal) relations, it is paradoxically maintained that problems of values (that is, of ethics) do not arise in this process.[1] Yet, in one sense, much of psychotherapy may revolve around nothing other than the elucidation and weighing of goals and values—many of which may be mutually contradictory—and the means whereby they might best be harmonized, realized, or relinquished.

The diversity of human values and the methods by means of which they may be realized is so vast, and many of them remain so unacknowledged, that they cannot fail but lead to conflicts in human relations. Indeed, to say that human relations at all levels—from mother to child, through husband and wife, to nation and nation—are fraught with stress, strain, and disharmony is, once again, making the obvious explicit. Yet, what may be obvious may be also poorly understood. This I think is the case here. For it seems to me that —at least in our scientific theories of behavior—we have failed to *accept* the simple fact that human relations are inherently fraught with difficulties and that to make them even relatively harmonious requires much patience and hard work. I submit that the idea of mental illness is now being put to work to obscure certain difficulties which at present may be inherent—not that they need be unmodifiable—in the social intercourse of persons. If this is true, the concept functions as a disguise; for instead of calling attention to conflicting human needs, aspirations, and values, the notion of mental illness provides an amoral and impersonal "thing" (an "ill-

ness") as an explanation for *problems in living* (Szasz, 1959). We may recall in this connection that not so long ago it was devils and witches who were held responsible for men's problems in social living. The belief in mental illness, as something other than man's trouble in getting along with his fellow man, is the proper heir to the belief in demonology and witchcraft. Mental illness exists or is "real" in exactly the same sense in which witches existed or were "real."

Choice, Responsibility, and Psychiatry

While I have argued that mental illnesses do not exist, I obviously did not imply that the social and psychological occurrences to which this label is currently being attached also do not exist. Like the personal and social troubles which people had in the Middle Ages, they are real enough. It is the labels we give them that concerns us and, having labeled them, what we do about them. While I cannot go into the ramified implications of this problem here, it is worth noting that a demonologic conception of problems in living gave rise to therapy along theological lines. Today, a belief in mental illness implies—nay, requires—therapy along medical or psychotherapeutic lines.

What is implied in the line of thought set forth here is something quite different. I do not intend to offer a new conception of "psychiatric illness" nor a new form of "therapy." My aim is more modest and yet also more ambitious. It is to suggest that the phenomena now called mental illnesses be looked at afresh and more simply, that they be removed from the category of illnesses, and that they be regarded as the expressions of man's struggle with the problem of *how* he should live. The last mentioned problem is obviously a vast one, its enormity reflecting not only man's inability to cope with his environment, but even more his increasing self-reflectiveness.

By problems in living, then, I refer to that truly explosive chain reaction which began with man's fall from divine grace by partaking of the fruit of the tree of knowledge. Man's awareness of himself and of the world about him seems to be a steadily expanding one, bringing in its wake an ever larger *burden of understanding* (an expression borrowed from Susanne Langer, 1953). *This burden, then, is to be expected and must not be misinterpreted.* Our only *rational* means for lightening it is *more understanding,* and appropriate *action* based on such understanding. The main alternative lies in acting as though the burden were not what in fact we perceive it to be and taking refuge in an outmoded theological view of man. In the latter view, man does not fashion his life and much of his world about him, but merely lives out his fate in a world created by superior beings. This may logically lead to pleading nonresponsibility in the face of seemingly unfathomable problems and difficulties. Yet, if man fails to take increasing responsibility for his actions, individually as well as collectively, it seems unlikely that some higher power or being would assume this task and carry this burden for him. Moreover, this seems hardly the proper time in human history for obscuring the issue of man's responsibility for his actions by hiding it behind the skirt of an all-explaining conception of mental illness.

Conclusions

I have tried to show that the notion of mental illness has outlived whatever usefulness it might have had and that it now functions merely as a convenient myth. As such, it is a true heir to religious myths in general, and to the belief in witchcraft in particular; the role of all these belief-systems was to act as *social tranquilizers,* thus encouraging the hope that mastery of certain specific problems may be achieved by means of substitutive (symbolic-magical) operations. The notion of mental illness thus serves mainly to obscure the everyday fact that life for most people is a continuous struggle, not for biological survival, but for a "place in the sun," "peace of mind," or some other human value. For man aware of himself and of the world about him, once the needs for preserving the body (and perhaps the race) are more or less satisfied, the problem arises as to what he should do with himself. Sustained adherence to the myth of mental illness allows people to avoid facing this problem, believing that mental health, conceived as the absence of mental illness, automatically insures the making of right and safe choices in one's conduct of life. But the facts are all the other way. It is the making of good choices in life that others regard, retrospectively, as good mental health!

The myth of mental illness encourages us, moreover, to believe in its logical corollary: that social intercourse would be harmonious, satis-

fying, and the secure basis of a "good life" were it not for the disrupting influences of mental illness or "psychopathology." The potentiality for universal human happiness, in this form at least, seems to me but another example of the I-wish-it-were-true type of fantasy. I do not believe that human happiness or well-being on a hitherto unimaginably large scale, and not just for a select few, is possible. This goal could be achieved, however, only at the cost of many men, and not just a few being willing and able to tackle their personal, social, and ethical conflicts. This means having the courage and integrity to forego waging battles on false fronts, finding solutions for substitute problems—for instance, fighting the battle of stomach acid and chronic fatigue instead of facing up to a marital conflict.

Our adversaries are not demons, witches, fate, or mental illness. We have no enemy whom we can fight, exorcise, or dispel by "cure." What we do have are *problems in livng*—whether these be biological, economic, political, or sociopsychological. In this essay I was concerned only with problems belonging in the last mentioned category, and within this group mainly with those pertaining to moral values. The field to which modern psychiatry addresses itself is vast, and I made no effort to encompass it all. My argument was limited to the proposition that mental illness is a myth, whose function it is to disguise and thus render more palatable the bitter pill of moral conflicts in human relations.

Notes

1. Freud went so far as to say that: "I consider ethics to be taken for granted. Actually I have never done a mean thing" (Jones, 1957, p. 247). This surely is a strange thing to say for someone who has studied man as a social being as closely as did Freud. I mention it here to show how the notion of "illness" (in the case of psychoanalysis, "psychopathology," or "mental illness") was used by Freud—and by most of his followers—as a means for classifying certain forms of human behavior as falling within the scope of medicine, and hence (by *fiat*) outside that of ethics!

References

Hollingshead, A. B., & Redlich, F. C. *Social Class and Mental Illness.* New York: Wiley, 1958.

Jones, E. *The Life and Work of Sigmund Freud.* Vol. III. New York: Basic Books, 1957.

Langer, S. K. *Philosophy in a New Key*. New York: Mentor Books, 1953.

Peters, R. S. *The Concept of Motivation*. London: Routledge & Kegan Paul, 1958.

Szasz, T. S. Malingering: "Diagnosis" or Social Condemnation? *AMA Arch Neurol. Psychiat.*, 1956, 76, 432–443.

Szasz, T. S. *Pain and Pleasure: A Study of Bodily Feelings*. New York: Basic Books, 1957. (a)

Szasz, T. S. The Problem of Psychiatric Nosology: A Contribution to a Situational Analysis of Psychiatric Operations. *Amer. J. Psychiat.*, 1957, 114, 405–413. (b)

Szasz, T. S. On the Theory of Psychoanalytic Treatment. *Int. J. Psycho-Anal.*, 1957, 38, 166–182. (c)

Szasz, T. S. Psychiatry, Ethics and the Criminal Law. *Columbia Law Rev.*, 1958, 58, 183–198.

Szasz, T. S. Moral Conflict and Psychiatry, *Yale Rev.*, 1959, in press.

Autonomy and Behavior Control

Gerald Dworkin

The advent of new modes of behavioral technology raises important issues for our understanding of human nature and our moral views about how people ought to influence one another. On the theoretical level we find claims that an adequate explanatory scheme for understanding human behavior can dispense with notions of free will, dignity, and autonomy. On the practical level we are faced with claims of effectiveness, efficiency, and moral legitimacy for methods of influencing people such as operant conditioning, psychotropic drugs, electrical stimulation of the brain, and psychosurgery. The theoretical and practical issues are, of course, linked. Our views as to what it is permissible to do to people reflect our views about the existence and desirability of various conditions. If autonomy is neither desirable nor possible then the question whether different methods affect autonomy in different ways will hardly be an interesting one. If, on the other hand, autonomy is both possible and desirable, then the possibility that various techniques of controlling behavior affect autonomy in distinctive ways, and to different degrees, may play a crucial role in our normative debates about such matters.

Are there significant differences, in terms of their impact on autonomy, among the various ways of influencing people? The ways of influence may be as varied as: offers of money, threats, hypnotism, argument, electrodes, providing information, lying, education, subliminal stimulation, psychotherapy, operant conditioning, and psychosurgery. Answering such a question would obviously require a good deal of very specific factual information about each technique, so my answer will be of the form: What would we want to know about such techniques in order to decide the issue? What information about their effects, our attitudes towards them, the causal mechanisms that explain their effects, and so forth, would we have to know to make reasonable judgments about their impact on autonomy? To answer this we must have a clearer understanding of the concept of autonomy.

Autonomy

There is a recurring theme that runs through most attempts to clarify the notion of autonomy. It is indicated by the etymology of the term: *autos* (self) and *nomos* (rule or law). The word was first applied to the Greek city-state. A city had *autonomia* when its citizens made their own laws, as opposed to being under the control of some conquering power. To leap two thousand years of intellectual history, we find the same basic notion expressed by Kant:

> The will is therefore not merely subject to the law, but is so subject that it must be considered as also making the law for itself and precisely on this account as first of all subject to the law (of which it can regard itself as the author).[1]

Hastings Center Report *Vol. 6 (February 1976), pp. 23–28. Reprinted with permission of The Hastings Center. © Institute of Society, Ethics and the Life Sciences, 360 Broadway, Hastings-on-Hudson, N.Y. 10706.*

For Kant the forces that contrasted with self-rule were not merely external forces (in the sense of other agents) but those of one's own phenomenal self, in particular one's empirical inclinations. The principles one adopted could not be accounted for by any contingent facts about the individual or his social and biological circumstances. Only by reference to one's nature as a rational being could their selection be explained.

Extending the Kantian notion to the political realm, Robert Wolff defines the autonomous man as follows: "The autonomous man, insofar as he is autonomous, is not subject to the will of another. He may do what another tells him, but not because he has been told to do it. . . . For the autonomous man, there is no such thing, strictly speaking, as a command."[2]

We find the same basic conception of self-rule or independence in all these formulations. It is clear then that some investigation of the notion of the self and that of rule or law is required to advance our understanding beyond that of what is essentially a metaphor.

Let us start with what appears to be the simpler of the two concepts, that of rule or law. In the political and moral context it is clear what one is being autonomous with respect to. As Wolff indicates, the problem is how a citizen relates to the commands of authority. The relation in question is one of compliance or non-compliance with an authoritative order or command (in its legal form a law or injunction or notice or rule). But it is more than just a matter of what the agent does; it is also a matter of why he does it. Only certain kinds of reasons for complying will preserve autonomy. Autonomous behavior is related to a particular explanation of why the person obeys a given command. Similarly, in the moral context the Kantian notion concerns the moral principles on which a person acts and the reasons which explain their adoption. In his *Moral Judgment of the Child*, Piaget comments upon the relationship between the rules of a game and the child's acceptance of the rules. "Autonomy follows upon heteronomy; the rule of a game appears to the child no longer as an external law, sacred insofar as it has been laid down by adults; but as the outcome of a free decision and worthy of respect in the measure that it has enlisted mutual consent."[3]

All these cases share the feature that what the self is acting on is some regulative device which can be represented propositionally. "Each player takes a turn." "Pay your taxes." "Keep one's promises." But this does not seem to be the same problem that we are concerned about. Those worried about whether drugs interfere with autonomy are not worried about the rules or commands or principles which the agent is obeying or adopting. They are concerned about a more general relationship between the way people behave and their motivational structure. True, they are also concerned with what explains people's specific behavior, but that explanation can (and usually does) refer to a much broader set of mental elements—beliefs, wishes, choices, judgments, desires, emotions, reasons, habits, compulsions, and so forth. We may explain behavior via upbringing, social class, culture, glands, genes, religion, etc. Autonomous behavior concerns the relationship between the "self" and these explanatory factors. Moral and political autonomy are special cases in which the behavior is to be explained by reference to explicitly formulated rules or commands.

I would argue that once the problem is viewed in this broader fashion, the traditional notion of autonomy I have outlined is inadequate and leads to paradoxes and other difficulties—chief among them that it makes autonomy impossible.

Consider this last point first. We all know that persons have a history. They develop socially and psychologically in a given environment with a given set of biological endowments. They mature slowly and are heavily influenced by their parents, siblings, peers, and culture. What sense does it make to speak of their convictions, motivations, principles, and so forth as "self-selected"? This presupposes a notion of the self as isolated from the influences just enumerated and, what is almost as foolish, that the self which chooses does so arbitrarily. For to the extent that the self uses canons of reason, principles of induction, judgments of probability, etc., these also have either been acquired from others or, what is no better from the standpoint of this position, are innate. We can no more choose *ab initio* than we can jump out of our skins. To insist upon this as a condition is to make autonomy impossible.

The same view leads to a paradox in the relationship between autonomy and moral goodness. Autonomy, in this view, demands that the agent choose his moral principles independently of external constraints. But for many moral philosophers the principles of morality are such that their correctness or truth is independent of whether they are chosen or not. So we have a conflict between being subject to the constraints of a correct set of principles and the notion of choosing whatever the self decides upon. This is more than a theoretical paradox since one of the tasks of education is to achieve both ends. Following the advice dictated by the view in question, educators are left with the frustrating task of urging their pupils both to "think for themselves" and to "think, thusly."

Both of these difficulties can be avoided by facing squarely the fact that in most cases we cannot be said to have adopted or chosen or selected our beliefs, desires, emotions, principles, and so forth. In some cases this idea doesn't even make sense. In other cases it is simply a contingent fact that we find ourselves moved in certain ways. Autonomy cannot be located on the level of first-order considerations, but in the second-order judgments we make concerning first-order considerations. If the autonomous man cannot adopt his motivations *de novo*, he can still judge them after the fact. The autonomous individual is able to step back and formulate an attitude towards the factors that influence his behavior.

Authenticity

Let me present a theory which may be characterized, in desperate brevity, by the formula autonomy = authenticity + independence. The autonomous person is one who does *his own* thing. So we need characterizations of what it is for a motivation to be *his*, and what it is for it to be his *own*. The first is what I shall call authenticity; the second, independence.

It is characteristic of persons that they are able to reflect on their decisions, motives, desires, habits, and so forth. In doing so they may form preferences concerning these. Thus a person may not only desire to smoke. He can also desire that he desire to smoke. He may not simply be motivated by jealousy or anger. He can also desire that his motivations be different (or the same).

A person may want to break the habit of smoking and prefer to stop smoking because he recognizes its harmful character and because that recognition alone is effective in changing his behavior. But if he sees that causal path closed he may, all things considered, prefer to have a causal

structure introduced which brings him to be nauseated by the taste or odor of tobacco. Even though his behavior is not then under his voluntary control, he may wish to be motivated in this way in order to stop smoking. When this is true he views the causal influences as "his." The part of him that wishes to stop smoking is recognized as his true self, the one whose wishes he wants to see carried out.

To give another example, a person might desire to learn to ski. He might believe he has no further motivation than this straightforward and simple desire, or he might believe that what causes the desire is the wish to test his courage in a mildly dangerous sport. Suppose he is now led to see (correctly) that he desires to ski because he is envious of a brother who has always excelled in sports. Having recognized the source of his desire, he can now either wish he were not motivated in this way or reaffirm the desire. If the latter, then he is acting authentically in that he identifies himself as the kind of person who wants to be motivated by envy.

Similarly, to return to the problem of moral autonomy, if one affirms one's moral principles, no matter how first acquired, because of their conformity with what one believes to be a correct moral theory, then this is an expression of the fact that they are indeed one's moral principles. For Thrasymachus, on the other hand, who views moral principles as inculcated by the powerful to enforce their rule, and who does not regard such considerations as ones he wishes to act in accordance with, to continue to act in accordance with such principles would be inauthentic.[4]

It is the attitude a person takes towards the influences motivating him which determines whether or not they are to be considered "his." Does he identify with them, assimilate them to himself, view himself as the kind of person who wishes to be motivated in these particular ways? If, on the contrary, a man resents his being motivated in certain ways, is alienated from those influences, resents acting in accordance with them, would prefer to be the kind of person who is motivated in different ways, then those influences, even though they may be causally effective, are not viewed as "his."[5]

So far I have not mentioned an obvious question—whether one can change the determinants affecting one's behavior. It might be objected that approval of a way of being moved to action which could not be changed, even indirectly, puts the agent in the position of the willing slave. Such an individual may approve of his master's orders, and indeed of the fact that he is ruled by a master, yet if he disapproved there might be nothing he could do about it. It is certainly true that the slave is not free. What about the man who is a drug addict, who cannot give up his physiological cravings for the drug, and yet who wants to be in the grip of his compulsion? In my view the agent is autonomous. He, like the slave, is not free since he will take the drug independently of whether he wishes to be motivated in this way. But important as that fact is, there is another fact which is also true and which is also important. Namely he identifies with his addiction. And it is this identification that I am designating as authenticity.

This view of authenticity is opposed to the traditional existentialist position with its emphasis on choice and decision. Given that we are born into societies at a particular stage of development, with given social roles which provide a framework for participation, with a body of knowledge built up over time, with moral and other assumptions built into the social framework, the notion of decision or choice is implausible as a description of how we acquire our motivational structures.

We simply find ourselves motivated in certain ways and the notion of choosing, from ground zero, makes no sense. Sooner or later we find ourselves, as in Neurath's metaphor of the ship in mid-ocean being reconstructed while sailing, in mid-history. But we always retain the possibility of stepping back and judging where we are and where we want to be.

Independence

Authenticity, while necessary for autonomy, is not sufficient. A person's motivational structure may be *his*, without being his *own*. This may occur in either of two ways. First, the identification with his motivations, or the choice of the type of person he wants to be, may have been produced by manipulation, deception, the withholding of relevant information, and so on. It may have been influenced in decisive ways by others in such a fashion that we are not prepared to think of it as his own choice. I shall call this a lack of procedural independence.

Concern about such procedural failures is not simply an expression of general worries about determinism. Even if some strong thesis of determinism is correct, we will still want to make a distinction between those forms of influence which contribute to the agent making his own decisions and those which make those decisions and choices in some sense that of others.

Another way of seeing this point is that the notion of authentic behavior leaves no room for "false consciousness." An individual may identify or approve of his motivational structure because of an inability to view in a critical and rational manner his situation.

Suppose, however, that the identifications and approvals are influenced in such a way that they are procedurally independent. Still, a person may decide to renounce his independence of action or thought because he wants (genuinely) to be that sort of person. A person may want to do whatever his mother, or his government, tells him to do, and do so in a procedurally independent manner. By giving up what I call substantive independence he has authentically abandoned something we are inclined to think of as an important part of autonomy.

We now have two distinct problems: to characterize procedural independence and to characterize substantive independence.

The problem of analyzing procedural independence is the task of characterizing those influences which in some way prevent the individual's decisions from being his own. It may be helpful to think of procedural independence as a generalization of the notion of liberty. The paradigm cases of interference with liberty have been those of coercion, and the analytical task is to offer an account of why certain ways of getting a person to do something other than he originally intended (incentives, information, argument) do not count as interferences, whereas others (threats, physical force) do infringe freedom. With respect to autonomy, conceived of as authenticity under conditions of procedural independence, the paradigms of interference are manipulation and deception, and the analytic task is to distinguish these ways of influencing people's higher order judgments from those (education, requirements of logical thinking, provision of role-models) which do not negate procedural independence. This is a difficult problem, but it looks as if a solution is possible.

With respect to autonomy conceived as authenticity plus substantive independence I believe matters are different. The problem here is to characterize when a person is giving up independence (perhaps authentically) and when he retains it. I cannot, however, think of a hypothesis which will at the same time classify obvious examples of non-autonomy correctly (the servile lackey, the conformer to group pressures) and yet not also classify the compassionate or loyal or moral man as non-autonomous. For the compassionate or loyal or moral man is one whose actions are to some extent determined by the needs and predicaments of others. He is not independent or self-determining. Again, any notion of commitment (to a lover, a goal, a group) seems to be a denial of substantive independence and hence of autonomy. There seems to be no way of conceptualizing substantive independence which avoids this classification.

One can adopt various conclusions at this point. The first, and most reasonable, is that we should keep looking for an adequate account. The second is that we should be prepared to accept the idea that the compassionate man is less autonomous than the selfish one. This would indicate that any account of autonomy describes a value possibly in direct conflict with other crucial values and desirable traits. To discover that a person cannot be moral and autonomous at the same time would certainly be an unsatisfactory outcome to our quest for a theory of autonomy. A third view is that the notion of autonomy is not simply descriptive; that we are only prepared to designate a particular kind of independence as autonomy when we value *that kind* of independence. The main drawback of this last position is that it makes the concept useless in trying to evaluate various methods of behavior control in terms of their effect on autonomy. For we would already have had to answer the question whether a given form of influence is desirable or not in order to decide the question of whether autonomy is affected or not.

My view at this point is that autonomy can be conceived as authenticity + independence (procedural and substantive). But since it is unlikely that the notion of substantive independence is a genuinely desirable one, the notion of autonomy which should play a role in the evaluation of various methods of behavior control is that which requires authenticity and procedural independence.

One reason for reluctance to abandon substantive independence is the fear that the link with moral responsibility may be broken. As Wolff argues, if men are to be responsible agents and to assume responsibility for their actions, it is necessary for them to ascertain what is right. So far, so good. But there is no reason to suppose that by considering autonomy as authenticity plus procedural independence men are able to avoid responsibility. The man who does what his mother tells him is no more nor less responsible for what he does than the man who thinks through each issue for himself. He cannot evade responsibility by saying, "She told me to do it," precisely because, on our account of autonomy, he affirmed his own desire to be motivated by her desires—and hence bears the responsibility for that determination of his will.

Guidelines for the Preservation of Autonomy

Given the second-order nature of autonomy as I have considered it, there is an immediate consequence concerning the kinds of methods it is legitimate to use to influence people. If one values autonomy (and though I shall not argue why we should I believe such reasons can be given), then methods which interfere with the ability of the individual to reflect on his first-order motivations should not be used. There are various ways, in principle, that such interference might take place. There might be methods which keep the agent in ignorance of the true determinants of his behavior. Methods which rely on causal influences of which the agent is not conscious are of this nature. Subliminal motivation, if such were indeed possible, would be a primary example. Since the agent does not know the real reasons for his actions, he cannot reflect on such reasons and make a favorable or adverse judgment concerning them. Another example of this type would be those methods of changing people's attitude and conduct which rely on the theory of cognitive dissonance. Consider the following experiment.

Children are asked to rank a number of toys in order of preference. The adult then leaves the room and warns them not to play with the most preferred toy. He then returns, and the children are asked again to order their preferences. It turns out, as predicted by the theory, that the children shift downward their previous first choice. The theory predicts this on the basis of a conflict between preference and action inconsistent with preference. The conflict is resolved by shifting preference. But the agent is not aware of this as the cause of his change in attitude, and hence cannot make an independent judgment of whether he wishes to be motivated in this fashion

Obviously, methods of influence which destroy the ability of the agent to reflect critically and intelligently on his motivations violate autonomy. The processes by which this might be accomplished can vary from those which destroy parts of the brain necessary for such reflective tasks to processes which make the psychic costs of such examination so painful that something analogous to coercion takes place. In general, however, I think autonomy is in greater danger from manipulative methods of influence than from those outright assaults on the individual associated with the notions of brainwashing and psychosurgery.

It follows from this analysis that there will be only a small number of methods of influence which are in themselves denials of autonomy. It remains true, nevertheless, that we have certain broad preferences concerning ways in which we would like to be motivated, and, though a contingent fact, it may be decisive in generalizing about autonomy. There are, I believe, certain general categories of influence whose link to second-order attitudes can be understood in light of the causal mechanisms by which the techniques work.

One of the things we know about ourselves is that we have varied interests and ideals, varied tastes and preferences, varied desires and wishes. There are various life plans that individuals may have, and there is no choosing between most of them in terms of some overall ideal or principle of rationality. The good for humans is irreducibly multiple and variegated. Given this knowledge, are there considerations which make it preferable for rational agents either to encourage and adopt, or to discourage and reject, certain techniques of influence on the ground that the former facilitate, and the latter make more difficult, our tasks of forming rational plans for our own lives?

Given these general considerations, what more specific guidelines can be deduced or, perhaps more accurately, be harmonized with the preceding? I say "more accurately" because it seems to me that, although some of the specific guidelines might be made deductions by the introduction of various premises, the relation will often be one of "expressing an ideal" or "reflecting a general conception."

1. We have favorable attitudes towards those methods of influence which support the self-respect and dignity of those who are being influenced. Ideally such methods should constitute a public expression of agents as equal and sovereign individuals.

Obviously at this level of abstraction not much guidance is provided concerning specific techniques. All depends on how the techniques work and what their effect on dignity is supposed to be. But it is important to be clear about the distinction between expressing and supporting self-respect, and being causally connected with producing a state of affairs which might be called increased self-respect or dignity. For example, it is often argued that certain drastic techniques such as psychosurgery or aversive conditioning may result in the agent's being able to leave an institution, or to no longer "act out" in various ways. Hence such techniques are promoting dignity. Be that as it may, it may still be the case that the methods used are not expressive of the dignity of the agent. They may treat him as an object rather than a subject. Though leading to increased self-respect they are not expressive of it. Of course it might be that methods which are expressive of self respect or dignity are not causally effective in producing it.

2. Methods of influence which are destructive of the ability of individuals to reflect rationally on their interests should not be used.

This approximation seems fairly uncontroversial. At one time I thought that a stronger principle might be reasonable—that ideally methods should be used which appeal to the reasoning capacities of individuals. I was persuaded that this represented a rather parochial view, one perhaps endemic to philosophers, of the role of reasons in determining action. Is it really preferable to appeal to an individual's ability to think that what he is doing is just rather than to his love of justice?

3. Methods should not be used which affect in fundamental ways the personal identity of individuals. To the extent that the effects of certain modes of influence are such as to raise questions about whether the individual is the same person, or in a less extreme version, whether the discontinuities between the person at two close points of time are sufficiently sharp, we would not agree to their use.

We need to maintain a coherent and unified conception of our own identity. Notions of personal responsibility, long-range plans, a connection with our past, all depend on our being sufficiently similar at various time-stages to be thought of as the same person. We may welcome change, but within a framework of continuity.

4. Methods which rely essentially on deception, on keeping the agent in ignorance of relevant facts, are to be avoided.

This is not to assert that more knowledge is always better than less. Sometimes knowledge does increaseth sorrow. There are times when we really "don't want to know." But we do resent being manipulated even in our own interest.

5. Modes of influence which are not physically intrusive are preferable to those which are. By physically intrusive is meant roughly those methods which penetrate the body. Hence, drugs, psychosurgery, electric shock treatment, monitoring devices, etc.

The argument for this condition relies on psychological assertions concerning the necessity of some realm of physical integrity which cannot be violated. This is related to notions of dignity and privacy. It is possible that these feelings may be primitive (not capable of being reduced to other kinds of considerations) or it may be the case that this is not an independent condition but may be derived from some other conditions.

6. There will be some restrictions on the time in which the changes take place and the ability of the agent to resist the effects of various modes of influence.

Given our knowledge of the possibility of changing tastes, desires, new knowledge and so forth, we wish to maintain some options for reversing our behavior. Thus changes which are reversible are preferable to those which are not. We wish to guard against error and mistake in our current judgments. Of course, in some cases, the possibility of error is so slight that we may not care very much about this condition. It is better to be rich and healthy than poor and sick.

Similarly we are concerned about the rapidity with which the effects take place, and the duration of the change. Both of these are connected with the notion of reversibility, with the question of whether the agent can bring about the initial status unaided or requires the aid of another party. With respect to duration, even if the effect eventually wears off it makes a difference whether its duration is five minutes or five years.

7. We prefer methods of influence which work though the cognitive and affective structure of the agent, which require the active participation of the agent in producing the change, to those which shortcircuit the desires and beliefs of the agent and make him a passive recipient of the changes.

This preference is partly explicable in terms of the previous condition—the ability of the agent to resist the changes—but is also a distinct condition. In the first place the two are not tightly linked. Very powerful incentives (you offer me a Mercedes-Benz for a nickel) may be almost impossible to resist, but there is no question of shortcircuiting the motivational apparatus of the agent. I accept the offer because I want to. On the other hand, I may be able to resist the effects of so-called truth serums although their influence is of the short-circuiting kind.

But even if the two were contingently related in a very strong fashion I believe our reasons for resenting them are distinguishable. To the extent that my participation is required to bring about the change I can identify with my changed self. To the extent that the changes are brought about via purely physiological mechanisms, or even psychological ones which bypass my normal reflective processes (perhaps hypnotism might serve as an example), I view my new self as less continuous with the old.

The matter is, however, complicated. It is plausible in some circumstances to regard the more rational parts of ourselves as obstacles to a genuine part of ourselves which is suppressed and waits to be released. So various drug induced states are thought of as no less "me" although (or even because) they are brought about by a short-circuiting process.

In Conclusion

There are, it should be noted, two parts to my argument which, at least theoretically, are independent of one another. One can accept my analysis of autonomy while rejecting the claims concerning considerations relevant to the preference for some means of influencing behavior over others; or one can reject the analysis while accepting the considerations, and then try to find another theory to explain their choice.

Such a theory may either be one which analyzes autonomy in a different manner or one which does not make use of autonomy at all. It may be that quite different factors such as liberty, privacy, dignity, or notions of capacity or power are adequate to explain our reasoned judgments about the legitimacy of various methods of behavior control.

Notes

1. Immanuel Kant, *Groundwork of the Metaphysic of Morals* (London: Hutchinson University Library, 1961), p. 98.

2. Robert Wolff, *In Defense of Anarchism* (New York: Harper & Row, 1970), p. 14.

3. Jean Piaget, *The Moral Judgment of the Child* (London: Routledge & Kegan Paul, 1932), p. 57.

4. This shows that one cannot identify as "his" motivations the ones which in fact explain a person's actions. That is necessary but not sufficient.

5. This notion is more fully worked out in my "Acting Freely," *Nous* 4, no. 4 (1970). See also H. Frankfort, "Freedom of the Will and the Concept of a Person," *Journal of Philosophy* 68, no. 1 (1971).

Legal and Ethical Aspects of Behavior Control

Seymour L. Halleck

For more than a decade, the practice of involuntary and indeterminate commitment of the mentally ill has been rigorously criticized by those who fear that psychiatrists are too arbitrary in depriving people of liberty. More recently the use of treatments such as lobotomy, behavior therapy, and drug therapy has been questioned on the grounds that such treatment deprives the patient of the right to choose his own course of action.[1-3] The new critiques go beyond questioning the imposition of treatment upon involuntary patients. Some treatments offered to voluntary patients are also being attacked as repressive and dehumanizing. A few critics even fear that the psychiatric profession has involved itself in a gigantic conspiracy to control the behavior of citizens who deviate from social norms.[4]

In the new climate of concern over the powers of psychiatrists to shape behavior, there is a real likelihood that treatment decisions psychiatrists have come to view as routine medical decisions will be rigorously challenged by the courts. In one jurisdiction, for example, a judge recently upheld the argument of a plaintiff who asked the court to restrain state hospital doctors from giving him phenothiazines. Decisions such as this, which I believe will become common, raise critical questions as to the future practice of psychiatry.

If psychiatrists wish to continue to practice in an effective manner, I am convinced they must develop a system of internal control and monitoring of psychiatric practices that will protect the rights of patients and still make it possible to treat those who will benefit from treatment.

The Potentialities of Behavior Control

The new fear of psychiatric treatment is best understood in terms of the concept of behavior control. Perry London has defined behavior control quite simply as getting people to do someone else's bidding.[5] I would like to expand slightly on this definition. Most psychiatric treatments are designed to change the patient's behavior. In its broadest sense behavior control can be viewed as a special form of behavioral change. It is treatment imposed on or offered to the patient that to a large extent is designed to satisfy the wishes of others. Such treatment may lead to the patient's behaving in a manner which satisfies his community or his society. Of course, behavioral change that satisfies the wishes of others may also satisfy many of the wishes of the patient. For reasons that will become clear later, it is sometimes necessary to include even this category of behavior change under the heading of behavior control.

The question of behavior control has been made more critical by the growing effectiveness of psychiatric treatment. The newer drugs and new behavior therapy techniques make it possible to change behavior in a relatively efficient and rapid manner. Long-term psychotherapeutic techniques can, of course, also modify behavior. However, traditional psychotherapy works slowly. It gives the patient time to contemplate the meaning of

The American Journal of Psychiatry, 131:4 (1974) 381–385. Copyright 1974, the American Psychiatric Association. Reprinted by permission of the author and publisher.

behavioral change and to resist such change. It also offers the patient the opportunity to learn to behave in ways which do not meet the needs of others. Some traditional psychotherapists even welcome changes that leave the patient more aggressive, more rebellious, and perhaps more abrasive to those around him. (This may, of course, just be a variant of behavior control in which the patient does the bidding of his therapist rather than the bidding of members of his community.)

Biological and behavior therapies, on the other hand, seem to be peculiarly adaptable to serving the needs of society. Lobotomy, electric shock, and tranquilization are likely to increase conformity and to decrease assertiveness. Behavior therapies are used somewhat more flexibly. Some forms of behavior therapy may help the patient develop greater assertiveness. In practice, however, there is little evidence that they have been used to promote assertiveness. Biological and behavior therapies also work quickly. They can be used without giving the patient a chance to contemplate the meaning of his behavior. Once the patient agrees to or is coerced into treatment, he is unlikely to consider the interpersonal or social causes of his behavior or the social consequences of his treatment.

While recognizing that almost any psychiatric treatment can be a form of behavior control, I will focus this discussion on some of the more ethically controversial therapies, including biological therapies (i.e., lobotomy, electric shock therapy, and drug therapy); behavior therapies (including aversive therapy, desensitization, and operant conditioning); and the use of physical or chemical restraint.

There are three classes of situations in which the implications of behavior control will be considered.

1. Situations in which the patient does not verbally consent to receive treatment. Sometimes the patient verbally (or physically) resists treatment. Sometimes he merely acquiesces without giving verbal consent. Usually these situations arise when the patient is civilly or criminally committed. However, treatments can also be imposed upon voluntary patients without their knowing about it.

2. Situations in which the patient consents to treatment under some duress. These situa-

tions are most blatant when the patient is involuntarily committed, civilly or criminally, and is informed that certain actions that he might consider punitive will take place unless he consents to treatment. They also arise in a more subtle form when the patient's family or community pressure him into accepting treatment either through threats of sanction or threats of withdrawal of love or status.

3. Situations in which the patient consents to treatment or may even request treatment. At present these situations are the least controversial, but in the long run they may raise the most complex ethical questions for our profession and our society.

The Nonconsenting Patient

Nonconsenting treatment is most likely to be imposed upon those who are civilly committed as mentally ill or who are criminally committed and are later certified psychotic. In such situations it is usually assumed that the patient desperately needs to be treated but is too confused to understand what is best for him.

Currently electric shock, lobotomy, and drug therapy are used with some frequency in treating nonconsenting patients. Behavior therapy is used somewhat less frequently. For example, aversive therapy (with some troubling exceptions) is not regularly used with nonconsenting patients. The use of operant methods with the nonconsenting patient, however, is more common. Some patients are required to live in units where a token system that rewards socially approved behavior is enforced without the patient's ever having agreed to participate in such a program. Behavior-shaping programs are also used in more traditional hospital wards without consultation with the patient and therefore without his consent. In such instances the staff merely decides what types of behavior it wishes to reinforce and creates an environment that provides such reinforcement. Since there is no informed consent here, the treatment can be viewed as coercive.

I do not feel there is ever any ethical justification for deceiving the patient. All patients, even the most disturbed, should be informed of what will be done to them, why it will be done, and what effects the treatment is likely to have. If after having such information, the patient still does not consent to treatment, coercive treatment is justified only if the following sets of conditions are met:

First, the patient must be judged to be dangerous to himself or others. In the case of civilly committed patients, this judgment has often been made in the process of commitment.

Second, those who are providing treatment must believe there is a reasonable probability that treatment will be of benefit to the patient as well as to those around him.

Third, the patient must be judged to be incompetent to evaluate the necessity for treatment.

It should be obvious that each of these criteria calls for highly value-laden and sometimes arbitrary judgments. Without embarking on a prolonged discussion of dangerousness, it may be sufficient to note that psychiatrists have modest skills in predicting dangerousness to self and quite limited skills in predicting dangerousness to others;[6] in both instances we tend to overdiagnose dangerousness.

With regard to the issue of treatment, too often the only criterion used in evaluating the helpfulness of a treatment is whether it makes the patient more placid. There is an implied assumption that if the patient ceases to be abrasive, he will benefit from the favorable reactions of others and will feel better. The words "help" or "treatment" in this context should mean something more than docility. As a result of treatment the patient should experience a greater sense of psychological well-being and his feeling better should not be totally dependent on the reactions of those who initially disapproved of his behavior. The doctor who treats should have a reasonable belief that the treatment imposed will produce changes that it can be assumed the patient might have sought if he had been more rational.

Decisions as to the patient's competency to evaluate the usefulness of treatment are also difficult to make. There are many patients who are too confused to understand that certain potentially frightening treatments might be helpful to them. But there is at the same time ample evidence that psychiatrists tend to overdiagnose incompetency.[7] Many patients who resist psychiatric treatment, including some severely handicapped persons, may be making quite rational decisions. The patient's competency to understand the usefulness of treatment should be evaluated in rather

straightforward terms. I would suggest that to be competent in this situation, the patient need only appreciate the possible results of being treated and the possible results of not being treated.

There is little problem justifying coercive treatment if all three criteria of dangerousness, treatability, and incompetence are obviously present. In some rare instances, however, imposition of treatment upon nonconsenting patients might be desirable if only two of the three criteria were met. This is a highly controversial issue. Should a very dangerous incompetent person be involuntarily treated even when considerable doubt exists as to the efficacy of treatment? Should a highly treatable incompetent person be involuntarily treated if he is not dangerous? Or should a highly dangerous, easily treatable person who is competent to resist treatment ever be treated against his will? Each of these questions could be debated endlessly. There can be no standard formula for answering them; the most that can be said here is that the psychiatric profession and society need to thoroughly consider these questions whenever an involuntary treatment decision is being made.

The decision to impose treatment upon a nonconsenting patient requires extraordinarily complex medical and ethical judgments. I do not believe that such decisions should be made by a single doctor except in emergencies. For that matter, such decisions should not be made by groups of doctors working in the same institutional setting *without* the benefit of some outside monitoring and feedback.

I propose that any treatment recommendation for nonconsenting patients involving brain surgery, electric shock therapy, prolonged use of tranquilizers, or behavior therapy be reviewed and approved by a monitoring agency. A board consisting of one of the therapists who recommended treatment, a psychiatrist who is affiliated with the institution (who ideally should represent a different school of thought than the doctor who made the recommendation), and an attorney should review and pass on the desirability of each therapeutic recommendation. Ideally, the consulting psychiatrist and the attorney should be replaced by new people at regular intervals so that there is less danger of stagnant attitudes and collusion.

Under this plan I would find nothing objectionable in the nonconsenting patient's requesting that his privately hired psychiatrist and/or attorney also participate in these proceedings. If the case for treatment is good, even the patient's own agents should concur in the recommendation. If the case for treatment is weak, an adversary procedure might help in making the right decisions.

The kind of review board I am recommending would certainly add to the administrative burdens of psychiatric treatments and could conceivably be expensive. However, its advantages outweigh these deficits. First of all, such an approach would give patients a greater sense of safety and security. It would serve as a message to society that even the most disturbed individuals are not to be subjected to behavior control without careful consideration. The existence of such a board would encourage doctors to be more precise and thoughtful in making recommendations for treatment. Finally, this approach would continue to leave medical decisions primarily in the hands of doctors and in the long run would diminish the possibility that treatment decisions might be made by the courts.

It must be emphasized that emergency situations would have to be excluded from committee review. When the patient is so disorganized that his life or the physical well-being of those around him is threatened, there is not time to review treatment decisions. The committee would become involved only if the physician wished to continue involuntary treatment after the emergency situation had passed. An arbitrary period of time for invoking committee review of what were initially emergency treatment decisions might be two weeks. In 14 days most "life or death" issues will have been resolved and treatment decisions can be reviewed with due regard to the patient's rights.

Consent Under Duress

The ethical problems involved in treating patients who consent to treatment under pressure are almost as excruciating as those involving patients who do not consent. One immediate problem is assessing the nature of the pressure imposed upon the patient. Pressure to consent may be quite subtle. Often the patient's family or community may threaten loss of love or sanctions if the patient does not enter a hospital and cooperate in receiving certain treatments.

The authority of the doctor is also a powerful influence. Most people will take the advice of doctors even if they fear that the consequences of such

passivity might not be in their own interests. Unfortunately, some doctors are unnecessarily authoritarian. Sometimes they enunciate or imply, without good reason, that terrible consequences will befall the patient if he does not consent to a certain treatment. Sometimes the patient is not fully informed as to alternative treatments that might be available.

The ethical issues involved in consent under subtle pressure are in many ways similar to those involved when the patient consents willingly. These will be discussed later. It should be stated here, however, that when the patient is reluctant to undergo treatment, the doctor has an ethical obligation not to frighten or threaten him. He should also provide the patient with all possible information as to the effects of the treatment he is recommending and as to the possibilities of alternative treatments.

Consent obtained under severe and direct pressure is a different matter. Sometimes patients in mental hospitals are told (or correctly perceive) that they must undergo certain treatments if they are ever going to be released. In some correctional programs, particularly indeterminate programs for sexual and "psychopathic" offenders, the patient knows that release is primarily dependent upon his cooperation in treatment. If he accepts treatment the meaning of such "consent" is difficult to ascertain.

The problem is poignantly illustrated in a recent film based on the novel *A Clockwork Orange*. A violent and sexually assaultive young man serving a long prison sentence is informed that he can be released in only a few weeks if he agrees to undergo a new treatment. He consents and is given a sophisticated form of aversive therapy that "cures" him of his sexuality and aggressiveness. He leaves the prison a free man but finds himself unable to enjoy life or even to function effectively when deprived of his old behavior patterns. Eventually he is driven to attempt suicide.

The film raises many ethical and political questions. Assuming that we can change people so drastically—and it is likely that we will soon be able to do so—do we have a right to alter human beings in a manner that so seriously impairs their capacity to choose? What if the patient's assaultiveness was politically motivated? What would be the political consequences of "curing" the aggressiveness of a Malcolm X or an Eldridge Cleaver?

These are fascinating questions, but for our purposes here the most important questions are: "To what extent can we view the patient's consent as freely chosen if the only alternative to consent is harsh punishment?" "Does the consent of a man who has no way of knowing what effect the treatment will have upon him really mean very much?"

As long as there are potentially dangerous individuals confined to prisons or hospitals and as long as new treatments are available that might change these individuals, the pressures of incarceration will motivate many of them to accept treatment, whether or not this is the conscious intent of social agencies. Since many patients can and probably will benefit from such treatment, consent under pressure is not altogether undesirable. It would help, however, if in the process of motivating and treating such patients, certain rules were carefully followed.

First, the patient should be given a clear explanation of the possible consequences of treatment.

Second, the patient should be told what other treatments are available and he should be given an opportunity to choose among them, rather than having only one treatment option open to him.

Third, no special punishment should be imposed on the patient if he refuses treatment. His conditions of confinement should never be made worse in order to persuade him to accept treatment, nor should he be denied release from an institution if he improves without undergoing treatment.

Fourth, treatments to which the patient consents under direct threat of sanction, like treatments imposed upon a nonconsenting patient, should be reviewed and approved by a committee that should include an attorney and at least one doctor not directly involved with the treatment.

The Voluntary Patient

The most fascinating and in some ways the most insidious aspect of behavior control involves truly voluntary patients who are neither treated without consent nor coerced into giving consent. People are usually unwilling to tolerate the psychological pain associated with anxiety or depression. If treatments that alleviate these unpleasant emotions are available, such treatments will be sought eagerly. The problem is that, while alleviation of suffering through treatment may serve the patient's short-term needs, the behavioral changes produced by treatment may not serve the patient's long-term needs and may eventually be of more value to those around him than to the patient himself. By gratifying a short-term need for comfort, the patient may find himself in a situation where his long-term needs for power, autonomy, and status are compromised.

This concept can be dramatized by considering the use of heroin in the ghetto. Heroin usage is a highly effective, albeit short-lived and dangerous, treatment for human despair. Many oppressed blacks use heroin to make life tolerable, to add meaning to life, or to blot out the psychological suffering resulting from poverty and discrimination. The drug is not forced upon them; rather, they seek it eagerly. The immediate effect of heroin is to make the user feel better. But in the long run the willing use of this drug strengthens the position of those who oppress blacks. The contentment and euphoria produced by heroin diminishes the militancy of the user and makes him less likely to do anything to change his situation.

The psychiatrist is usually called upon to treat symptoms that have less powerful political implications than the militancy of oppressed blacks. Nevertheless, treatment of common psychiatric symptoms has important implications for the patient's relationship to his environment and to the ethics of behavior control. Symptoms can be viewed as signals or as efforts on the part of the individual to communicate personal distress to his environment. A person is viewed as having a symptom if he behaves in a manner that reveals he is anxious, depressed, confused, or angry. The behavior tends to be viewed as abnormal because the basis for the behavior is not apparent either to the patient or to those around him. Yet such behavior often arises from a need to influence and attempt to change what the patient perceives as an oppressive environment.

Symptoms always elicit some response from the patient's environment. Often they have a powerful influence. The husband of the frigid wife must deal with his partner's unresponsiveness. The community must respond to the aggressive child's delinquency. There is no way of knowing the extent to which any symptomatic behavior is an effort to influence an oppressive environment and to what extent it is an autonomous happening that has little social meaning. It is likely, however, that even the sickest person who suffers profoundly is in part seeking to change his environment. To the extent that we treat and extinguish behaviors that are designed to influence the environment which is bothering the patient, we tend to preserve the stability of social systems and risk becoming agents of the status quo.

In the case of voluntary as well as involuntary treatments, it is the biological and behavioral therapies that have the most significant ethical implications. In traditional psychotherapy (individual, family, or group) considerable effort is made to help the patient understand the meaning of his symptom. If he is aware of the manner in which his environment may be oppressing him, the patient at least has the option to do something about changing his environment. Biological therapies and behavior therapies, however, do not expand awareness. As a matter of fact, their principal merit is that they can be used efficiently and impersonally without the necessity to deal with the troubling implications of what the patient's behavior might mean. They can be superior instruments of behavior control without the slightest pretense of coercion.

This issue has profound implications for psychiatric practice. The overwhelming majority of patients accept biological and behavioral treatments without having sufficient information as to how these treatments may affect their future capacities. I believe the psychiatrist has an ethical responsibility to help the patient find this information.

Except in emergencies, if the therapist is to use drugs or behavior therapy he should accompany such treatment with an effort to help the patient explore the meaning of his symptom. The patient should be encouraged to seek an awareness of the extent to which his symptom is an effort to influence the environment and also to become aware of how the alleviation of the symptom might change his relationship to his environment. If a reasonable effort (perhaps only an hour or two of investigation) has been made to help the patient explore these variables, and if he still wants the biological or behavioral treatment, he should receive it. All of this is of course time-consuming and might impress some "hard-thinking" clinicians as too compulsively ethical. I would argue, however, that efforts to increase the patient's awareness of a social situation are not merely an

ethical necessity but are also an essential part of good psychiatric treatment. The patient's capacity to understand and then either to try to accept or to change his environment may in the long run be a greater force in promoting his psychological well-being than the sometimes temporary comfort he might obtain from symptomatic treatment.

This does not mean that the physician should withhold treatment on the basis of the unproven assumption that to withhold it might be best for the patient in the long run. Rather, physicians should be committed to helping the patient make a rational choice as to the desirability of the treatment. I am convinced that the usefulness and reasonableness of the patient's choice will be positively correlated with the amount of accurate information he has about himself and about the stressful factors in his environment.

Conclusions

While there are many people in our country who are wary of the psychiatrist's power to control behavior, there are also many who would encourage psychiatrists to use their power to shape citizens in such a way that they are more conforming. I predict that psychiatrists will soon experience an increase in pressure from both groups. If we are to respond to these pressures rationally and humanistically, we must familiarize ourselves with the legal and ethical implications of behavior control. And we must develop a system of internal regulations of our activities that will satisfy the needs of our patients, ourselves, and the general public.

Notes

1. Szasz, T. *Psychiatric Justice.* New York, Macmillan, 1965.

2. Halleck, S. *The Politics of Therapy.* New York, Science House, 1971.

3. Kittrie, N. *The Right To Be Different.* Baltimore, Johns Hopkins Press, 1971.

4. Ennis, B. *Prisoners of Psychiatry: Mental Patients, Psychiatry, and the Law.* New York, Harcourt, Brace, Jovanovich, 1972.

5. London, P. *Behavior Control.* New York, Harper & Row, 1970.

6. Wenk, E.; Robinson, O.; Smith, G. "Can Violence Be Predicted?" *Crime and Delinquency* 18:393–402, 1972.

7. Szasz, T. *Law, Liberty, and Psychiatry.* New York, Macmillan, 1963.

Brain Surgery in Aggressive Epileptics

Vernon H. Mark

A little over two years ago Frank Ervin, a psychiatrist, and I, a neurosurgeon, wrote a book called *Violence and the Brain,* detailing the application of brain surgery to problems of violent behavior. The public response to that book underscores with great vividness the fact that the medical issues of neurosurgery are no more interesting or vital than the issues of neurosurgery's *social role.* I would like here to offer some reflections about those social issues.

The most important problem to conjure with, from the standpoint of the sciences of human behavior, is the unfortunate dichotomy in basic approaches to behavior. Certain kinds of behavior (for instance, paralysis, blindness and dementia) were put into the province of *organic neurology.* Physicians working in this field have been increasingly reluctant to examine other kinds of abnormal behavior, even when they are associated with obvious brain abnormalities.

On the other hand, social psychiatrists, sociologists, criminologists, and many psychologists tend to view the other behavioral abnormalities, for instance intractable depressions and aggressive assaultive behavior, as pure reflections of unusual or abnormal environmental stress. They believe that brain function or dysfunction is not an important determinant as far as abnormal behavior is concerned. To them, all human beings function with the same "normal" brains. Even those few social scientists who admit that brain function might be important in abnormal behavior feel that so little is known about brain function that it is useless to spend time and money investigating it.

Now whatever the sociological reasons for this division of labor in the scientific vineyard, any high school student can see that it results in absurd theoretical suppositions. No human behavior whatever, be it normal or abnormal, can be the consequence of the brain alone without the environment. Nor can any behavior, whatever its environmental determinants, take place without the brain freighting its mechanical impulses with emotion and culture. Therefore any thorough investigation of abnormal, violent behavior should look not only to the environment for causes but also to the brain itself.

Yet when President Lyndon Johnson and Milton Eisenhower convened the Commission on Violence, there were over fifty consultants representing various fields of sociology, criminology, history, government, law, social psychiatry, and social psychology, but only two representing the brain!

Let me stress that recognition of the brain in behavior does not entail, as some critics might fear, that all behavior should be controlled through the brain. Rather it is precisely because any behavior, normal or abnormal, *could be* modified through altering the brain, at least in principle, that it is absolutely crucial to make *moral* decisions about the sort appropriate for neurosurgery and other direct brain manipulations. There are important moral issues at stake, for example, in the very definition of a problem as a medical one, for which medical therapy is appropriate. This problem is pressed further when a behavior problem is defined as a neurological one.

My own position regarding the appropriateness of neurosurgery can be illustrated in terms of three alternatives. The first two of these I unequivocally reject:

The first of these positions holds that medical means should be undertaken to improve *any* behavior, wherever possible, be the behavior normal or abnormal. Although neurosurgery is not in a position now to improve normal behavior, some people advocate the use of drugs—amphetamines, for instance—for that purpose. The advantage of this position is that it avoids the obvious difficulties in defining normality. The grave disadvantage is that it makes the medical men authorities on improvement and the good life, which they are not, at least under our present social arrangement. Moral values are social concerns, not medical ones in any presently recognized sense.

Reprinted by permission of the author and the publisher from the Hastings Center Report *3 (February 1973).*
© *Institute of Society, Ethics and Life Sciences, 360 Broadway, Hastings-on-Hudson, New York.*

A second position holds that any *abnormal* behavior should be treated by whatever medical means are available. Often argued by psychotherapists, this position says that, regardless of any *organic* abnormality, what is undesirable in abnormal behavior is the behavior, not its organic base. The criteria for alteration should refer to the behavior, irrespective of whether the organic base is normal or abnormal. Should an unusual brain abnormality produce a 50 point I.Q. rise, no one would suggest ablating it: its behavioral product is desirable. (With regard to neurosurgical control of violent behavior, I am *against* the principle that it could be used to treat abnormal behavior when there is no organic abnormality of the brain.)

A third position, then, is that medical procedures like neurosurgery should be used only when behavior is abnormal, and bad, as the result of an abnormality in the brain. As I shall repeat below, violent behavior *not* associated with brain disease should be dealt with politically and socially, not medically.

With this brief positioning of what I take to be support for a very circumscribed domain for neurosurgical procedures, I now want to deal with some common criticisms of neurosurgery. Most of the criticisms either construe neurosurgery to be capable of more than it is, or assume that it would be used in areas I believe to be inappropriate. Like any technological power, neurosurgery can be misused, and setting the limits of its use is more than a medical problem.

Political Versus Personal Violence

Implicit in many of the criticisms of the surgical treatment of violent epileptics is the fear that this treatment will be used against political protestors. This fear is based on an semantic confusion about the word "violence." Many activities in our society are called violent. The "establishment" tends to view as violent any protest movement against the war, unfair living conditions, or the prison system. Protestors view the reaction of police and the National Guard as violent. Minority groups have indicated that social or job discrimination is a form of violence.

The kind of violent behavior for which I might approve neurosurgery, however, has a much narrower definition: *personal violent behavior; unwarranted and usually unprovoked acts that directly attempt to, or actually do injure or destroy another person or thing.* And, as I have said, I would not approve neurosurgery even in such cases unless the personal violence could be traced to organic brain disease and could not be treated by non-surgical methods.

Some political psychiatrists have argued that social injustice provokes individual acts of violence which seem "senseless" but which, in reality, are political protests against the social system. As Goebbels showed, political violence of mass proportions can be culled up without counting on people with diseased brains. However, the person whose violence is related to brain disease and is used by a Hitler or Goebbels is a danger to himself and his loved ones, and cannot be counted on to rage only in politically strategic situations. Thus, the morality of preventing such an individual from seeking proper medical diagnosis and care is certainly in question.

Biological Factors in Personal Violence

Many sociologists believe that brain dysfunction does not have a role in such behavioral abnormalities as intractable depression, thought disorders, paranoia, or aggressive assaultive behavior of the sort I am concerned with. In the last case, however, there is *solid* medical evidence to link aggressive behavior to focal brain disease. This behavioral symptom is often present in such clinical disorders as temporal lobe epilepsy, temporal lobe tumors, infections of the brain (such as rabies and post-encephalitic syndromes), and serious brain injuries which affect the under-surfaces of the frontal lobes and the anterior tips of the temporal lobes (usually a transient phenomenon in the last disorder).

The most frequent occurrence of brain dysfunction in violent behavior is in brain poisoning, the most serious and ubiquitous of which is caused by alcohol. Alcohol is a specific brain poison and individuals acutely poisoned with alcohol may have as much dysfunction during the poisoning as would be caused by a brain tumor, infection or injury. The only difference between the former and the latter is that alcohol poisoning is temporary.

The violence in automobile accidents caused by drunk drivers takes a far greater toll than the violence in political protest or repression. A drunk driver suffers from a temporary brain abnormality. Although I certainly do not advocate neurosurgery for the treatment of alcoholism, nor for all kinds of organic brain disease, it is clear that violence is sometimes a function of brain abnormalities, and should be viewed as such.

Racism

In the most *avant garde* circles today the favorite critical epithet is "chauvinist." Neurosurgery seems to draw its critics from a somewhat stodgier class: neurosurgical treatment of violent epileptics has been called "racist."

Speaking to a national group of psychiatric investigators about our approach to the problem of violent behavior, a major professor of psychiatry conceded that the biological-social model of violence and the investigation of brain disease associated with violence had some merit. But he classified our project with the proposal of those psychologists who claim that black people have a constitutionally inferior IQ compared to white people. Admitting that the racial idea might have some merit too, he felt that nevertheless funding and research should not be given to such projects until all possible avenues of social and educational rehabilitation have been exhausted.

It seems to me there are really two issues here. The first concerns the political implications of a theory about violence. One of the functions of a theory is that it tells you where to look to find the phenomenon in question. Does the theory that some violence is caused by brain disease lead us to expect it is a characteristic mainly of black people? Certainly not. On the other hand, the theory that personal violence is caused exclusively by social conditions might very well lead us to look at the black ghettos. The environmental cues to personal violence may very well cluster around racially differentiated areas.

The second issue is whether there is any empirical evidence that organically based personal violence is more common among blacks than whites. In my experience there is no special correlation of violence with race. Domestic personal violence occurs in upper- and middle-class homes as well as in the ghettos. When it occurs in the ghetto, however, it may be more visible, spilling out into the streets from the very pressures of overcrowding. It may very well be that violence in ghettos more often gets reported in police records and other data available to the sociologist. But the perspective of the physician is the emergency room and clinic where the products of violence are immediate. From this perspective, claret is the predominant color, not black or white.

It is my perception that the biological-social model of violence will not concentrate on one race, ethnic group, or other social segment of our population as do the subculture theories of violence. In fact, I feel it is important in cases of violence related to brain disease to study the violent act primarily and to consider the style of violence, which is socially determined, as a secondary phenomenon.

Dangers in a Medical Model of Violence

All sorts of dire predictions have been made about the outcome of brain research directed toward the understanding and treatment of emotional disorders, and especially those related to violent behavior. Shades of 1984! "The neurosurgeons want to put electrodes in everyone's brain to keep them from protesting!" "They're going to develop a new drug that will completely destroy the will!" "Man's dignity will be shattered and his innate human quality will be destroyed!" These would indeed be serious statements if they were true. But it is important to see just what the issues are.

It is one thing to advocate neurosurgical procedures for certain kinds of violent behavior caused by organic brain disease or dysfunction. It is quite another to advocate them as general methods of behavior control. My own belief is that no form of conditioning, drug therapy, or surgery is necessary or desirable to control normal-brained members of our society, no matter what their political views are or how they express them.

Of course it is true that behavior control techniques developed to be used in a circumscribed sphere might be adapted to widespread and immoral ends by unscrupulous people. No greater lesson is needed than that provided by Nazi Germany.

But interestingly enough, the controls Goebbels used were environmental ones, not direct alterations of the brain. No drugs were needed to seduce the German population. The S.S. storm troopers did not have little electrodes implanted in their limbic systems.

Although Joseph Goebbels might have reduplicated Skinner's experiments in the best conditioning traditions, he did so before, rather than after, the fact. As a clinician living among the German people for two years after the war, I could find nothing in them that would distinguish them from other human beings.

Can one imagine the most advanced brain electrode technology of the future, or even a new and much more sophisticated group of psychic drugs, that could produce a more perfect form of behavior control than that initiated by environmental "natural" factors in the Third Reich?

One of the important factors to emerge from our own research on the relative influence of deep electrical brain stimulation versus environmental "natural" stimuli is the importance, in terms of effectiveness, of the latter. Of course, effective electrical brain stimulation in target areas can produce pronounced behavioral effects. However, even in susceptible individuals with brain disease, the effect of non-convulsing doses of electrical stimulation can be remarkably altered and suppressed by giving the subject a demanding and attention-absorbing task during electrical brain stimulation.

My thesis that behavior control through the direct manipulation of the brain is not as dangerous for mass abuse as environmental forms of control should not be taken to imply that it has no dangers whatsoever for mass abuse. But the social limitations on who performs neurosurgery or administers drugs, on whom, and for what reasons, ought to be set through public discussion and social decision. My own claim is that the dangers of mass abuse are not sufficient to warrant preventing the very development of the techniques that might have very great therapeutic value for patients with organic brain disease.

Moral Problems in Neurosurgery

If neurosurgery is not much of a danger as a political tool, there still are serious problems with its medical use. I would like to address two of these.

First is the problem of neurological diagnosis. The emphasis I have been placing on the neurological side of the problem of violence ought not be taken out of the context of environmental factors also. Due to the very fundamental problem of specialization in medicine, it is very difficult to maintain a biological-social model of violence in actual practice. The neurologists are in one place and the psychiatrists and social workers are in another.

Yet if the model is worthwhile, treatment of a patient should involve not only his brain but his family, living conditions, job and role in society. It is very important, therefore, to imbed a neurological diagnosis of problems of violence into a larger integrated approach to human behavior. The social forms for this holistic therapy are yet to be worked out, although my own group has tried to include psychiatric and social psychiatric diagnosis along with the neurological.

From my reading of the present situation, however, I believe the greater danger is that the neurological side will be left out. Recently, for example, an airplane hijacker killed one pilot and shot another before he himself was subdued with a blow to the head. Examination of this man afterward revealed he had been a neurological cripple for eleven years, ever since receiving a gunshot wound of the brain. Yet repeated tests, including hours of brainwave examinations, psychological testing, psychiatric and neurological assessment, failed to reveal the tremendous damage that had occurred in this man's emotional center or limbic brain.

The difficulties of diagnosis had their classic but tragic expression in the case of George Gershwin. This talented composer was seen and treated psychiatrically for a long time while a tumor in the limbic system of his brain grew to an unmanageable and untreatable size. The George Gershwin syndrome of the thirties is still being treated in the seventies. Recently eighteen patients were committed to a mental hospital at one of our best university centers who turned out to have tumors of their limbic brains. In some cases, the true nature of this illness was not recognized until the tumor had caused the patient's death.

Second, after the diagnosis of brain disease has been confirmed, *what are the problems of proper consent to treatment?* Does the patient consent to the treatment? Does he know the dangers of the treatment, and how those dangers compare with letting him pass without treatment? What are the wider factors involved in informed consent when the patient is mentally incompetent?[1]

Usually close members of their families are the sources of consent. But in cases of surgery for violence, I believe the patient and his family should have the assistance of an impartial, noninvolved professional group to determine whether surgery or other forms of treatment should be undertaken. In practical terms, this means that a committee of some sort, composed of physicians, or in some cases, physicians and informed laymen, should be present to monitor the medical, psychiatric, and/or surgical treatment.[2]

In my own practice, I and my group do not accept patients for treatments who do not want therapy, and we do not believe that the public good or public interest should intrude upon the personal medical model in terms of protecting the public against violent individuals.

Free Will and Behavior Control

Radical critics of the biological-social model of violence often construe human violence to be an expression of free will. In line with this they consider the medical correction of brain disease that would, as a secondary result, stop violent episodes, to have an unnatural and degrading effect on human dignity. As a physician I find this view particularly inappropriate, not because I deny free will, but because I prize the quality of human life.

Many of the patients who come to us with focal brain disease associated with violent behavior are so offended by their own actions they have attempted suicide. They feel their human dignity has been lost precisely because of uncontrollable behavior patterns they find unnatural and repugnant.

Because our work, and that of other physicians, has indicated a clinical relationship between limbic brain disease, such as temporal lobe epilepsy, and aggressive assaultive behavior, *I believe the correction of that organic condition gives the patient more rather than less, control over his own behavior.* It enhances, and does not diminish, his dignity. It adds to, and does not detract from, his human qualities.

Finally, it is appropriate to return to the spec-ter of a tyrannical government controlling a submissive population through neurosurgery and electrical brain stimulation. Even though this is technically unlikely now, it is a possibility to be conjured with. In the face of this possibility I still have great confidence that the neurological research in behavior control now being done will lead to a better understanding of brain mechanisms, and that when this occurs, *it should be possible for brain scientists to devise techniques for making behavior control of one individual by another more difficult or even impossible.*

In other words, one of the expected benefits of increased brain research will be the creation of new techniques enabling each individual better to control or govern his or her behavior, without unwarranted or unwanted interference by other individuals or devices.

There is already enough knowledge of environmental and psychopharmacological drugs to control a vast segment of our population, without invoking brain surgery or electrical brain stimulation. The great hope of emotional brain research is that it will free us from our present tyrannies and future dangers of control. To this end brain scientists need the help of philosophers, ethicists, theologians, social scientists and jurists, working in concert.

Notes

1. Prison inmates suffering from epilepsy should receive only medical treatment; surgical therapy should not be carried out, because of the difficulty in obtaining truly informed consent.

2. In conjunction with Dr. David Allen, we are exploring "consumer advocacy" utilizing a group with religious, legal and community representatives in addition to physicians.

Psychosurgery: A Neuropsychological Perspective

Stephan L. Chorover

Introduction

We are still far from understanding how our brains give rise to the varied phenomena of our subjective experience. But despite our relative ignorance, we biologists and behavioral scientists stand today in a position comparable to that occu-

Reprinted with permission of the publisher from Boston University Law Review 54, no. 2(March 1974), pp. 231, 239–48.

pied by our colleagues in nuclear physics almost 30 years ago. In 1945, developments in that field led to the atomic bomb and ushered in a new world of ethical and social problems. During the past few decades, developments in the biobehavioral sciences have spawned a wide-ranging psychotechnology, a varied arsenal of tools and techniques for predicting and modifying human social behavior. The continued development and deployment of this psychotechnology has also engendered serious ethical and social problems that can no longer be ignored.

Psychosurgery is among the more controversial forms of psychotechnology. Also known as "psychiatric neurosurgery," "mental surgery." "functional neurosurgery," and "sedative neurosurgery," psychosurgery may be defined as brain surgery that has as its primary purpose the alteration of thoughts, social behavior patterns, personality characteristics, emotional reactions, or some similar aspects of subjective experience in human beings.[1]. . .

Psychosurgery for Violence

It has long been popularly believed that there is a close association between epilepsy and violence. The phrase "a fit of anger" nicely epitomizes this view. Over the years, a large number of clinical studies have dealt with this question. After reviewing the available literature and assessing the clinical experience of neurologists who have cared for many patients with seizure disorders, a recent study sponsored by the National Institute of Neurological Diseases and Stroke concluded that "violence and aggressive acts do occur in patients with temporal lobe epilepsy but such are rare, perhaps no more frequent than in the general population."[2]

Two of the best known cases of this kind are "Thomas R." and "Julia S." Their pseudonyms have entered the vocabulary of psychosurgery, their cases have been fictionalized in a best-selling novel,[3] and they continue to arouse public interest as purported successes of Drs. Vernon H. Mark and Frank R. Ervin, the authors of the controversial *Violence and the Brain*. Bearing in mind that the existence of a causal connection between epilepsy and violence remains an open question in the view of most neurologists, let us consider each of these cases in turn.

The Case of Thomas R.

The presentation by Mark and Ervin. Thomas is introduced to Mark and Ervin's readers in the following passages:[4]

> He was a brilliant [*sic*] 34-year-old engineer with several important patents to his credit. Despite his muscular physique it was difficult to believe he was capable of an act of violence when he was not enraged, for his manner was quiet and reserved, and he was both courteous and sympathetic.

Despite a history of physical illness, Thomas managed to educate himself as an engineer.

> He was an extremely talented, inventive man, but his behavior at times was unpredictable and even frankly psychotic. He was seen and treated by psychiatrists over a period of 7 years with no effect on his destructive outbursts of violence.
>
> Thomas's chief problem was his violent rage; this was sometimes directed at his co-workers and friends, but it was mostly expressed toward his wife and children. He was very paranoid, and harbored grudges which eventually produced an explosion of anger. He often felt that people were gratuitously insulting to him. . . .

For example, during a conversation with his wife,

> he would seize upon some innocuous remark and interpret it as an insult. At first, he would try to ignore what she had said, but could not help brooding; and the more he thought about it, the surer he felt that his wife no longer loved him and was "carrying on with a neighbor." Eventually he would reproach his wife for these faults, and she would hotly deny them. Her denials were enough to set him off into a frenzy of violence.

Thomas was referred to Mark and Ervin by a psychiatrist who they say had concluded that "prolonged psychiatric treatment did not improve his behavior and . . . that his spells of staring, automatisms and rage represented an unusual form of temporal lobe seizure."[5] An electro-encephalographic examination revealed electrical brain activity considered by them to be indicative of epilepsy, and additional tests suggested the presence of other brain abnormalities. After experimenting with a wide range of pharmacological agents, none of which proved therapeutic, they decided to proceed with stereotaxic surgery.

Arrays of electrodes were implanted in both temporal lobes with their ends reaching the nucleus amygdala. The "optimal site for destructive lesions"[6] was sought through repeated stimulation and recording. Stimulation in one portion of the amygdala "produced a complaint of pain, and a feeling of 'I am losing control'," two reactions that marked the onset of Thomas's periods of violence. However, stimulation of a portion of the amygdala just four millimeters to the side produced the opposite reactions of detachment, "hyperrelaxation" and a "feeling like Demerol."[7]

Mark and Ervin's account of how they obtained Thomas's consent to their proposed surgery is revealing both in terms of what is said and what is left unsaid. They viewed Thomas as keenly aware of personal insults and highly sensitive to threats, and found that "the suggestion that the medial portion of his temporal lobe was to be destroyed . . . . would provide wild, disordered thinking."[8] At this point in their discussion, they acknowledge in a footnote the physician's "extraordinary responsibility" of safeguarding the rights of the patient and of securing his free and informed consent.[9] But, they continue, "[u]nder the effects of lateral amygdala stimulation, [Thomas] showed bland acquienscence to the suggestion" that psychosurgery be performed.[10]

> However, 12 hours later, when this effect had worn off, Thomas turned wild and unmanageable. The idea of anyone's making a destructive lesion in his brain enraged him. He absolutely refused any further therapy, and it took many weeks of patient explanation before he accepted the idea of bilateral lesions [sic] being made in his medial amygdala.[11]

Since Mark and Ervin considered Thomas's rage inappropriate and were, by their own account, able to blunt it by lateral amygdala stimulation, it is perhaps not surprising to learn that Thomas finally "accepted the idea." Directly following this quoted passage, we are informed of the success of the procedure in these brief sentences: "Four years have passed since the operation, during which time Thomas has not had a single episode of rage. He continues, however, to have an occasional epileptic seizure with periods of confusion and disordered thinking."[12]

The reader, recalling Mark and Ervin's original assertion that Thomas's "chief problem was his violent rage"[13] and that he exhibited some preoperative seizures and confused or disordered thinking, may reasonably conclude from this account that bilateral amygdalectomy has not only improved Thomas's condition, but has also effected a specific and total cure of his chief complaint. The rage is allegedly gone, the other preoperative symptoms remain essentially unchanged, and no postoperative side effects are mentioned. In light of the devastating effects of bilateral amygdalectomy on the social behavior of nonhuman primates, the apparently successful outcome of Thomas's case seems remarkable indeed. The implied absence of any adverse social reactions appears especially unexpected. Is it sufficient, however, to rely on mere implications? Highly relevant information is not provided by the published case histories. Prior to his operation, Thomas was married and supported his family through his work as an engineer. It would seem that a full account of the effects of his psychosurgery should include, for example, information concerning his marriage and his employment.

Contradictory reports. At the request of Thomas's family an independent follow-up of Thomas's case has been performed by Dr. Peter R. Breggin, a psychiatrist and well-known critic of psychosurgery.[14] Dr. Breggin interviewed the patient and his family, reviewed the hospital charts made before and after surgery and discussed the case with several well-informed individuals.

According to Dr. Breggin, Thomas was continuously employed through December 1965. During that year he began to have serious marital problems which prompted visits to his wife's psychiatrist. Breggin conducted a telephone interview with this psychiatrist during which he was told that Thomas's wife was indeed afraid of him, but that no actual harm was done to her.[15] Moreover, writes Breggin:

> [the] psychiatrist remembers that Thomas was depressed, but not sufficiently depressed to warrant electroshock or drugs. His memory is entirely consistent with the hospital records which report no hallucinations, delusions, paranoid ideas or signs of difficulty with thinking. In the charts, his most serious psychiatric diagnosis is "personality pattern disturbance," [a classification] reserved for mild problems with no psychotic symptomatology.[16]

Finally, certain hospital charts state that "[h]e has never been in any trouble at work or otherwise for aggressive behavior,"[17] In short, Dr. Breggin's account stands in sharp contrast to the published assertions of Drs. Mark and Ervin. Indeed, Breggin claims that the only incidence of violence mentioned in Thomas's hospital files were those provoked by Mark and Ervin themselves.

Thomas was treated by Mark and Ervin from October 1966 until his release from Massachusetts General Hospital on August 27, 1967. He subsequently returned with his mother to the west coast, unable to rejoin his wife and children because his wife had, during his treatment, filed for divorce. Eventually, she married the man about whom Thomas had allegedly been paranoid.[18] Shortly after the operation, it became apparent that Thomas was socially confused and unable to cope with the complexities of normal life. He was soon admitted to a west coast Veterans Administration hospital where he was placed on a locked ward and given heavy doses of medication. Breggin's account suggests that Thomas's new physicians did not have access to his medical records from Massachusetts General Hospital. Indeed, they regarded his comments concerning Mark and Ervin's procedures as evidence of his delusional state of mind.[19] After six months of confinement, he was discharged with a diagnosis of "schizophrenic reaction, paranoic type."[20] At present, Breggin claims, Thomas is totally unable to work, is incapable of caring for himself, and must periodically be rehospitalized as assaultive and psychotic.

Dr. Breggin is not the only available source of information about Thomas's postoperative history. His follow-up study has recently been supplemented by a complaint filed in behalf of the patient[21] and is generally consistent with information the author has obtained from other sources.[22] In August 1972, Dr. Ernst Rodin, a Detroit neurosurgeon, visited Dr. Mark's project in Boston. Rodin, at that time a co-author of a proposal to perform psychosurgery on involuntarily incarcerated individuals,[23] made the visit "to obtain the most up-to-date information on the results of surgery for aggressive behavior in human beings. . . ."[24] Hoping that this inquiry would strengthen his proposal, Rodin was all the more disturbed by the disparities he discovered between the published accounts and the information available at first hand. Specifically, Dr. Ira Sher-win, a neurologist involved with the project, told Rodin that "he was not aware of any genuinely successful cases"[25] and that Thomas R. "will never be able to function in society."[26]

The Case of Julia S.

The presentation by Mark and Ervin.   Julia S., another one of Mark and Ervin's celebrated patients, is the daughter of a well-to-do physician. She is described as being "an attractive, pleasant, cherubic blonde who looked much younger than her age of 21."[27] Starting with an attack of encephalitis before the age of two, she had a long history of brain disease. Her epileptic seizures began at about the age of 10, some being grand-mal convulsions, but most appearing to be petit-mal, or psycho-motor, seizures characterized by "brief lapses of consciousness, staring, lip smacking, and chewing."[28] Between seizures, Julia's behavior was marked by "severe temper tantrums followed by extreme remorse."[29] She also experienced "racing spells," which began with terrifying feelings of panic and ended in her rapidly running aimlessly about the streets. At least 12 people are said to have been assaulted by her, and, when she was 18, she seriously injured other women in two separate stabbing incidents.[30]

Because Julia failed to respond to extensive psychotherapy, drugs, and electroshock, Mark and Ervin concluded that her case "clearly illustrates the point that violent behavior caused by brain dysfunction cannot be modified except by treating the dysfunction itself."[31] Accordingly, they explored Julia's brain, producing rage reactions with the aid of amygdala electrodes and a telemetry device called a "stimoceiver." Finally, lesions were made in the "appropriate areas." *Violence and the Brain*, which was published two years after Julia's operation, contains the following evaluation by Mark and Ervin:

> It is still too early to assess the results of the procedure, but she had only two mild rage episodes in the first postoperative year and none in the second. Since she had generalized brain disease and multiple areas of epileptic activity, it is not surprising that epileptic seizures have not been eliminated, or that her psychotic episodes have continued at the postoperative level.[32]

Contradictory reports   The author is aware of no independent and detailed follow-up studies that may have been made of Julia's case. However, a former member of the project staff, a professional person who was particularly concerned about Julia and in a position permitting almost constant observation of her, recalls that Mark and Ervin's treatments made Julia more despondent and brought an end to her guitar playing and to her desire to engage in intellectual discussion.[33]

Psychosurgery and Deviance Control

Results obtained in both animals and human beings raise serious doubts about the purported merits of psychosurgery. The continued performance of the procedure when its scientific foundations remain dubious and its therapeutic value has yet to be established may justifiably be considered questionable or even irresponsible. What is more ominous, however, is the increasing promotion and practice of psychosurgery as a technique of deviance control. The development of psychosurgery is another example of the time-honored practice of reducing complex social problems to the status of personal infirmities.[34] The authors of *Violence and the Brain* are among those who have advanced the view that social deviance and interpersonal violence in our society may be attributable to some kind of "brain dysfunction." It follows from this view that amygdalectomy may be an appropriate treatment for individuals whose brain dysfunction results in "a low threshold for impulsive violence."[35]

Other psychosurgeons have also advocated their medical procedures as an approach to social policy planning in the area of deviance control. At the Second International Conference of Psychosurgery in 1970, for example, Dr. M. Hunter Brown, a California psychosurgeon, urged his colleagues "to initiate pilot programs for precise rehabilitation of the prisoner-patient who is often young and intelligent, yet incapable of controlling various forms of violence."[36] Jessica Mitford has recently noted, however, that the increasing popularity of behavior alteration programs among penologists is in part due to their interest in suppressing those prisoners who interpret prison life in socioeconomic or racial terms.[37] These suggested uses for psychosurgery clearly involve more than medical considerations.

Foreign psychosurgeons, it would seem, have been at least as devoted to deviance control as their American counterparts. During 1972, a group of German neurosurgeons performed stereotaxic psychosurgery involving the destruction of a portion of the hypothalamus upon "22 male patients, 20 of them being sexual deviants, one suffering from neurotic 'pseudo homosexuality' and one from intractable addiction to alcohol and drugs."[38] According to their report, "15 of the sexual deviants obtained a good result which was in most cases excellent with complete harmonization of sexual and social behavior."[39] In only one case were poor results acknowledged, and no cases of serious side effects were reported. In an earlier report, however, these same researchers found that their first three patients suffered a postoperative "incapacity to indulge in erotic fantasies and stimulating visions."[40] This obliteration of the patients' fantasy lives inexplicably failed to qualify as an untoward side effect in the more recent description of the same operations.

Psychosurgery explicitly aimed at taming hyperactive children has been performed in India, Thailand, Japan, and the United States. In a summary of 115 patients,[41] including 39 children under the age of 11, one team recently claimed that the destruction of the cingulate gyrus, amygdala, and regions of the hypothalamus "proved to be useful in the management of patients who previously could not be managed by other means."[42] An American psychosurgeon who favors the selective destruction of the thalamus in such cases has claimed to have obtained "good" or "fair" results in a majority of operations.[43] It is impossible to assess his findings in an objective fashion because of his characteristically unilluminating case reports, of which the following is typical:

> A seven-year-old mentally retarded child had sudden attacks of screaming, yelling, running and beating his head against the wall. The walls were actually indented by the blows.
> Following thalamotomy three years ago, the patient did not display the wild, aggressive and screaming behavior. The improved behavior was an enjoyment for both the child and the parents.[44]

Conclusion

Because the weight of the available evidence indicates that limbic system psychosurgery produces a marked deterioration in behavior, serious impairments of judgment, and other disastrous social adjustment effects, and because psychosurgeons have failed to provide balanced accounts of their cases, it would appear prudent for the medical profession and the relevant regulatory agencies of state and federal government to act promptly along the following lines. First, there should be an explicit recognition that psycho-surgery is a highly experimental procedure and not a proven therapeutic one as is so often alleged by its contemporary proponents. Second, psycho-surgery should not be performed upon children, prisoners, involuntarily held or committed mental patients, or those deemed to be mentally retarded. Third, a registry and assessment mechanism should be established to collect and disseminate information on present and past practices in psychosurgery. One function of such an agency might be the systematic psychological assessment of surviving psychosurgery patients and post-mortem examinations of their brain tissue when they die. Fourth, there should be a temporary moratorium on all further psychosurgical opera-tions until the risks can be weighed against the benefits descovered by a systematic and impartial review of the field.[45] Finally, basic research on brain mechanisms and behavior should be sup-ported and extended. Carefully pursued and properly interpreted, such research offers the only reliable course of action for increasing our under-standing of human brain function and its relation to behavior. A better understanding of this kind, coupled with broader public education in the brain sciences, should ultimately provide the best possi-ble defense against the simplistic theories upon which much of contemporary psychosurgery has been built.

It would be a mistake, however, to view psy-chosurgery in a social vacuum. Although it has unique characteristics, psychosurgery is, in terms of social policy, merely one of a large number of psychotechnological means that are continually being advanced to deal with troublesome indi-viduals or groups. The relevant "target popula-tions" are vaguely defined as "aggressive," "assaultive," "volatile," "acting-out," "disrup-tive," "incorrigible," "uncooperative," or "dan-gerous." The possibility that such behavior may be justifiable is generally ignored as are the social consequences of discouraging diversity. Indeed, the physical and chemical control of disruptive be-havior has been suggested in every futuristic

model of technological fascism. Insofar as the causes of social conflict actually lie in the domain of social affairs, psychotechnological treatment of deviants should be regarded as a perversion of medicine and a distinct threat to individual liberty. The time has come to examine the entire spectrum of psychotechnology and to question the prevalent ideologies of behavioral prediction, modification, and control. We must try, most of all, to assess the impact and social consequences of psychotechnol-ogy in the broad contexts of politics and public policy. For to deny the power and political appeal of repressive psychotechnology is to expedite its encroachment, and to refrain from combating it is to surrender not only our constitutional freedom, but also our human dignity.

Notes

1. This is essentially the definition given by Dr. Bertram S. Brown, Director of the National Institute of Mental Health. See *Hearings on S. 974, S. 878 and S. J. Res. 71 before the Subcomm. on Health of the Senate Comm. on Labor and Public Welfare*, 93d Cong., 1st Sess., pt. 2, at 339 (1973).

2. Goldstein, "Brain Research and Violent Behavior," 30 *Arch. Neurol.* 1, 28 (1974).

3. *See* M. Crichton, *The Terminal Man* (1972). Thomas appears to be the model for Harry Benson, the title character in Crichton's novel. Ellis, the fictional neurosurgeon in the book, expresses with some literary license Mark and Ervin's view that psychomotor epilepsy and other brain damage are major factors in contemporary social violence and that psychosurgery offers a rational approach to the prevention of such violence. In this connection, it is of interest to note that Crichton has added a postscript to the paperback edition of the book which reveals: "In the face of considerable controversy among clinical neuroscientsts, I am persuaded that the understanding of the relationship between organic brain damage and violent behavior is not so clear as I thought at the time I wrote the book." *Id.* at 282 (1973 ed.).

4. Mark & Ervin, *Violence and the Brain*, 93-94 (1970).

5. Mark & Ervin, "Is There a Need to Evaluate the Individuals Producing Human Violence?" *Psychiat. Opinion.* Aug. 1968, at 32, 33.

6. Id. at 33.

7. Mark & Ervin 96.

8. Mark & Ervin, *supra* note 5 at 34.

9. Id.

10. Id.

11. Mark & Ervin 96-97.

12. Id. at 97.

13. Id. at 93.

14. Breggin, "An Independent Followup of a Person Operated upon for Violence and Epilepsy by Drs. Vernon Mark, Frank Ervin and William Sweet of the Neuro-Research Foundation of Boston," *Rough Times*, Nov.-Dec. 1973, at 8, col. 1.

15. Id. at 8, col. 3.

16. Id.

17. Id.

18. Id. at 9, col. 2. For a description of this aspect of his "paranoia" see Mark & Ervin 93-94.

19. Thomas's discharge summary from the Veterans Administration Hospital reads: "Patient stated that . . . Massachusetts General Hospital were [*sic*] controlling him by creating lesions in his brain tissue some time before. Stated that they can control him, control his moods and control his actions, they can turn him up or turn him down." Breggin, *supra* note 22, at 9, col 2. See also Memorandum, note 14 *infra*, at 4.

20. Breggin, *supra* note 14, at 9, col. 3.

21. Kille v. Mark, Civil No. 681998 (Super. Ct., Suffolk County, Mass., filed Dec. 3, 1973).

22. Hunt, "The Politics of Psychosurgery," Part I, *Real Paper* (Boston), May 30, 1973, at 1, col. 1, *reprinted in Rough Times*, Sept.-Oct. 1973, at 2, col. 1; Hunt, "The Politics of Psychosurgery," Part II, *Real Paper* (Boston) June 13, 1973, at 6, col. 1, reprinted in *Rough Times*, Nov.-Dec. 1973, at 6, col. 1; Trotter, Violent Brains (unpublished manuscript written for Ralph Nader's Center for Responsive Law, Washington, D.C.); Memorandum from Dr. Ernst Rodin to Dr. J. S. Gottlieb, Aug. 9, 1972, submitted as Exhibit AC-4 in Kaimowitz v. Department of Mental Health, Civil No. 73-19434-AW (Cir. Ct., Wayne County, Mich., July 10, 1973).

23. This proposed research was ultimately blocked in Kaimowitz v. Department of Mental Health Civil No. 73-19434-AW (Cir. Ct., Wayne County, Mich., July 10, 1973), discussed elsewhere in this symposium. See comment, *Kaimowitz v. Department of Mental Health: A Right to Be Free from Experimental Psychosurgery?*," 54 B.U.L. Rev. 301 (1974).

24. Memorandum, *supra* note 22, at 1.

25. Id. at 4.

26. Id.

27. Mark & Ervin 97.

28. Id.

29. Id.

30. Id. at 97-98.

31. Id. at 98.

32. Id. at 107-08. As late as 1972, the authors were similarly uninformative: "It is still too early to assess the results of the procedure, but the frequency of both the rage attacks and epileptic seizures has been markedly decreased since operation." Mark, Ervin & Sweet, "Deep Temporal Lobe Stimulation in Man," in *The Neurobiology of the Amygdala*, *supra* note 23, [in original text] at 485, 494. *See also* Trotter, *supra* note 22, at 12 [in original text].

33. The author is in possession of an extensive record of personal observations made by this member of the project staff, who wishes to remain anonymous.

34. See Chorover, "Big Brother and Psycho-technology," *Psychology Today*, Oct. 1973, at 43, 45.

35. Mark & Ervin 2.

36. E. Valenstein, *Brain Control: A Critical Examination of Brain Stimulation and Psychosurgery*, 255 (1973).

37. See Mitford, "The Torture Cure," *Harper's*, Aug. 1973, at 16. See also J. Mitford, *Kind and Usual Punishment* (1973).

38. Müller, Roeder & Orthner, "Further Results of Stereotaxis in the Human Hypothalamus in Sexual Deviations, First Use of This Operation in Addiction to Drugs," 16 *Neurochirurgia* 113 (1973).

39. Id.

40. Roeder & Miller, "Zur Stereotaktischen Heilung der Pädophilin Homosexualität," 94 *Deutsch. Med. Wochnschr.* 409 (1969).

41. Balasubramaniam, Kanaka, Ramanugam & Ramanurthi, "Surgical Treatment of Hyperkinetic and Behavior Disorder," 54 *Int'l. Surgery* 18 (1970).

42. Id. at 22.

43. *Hearings, supra* note 1, at 353 (testimony of Dr. Orlando J. Andy).

44. Id. at 348. See also Andy, "Neurosurgical Treatment of Abnormal Behavior," 252 *Am. J. Med. Sci.* 232, 236-37 (1966), reprinted in *Hearings, supra* note 1, at 417, 421-22.

45. See S. J. Res. 86, 93d Cong., 1st Sess. (1973). This resolution, introduced by Senator Beall, calls for a two-year moratorium during which the Secretary of Health, Education and Welfare would compile and analyze the available data.

Decision Scenario 1

"Doris Jenkins is a thirty-two-year-old white typist and file clerk," Dr. Faberge said to the three men and one woman gathered around the table. "Her presenting complaints were recurrent headaches, periods of dizziness, and a few blackouts. We were unable to confirm any evidence of brain dysfunction, and her physical signs are within the range of the normal."

"How bad are the headaches?" Dr. Judith Boscovitz asked.

"She describes them as very severe," said Dr. Faberge. "They last for a period of seven or eight hours once or twice a month. She's been on several standard treatment modalities and they offer her no relief." Dr. Faberge paused. "That's why," he said, "I want to try something quite different with her."

"A surgical procedure?" asked Dr. Wannan Smith.

"That's right. I want to do a stereotactic procedure that will destroy part of the sensation integration center in the thalamus. The mortality and morbidity rates for the procedure are well within acceptable limits of risk."

"And you want us to give approval for that?" asked Dr. Boscovitz. "It sounds like to me that you're dealing with a nut case. Those headaches and blackouts are probably psychogenic."

"She has consented to the surgery," said Dr. Faberge. "And I would like to try it."

"I won't give my approval," said Dr. Boscovitz. "That poor woman might approve anything if somebody in authority asked her to."

"What are the risks compared to the gains?" asked Dr. Smith.

"The gain hoped for is pain relief. If we destroy too much, she may lose pain sensation from her limbs, but death is not very likely."

"And you want to do this procedure?" asked Dr. Smith.

"That's right. I think it could help her. I also think that we might be able to learn something new about treatment in these cases of uncontrollable headache."

"She's given her consent, you say?" asked Dr. Smith.

"That's right. I explained the risks and the possibility of eliminating the headache symptom."

"I will not be a party to this," said Dr. Boscovitz. "The risks are too great to run for a possible and very uncertain gain. Besides, Ms. Jenkins is not a good candidate for surgery of this type. She needs psychiatric help."

Dr. Faberge smiled. "I think that I know how you'll vote on this case, Judith. But perhaps others are not so opposed to trying new treatments as you are."

"This is not treatment, it's butchery."

Would Mark consider Ms. Jenkins a good candidate for any type of psychosurgery?

If she has given her informed consent, why should the surgery recommended by Dr. Faberge not be performed?

Would Kant's principles require that the surgery agreed on be performed?

Would utilitarianism permit it?

What view might be taken by the natural law theory of Catholicism?

Decision Scenario 2

"It's all very humane," Dr. Solder said. "So far as I can see, no genuine moral issue is involved. We are doing what prisons are supposed to do—rehabilitating."

"If I understand correctly," said Professor Ross, "people are not allowed to choose whether to participate in the behavior modification program."

"That's correct," said Dr. Solder. "Most of them are anxious to participate though. Only a few raise any objection."

"And you force them to participate?"

"Not at all. We do deprive them of the usual privileges that the other prisoners share such as attending movies, buying things at the commissary, minor things like that. But we don't punish them if they don't participate." Dr. Solder paused a moment. "What you don't seem to realize," he went on, "is that all the men were sentenced to prison after having been convicted of sexual crimes against children. We are just re-educating them."

"But," Professor Ross said, "your re-education involves showing them pictures of nude children and administering rather painful electric shocks."

"It's an effective technique and basically harmless."

"No doubt," said Ross. "But still you are forcing some people to change against their will. You are making them into different people without their permission or wish."

"We don't recognize such things as will," said Dr. Solder. "That's an outmoded philosophical notion. What we're concerned with is behavior. These men are conditioned to respond to children as desirable sexual objects. We just change the conditioning."

"I consider what you are doing as morally objectionable," said Professor Ross.

"I think you are being ridiculous," said Dr. Solder. "We are doing no more than carrying out the wishes and aims of society. In doing so we are also benefitting the individuals we treat, whether they are aware of it or not."

Restate the arguments that are involved in this dispute.

What kind of moral principles might Dr. Solder appeal to in order to justify the position he has taken?

What principles might Professor Ross invoke as the basis of her criticism?

Would Seymour Halleck endorse either point of view?

What conditions would Halleck require be met before such a program as the one conducted by Solder could be regarded as justifiable?

If Solder's proposal involved only mandatory attendance of vocational training classes and counseling sessions, would the same objections that might apply to his behavior modification proposal also apply?

Decision Scenario 3

"It's definitely a condition that we call temporal lobe epilepsy," Dr. Sanders said. "Now we don't know this for sure, but we think that this is what's causing your violent outbursts of temper."

"Can you tell me for sure that that's why I attacked that cop at the demonstration?" Carver Clay asked.

"Not for sure. But since you say you just 'lost your head' and 'everything just blanked out,' I think it's a good possibility."

"I'd sure like to get out of this jail," Clay said. "Can you cure me?"

"We can try. There's a small brain operation we can perform. If we can locate an area that seems to be giving off abnormal electrical discharges, we can go in and destroy a little of the tissue in that area."

"You're not talking about doing some kind of experiment on me, are you?" Clay asked. "I don't want to be no guinea pig."

"We don't know all there is to know," said Dr. Sanders. "But I wouldn't call it experimental. There's good reason to believe that uncontrollable violence is associated with the kind of brain disease that you have."

"Isn't there any other way? I mean, cutting up a man's brain is a terrible thing to do. Couldn't I just talk to a psychiatrist or something like that?"

"We don't think it would be effective," Dr. Sanders said. "Not for somebody like you. You came close to killing that policeman, you know."

"I know," Clay said. "I feel real bad about that now. Maybe there is something the matter with my head. What if this operation doesn't work out?"

"Even if it's not effective in curing your tendency towards violence, the chances are good that there wouldn't be any serious after effects. But to be honest, we don't really know exactly what might happen."

"Let me think about it some more," Clay said. "I'd sure like to get out of this place, and they won't let me out until I prove to them I'm not crazy anymore."

Would Mark consider Clay a good candidate for psychosurgery? If not, why not?

What are some of the difficulties in determining whether violence (such as that which occurs in the course of political demonstrations) is genuinely "pathological?" What is Chorover's view?

What are some of the difficulties in establishing whether such violence is "caused" by a brain dysfunction?

If it could be shown that brain disease is the cause of "unacceptable violence,"
would the most morally justifiable form of treatment for those found guilty of crimes
involving such violence be psychosurgery? Why or why not?

Decision Scenario 4

"I'll have to be honest with you and tell you that we really don't know how it works," Dr. Mabbot said. "But the statistics show that it does work, particularly in people like you."

"Shock treatments," Carlo Bulgari said. "That's what they call them, isn't it?"

"That's the popular name," Dr. Mabbot admitted. "We call it ECT—electro-convulsive therapy. It's a simple procedure, really. We place electrodes on your temples, then pass a current of about a hundred volts through your head. It doesn't hurt at all. You're anesthetized, and we give you muscle relaxants so your muscles don't tighten up and make you hurt yourself."

"It sounds terrible."

"It's not. The only bad side effects we know about are temporary disorientation that lasts usually no longer than a day and some short-term memory loss. How old are you now?"

"Seventy-three."

"You've been severely depressed for over six weeks now, and you're in the age group that can benefit most from ECT. Sometimes it works almost like magic."

"I just get shocked once?"

"A course of three to five treatments is usual. And you really don't get shocked, you know."

"This will help me get to feeling better?"

"I can't promise that it will, but it holds out a good chance of helping. For you, it offers a better chance than drugs or psychotherapy."

"I have to give my permission?"

"Yes."

"All right," Mr. Bulgari said. "Give me the paper. I'll sign it."

Assuming Mr Bulgari is severely depressed, would Szasz be prepared to say that he is suffering from a mental illness? If not, why not?

Suppose that Mr. Bulgari can reasonably expect to be helped by ECT, in Szasz's view would it be wrong for Dr. Mabbot to recommend it?

In which of the three classes of situations distinguished by Halleck can Mr. Bulgari best be classified?

In Dworkin's view, assuming that Mr. Bulgari is severely depressed, is he capable of acting autonomously?

Using Dworkin's seven criteria for comparing behavior-control techniques, what conclusion can be reached about the moral status of ECT?

Decision Scenario 5

"I'm really surprised that I don't have low blood sugar," Mrs. Morris said. "I feel so tired in the morning that after I get my husband and children out of the house, I usually just go back to bed."

"All your tests check out to be quite normal," Dr. Comtom said. "Do you get any exercise?"

"I work hard around the house, but I don't jog or anything like that."

"Are you involved in any clubs or church activities or anything like that?"

"Not really. I've got a good friend who's a neighbor, and I usually talk to her every day. I sometimes think I'd go crazy if I didn't have her to pass some time with."

"You're not into gardening, cooking, sewing, or anything?"

"I just don't have the time or energy to do things like that. By the time I do the housework, it's time for the children to come home. Then it's time for me to cook dinner. Every day it's a real struggle."

"Physically, so far as I can tell, you're in very good health," Dr. Comtom said. "I think your problem is that you're depressed."

"I agree with that," Mrs. Morris said. "Is there something you can give me to make me feel better?"

"I'm going to prescribe an antidepressant for a while and see if that doesn't make you feel better."

"That sounds like something I need," Mrs. Morris said.

Would Szasz be likely to approve of this way of dealing with Mrs. Morris's complaint?

How would Halleck be likely to assess such short-term therapy?

What disadvantages do you see in the therapeutic approach to Mrs. Morris taken by Dr. Comtom?

Why might a utilitarian or a Kantian object to such therapy?

7

GENETICS: INTERVENTION, CONTROL, AND RESEARCH

CASE PRESENTATION
The Recombinant DNA Debate

In 1971 a research worker named Robert Pollack at the Cold Spring Harbor Laboratory learned that Stanford biochemist Paul Berg intended to conduct an experiment in which a monkey virus (SV40) would be inserted in the bacterium *E. coli*. The virus is known to cause tumors when injected into animals and to make cultures of human cells turn cancerous. Yet there is no evidence that SV40 produces cancer in either people or monkeys under ordinary conditions. *E. coli* is found by the billions in every human intestine, however, and Pollack questioned the wisdom of inserting genes known to cause cancer in such a common organism.

Pollack called Berg and expressed his doubts. Berg had not been particularly concerned because he knew that SV40 had long been used as an experimental material and had a perfect safety record. He knew of course that SV40 possessed genes that could transform normal cells into cancerous ones. It was, in fact, this feature that led him to want to study the virus. But when Berg consulted his colleagues in the field of molecular genetics, they expressed doubts similar to Pollack's. Some mentioned the possibility that *E. coli* with attached viral genes might reproduce in human intestines for a long period and then, for reasons unknown, transform the normal cells into cancerous ones. Berg was convinced enough of the danger to postpone his plans to carry out the experiments with SV40.

While Berg was deciding what to do, research into recombinant technology was moving ahead at an incredible rate. Two discoveries in particular made recombination a comparatively simple process. Herbert Boyer's research group at the University of California, San Francisco, isolated a restriction enzyme that would sever double-stranded DNA so as to leave "jagged" ends. That is, the ends of the two strands were chemically cut at different places. DNA segments from another source would bond to these "sticky" ends more quickly than to strands cut at the same place. Also, Stanley Cohen's group at Stanford identified a plasmid that would accept new DNA readily and would easily pass through the cell membrane of *E. coli*.

As the search for other plasmids and other restriction enzymes continued in research groups throughout the world, Berg, Cohen, and others realized that there was a pressing need to assess the risks that might be involved in recombinant DNA experiments. The issue was discussed at a meeting of molecular biologists in New Hampshire in 1973, and those present voted to ask the National Academy of Science to set up a committee to investigate the hazards of recombinant research. They also agreed to make their concerns known to the scientific community by means of a letter in *Science*, the widely read journal of the American Association for the Advancement of Science.

The Academy responded by establishing a committee, with Berg as chairman, and charging it to look into the recombinant issue. At a meeting at MIT in April, 1974, the committee decided that immediate action was required to keep recombinant research from expanding beyond the capacity for review and control. They concluded that scientists should be asked to voluntarily suspend work on recombinant experiments involving tumor viruses, increase in drug resistance in harmful bacteria, and increase in toxicity in bacteria. The request was published in *Science* and in the British journal *Nature*.

This was a step unprecedented in the history of science. Never before had a professional group asked that the scientific community halt research in a particular area for essentially moral reasons—the belief that it would be wrong to subject people to the unknown hazards associated with recombinant DNA.

In February of 1975, a group of scientists was called together by Berg at the Asilomar Conference Center in California to discuss the potential hazards of recombinant DNA research and how they might be dealt with. This group voted to maintain the voluntary restrictions on research and to push the National Institutes of Health (the major federal agency involved in molecular biological research and funding) to formulate guidelines for research. Berg's committee, in its report to the National Academy, also presented its own recommendations concerning safety standards for dealing with potentially hazardous biological materials.

In June of 1976, an NIH subcommittee headed by David Hogness of Stanford released a set of guidelines. They established four levels of physical containment (P-1–P-4). The lowest level required following procedures usual in microbiological laboratories for work with well-understood organisms that involve little risk. The P-4 level included a negative-pressure environment and air locks. These most-secure precautions were mandated for work with such materials as animal tumor viruses. In addition, the guidelines required that the host cells used in recombinant experiments be specially weakened forms of bacteria that have little chance of living and multiplying outside of carefully controlled laboratory conditions.

The NIH guidelines placed primary responsibility on individual researchers. But they also required establishing special monitoring committees by sponsoring institutions and funding agencies.

The NIH guidelines did not put an end to the debate over recombinant DNA experiments. The guidelines balanced possible risk against specific safety measures for minimizing risk. But because so little is understood about DNA recombinants, there was much room for disagreement about the nature and severity of the risks posed by research. Furthermore, commercial laboratories (such as those of pharmaceutical companies) are bound by NIH regulations. For these reasons, critics of recombinant research made its regulation an issue at local, state, and national levels.

The most sustained and virulent controversy occurred in Cambridge, Massachusetts. As the site of the Harvard Biological Laboratories, the Harvard Medical School, and MIT, Cambridge is one of the world's centers of molecular genetic research. The opposition to recombinant work in Cambridge was led by George Wald of Harvard, winner of the Nobel Prize for his work on the biology of vision. Wald and his supporters convinced Cambridge Mayor Alfred Velluci that the hazards of recombinant work were so serious a threat to the public that they should be stopped. The city council, at the mayor's urging, asked Harvard and MIT to declare a moratorium on P-3 research until an eight-member citizen's review board could consider the problem. The institutions consented to the request.

The public debate that followed was long and acrimonious. It concerned both the nature and seriousness of the biohazards and also the wisdom and legitimacy of allowing a local government to regulate scientific research. In February of 1977, the council rejected the mayor's recommendation that P-3 work be permanently banned and passed an ordinance allowing research under guidelines only somewhat stricter than those of NIH.

Other communities also became involved in the recombinant issue. San Diego, California, Madison, Wisconsin, and Bloomington, Indiana all held local hearings and debated the regulation of research. States also showed concern. The New York State Attorney General held a public hearing, and legislation governing DNA research was introduced in the California Assembly.

Both the Senate and the House of Representatives held hearings on the issue. In April, 1977, Secretary of Health, Education, and Welfare Joseph Califano asked the Senate Committee on Health to recommend legislation to regulate DNA research. According to Califano, potential but still unidentified hazards posed by such research led to the conclusion that "there is no reasonable alternative regulation under law." In the fall of 1977, two bills regulating research were before Congress, but neither was approved.

Since the formulation of the original guidelines in 1976, a great deal of recombinant DNA research has taken place. Hundreds of universities, research institutes, and commercial laboratories have performed literally thousands of recombinant DNA experiments. So far, no biological catastrophies have occurred. Not only have there been no epidemics, but not a single person has been reported as harmed as a result of such research.

The apparent safety of the research has led to a modification of the guidelines. Since 1976, they have been revised three times. The federal Recombinant

DNA Advisory Committee recommended in 1981 that all guidelines be made voluntary. This recommendation was not taken, and in 1982 the National Institutes of Health adopted guidelines that are binding on all research receiving federal support.

Although the new guidelines continue to be mandatory, they are much less restrictive than the original ones. They eliminate the requirement that production involving more than ten liters of a substance receive prior federal approval. By placing approval in the hands of a local biosafety committee, they encourage the development of industrial processes. Most important, the guidelines exempt from federal approval (except in special cases) experimental systems that involve *E. coli* (the most common organism in recombinant DNA research), yeast, and the bacterium *bacillus subtilis*.

Was the great controversy over recombinant DNA research that peaked in the late 1970s an overreaction by society? Some believe that it was and that such research poses no more danger than does traditional microbiological research.

Yet not all believe that the concern was excessive or that we can now allow research to proceed virtually unregulated. In the view of some critics, recombinant DNA continues to pose a potential threat both to our health and to our society. The fact that no biological catastrophe has yet occurred does not mean that one is impossible.

Furthermore, many are worried by the kinds of changes that the technology of recombinant DNA may make possible. If we are able to control and predict the expression of genes in humans, then the way is clearly open to design and produce people in accordance with some imagined ideal. What will happen then to such traditional and moral values as autonomy, diversity, and the inherent worth of the individual? In the opinion of some, this is a technological power we should never attempt to possess.

But to what extent should recombinant DNA research be legislated? Should safety alone be the only consideration? Or should research be stopped before we are presented with a power it is perhaps better not to have?

Many scientists see the freedom of scientific inquiry severely compromised by any laws or regulations imposed by nonscientists with little understanding of the nature and importance of basic research. Furthermore, many see regulation as posing the danger of political interference in all research. A political pressure group or a demagogue, they suggest, might be able to force scientists to stop research in any "unapproved" area.

Proponents of some form of legislative or regulatory control argue that biology is now at the stage physics was when it first split the atom. As with physics, biology is acquiring powers hardly dreamed of. Yet those powers also pose potential dangers to people, the environment, and indeed to all of civilization. For this reason, research without supervision and regulation cannot be permitted. Government owes to its citizens protection from dangers that are still largely unknown.

Yet even those in favor of regulation are rarely wholehearted advocates. They see it merely as an evil necessity, and they too warn about its dangers. Molecular biologist Norton Zinder expresses this concern: "We are moving into a precedent-making area—the regulation of an area of scientific research—and I must plead that this be done with extreme care and without haste. The record of past attempts of authoritative bodies, either church or state, to control intellectual thought and work have led to some of the sorriest chapters of human history."

Introduction

The two great triumphs of nineteenth-century biology were Darwin's formulation of the theory of organic evolution and Mendel's statement of the laws of transmission genetics. One of the twentieth century's outstanding accomplishments has been the development of an understanding of the molecular structures and processes that are involved in genetic inheritance. All three great achievements give rise to moral and social issues of considerable complexity. The theories are abstract, but the problems they generate are concrete and immediate.

Two major sorts of problems are associated with our increased knowledge of inheritance and genetic change. One kind has to do with the use we make of the knowledge that we possess. We now know a great deal about the ways in which genetic diseases are transmitted and about the sorts of errors that can occur in human development. We have the means to make reliable predictions about the chances of a disease in a particular case, and we have the medical technology to detect some disorders before birth.

To what extent should we employ this knowledge? One possibility is that we might use it to detect, treat, or prevent genetic disorders that may occur in particular cases. Thus, we might require that everyone submit to screening and counseling before having children. Or we might require that children be tested either prenatally or immediately after birth. In this way, it might be possible to bring genetic defects under control in much the same way that we have brought contagious diseases under control.

Requiring screening and testing suggests another possibility, one that involves taking a broader view of human genetics. In this view, eliminating genetic disease might simply become one part of a much more ambitious plan for deliberately improving the entire species. Shall we attempt to control human evolution by formulating policies and practices that are designed to alter the genetic composition of the human population? That is, shall we practice some form of eugenics?

Problems of the second kind are those connected with the acquisition of knowledge. Increasing scientific understanding requires conducting research. But the fact that research must be conducted in a social context creates difficulties. When research poses possible threats to the safety and well-being of the community, we must decide whether we are willing to assume the risk for the sake of the promised outcome of increasing knowledge. Are we willing to seek knowledge at any price? If not, what justification can we offer for restricting inquiry, for limiting the scientific freedom that we have traditionally supported?

These two sorts of problems are not unrelated. Research in molecular genetics that is concerned with recombinant DNA may well reveal to us ways in which the machinery of cells can be altered in beneficial ways. Not only will we be able to synthesize such important biological products as insulin, but we may be able to correct certain kinds of inborn errors in human cells. "Genetic engineering" and "genetic surgery" thus may offer the possibility of direct genetic intervention and control.

In the following three sections, we shall focus attention on the issues that are raised by the actual and potential use of genetic information and by the research required to obtain it. Our topics are these: genetic intervention (screening, counseling, and prenatal diagnois), eugenics, and recombinant-DNA research.

Genetic Intervention: Screening, Counseling, and Diagnosis

Our genes play a major role in making us what we are. Biological programs of genetic information work amazingly well to produce normal, healthy individuals. But sometimes things can go wrong, and when they do, the results can be tragic.

Almost two thousand human diseases have been identified as involving genetic factors. Some of the diseases are quite rare, while others are relatively common. Some are invariably fatal, while others are comparatively minor. Some respond well to treatment, while others do not.

The use of genetic information in predicting and diagnosing diseases has significantly increased during the last two decades. New scientific information, new medical techniques, and new social programs have all contributed to this increase.

Three approaches in particular have been adopted by the medical community as means of acquiring and employing genetic information related to diseases: genetic screening, genetic counseling, and prenatal genetic diagnosis. Each approach has been the source of significant ethical and social issues, but before examining the approaches and the problems they present, we need to consider what is usually meant in talking about genetic disease.

Genetic Disease

The concept of a "genetic" disease is far from being clear. Generally speaking, a genetic disease is one in which genes or the way in which they are expressed are causally responsible for particular biochemical, cellular, or physiological defects. Rather than rely upon such a general definition, it is more useful for the purpose of understanding genetic diagnosis to consider some of the ways in which genes may play a role in producing diseases.

Gene defects.   The program of information that is coded into DNA (the genetic material) may in some way be abnormal because of the occurrence of a mutation at some time or other. (That is, a particular gene may have been lost or damaged, or a new gene added.) Consequently, when the DNA blueprint is "read" and its instructions followed, the child that develops will have defects.

For example, a number of diseases (such as PKU and Tauri's disease) are the result of so-called "inborn errors of metabolism." The diseases are produced by the lack of a particular enzyme necessary for ordinary metabolic functioning. In each case, the genetic information required in coding for the production of the enzyme is simply not present. The gene for the enzyme is missing.

A missing or defective gene may be due to a new mutation, but more often the condition has been inherited. It has been transmitted to the offspring through the genetic material contributed by its parents. Because defective genes can be passed on in this way, the diseases that they produce are themselves described as heritable. (Thus, PKU is a genetically transmissible disease.) The diseases follow regular patterns through generations, and tracing out those patterns has been one of the great accomplishments of modern biology and medicine.

Developmental defects. The biological development of a human being from a fertilized egg to a newborn child is an immensely complicated process. It involves an interplay among both genetic and environmental factors, and the possibility of the occurrence of errors is quite real.

Mistakes that result as part of the developmental process are ordinarily called "congenital." Such defects are not in the original blueprint (genes) but result either from genetic damage or from the reading of the blueprint. When either happens, the manufacture and assembly of materials required for normal fetal development are affected.

Radiation, drugs, chemicals, and nutritional deficiencies can all cause changes in an otherwise normal process. Also, biological disease agents, such as certain viruses, may intervene in development. They may alter the machinery of the cells, interfere with the formation of tissues, and defeat the carefully programmed processes that lead to a normal child.

Finally, factors internal to fetal development may also alter the process and lead to defects. The most common form of Down's syndrome, for example, is known to be caused by a failure of chromosomes to separate normally. (However, the cause of this failure is presently unknown.) The result is a child that has failed to develop properly and displays physical anomalies and some degree of mental retardation.

Defects that occur during the developmental process are not themselves the results of inheritance and they cannot be passed on to the next generation.

Genetic carriers. Some diseases are produced only when an individual inherits both genes (alleles) for the disease from his or her parents. The parents themselves possess only one gene for the disease, and generally show none of its symptoms. However, sometimes a parent may have symptoms of the same kind that are associated with the disease, although to a much lesser degree of severity.

In the metabolic disease PKU, for example, individuals who have inherited only one of the genes (that is, the offspring are heterozygous, rather than homozygous) may show a greater than normal level of phenylalanine in their blood. Such people are somewhat deficient in the enzyme required to metabolize this substance. The level of the substance may not be high enough to have caused any damage to them. Yet they are the carriers of a gene which, when passed on with the same gene from the other parent, can cause the disease PKU in their offspring. (As we will see later, the same is also true for those who are carriers of sickle-cell trait.) The individual who receives both genes for PKU obviously has the disease, but what about the parents? Clearly, the point at which a condition becomes a disease is often a matter of degree.

Genetic predisposition.   It has been suggested that virtually every disease involves a genetic component in some way or other. Whether or not this is true, there is good evidence that hypertension, heart disease, various forms of cancer, and differential responses to environmental agents (such as sunlight, molds, or chemical pollutants) run in families. This suggests that the genetic makeup of particular individuals may predispose them to specific diseases.

At present, it is not possible to say just what genetic factor might be partly responsible for a particular disease, just what role it plays, or through what mechanism it expresses itself. It is important to keep in mind that predispositions are not themselves diseases. At best, they can be regarded only as causal conditions which, in conjunction with other conditions, can produce disease.

The actions of genes in disease processes is much more complicated than we have been able to discuss here. Nevertheless, our general categories are adequate to allow us to talk about the use made of information in genetic diagnosis.

Genetic Screening

In 1962 Dr. Robert Guthrie of the State University of New York developed an automated procedure for testing the blood of newborn children for the disease PKU. Although a diagnostic test for PKU had been available since 1934, it was time-consuming and labor-intensive. The Guthrie test made it practical to diagnose a large number of infants at a relatively low price.

PKU (phenylketonuria) is a serious metabolic disorder. Infants affected are deficient in the enzyme phenylalanine hydroxylase. Since the enzyme is necessary to convert the amino acid phenylalanine into tyrosine, as part of the normal metabolic process, a deficiency of the enzyme leads to a high concentration of phenylalanine in the infant's blood. The almost invariable result is severe mental retardation.

However, if the high level of phenylalanine in an infant's blood is detected very early, the infant can be put on a diet that is very low in that particular amino acid. Keeping children on the diet until they are around the age of six significantly reduces the severity of the retardation that is otherwise inescapable.

The availability of the Guthrie test and the prospects of saving newborn children from irreparable damage encouraged state legislatures to pass mandatory screening laws. Massachusetts passed the first such law in 1963, and by 1967 similar legislation had been adopted by forty-one states.

The term "genetic screening" is sometimes used to refer to any activity having to do with locating or advising people with genetically connected diseases. In our discussion, we will restrict the term's application and use it to refer only to public health programs which survey or test target populations with the aim of detecting individuals who are at risk of disease for genetic reasons.

The Massachusetts PKU law pointed the way for the development of public screening programs. PKU was the first disease tested for, but before long others were added to the list. For example, New York state law requires that an infant be tested for seven diseases. A number of public health programs now screen particular populations for such conditions as sickle-cell anemia, sickle-cell trait, metabolic disorders, hypothyroidism, and chromosome anomalies.

Although genetic screening is relatively new as a social program, the concept is historically connected with public health measures for the detection of communicable diseases like tuberculosis and syphillis. If an individual with such a disease is identified, then he or she can receive treatment. Furthermore, the diseased individual can be prevented from spreading the disease to other members of the population.

Similarly, it is possible to think of diseases with a genetic basis as resembling contagious diseases. Individuals are affected, and they can pass on the disease. But with genetic diseases, the potential spread is not horizontal through the population, but vertical through the generations.

In terms of this model, public health measures similar to the ones that continue to be so effective in the control of contagious diseases might be used to help bring genetic diseases under control. When screening locates an individual with a genetic disorder, then steps can be taken to ensure that he receives appropriate therapy. Furthermore, when carriers of genes that produce diseases are identified, then they can be warned about their chances of having children that are genetically defective. Thus, at least a limited amount of control over the spread of genetic disease can be exercised, and the suffering of at least some individuals can be reduced or eliminated.

The justification of laws mandating screening programs can be sought in the power and responsibility of government to see to the welfare of its citizens. Here again, the public-health measures employed to control contagion might be looked to as a model. We do not permit the parents of a child to decide on their own whether the child should be vaccinated against smallpox. We believe that the society, operating through its government, has a duty to protect the child. Similarly, it can be argued that the society owes it to the child with PKU to see to it that the condition is discovered as quickly as possible so that appropriate treatment can be instituted.

Critics of screening programs have not been convinced that the contagious-disease model is at all appropriate in dealing with genetic diseases. Because the way in which genetic diseases are spread is so different, only a very small part of the population can be said to suffer any risk at all. By contrast, an epidemic of smallpox may threaten millions of people. Furthermore, some genetic screening programs do not have follow-up or counseling services attached to them so often nothing is done that benefits participants. By being told that they are the carrier of a genetic disease, people may be more harmed than helped by the programs.

In general, there are serious questions about whether the benefits of screening programs are sufficient to outweigh the liabilities. In particular, are screening programs so worthwhile that they justify the denial of individual choice entailed by required participation?

These issues and others related to them are easier to appreciate when they are considered in the context of particular kinds of screening programs. We will discuss briefly two programs that have been both important and controversial.

PKU screening.   As we pointed out earlier, screening for PKU was the first mass testing program to be mandated by state laws. It is generally agreed that it has also been the most successful program.

PKU is a relatively rare disease. It accounts for only about 0.8 percent of mentally retarded people who are institutionalized, and among the infants screened during a year in a state like Massachusetts, only about three of four cases of PKU may be discovered. (The incidence is 5.4 per 100,000 infants.) Given this relatively low incidence of the disease, some critics have argued that the abrogation of the freedom of choice required by a mandatory program does not make the results worthwhile.

This is particularly true, they suggest, because of the difficulties with the testing procedure itself. The level of phenylalanine in the blood may fluctuate so that not all infants with a higher than normal level at the time of the test actually have PKU. If they are put on the restricted diet, then they may suffer consequences from the diet that are harmful to their health. Thus, in attempting to protect the health of some infants, a mandatory program may unintentionally injure the health of other infants.

Tests more refined than the Guthrie one are possible. However, their use increases considerably the cost of the screening program, even if they are employed only when the Guthrie test is positive for PKU. In social terms, then, the financial cost of preventing a few cases of PKU may be much greater than allowing the cases to remain undetected and untreated.

Furthermore, there are additional hidden social costs. Female infants who are successfully treated for PKU may grow into adults and have children of their own. Their children run a very high risk of being born with brain damage. The reason for this in not genetic but developmental. The uterine environment of PKU mothers is one high in phenylalanine, and in high concentrations it causes damage to the infant. Thus, one generation may be saved from mental retardation by screening only to cause mental retardation in the next.

Sickle-cell.   Sickle-cell disease is a disorder of the hemoglobin in red blood cells. The cells assume a characteristic sickle shape and do not transport oxygen as well as normal red cells. They are also fragile and break apart more frequently. The result is anemia and, often, the blocking of blood vessels by fragments of ruptured cells.

The disease occurs only in those who have inherited both genes for the disease from their parents. (That is, the gene for the disease is recessive, and those who are homozygous for the gene are the ones who develop the disease.) Those with only one gene for the disease (that is, are heterozygous) are said to have sickle-cell trait.

Sickle-cell disease may develop at infancy or it may manifest itself later in life in painful and debilitating symptoms. Those with sickle-cell trait rarely show any of the clinical symptoms.

In the United States, the disease is most common among blacks and those of Mediterranean ancestry. The trait is carried by about 7–9 percent of the black population, and the disease occurs in about 0.3 percent of the population. Many people with the disease are not severely affected and can live relatively normal lives. However, the disease may also be fatal, and at the present there is no adequate therapy for it. There is no cure, nor is there a satisfactory means of diagnosing the disease prenatally. (However, a new test based on an examination of chromosomes from the fetal membrane is regarded as promising.)

In 1970 a relatively inexpensive and accurate test for sickle-cell hemoglobin was developed, making it possible to identify the carriers of sickle-cell trait. This technological development combined with political pressures generated by rising consciousness in the black population was to lead to the passage of state laws mandating sickle-cell screening. During 1971 and 1972, twelve states enacted sickle-cell legislation.

The results were socially disastrous. Some laws required blacks who applied for a marriage license to undergo screening. Since the only way to reduce the incidence of the disease is for two carriers to avoid having children, many blacks charged that the mandatory screening laws were a manifestation of a plan for genocide.

Medical reports that carriers of sickle-cell trait sometimes suffered from the pain and disability of sickling crises came to serve as a new basis of discrimination. Some employers and insurance companies began to require tests of black employees, and as a result some job possibilities were closed off to blacks with sickle-cell trait.

In 1972, Congress passed the National Sickle-Cell Anemia Control Act. In order to qualify for federal grants under the act, states were required to make sickle-cell screening voluntary, provide genetic counseling, and take steps to protect the confidentiality of participants. The most significant impact of the act was to force states to modify their laws to bring them into conformity with the act's requirements. In response, the seventeen states with sickle-cell screening laws now require only voluntary programs.

The National Genetic Diseases Act, passed in 1976 and funded annually since then, provides testing and counseling for the diagnosis and treatment of a number of genetic diseases. The act further strengthens the commitment to voluntary participation and to guarantees of confidentiality.

The lesson learned from the public controversy over the first sickle-cell screening programs is that genetic information can be used in ways that are harmful to the interests of individuals. Furthermore, the information can be used as a basis for systematic discrimination.

Genetic Counseling

Much is known about the ways in which a number of genetic diseases are inherited. Ones like PKU, sickle-cell, and Tay-Sachs follow the laws of Mendelian transmission genetics. Accordingly, given the appropriate information, it is often possible to determine how likely it is that a particular couple will have a child with a certain disease.

Suppose, for example, that a black couple is concerned about the possibility of having a child with sickle-cell disease. They will be tested to discover whether either or both of them is a carrier of sickle-cell trait.

Sickle-cell disease occurs only when two recessive genes are both present—one inherited from the mother, one from the father. If only one of the parents is a carrier of the trait (is heterozygous), then no child will have the disease. However, if both parents are carriers of the trait, then the chances are one out of four that their child will have the disease. (This is determined simply by considering which combinations of the two genes belonging to each parent will produce a combination that is a homozygous recessive. The combination of *Ss* and *Ss* will produce *ss* in only 25 percent of the possible cases.)

Such information can be used to explain to potential parents the risks they might run in having children. But, as the case of sickle-cell disease illustrates quite well, it is often very difficult for individuals to know what to do with such information.

Is a 25-percent risk of having a child with sickle-cell disease sufficiently high that a couple ought to decide to have no children at all? Because there is no safe and effective prenatal test for the disease, this question is one that is best considered in advance of a pregnancy. Answering it is made more difficult by the fact that sickle-cell disease varies greatly in severity. A child with the disease may be virtually normal, or doomed to a short life filled with suffering. No one can say in advance of its birth which possibility is more likely.

It is generally agreed that the question of whether to have a child when a serious risk is involved is a decision that must be made by the couple. The counselor may provide information about the risk, and just as important, the counselor may provide information about medical therapies that are available for a child born with a hereditary disease.

In diseases in which prenatal diagnosis is possible, the option of abortion may be open to potential parents. Here, too, the object of counseling is to see to it that the couple is educated in ways relevant to their needs.

Prenatal Genetic Diagnosis

A variety of new technological developments now make it possible to secure a great amount of information about the developing fetus while it is still in the uterus. Ultrasound, radiography, and fiber optics allow examination of soft-tissue and skeletal development. Anatomical abnormalities can be detected early enough to permit an abortion to be safely performed, if that is the decision of the woman carrying the fetus.

Yet the most common method of prenatal diagnosis continues to be amniocentesis. The amnion (the membrane surrounding the fetus) is filled with a fluid that contains fetal cells, urine, and metabolic products. By means of a needle puncture through the woman's abdomen, some of the amniotic fluid can be removed for study.

The procedure cannot be usefully performed until fourteen to sixteen weeks into the pregnancy. Until that time, there is an inadequate amount of fluid. The risk to the woman and to the fetus from the procedure is relatively small, something less than 1 percent.

Amniocentesis came into wide use only in the early 1960s. At first, it was mostly restricted to testing fetuses in cases in which there was a risk of Rh incompatibility. When the mother lacks a group of blood proteins called the Rh (or Rhesus) factor, and the fetus has it, then the immune system of the mother may produce antibodies against the fetus. The result for the fetus may be anemia, brain damage, and even death.

It was soon realized that additional information about the fetus could be gained from further analysis of the amniotic fluid and the fetal cells in it. The fluid can be chemically assayed, and the cells can be grown in cultures for study.

An examination of the chromosomes from the cells will show whether there are any known abnormalities that are likely to cause serious physical or mental defects. The presence or absence of the X chromosome will also show the sex of the fetus. (Only males have an X chromosome, so it is impossible to examine the chromosomes without discovering the sex of the fetus.)

Some metabolic disorders (such as Tay-Sachs disease) can be detected by chemical analysis of the amniotic fluid. However, some of the more common ones, such as PKU and cystic fibrosis, cannot be diagnosed in this way. Furthermore, at the present time there is no safe and effective way of diagnosing blood disorders like sickle-cell anemia using amniotic materials.

Amniocentesis does have some hazard attached to it. Accordingly, it is not at all regarded as a routine procedure to be performed in every pregnancy. There must be some indication that the fetus is at risk from a genetic or developmental disorder.

One indication is the age of the mother. Down's syndrome is much more likely to occur in fetuses conceived by women over the age of thirty-five. Since the syndrome is produced by a chromosome abnormality, an examination of the chromosomes in the cells of the fetus can reveal the defect. (See the Introduction to Chapter 2 for a fuller discussion.)

Genetic screening can also provide an indication of a need to perform amniocentesis. For example, Tay-Sachs disease is a metabolic disorder that occurs ten times as often among Jews originating in central and eastern Europe (the Ashkenazy) as in the general population. (The disease is invariably fatal and follows a sad course. An apparently normal child progressively develops blindness and brain damage, then dies at an early age.) Carriers of the Tay-Sachs gene can be identified by a blood test, and couples who are both carriers of the trait run a 25-percent risk of having a child with the disease. In such a case, there would be a good reason to perform amniocentesis.

If a woman has already had a child with a genetic disease, then this is also an indication that amniocentesis might justifiably be performed. For example, Huntington's chorea is a disorder of the central nervous system that produces loss of muscular control and eventually dementia. The gene for the disease is carried as a dominant so the risk of having a child with the disease is 50 percent for the carrier. Since there is no screening method for the disease, if a woman has already had a child with the disease, amniocentesis would be in order.

Until recently, there was no way to use amniocentesis to determine whether a fetus was affected with a neural-tube defect. (See Chapter 2 for a discussion of such defects as spina bifida.) The situation has now changed quite dramatically.

The cause of neural-tube defects is unknown, and they occur in about one out of every 500 births in the United States. They follow no known family patterns, have no known genetic basis, and cannot be predicted by genetic screening. They are also considered to be among the worst of all birth defects.

However, a test is available to indicate the presence of a neural-tube defect in a developing fetus. In 1972 David H. Brock of Edinburgh discovered that there is an unusually large amount of the substance alpha-fetoprotein (AFP) in the amniotic fluid taken from women who give birth to children with neural-tube defects.

The reason for this, Brock decided, is that the open spine or skull of the fetus allows the AFP it normally contains to leak into the amniotic fluid. Through additional research, Brock determined that there is also a greater level of AFP in the blood of women carrying a fetus with the defect than in that of women with normal fetuses. The AFP enters the mother's circulatory system by passing through the umbilical cord and the placenta.

The blood test is not wholly reliable. Because the level of AFP varies in all women, the test produces many false positives. Also, women with twins or triplets have a level of AFP that is higher than women carrying a single fetus. Consequently, the blood test must be supplemented by ultrasound examination to determine whether only one fetus is present. If so, then amniocentesis is performed to get a more accurate measurement of the AFP present.

Selective Abortion

In most cases in which prenatal diagnosis indicates that the fetus suffers from a genetic disorder or developmental defect, the only means of avoiding the birth of a defective child is abortion.

Because those who go through the tests required to determine the condition of the fetus are concerned with having a child, abortion performed under such circumstances is called *selective*. That is, the woman decides to have an abortion to avoid producing a child with birth defects, not just to avoid having a child.

Those who oppose abortion in principle (see Chapter 1) also oppose selective abortion. In the view of some, the fact that a child will be born defective is in no way a justification for terminating the life of the fetus.

Those who are prepared to endorse abortion at all typically approve of selective abortion as an acceptable way of avoiding suffering. In their view, it is better that the potential person that is the fetus not become an actual person, full of pain, disease, and disability.

At this time, there is some hope that the painful decision between having an abortion or giving birth to a defective child may someday be avoided. In the last few years, techniques of fetal surgery have been employed to correct certain abnormal physical conditions.

Repairs to the heart, the insertion of shunts to drain off excess brain fluids, and the placement of tubes to inflate collapsed lungs are some of the intrauterine surgical procedures now being performed. It is believed that it may be possible to expose the fetus within the uterus, perform surgery, then close up the amnion again. This would make possible more extensive surgery for a greater variety of conditions.

The present hope is that as new surgical techniques for the treatment of fetuses are perfected and expanded, the need to rely on abortion to avoid the birth of defective children will significantly decline. Of course, surgery cannot, even in principle, provide a remedy for a large number of hereditary disorders. Surgery can do nothing for a child with Tay-Sachs disease or PKU.

Helplessness in this regard is matched by another hope. Perhaps in future years pharmaceutical and biochemical therapies will be available to employ in cases involving missing enzymes. Or perhaps "gene surgery" will make it possible to insert the proper gene for manufacturing a needed biochemical into the DNA of the cells of a fetus.

Hopeful though we may be, the painful present reality is that for most children born with genetic diseases or defects very little can be done. Selective abortion continues to be the primary means to avoid the birth of a child known to be genetically defective.

Difficulties with Genetic Intervention

Genetic screening, counseling, and prenatal diagnosis present bright possibilities for those who believe in the importance of exercising control through rational planning and decision making. The prospect of avoiding the birth of children with crippling defects is seen by them as one of the triumphs of contemporary medicine.

Furthermore, the additional prospect of wholly eliminating some genetic diseases by counseling and control holds the promises of an even better future. For example, if people who are carriers of diseases caused by a dominant gene (such as Huntington's chorea) produced no children with the disease, the disease would soon disappear entirely. The gene causing the disease would simply not be passed on to the next generation.

A vision of a world without the misery caused by genetic defects is a motivating factor among those who are strong advocates of programs of genetic intervention. (See the section on eugenics in this chapter for more details.) The vision must have its appeal to all who are moved by compassion in the face of suffering. Yet whether or not one shares this vision and is prepared to use it as a basis for social action, there are serious ethical questions about genetic intervention that must be faced.

We have already mentioned some of the issues in connection with particular programs and procedures. We can now add some more general questions to that list, but it should be kept in mind that our discussion cannot be complete. The moral and social issues connected with genetic intervention are woven into a complicated fabric of personal and social considerations. We can merely sketch the main outline of the pattern.

1. Is there a right to have children who are likely to be defective? Suppose that a woman is informed, after the AFP test and amniocentesis, that the child she is carrying will be born with a neural-tube defect. Does she have the right to refuse an abortion and have the child anyway?

Those who are opposed to all abortion on the grounds of natural law would favor the woman's right to decide to have the child. By contrast, a utilitarian might well argue that the decision would be wrong. The amount of suffering the potential child might be expected to undergo outweighs any parental loss. For different reasons, a Kantian might endorse this same point of view. Even if we assume the fetus is a person, a Kantian might argue that we are obliged to prevent its suffering. (For more details of these and similar arguments, see Chapters 1 and 2.)

Suppose we decide that a woman does have a right to have a child that is almost certain to be defective. If so, then is the society obligated to bear the expense of caring for such a child? On the natural law view, the answer is almost certainly yes. The child, defective or not, is a human person, and, as such, is entitled to the support and protection of the society. If we agree that the defective child is a person, then he or she is also a disadvantaged person. Thus, an argument based on Rawls' principles of justice would support the view that the child is entitled to social support. (Again, see Chapter 2 for more detail.)

2. Is the society justified in requiring that people submit to genetic screening, counseling, and prenatal diagnosis? Children born with genetic diseases and defects require the expenditure of large amounts of public funds. Mandatory diagnosis need not be coupled with mandatory abortion or abstention from bearing children.

On utilitarian grounds, it might be argued that society has a legitimate interest in seeing to it that, no matter what people ultimately decide, they should at least have the information about the likelihood that they will produce a defective child.

If this view is adopted, then a number of specific medically related questions become relevant. For example, who should be screened? It is impractical and unnecessary to screen everyone. Why should we screen schoolchildren or prisoners, those who are sterile, or those past the age of childbearing?

This is closely connected with a second question: What should people be screened for? Should everyone be screened for Tay-Sachs disease, even thought it is the Jewish population that is most at risk? Should everyone be screened for sickle-cell trait, even though it is primarily the black population that is at risk?

Those who accept the contagious-disease model of genetic screening frequently defend it on the utilitarian grounds that screening promotes the general social welfare. However, one might argue that screening can also be justified on deontological grounds. It could be claimed that we owe it to developing fetuses, regarded as persons, to see to it that they receive the opportunity for the most effective treatment. For example, it might be said that we have an obligation to provide a PKU child with the immediate therapy required to save him or her from severe mental retardation. The restriction of the autonomy of individuals by requiring screening might be regarded as justified by this obligation. If screening is voluntary, then the welfare of the child is made to depend on ignorance and accidental opportunity.

3. Do physicians have an obligation to inform their patients who are prospective parents about the kinds of genetic tests that are available? A study of one population of women screened for Tay-Sachs disease showed that none had sought testing on the recommendation of her physician.

If the autonomy of the individual is to be preserved, then it seems clear that it is the duty of a physician to inform patients about genetic testing. A physician who disapproves of abortion might be reluctant to inform patients about tests that might encourage them to seek an abortion. Nevertheless, to the extent that abortion is a moral decision, it is a decision properly made by the individual, not by someone acting paternalistically in her behalf.

The duty of a physician to inform patients about the possibility of genetic tests seems quite straightforward. Yet the issue becomes more complicated in light of the next question about truth telling.

4. Do patients have a right to be informed of all of the results of a genetic test? Ethical theories that are based on respect for the autonomy of the individual (such as Kant's and Ross's) suggest that patients are entitled to know what has been learned from the tests.

But what if the test reveals that the fetus has only a quite minor genetically transmissible disease? Should the physician run the risk of the patient's deciding to have an abortion merely because she is committed to the ideal of a "perfect" baby? A utilitarian answer would suggest not.

Furthermore, what about the matter of sex determination? Screening tests that involve chromosome examination also reveal the sex of the fetus. Are prospective parents entitled to know this information? When abortion is elective, it is quite possible for the woman to decide to have an abortion to avoid giving birth to a child of a particular sex.

It might be argued on both utilitarian and deontological grounds that the sex of the fetus is information that is not relevant to the health of the fetus. Accordingly, the physician is under no obligation to reveal the sex of the fetus. Indeed, the physician may be under an obligation *not* to reveal the sex of the fetus in order to avoid the possibility of its destruction for a basically trivial reason.

5. Should public funds be used to pay for genetic tests when an individual is unable to pay? This is a question that holders of various ethical theories may not be prepared to answer in a simple yes or no fashion. Those who oppose abortion on natural law grounds might advocate providing funds only for genetic screening and counseling. That is, they might favor providing prospective parents with information that they might then use to decide whether to refrain from having children. Yet opponents of abortion might be against spending public money on tests that might encourage the use of abortion to prevent the birth of a defective child.

The views of Rawls and of utilitarianism might well support the use of public funds for genetic testing as part of a more general program of providing for health-care needs. Whether genetic testing programs are funded and the level of funding would then depend on judgments about their expected value in comparison with other health-care programs.

A present ethical and social difficulty is caused by the fact that federal funds may be employed to pay for genetic screening and testing, yet federal money cannot legally be used to pay for abortions. Consequently, it is possible for a woman to discover that she is carrying a fetus with a serious genetic disease, wish to have an abortion, yet lack the financial means to pay for it.

Issues about the confidentiality of test results, informed consent, the use of genetic testing to gather epidemiological information, and a variety of other matters might be mentioned here in connection with genetic intervention. Those that have been discussed are sufficient to indicate that the difficulties presented by genetic intervention are at least as numerous as the benefits it promises.

Eugenics

Like other organisms, we are the products of millions of years of evolutionary development. This process has taken place through the operation of natural selection on randomly produced genetic mutations. Individual organisms are successful in an evolutionary sense when they contribute a number of genes to the gene pool of their species proportionately greater than the number contributed by others. Most often, this means that the evolutionarily successful individuals are those with the largest number of offspring. These are the individuals favored by natural selection. That is, they possess the genes for certain properties that are favored by existing environmental factors. (This favoring of properties is natural selection.) The genes of "favored" individuals will occur with greater frequency than the genes of others in the next generation. If the same environmental factors continue to operate, these genes will spread through the entire population.

Thanks to Darwin and the evolutionary biologists who have come after him, we now have a sound understanding of the evolutionary process and the mechanisms by which it operates. This understanding puts us in a position to intervene in the process. That is, we no longer have to consider ourselves subject to the blind workings of natural selection. If we choose to do so, we can modify the course of human evolution. As the evolutionary biologist Theodosius Dobzhansky expressed the point: "Evolution need no longer be a destiny imposed from without; it may conceivably be controlled by man, in accordance with his wisdom and values."

Those who advocate eugenics accept just this point of view. They favor social policies and practices which, over time, offer the possibility of increasing the number of genes in the human population responsible for producing or improving traits (for example, intelligence) that we value.

The aim of increasing the number of favorable genes in the human population is called *positive eugenics*. By contrast, *negative eugenics* aims at decreasing the number of undesirable or harmful genes. Those who advocate negative eugenics are generally most interested in eliminating or reducing the number of those genes that are responsible for various kinds of birth defects and sex-linked diseases.

Both positive and negative eugenics require instituting some sort of control over human reproduction. Several kinds of policies and procedures have been advocated, and we will discuss a few of the possibilities below.

Genetic Intervention

The discussion in the preceding section of genetic screening, counseling, and prenatal genetic diagnosis makes it unnecessary to repeat here information about the possibilities and procedures we currently possess for predicting and diagnosing genetic diseases. It is enough to recall that, given information about the genetic makeup and background of potential parents, a number of genetic diseases can be predicted with a certain degree of probability as likely to occur in a child of such parents. This is true of such diseases as PKU, sickle-cell anemia, hemophilia, Huntington's chorea, and Tay-Sachs disease.

When genetic information is not adequate to serve as a basis for a reliable prediction, then information about the developing fetus can often be obtained by employing one of several procedures of prenatal diagnosis. Even when genetic information is adequate for a statistical prediction, whether the fetus has a certain disease can be determined by prenatal testing. Thus, in addition to the disorders named above, prenatal tests can be performed for such other defects as neural-tube anomalies and Down's syndrome.

A proponent of negative eugenics might advocate that a screening process for all or some currently detectable genetic diseases be required by law. When the probability of the occurrence of a disease is high (whatever figure that might be taken to be), then the potential parents might be encouraged to have no children. Indeed, the law might *require* that such a couple abstain from having children and prescribe a penalty for going against the decision of the screening board. If those carrying the genes for some genetic diseases could be prevented from having children, then over time the incidence of the diseases in the population would decrease. In some cases, when the disease is the result of a dominant gene (as it is in Huntington's chorea), the disease would eventually disappear.

When the disease is of a kind that can be detected only after a child is conceived, then if the results of a prenatal diagnosis show that the developing fetus has a heritable disease, an abortion might be encouraged. Short of a law requiring abortion, a variety of social policies might be adopted to make abortion an attractive option. (For example, the cost of an abortion might be paid for by government funds or women choosing abortion might be financially rewarded.) The aborting of a fetus found to have a transmissible genetic disease would not only prevent the birth of a defective infant, it would eliminate a potential carrier of the genes responsible for the disease.

Similarly, the sterilization of people identified as having genes that are responsible for certain kinds of physical or mental defects would prevent them from passing on these defective genes. (See Chapter 8 for a discussion of sterilization.) In this way, the number of such genes in the population would be proportionately reduced.

Currently, there are no state or federal laws that make it a crime for couples who are genetically a bad risk to have children. Yet there may be developing a tendency toward more genetic regulation. As we mentioned earlier, several states now require the screening of newborn infants in order to detect the presence of certain genetic diseases that respond well to early treatment. Also, genetic screening programs are frequently offered in communities to encourage people to seek information about particular diseases.

At present, genetic screening (for adults) and genetic counseling are voluntary. They aim at providing information and then leave reproductive decisions up to the individuals concerned. Most often, they are directed toward the immediate goal of decreasing the number of children suffering from birth defects and genetic diseases. Yet genetic screening and counseling might also be viewed as a part of negative eugenics. To the extent that they discourage the birth of children carrying deleterious genes, they also discourage the spread of those genes in the human population.

Obviously, screening programs and genetic counseling might also be used to promote *positive* eugenics. Individuals possessing genes for traits that society values might be encouraged to have large numbers of children. In this way, genes for traits that are considered worthwhile would increase in relative frequency within the population.

There are no programs of positive eugenics. Yet it is easy to imagine a variety of social and economic incentives (for example, government bonuses) that might be introduced as part of a plan to promote the spread of certain genes by rewarding favored groups of people for having children.

Use of Desirable Germ Cells

Artificial insemination by the use of stored sperm is already a reality. The implantation of a donor ovum in the wall of the uterus is also possible, and we can imagine the development of a biotechnology that would permit the long-term storage of ova. In such a situation, then, a man or woman might choose to have a child by selecting stored germ cells contributed by individuals possessing traits that they admire. Sperm banks and ova banks would then provide a way for the human population to improve itself—that is, to increase the number of genes for desirable traits in the population.

Difficulties with Eugenics

Critics have been quick to point out that the proposals we have discussed suffer from serious drawbacks. First, negative eugenics is not likely to make much of a change in the species as a whole. Most hereditary diseases are genetically recessive and so occur only when both parents possess the same defective gene. Even though a particular couple might be counseled (or required) not to have children, the gene will still be widespread in the population among people we would consider wholly normal. For a similar reason, sterilization would have few long-range effects. Also, there is the uncomfortable fact that geneticists have estimated that on the average, everyone carries recessive genes for five genetic defects or diseases. Genetic counseling may help individuals, but negative eugenics does not promise much for the population as a whole.

Positive eugenics can promise little more. It is difficult to imagine that we would all agree on what traits we would like to see increased in the human species. But even if we could, it is not clear that we would be able to increase them in any simple way. For one thing, we have little understanding of the genetic basis of traits such as "intelligence," "honesty," "musical ability," and so on. It is clear, however, that there is not just a single gene for them, and the chances are that they are the result of a complicated interplay between genetic endowment and social and environmental factors. Consequently, the task of increasing their frequency is quite different from that of, say, increasing the frequency of short-horned cattle. Furthermore, the desirable traits may well be accompanied by less desirable traits, and we may not be able to increase the first without also increasing the second.

Quite apart from biological objections, eugenics also raises questions of a moral kind. Have we indeed become the "business manager of evolution" as Julian Huxley once claimed? If so, then do we have a responsibility to future generations to improve the human race? Would this responsibility justify our requiring genetic screening? Would it justify our establishing a program of positive eugenics? Affirmative answers to these questions may generate conflicts with notions of individual dignity and self-determination.

Of the ethical theories we have discussed, it seems likely that only utilitarianism might be construed as favoring a program of positive eugenics. The possibility of increasing the frequency of desirable traits in the human species might, in terms of the principle of utility, justify present restrictions on reproduction. It is not clear that this is so, however. The goal of an improved society or human race might well be regarded as too distant and uncertain to warrant the imposition of restrictions that would increase current human unhappiness.

So far as negative eugenics is concerned, the principle of utility could certainly be appealed to in order to justify social policies that would discourage or prohibit parents who are serious genetic risks from having children. The aim here need not be the remote one of improving the human population but the more immediate one of preventing the increase in sorrows and pains that would be caused by a defective child.

Natural law doctrines of Roman Catholicism forbid abortion (see the introduction to Chapter 1 and the introductory chapter) and sterilization. Thus, these means of practicing negative eugenics are ruled out. Also the natural law view that reproduction is a natural function of sexual intercourse seems, at least prima facie, to rule out negative eugenics as a deliberate policy altogether. It could be argued, however, that voluntary abstinence from sexual intercourse or some other acceptable form of birth control would be a legitimate means of practicing negative eugenics.

Ross's prima facie duty of causing no harm might be invoked to justify negative eugenics. If there is good reason to believe that a child is going to suffer from a genetic disease, then we may have a duty to prevent the child from being born. Similarly, Rawls's theory might permit a policy that would require the practice of some form of negative eugenics for the benefit of its immediate effects of preventing suffering and sparing all the cost of supporting those with genetic diseases.

It is difficult to determine what sort of answer to the question of negative eugenics might be offered in terms of Kant's ethical principles. Laws regulating conception or forced abortion or sterilization might well be considered to violate the dignity and autonomy of individuals. Yet moral agents as rational decision makers require information on which to base their decisions. Thus, programs of genetic screening and counseling might be considered to be legitimate.

Genetic Research, Therapy, and Technology

By replacing natural selection with artificial selection that is directly under our control, we can, over time, alter the genetic composition of populations of organisms. This has been done for thousands of years by animal and plant breeders, and our improved understanding of genetics allows us to do it today with more effectiveness and certainty of results. Yet such alterations require long periods of time. Molecular genetics holds out the possibility of immediate changes. Bacteria continue to be the major organisms of research, but genetic technology is already being applied to plants and animals. Many scientists believe it is only a matter of time before the same technology can be applied to humans. But the time will be short, they say, only if DNA research is allowed to continue at its present pace.

Recombinant DNA

The information required for genetic inheritance is coded in the two intertwined strands of DNA (deoxyribonucleic acid) found in plant and animal cells—the double helix. The strands are made up of four kinds of chemical units called nucleotides, and the genetic message is determined by the particular sequence of nucleotides. Three nucleotides in sequence form a triplet codon. Each codon directs the synthesis of a particular amino acid and determines the place that it will occupy in making up a protein molecule. Since virtually all properties of organisms (enzymes, organs, eye color, and so on) depend on proteins, the processes directed by DNA are fundamental.

Alterations in the nucleotide sequence in DNA occur naturally as mutations—random changes introduced as "copying errors" when DNA replicates (reproduces) itself. These alterations result in changes in the properties of organisms since the properties are under the control of DNA. Much research in current molecular genetics is directed toward bringing about desired changes by deliberately manipulating the nucleotide sequences in DNA. The major steps toward this goal have involved the development of techniques for recombining DNA from different sources. A basic understanding of how and why this is done is crucial for grasping the issues that are central in the current debates about recombinant DNA research and its potential significance. (Some of the details of one aspect of the debate are given in the Case Presentation of this chapter.)

The recombinant process begins by taking proteins known as restriction enzymes from bacteria and mixing them with DNA that has been removed from cells. These enzymes cut open the DNA strands at particular nucleotide locations. DNA nucleotide sequences from another source can then be added, and certain of these will attach to the cut ends. Thus, DNA from two distinct sources can be recombined to form a single molecule.

This recombinant DNA can then be made to enter a host cell. The organism almost universally employed as a host is the one-celled bacterium *E. coli* that inhabits the human intestine by the billions. In addition to the DNA that makes up the chromosome of the cell, *E. coli* also possesses small circular strands of DNA known as plasmids. The DNA of a plasmid can be recombined with the DNA of a foreign source and returned to the cell. There the plasmid will start replicating again. It will make copies of the original nucleotides *plus* copies of the added segments. Thus, a strain of bacteria can be produced that will make limitless numbers of copies of the foreign DNA.

The obvious question is, what benefits might this recombinant technique produce? It might lead to the understanding and control of the molecular processes involved in such diseases as cancer, diabetes, and hemophilia. It might provide more effective treatment for metabolic diseases like PKU and Tay-Sachs.

From the more commercial standpoint, recombinant DNA technology might lead to the development of new breeds of plants that are able to utilize nitrogen from the air and thus require no fertilizer. Specially engineered bacteria might be used to clean up the environment by breaking down currently nonbiodegradable compounds like DDT and Agent Orange. Other bacteria might be used to convert petroleum into other useful chemical compounds, including plastics.

The most immediate benefits of recombinant DNA are likely to be the use of modified bacteria as chemical factories to produce biological materials of medical importance. In addition, the transplanting of human genes into nonhuman embryos promises to lead to an understanding of the ways in which genes can be made to reproduce themselves and be passed on to succeeding generations.

Just a glance at a few of the many recent research developments is enough to gain an appreciation of the powerful potentials of genetic technology:

In 1977 the DNA sequence responsible for producing insulin was taken from rat DNA and combined with *E. coli* plasmid. The recombinant DNA replicated, but in the absence of a biochemical stimulus to "turn on" the gene, no insulin was manufactured. Yet most molecular biologists believe that the large-scale production of insulin by bacteria is not far away.

In April, 1982 Dr. John D. Baxter and his associates at the University of California in San Francisco succeeded in developing a bacterial strain capable of producing endorphin. Because endorphin is a natural opiate, the hope is that it can be used as an effective substitute for such addictive drugs as morphine. The gene involved was obtained from a culture of mouse pituitary tumor cells.

A group of researchers from the U.S. and Switzerland has been able to insert the gene for human insulin into mouse embryos and to get the gene incorporated into the genetic code of the embryos.

The human gene for interferon has been transplanted into fertilized mouse ova and passed on to the next generation. Because interferon is an antiviral agent thought to be effective in the treatment of some forms of cancer, this accomplishment promises to hold significant therapeutic benefits.

The viral gene for the enzyme thymidine kinase has been incorporated into mouse embryo cells. The gene was active in its new environment, and the fetal mice produced the enzyme. The enzyme is one of those required for the production of DNA.

Gene Therapy

None of the experimental techniques used in the research mentioned above is currently employed to treat any human genetic or developmental problem. Genetic knowledge has advanced considerably in the last decade, but most experts believe that the use of recombinant DNA techniques as part of a program of medical therapy is not likely in the foreseeable future.

Nonetheless, the possibility of performing some sort of gene surgery, in which a defective gene is cut out or a needed gene is inserted, is a compelling prospect. The ability to alter the basic machinery of life to correct its malfunctioning is surely the most powerful form of therapy imaginable. However, at the moment, the generally accepted view is that our knowledge is still too partial to attempt to apply it to humans.

This is the view that led many molecular geneticists to consider as premature an experimental attempt at gene therapy conducted by Dr. Martin J. Cline of UCLA and his associates. The effort was unsuccessful, but it provides an example of what might be possible if our knowledge of molecular genetics were commensurate with our aims, if our reach did not exceed our grasp.

In 1980, Dr. Cline treated two patients suffering from an incurable blood disorder called beta-zero thalassemia. The disease is one in which the gene for beta globulin, one of the constituents of the hemoglobin in red blood cells, is either missing or unexpressed. Those with the disease usually die very early.

The use of viruses to insert genes into cells is clearly not suitable when dealing with humans, for the viruses may cause disease or death. So Dr. Cline relied on another technique that had been developed through research with animals. The technique, called *transformation,* is one that depends on the chemical properties of DNA and on the fact that cells take in calcium from their environment. Under proper conditions, the cell will take up DNA fragments along with the calcium.

Cells in the bone marrow (stem cells) are among those responsible for the production of red blood cells. Thus Cline and his associates took bone marrow from the patients and added the appropriate DNA segments to a cell culture of that material. The hope was that the DNA would be incorporated into the genetic code of the cells—that the cells would be transformed.

Afterwards, the treated cells were injected into the patients. According to the theory, the cells would then multiply and their copies would include the new genes. The patients would thus be supplied with the cells necessary to produce beta globulin.

Unfortunately, the plan was not successful. Transformation is a very ineffective process, and very few cells in a culture actually incorporate the foreign DNA. Perhaps the material injected into the patients did not contain enough transformed cells to make a difference. Or perhaps the transformed cells did not multiply sufficiently or otherwise perform as expected. In any case, the patients were not helped by the attempt at therapy, although there was no indication that they were harmed either.

Dr. Cline was reprimanded by the National Institutes of Health for engaging in medical experiments without securing the approval of the appropriate UCLA committees. In his own view, the experiments were both scientifically sound and morally justifiable.

Cline's effort in employing a wholly new therapeutic technique raises clearly and forcefully the question of when it is morally legitimate to use an experimental procedure in treating humans. If a disease condition is regarded as hopeless, is it proper to attempt a therapy which will do no harm and may help? Or must the safety and effectiveness of the therapy be established first by animal experiments?

Whatever view may be taken of these questions, it is clear that eventually gene therapy, based on recombinant-DNA techniques, will be added to the medical arsenal. The promise is too great to ignore.

Commercial Applications

Commercial uses of recombinant-DNA technology are much closer at hand than gene therapy, and an entire industry of biotechnology has already emerged. Large-scale production of drugs, hormones, and enzymes is expected to begin during this decade, and some financial analysts have estimated that by 1990 the market for such biological goods will amount to some three billion dollars. More than 150 companies have already been formed to develop and sell the products of recombinant technology.

The great commercial expansion has brought with it a number of legal, moral, and social problems. In 1981, the Supreme Court ruled that new organisms created by recombinant techniques can be patented in the same way as other commercial products or processes. Many members of the scientific community have been critical of this decision. Some object that it is simply wrong to grant exclusive rights to life forms that should belong to all.

Others have argued that the information used to create new forms is the result of scientific research paid for through public grants to universities and research establishments. Consequently, the fruits of that research ought to belong to everyone.

This issue is clearly seen in a case involving Genentech, one of the first and largest of the biotechnology companies. Genentech obtained cells from the National Cancer Institute. From those cells, Genentech workers were able to extract the gene responsible for the production of interferon and splice it into bacterial genes. Scientists at UCLA who had identified the cells as ones producing interferon and sent samples of them to the NCI objected to Genentech's being given the cells. They claimed that the commercial organization had no right to use the cell line they had identified for the purposes of profit.

The traditional character of universities has also been challenged by the prospect of being directly involved with the development of commercially valuable organisms and organic products. For example, Stanford is one of the holders of a patent which it has licensed on the condition of royalty payments by users. Some have questioned whether universities, which have traditionally been committed to the pursuit of knowledge for its own sake, ought to be permitted to profit from research done by faculty members. The suggestion is that universities ought to be functioning for the benefit of society and humanity, not for their own welfare.

In addition, new commercial alliances call into question the impartiality of universities and their faculties. In 1981, MIT accepted one hundred million dollars from a commercial concern to establish an independent research institute in molecular biology. Although a variety of safeguards have been built into the agreement, some critics are still of the opinion that there is substantial risk that academic values (such as independent research and the transmission of free information) run a high risk of being compromised.

Similarly, a number of scientists on the faculties of universities have become personally involved with biotechnology companies. In the view of some, such personal and financial interests may result in scientists losing their credibility with the public and with the government. Such a loss of trust may mean that we will no longer be able to rely on the impartiality of scientific experts in attempting to decide matters affecting public interest and policy.

Biohazards

The issues connected with genetic therapy and with the commercial development of genetic technology may be overshadowed in significance by questions concerning the dangers inherent in the very process of recombinant-DNA research. Suppose that a nucleotide sequence for manufacturing a lethal toxin were combined with the DNA of *E. coli*. This currently harmless inhabitant of the intestine might be transformed into a deadly organism that would threaten the existence of the entire human population. Or perhaps a nucleotide sequence that transforms normal cells into cancerous ones might trigger an epidemic of cancer. Without a thorough knowledge of the molecular mechanisms involved, little could be done to halt the outbreak. Indeed, it is not clear what would happen if an insulin-producing strain of bacteria spread through the human population.

No one knows how real these and similar dangers are. Some have suggested that they are very real, while others have dismissed them as unrealistic horror stories. It cannot be denied that over a decade of recombinant-DNA research has passed without the occurrence of any biological catastrophes. A number of observers regard this as sufficient proof of the essential safety of the research. Yet in the view of others, the fact that no catastrophes have yet occurred serves only to give us a false sense of security. Few people now advocate that the research be abandoned, but several molecular geneticists have argued that the very fact that we still do not know enough to estimate the risks involved in recombinant-DNA research is a good reason for continuing to control it severely.

Quite apart from the possible hazards associated with recombinant DNA, many molecular biologists continue to be uneasy about the general direction of their research. A number of biotechnological possibilities are on the horizon, and some of them might have far-reaching consequences. Genetic surgery, for example, offers more possibilities than just medical therapy. If undesirable DNA segments can be sliced out of the genetic code and replaced by others, then this would permit the "engineering" of human beings to an extent and to a degree of precision never before imagined. The eugenic dream of producing people to match an ideal model would be a reality.

The same techniques employed to manufacture the ideal person might also be used to engineer others to fit special needs. It is not difficult to imagine using genetic surgery to design a subhuman race to serve as a slave class for the society. The scenarios of cautionary science fiction might be acted out in our own future.

In addition, the biological technique of asexual reproduction known as cloning might be employed to produce individuals that are exact genetic copies of the DNA donor. These "Xeroxed" organisms—including human beings—are within the scope of technological imagination.

To mention just one last possibility, virtually new organisms might be produced by splicing together DNA from two or more sources. Thus, the world might be faced with creatures of an unknown and unpredictable nature that are not the product of the natural processes of evolution.

It is little wonder that molecular biologists have become concerned about the nature and direction of their research. As Robert Sinsheimer of the California Institute of Technology says, "Biologists have become, without wanting it, custodians of great and terrible power." Such power in the hands of a tyrannical government could be used with irresistible effectiveness to control its subjects.

Societies might create a race of semihuman slaves or armies of genetically engineered soldiers. The possibilities are both fantastic and unlimited.

Difficulties with Genetic Research, Therapy, and Technology

The risks involved in gene therapy are not unique ones. In most respects, they exactly parallel those involved in any new medical treatment. Accordingly, it seems reasonable to believe that the same standards of safety and the same consideration for the welfare of the patient that are relevant to the use of other forms of therapy should be regarded as relevant to gene therapy.

The natural law view and the principles of Kant and Ross would suggest that the autonomy of the individual be respected and preserved. In particular, the individual ought not be viewed as an experimental case for testing out a procedure that may later prove helpful. If the person is well enough to be adequately informed and to give consent, and if there is no alternative therapy likely to be effective, it would be morally legitimate for the patient to be given the opportunity to benefit from the therapy. However, if the hazards are great or if they are completely unknown, then it is doubtful whether the patient would be justified in risking his or her life.

By contrast, on utilitarian principles, if the outcome of gene therapy can be reasonably expected to produce more benefit than harm, then the use of the therapy might be considered justifiable. If we assume that a person is likely to die anyway, then that in itself might be enough to warrant the use of the therapy. In addition, since each case treated is likely to contribute to increased understanding and to benefit others, this tends to support the use of gene therapy, even in cases in which it is of doubtful help to the individual. (See Chapter 5 for a fuller discussion.)

Genetic research and its associated technology present issues that are much greater in scope than those raised by gene therapy. They are issues that require us to decide what sort of society we want to live in.

Should work in molecular genetics be halted? Are the dangers of recombinant DNA too great to be chanced? Are the possibilities of genetic engineering too frightening and threatening to deal with? Is it better to call a halt to their development before matters get out of hand?

These questions bring up the more general problem of whether it is ever legitimate to end or restrict free scientific inquiry to achieve general social goals. Certainly there is general agreement that research must not violate the rights of individuals. But what about potential dangers? And what about merely possible long-range difficulties, such as are posed by genetic engineering?

The natural law view of ethics would not, in general, support any policy of ending scientific research. For on this view, there is a natural inclination (and hence a natural duty) to seek knowledge. Yet certain types of experiments and engineering possibilities would be ruled out. Those that aim at altering human beings or creating new life forms would likely be considered, on the Roman Catholic view, to violate nature. By doing so, they would run counter to God's plan and purpose and so be immoral.

The principle of utility might be invoked to justify limiting, directing, or even ending scientific research. If research or its pursuit is likely to bring about more harm than benefit, then regulation would be called for. Yet if the promise of relieving misery or increasing well-being is great, then the risks might be acceptable. Such an analysis also seems to be consistent with Rawl's principles. There is not, for Rawls, an absolute right to seek knowledge, and restrictions might well be imposed on scientific research if the good of society seems to demand it.

The Selections

In the first selection, Robert F. Murray, Jr. is most concerned with the effects that mass genetic screening programs can have on individuals. Murray admits that screening can bring genuine benefits to those who are discovered to have a treatable disease like PKU, but the results are far from beneficial for those who are told that they or their children have a disease for which there is no effective therapy. Such information is basically useless to them, and it may destroy their pleasure and sense of well-being without substituting anything of value.

Similarly, Murray asks, when carriers of hereditary diseases are told of their condition, what benefits do they derive? If the disease is one like Tay-Sachs, then prenatal diagnosis may be performed and selective abortion chosen if it seems indicated. But what about carriers of sickle-cell trait? Since no effective prenatal test is in general use and since the disease itself shows wide variation in severity, the individual can learn little that is helpful. What is more, he or she may feel stigmatized by being identified as a carrier.

For Murray, such considerations suggest that the development of new screening programs should take into account the needs of the individual and that pressure to make screening mandatory should be resisted.

Leon R. Kass, in "Implications of Prenatal Diagnosis for the Human Right to Life," expresses concern that the practice of "genetic abortion" will strongly affect our attitudes toward all who are "defective" or abnormal. Those who escape the net of selective abortion might receive less care and might even come to think of themselves as second-class specimens. Furthermore, on Kass's view, genetic abortion might encourage us to accept the general principle that defectives of any kind ought not be born. This, in turn, would threaten our commitment to the basic moral principle that each person, despite any physical or mental handicap, is the inherent equal of every other person.

Kass presents six criteria that he suggests ought to be satisfied to justify the abortion of a fetus for genetic reasons. In the remainder of his paper, he focuses on the question raised by the last criterion: According to what standards should we judge a fetus with genetic abnormalities unfit to live? As candidates for such standards, Kass examines the concepts of social good, family good, and the "healthy and sound" fetus. He finds difficulties with all, and in the end, he professes himself unable to provide a satisfactory justification for genetic abortion.

Critics of genetic screening and selective abortion have often charged that it is only a small social step from such programs to the practice of positive eugenics. Martin Golding in his essay reviews some of the arguments that have been presented by advocates of eugenics. He argues that it is doubtful that we have an obligation to establish social programs that would benefit the distant future.

The existence of such an obligation is the usual assumption underlying eugenics programs. Golding then points to some of the specific difficulties that face all eugenic proposals. Apart from the biological difficulties that stand in the way of delivering what is promised, Golding raises the doubt that a eugenic program could be successful without relying upon totally unacceptable authoritarian methods.

In "Inquiring into Inquiry," Robert L. Sinsheimer raises the question of when scientific inquiry might be halted. He suggests that we might wish to limit inquiry when human dignity is threatened, when research poses unacceptable risks, or when it becomes too expensive. Most important, on Sinsheimer's view, we need to ask whether the secondary consequences of the knowledge we gain are likely to be beneficial. That is, given the nature of human beings and of our society, are we willing to accept the results that the acquisition of new knowledge may bring about?

Although Sinsheimer merely alludes to recombinant-DNA research and technology, the questions he raises about research in general are especially relevant to that area. Answering the questions in a particular way would suggest that we call a halt to DNA research and to the development of much biotechnology.

The moral and social problems associated with recombinant-DNA research are dealt with directly by Carl Cohen, who endorses, in general, the principles that "freedom of inquiry is of such profound importance that it must not be abridged without the most compelling reasons" and that "some research undertakings should properly be restricted." Cohen examines the implicit argument in Sinsheimer's suggestion that inquiry might be restricted if its results are not likely to be beneficial and gives reasons for rejecting it. Cohen points out that the result of Sinsheimer's principle would be to restrict all scientific research and condemn us to ignorance in every sphere of inquiry.

Altogether, Cohen considers six proposals (with variants) for justifying restriction of scientific research. He argues that no one has succeeded in both establishing a principle for limiting research as hazardous and intolerable and also showing that DNA research is hazardous and intolerable in the relevant ways.

Problems Behind the Promise: Ethical Issues in Mass Genetic Screening

Robert F. Murray, Jr.

I will follow that system of regimen which according to my ability and judgment, I consider for the benefit of my patients, and abstain from whatever is deleterious and mischievous. *The Hippocratic Oath*

There are occasions when in the act of abstaining "from whatever is deleterious and mischievous" the physician may withhold from a given patient information or even treatment which he judges would do more harm than good. But always at the

Reprinted with permission of the author and The Hastings Center from Hastings Center Report, 2 (April 1972): 10–13. © Institute of Society, Ethics and the Life Sciences, 360 Broadway, Hastings-on-Hudson, NY 10706.

center of the clinician's concern is the individual—that particular patient with whom he is immediately concerned. His interests have, in the past, extended beyond the individual usually only when communicable infectious diseases or toxic environmental agents have been involved which might have constituted immediate danger to members of the larger community.

Large-scale screening for genetic disorders is another instance in which the focus of attention of the physician has extended beyond the individual to the group. The group may be the family, a community, or all of mankind. The difference here is that the conditions about which the physician is concerned are not communicable or dangerous in the immediate sense but rather in a futuristic sense, and only a minority, and in many cases a small minority, of the total population is usually threatened. But just as the emphasis when working with the community on communicable disorders is on prevention, the emphasis in screening for genetic disorders is *not* primarily on treatment, but on prevention of disease and even on prevention of the birth of the potentially diseased individual.

In the past the clinician has thought of the prevention of disease in a positive sense. Disease has been prevented by treating the living patient or his environment in a specific manner rather than by eliminating him. The mental retardation that will almost always occur in phenylketonuria or galactosemia is prevented by removing phenylalanine in the first instance, and galactose in the second instance, from the environment of infants who have the specific mutations that produce these metabolic errors.

It is the treatment and possibly the prevention of disease in this latter sense that has excited intense interest in and promoted the development of massive programs of screening large populations for diseases that are presumably the result of mutant genes or other aberrations in the genetic material. The dream of the physician is, after all, the prevention of the manifestation of disease rather than its cure after it has been found.

What, then, could be better than to check all newborn infants at birth for as many known biochemical and chromosomal defects as possible? One would not only identify those neonates who are diseased, but would be able to assure the parents of those who are not affected that they need not worry, at least about conditions that have been tested for. It is essential in those cases where ge-

netic disease or a mutant gene product has been identified, that there be therapy or a positive course of action for the condition. And herein lies a part of the dilemma of the clinician.

In most of the cases where genetic disease or potential for disease is detected, there is no effective therapy or direct course of action available for the patient. If the condition is chronic, debilitating, and slowly progressive, like, for example, muscular dystrophy of the Duchenne type, or sickle-cell disease, and there is no effective therapy available, knowing about the condition prior to its clinical manifestation may merely provoke increased patient or parental anxiety without offering them any positive reassurance. There will be little benefit to the patient and, for a time, at least, some possible degree of harm to the parents and patient, depending upon their emotional stability.

Prior knowledge of the defect supports the ethical value of truth telling, but it does so at the expense of other very important ethical values.

Now, to the physician as with other scientists and scholars, knowledge is in and of itself a value. This is a purist's point of view. Many utilitarians and many of today's modern youth ask of knowledge, "What good is it?" This is a valid question asked by many parents. Knowing ahead of time without there being some way of altering the course of the disorder is to them more an academic exercise than a benefit. Knowing might, for example, infringe on whatever pleasure and well-being parents might enjoy. In some cases ignorance may well be bliss!

It is, in this instance, that one special aspect of genetic counseling assumes importance. For where, on one hand, the physician takes away from the well-being of parents by informing them of their child's condition, he can enhance their well-being by reassuring them of their innocence in the causation of the condition. He can make it clear that it was a consequence of fate and help them appreciate what they can do for the child, even when there is no effective treatment for the condition. He can help them look at their child as a human being to be helped, not pitied. And he can help them avoid the self-pity that frequently ensues.

The fact that most hereditary disorders now detected by screening have no effective therapy has been responsible for the emphasis on intrauterine diagnosis followed by therapeutic abortion. Therapeutic, in this instance, is to the mother and father, not the embryo, which has the disease. Furthermore, it has emphasized the necessity for the identification of those clinically normal carriers of mutant genes, more specifically those that are autosomal recessives, so that the conception of individuals with genetic disease might be prevented.

The Dilemma of the Carrier

The clinician who is vitally interested in the development of screening programs to detect the clinically normal, heterozygous carriers of hereditary biochemical abnormalities must consider the process from the point of view of both the carrier and the noncarrier. Subjects who are identified as noncarriers will have their state of well-being enhanced, their freedom increased, and their faith in science and medicine bolstered by such screening, since they have received "genetic good news." But what of the person detected as the carrier? He is usually unprepared for the disappointing news that he receives unless he already knows that he has a positive family history. Even individuals who are knowledgeable about a particular condition, like for example sickle-cell trait, may well be unable to readily accept the news that they are a carrier.

An example of this occurred on a recent Washington, D.C. television program on sickle-cell anemia. One enthusiastic volunteer worker was emphasizing the importance of everyone's knowing whether or not he or she had the sickle-cell trait. To dramatize this the volunteer, who didn't know her hemoglobin type, had a sample of blood taken at the beginning of the program and a sickling test was performed during the show. She was shocked into speechlessness when she was told that the test was definitely positive.

What options are open to the individual identified as a carrier? Let us assume that the carrier of this trait, say sickle-cell trait, wishes to act in a positive way on the information provided to prevent the possible birth of a child with sickle-cell anemia.

1. Since the freedom of mating of the carrier is compromised, he or she might inquire of all prospective mates (perhaps on the first date) of his or her carrier status. In the U.S.A. roughly one in ten black men will be eliminated as a mate for a black female carrier of sickle-cell trait. Other persons carrying hemoglobin C or beta thalassemia genes will also be eliminated since offspring double heterozygous for these conditions will have serious clinical disease. Of course, this kind of practice might tend to inhibit social relationships.

2. The carrier might just take a chance and then check the carrier status of the spouse after marriage. The chances are roughly nine in ten for a carrier-noncarrier marriage in sickle-cell trait. If they have not had this good fortune, and two carriers have by chance mated they must either: (a) not have children of their own, or (b) use artificial insemination with noncarrier donor semen, or (c) be able to detect the potential disease condition before birth in order to prevent the birth of the child through therapeutic abortion. This is not yet possible with sickle-cell anemia, and I am not as optimistic as some are that we will soon have a reliable method of intrauterine diagnosis.

3. If there should be some effective way to treat the condition (and in the case of sickle-cell anemia there is not), they need worry only about the exorbitant costs of medical care.

The practitioner is confident when he is able to detect the carrier state of an hereditary disease for which there is specific medical therapy or where therapeutic abortion might be employed as a preventive measure. The mass screening program of Kaback and his colleagues to detect carriers of Tay-Sachs disease in a Baltimore Jewish population is such an example. There is ethical support for screening in cases like this because the well-being and freedom of the parents and even to some degree the general welfare of the community may be enhanced.

On the other hand, there is ethical conflict for the practitioner when he detects the carrier state in disorders like sickle-cell trait where there are no medical therapeutic alternatives and the freedom and well-being of the patient as well as the general welfare of the community may be reduced. After all, an effective program of preventive counseling of sickle-cell trait subjects will actually result in an increase in the frequency of the sickle gene in the population.

Mass Screening Programs for Carriers

Among the questions that must be answered before effective screening programs are instituted are: Who is to be tested? Should testing be voluntary or compulsory? What should be done with the information obtained from testing? What will be the attitude of the public and their peers toward the individual who is identified as a carrier?

At first glance it would seem logical that testing should be done only in high-risk populations where the carrier frequency is significantly high. Jewish groups would be tested for the carrier state for the ethnically frequent conditions like Tay-Sachs disease. Blacks would be tested for sickle-cell trait. And if testing is voluntary, this might be an ethically acceptable approach to screening. But if testing for traits like these should be made compulsory, especially in preschools or elementary schools, it might happen that children identified as carriers could be stigmatized as different or as having undesirable parents or as being weaker or less fit. Furthermore, compulsory screening only in specific ethnic groups might also tend to reinforce racist doctrines.

A recent advertisement placed in *Ebony* magazine for the purpose of raising money for sickle-cell research characterized carriers of sickle-cell trait as being weak. This kind of exaggeration and misinformation will help promote the kind of stigmatization that might occur. If there is to be compulsory testing for traits like Tay-Sachs disease or sickle-cell trait *everyone* should be tested, since some Caucasian individuals of Mediterranean descent will also carry the sickle-cell trait.

The large-scale screening programs must be combined with extensive educational programs in order to avoid the misinformation and ''negative'' labeling of carriers of hereditary traits that might result. There might also be a tendency to extrapolate from recent reports of possible death associated with sickle-cell trait that have appeared in the medical literature.

The information from screening must be transmitted to the individual, depending upon his age, or his parents, but it is not enough to report that the screening test is positive or negative. The patient must be educated about the meaning of the carrier state from a medical and genetic point of view. He should also learn about the disease and the range of severity that occurs in the homozygous state. He must understand the condition well enough to make an intelligent decision based on the information he has been given. If this is to be the *patient's* decision (and I believe it should be), the physician must be careful not to knowingly directly influence the patient's decision unless he has a very good reason to do so.

I do not believe that this data should be placed in large centralized computers, as has been suggested by some, because of the problems of maintaining the privacy of the data in the computer.

Illustrative Cases

I should like to illustrate the kinds of conflicts that might arise in the course of genetic screening. These actual cases did not really occur from a screening program, but they show the kinds of problems with which one might be confronted as a consequence of such a program. All of them involved the detection of the sickle-cell trait.

Case 1

The husband of a childless young black couple came to the Heredity Clinic at Howard for genetic counseling because he had learned that he and his wife both carried the sickle-cell trait. His wife, who wanted her own natural child very much, was so disheartened by this news that she refused to come to the clinic. They were under the impression that sickle-cell disease was a horrible, crippling, rapidly fatal disease about which nothing could be done. After a thorough discussion of the range of severity of the disease, the origin and significance of the sickle-cell gene, and what the genetic possibilities were, we reviewed the husband's perception of the situation. He was much less discouraged and said that he would talk to his wife about taking a chance and trying for one natural child. If they were to have a child, regardless of its phenotype, he thought that they would adopt other children. It was clear to me when he left that this young man still had a great deal of the emotional conflict to work out in his own mind.

Case 2

A twenty-seven-year-old black female brought her year-old infant to the hospital because of anemia and failure to thrive. During this workup the child was found to have sickle-cell anemia. Sickling tests were done on the mother and the putative father, the woman's common-law husband. The mother was positive, but the father was negative. The mother was told that the test was inconsistent with her common-law husband being the father of the child. The woman swore ''on her mother's grave'' that he had to be the father. This is a very strong oath in the black community, and rather than dismiss this as just another case of nonpaternity, hemoglobin electrophoresis was performed. The common-law husband's red cells did in fact contain a small amount (only 5 percent) of sickle-cell hemoglobin.

In this instance the physician avoided producing family discord by heeding the mother's insistence and performing more careful studies. This case further illustrates the kind of serious errors that can occur when a screening test has false negative results. The physician must be extremely cautious in cases where nonpaternity appears to be involved.

Where there is a conflict between human relations, well-being, and total scientific truth, I have tended to sacrifice the truth, as in this next case.

Case 3

A black couple was being interviewed to determine the psychological effects of sickle-cell anemia on their four-year-old child. The mother volunteered that only she had the sickle-cell trait. This was verified by hemoglobin electrophoresis. It was clear from subsequent discussions that this couple did not understand the genetics of sickle-cell anemia. It seemed that an entirely lucid explanation of the genetics would raise the question of nonpaternity and perhaps lead to the disruption of what appeared to be a very compatible family relationship. It was explained to them that an egg from the mother containing a sickle-cell gene was fertilized by a sperm in which a fresh mutation also producing a sickle-cell gene had occurred. It was *not* pointed out that mutations are extremely rare. They were not interested in further genetic counseling since they had already completed their family.

Summary

The physician should consider the needs of the community in developing new programs of genetic screening, but the ethical considerations and the needs of the individual patient or couple must still come first. It is probably unjustified on ethical grounds to mount large-scale screening programs for disease or carrier detection in conditions where the patients and carriers cannot be offered specific effective medical therapeutic alternatives, including intrauterine diagnosis and abortion.

It is on the one hand unfair that everyone cannot yet know his or her "mutant gene carrier status," since all of us are heterozygous for at least several mutant genes, and also unfair that those whose mutant carrier status can be determined may be stigmatized by their peers. It is probably also unjustified at this time to make screening programs compulsory. Even large-scale educational programs can result in a kind of indirect coercion from peer group pressure that might be exerted. The current state of genetic knowledge is such that we cannot and, I feel, should not use any kind of coercive methods either direct or indirect to insist that carrier couples should not have children in those cases where intrauterine diagnosis is not yet available.

Finally, as important as our concern about the correct application of genetic advances continues to be, it must be kept in its proper perspective. There exist even more pressing problems of high infant mortality in the black population, as well as malnutrition, overcrowding, and social and economic unrest which are largely the result of social inequities that we now have the power to correct if we but apply ourselves to the task. If we do not devote at least a significant portion of our energies to these more serious problems, we shall be acting unethically and inhumanely.

Implications of Prenatal Diagnosis for the Human Right to Life

Leon R. Kass

Any discussion of the ethical issues of genetic counseling and prenatal diagnosis is unavoidably haunted by a ghost called the morality of abortion. This ghost I shall not vex. More precisely, I shall not vex the reader by telling ghost stories. However, I would be neither surprised nor disappointed if my discussion of an admittedly related matter, the ethics of aborting the genetically defec-

Reprinted from Ethical Issues in Human Genetics: Genetic Counseling and the Use of Genetic Knowledge, *edited by Bruce Hilton, Daniel Callahan, Maureen Harris, Peter Condliffe, and Burton Berkley (New York: Plenum Press; 1973), pp. 185–199.*

tive, summons that hovering spirit to the reader's mind. For the morality of abortion is a matter not easily laid to rest, recent efforts to do so notwithstanding. . . .

Yet before leaving the general question of abortion, let me pause to drop some anchors for the discussion that follows. Despite great differences of opinion both as to what to think and how to reason about abortion, nearly everyone agrees that abortion is a moral issue.[1] What does this mean? Formally, it means that a woman seeking or refusing an abortion can expect to be asked to justify her action. And we can expect that she should be able to give reasons for her choice other than "I like it" or "I don't like it." Substantively, it means that, in the absence of good reasons for intervention, there is some presumption in favor of allowing the pregnancy to continue once it has begun. A common way of expressing this presumption is to say that "the fetus has a right to continued life."[2] In this context, disagreement concerning the moral permissibility of abortion concerns what rights (or interests or needs), and whose, override (take precedence over, or outweigh) this fetal "right." Even most of the "opponents" of abortion agree that the mother's right to live takes precedence, and that abortion to save her life is permissible, perhaps obligatory. Some believe that a woman's right to determine the number and spacing of her children takes precedence, while yet others argue that the need to curb population growth is, at least at this time, overriding.

Hopefully, this brief analysis of what it means to say that abortion is a moral issue is sufficient to establish two points. First, that the fetus is a living thing with some moral claim on us not to do it violence, and therefore, second, that justification must be given for destroying it.

Turning now from the general questions of the ethics of abortion, I wish to focus on the special ethical issues raised by the abortion of "defective" fetuses (so-called "abortion for fetal indications"). I shall consider only the cleanest cases, those cases where well-characterized genetic diseases are diagnosed with a high degree of certainty by means of amniocentesis, in order to sidestep the added moral dilemmas posed when the diagnosis is suspected or possible, but unconfirmed. However, many of the questions I shall discuss could also be raised about cases where genetic analysis gives only a statistical prediction about the genotype of the fetus, and also about cases where the defect has an infectious or chemical rather than a genetic cause (e.g., rubella, thalidomide).

My first and possibly most difficult task is to show that there is anything left to discuss once we have agreed not to discuss the morality of abortion in general. There is a sense in which abortion for genetic defect is, after abortion to save the life of the mother, perhaps the most defensible kind of abortion. Certainly, it is a serious and not a frivolous reason for abortion, defended by its proponents in sober and rational speech—unlike justifications based upon the false notion that a fetus is a mere part of a woman's body, to be used and abused at her pleasure. Standing behind genetic abortion are serious and well-intentioned people, with reasonable ends in view: the prevention of genetic diseases, the elimination of suffering in families, the preservation of precious financial and medical resources, the protection of our genetic heritage. No profiteers, no sex-ploiters, no racists. No arguments about the connection of abortion with promiscuity and licentiousness, no perjured testimony about the mental health of the mother, no arguments about the seriousness of the population problem. In short, clear objective data, a worthy cause, decent men and women. If abortion, what better reason for it?

Yet if genetic abortion is but a happily wagging tail on the dog of abortion, it is simultaneously the nose of a camel protruding under a rather different tent. Precisely because the quality of the fetus is central to the decision to abort, the practice of genetic abortion has implications which go beyond those raised by abortion in general. What may be at stake here is the belief in the radical moral equality of all human beings, the belief that all human beings possess equally and independent of merit certain fundamental rights, one among which is, of course, the right to life.

To be sure, the belief that fundamental human rights belong equally to all human beings has been but an ideal, never realized, often ignored, sometimes shamelessly. Yet it has been perhaps the most powerful moral idea at work in the world for at least two centuries. It is this idea and ideal that animates most of the current political and social criticism around the globe. It is ironic that we should acquire the power to detect and eliminate the genetically unequal at a time when we have finally succeeded in removing much of the stigma and disgrace previously attached to victims of congenital illness, in providing them with improved care and support, and in preventing, by means of education, feelings of guilt on the part of their parents. One might even wonder whether the development of amniocentesis and prenatal diagnosis may represent a backlash against these same humanitarian and egalitarian tendencies in the practice of medicine, which, by helping to sustain to the age of reproduction persons with genetic disease has itself contributed to the increasing incidence of genetic disease, and with it, to increased pressures for genetic screening, genetic counseling, and genetic abortion.

No doubt our humanitarian and egalitarian principles and practices have caused us some new difficulties, but if we mean to weaken or turn our backs on them, we should do so consciously and thoughtfully. If, as I believe, the idea and practice of genetic abortion points in that direction, we should make ourselves aware of it. And if, as I believe, the way in which genetic abortion is described, discussed, and justified is perhaps of even greater consequence than its practice for our notions of human rights and of their equal possession by all human beings, we should pay special attention to questions of language and in particular, to the question of justification. . . .

Genetic Abortion and the Living Defective

The practice of abortion of the genetically defective will no doubt affect our view of and our behavior toward those abnormals who escape the net of detection and abortion. A child with Down's syndrome or with hemophilia or with muscular dystrophy born at a time when most of his (potential) fellow sufferers were destroyed prenatally is liable to be looked upon by the community as one unfit to be alive, as a second-class (or even lower) human type. He may be seen as a person who need not have been, and who would not have been, if only someone had gotten to him in time.

The parents of such children are also likely to treat them differently, especially if the mother would have wished but failed to get an amniocentesis because of ignorance, poverty, or distance from the testing station, or if the prenatal diagnosis was in error. In such cases, parents are especially likely to resent the child. They may be disinclined to give it the kind of care they might have before the advent of amniocentesis and ge-

netic abortion, rationalizing that a second-class specimen is not entitled to first-class treatment. If pressed to do so, say by physicians, the parents might refuse, and the courts may become involved. This has already begun to happen.

In Maryland, parents of a child with Down's syndrome refused permission to have the child operated on for an intestinal obstruction present at birth. The physicians and the hospital sought an injunction to require the parents to allow surgery. The judge ruled in favor of the parents, despite what I understand to be the weight of precedent to the contrary, on the grounds that the child was Mongoloid, that is, had the child been "normal," the decision would have gone the other way. Although the decision was not appealed to and hence not affirmed by a higher court, we can see through the prism of this case the possibility that the new powers of human genetics will strip the blindfold from the lady of justice and will make official the dangerous doctrine that some men are more equal than others.

The abnormal child may also feel resentful. A child with Down's syndrome or Tay-Sachs disease will probably never know or care, but what about a child with hemophilia or with Turner's syndrome? In the past decade, with medical knowledge and power over the prenatal child increasing and with parental authority over the postnatal child decreasing, we have seen the appearance of a new type of legal action, suits for wrongful life. Children have brought suit against their parents (and others) seeking to recover damages for physical and social handicaps inextricably tied to their birth (e.g., congenital deformities, congenital syphilis, illegitimacy). In some of the American cases, the courts have recognized the justice of the child's claim (that he was injured due to parental negligence), although they have so far refused to award damages, due to policy considerations. In other countries, e.g., in Germany, judgments with compensation have gone for the plaintiffs. With the spread of amniocentesis and genetic abortion, we can only expect such cases to increase. And here it will be the soft-hearted rather than the hard-hearted judges who will establish the doctrine of second-class human beings, out of compassion for the mutants who escaped the traps set out for them.

It may be argued that I am dealing with a problem which, even if it is real, will affect very few people. It may be suggested that very few will escape the traps once we have set them properly and widely, once people are informed about amniocentesis, once the power to detect prenatally grows to its full capacity, and once our "superstitious" opposition to abortion dies out or is extirpated. But in order even to come close to this vision of success, amniocentesis will have to become part of every pregnancy—either by making it mandatory, like the test for syphilis, or by making it "routine medical practice," like the Pap smear. Leaving aside the other problems with universal amniocentesis, we could expect that the problem for the few who escape is likely to be even worse precisely because they will be few.

The point, however, should be generalized. How will we come to view and act toward the many "abnormals" that will remain among us— the retarded, the crippled, the senile, the deformed, and the true mutants—once we embark on a program to root out genetic abnormality? For it must be remembered that we shall always have abnormals—some who escape detection or whose disease is undetectable *in utero*, others as a result of new mutations, birth injuries, accidents, maltreatment, or disease—who will require our care and protection. The existence of "defectives" cannot be fully prevented, not even by totalitarian breeding and weeding programs. Is it not likely that our principle with respect to these people will change from "We try harder" to "Why accept second best?" The idea of "the unwanted because abnormal child" may become a self-fulfilling prophecy, whose consequences may be worse than those of the abnormality itself.

Genetic and Other Defectives

The mention of other abnormals points to a second danger of the practice of genetic abortion. Genetic abortion may come to be seen not so much as the prevention of genetic disease, but as the prevention of birth of defective or abnormal children—and, in a way, understandably so. For in the case of what other diseases does preventive medicine consist in the elimination of the patient-at-risk? Moreover, the very language used to discuss genetic disease leads us to the easy but wrong conclusion that the afflicted fetus or person is rather than has a disease. True, one is partly defined by his genotype, but only partly. A person is more than his disease. And yet we slide easily

from the language of possession to the language of identity, from "He has hemophilia" to "He is a hemophiliac," from "She has diabetes" through "She is diabetic" to "She is a diabetic," from "The fetus has Down's syndrome" to "The fetus is a Down's." This way of speaking supports the belief that it is defective persons (or potential persons) that are being eliminated, rather than diseases.

If this is so, then it becomes simply accidental that the defect has a genetic cause. Surely, it is only because of the high regard for medicine and science, and for the accuracy of genetic diagnosis, that genotypic defectives are likely to be the first to go. But once the principle, "Defectives should not be born," is established, grounds other than cytological and biochemical may very well be sought. Even ignoring racialists and others equally misguided—of course, they cannot be ignored—we should know that there are social scientists, for example, who believe that one can predict with a high degree of accuracy how a child will turn out from a careful, systematic study of the socioeconomic and psychodynamic environment into which he is born and in which he grows up. They might press for the prevention of sociopsychological disease, even of "criminality," by means of prenatal environmental diagnosis and abortion. I have heard rumor that a crude, unscientific form of eliminating potential "phenotypic defectives" is already being practiced in some cities, in that submission to abortion is allegedly being made a condition for the receipt of welfare payments. "Defectives should not be born" is a principle without limits. We can ill-afford to have it established.

Up to this point, I have been discussing the possible implications of the practice of genetic abortion for our belief in and adherence to the idea that, at least in fundamental human matters such as life and liberty, all men are to be considered as equals, that for these matters we should ignore as irrelevant the real qualitative differences amongst men, however important these differences may be for other purposes. Those who are concerned about abortion fear that the permissible time of eliminating the unwanted will be moved forward along the time continuum, against newborns, infants, and children. Similarly, I suggest that we should be concerned lest the attack on gross genetic inequality in fetuses be advanced along the continuum of quality and into the later stages of life.

I am not engaged in predicting the future; I am not saying that amniocentesis and genetic abortion will lead down the road to Nazi Germany. Rather, I am suggesting that the principles underlying genetic abortion simultaneously justify many further steps down that road. The point was very well made by Abraham Lincoln (1854):

> If A can prove, however conclusively, that he may, of right, enslave B—Why may not B snatch the same argument and prove equally, that he may enslave A?
>
> You say A is white, and B is black. It is color, then; the lighter having the right to enslave the darker? Take care. By this rule, you are to be slave to the first man you meet with a fairer skin than your own.
>
> You do not mean color exactly? You mean the whites are intellectually the superiors of the blacks, and, therefore have the right to enslave them? Take care again. By this rule, you are to be slave to the first man you meet with an intellect superior to your own.
>
> But, say you, it is a question of interest; and, if you can make it your interest, you have the right to enslave another. Very well. And if he can make it his interest, he has the right to enslave you.

Perhaps I have exaggerated the dangers; perhaps we will not abandon our inexplicable preference for generous humanitarianism over consistency. But we should indeed be cautious and move slowly as we give serious consideration to the question "What price the perfect baby?"[3]

Standards for Justifying Genetic Abortion

The rest of this paper deals with the problem of justification. What would constitute an adequate justification of the decision to abort a genetically defective fetus? Let me suggest the following formal characteristics, each of which still begs many questions. (1) The reasons given should be logically consistent, and should lead to relatively unambiguous guidelines—note that I do not say "rules"—for action in most cases. (2) The justification should make evident to a reasonable person that the interest or need or right being served by abortion is sufficient to override the otherwise presumptive claim on us to protect and preserve the life of the fetus. (3) Hopefully, the justification would be such as to help provide

intellectual support for drawing distinctions between acceptable and unacceptable kinds of genetic abortion and between genetic abortion itself and the further practices we would all find abhorrent. (4) The justification ought to be capable of generalization to all persons in identical circumstances. (5) The justification should not lead to different actions from month to month or from year to year. (6) The justification should be grounded on standards that can, both in principle and in fact, sustain and support our actions in the case of genetic abortion and our notions of human rights in general.

Though I would ask the reader to consider all these criteria, I shall focus primarily on the last. According to what standards can and should we judge a fetus with genetic abnormalities unfit to live, i.e., abortable? It seems to me that there are at least three dominant standards to which we are likely to repair.

The first is societal good. The needs and interests of society are often invoked to justify the practices of prenatal diagnosis and abortion of the genetically abnormal. The argument, full blown, runs something like this. Society has an interest in the genetic fitness of its members. It is foolish for society to squander its precious resources ministering to and caring for the unfit, especially for those who will never become "productive," or who will never in any way "benefit" society. Therefore, the interests of society are best served by the elimination of the genetically defective prior to their birth.

The societal standard is all-too-often reduced to its lowest common denominator: money. Thus one physician, claiming that he has "made a cost-benefit analysis of Tay-Sachs disease," notes that "the total cost of carrier detection, prenatal diagnosis and termination of at-risk pregnancies for all Jewish individuals in the United States under 30 who will marry is $5,730,281. If the program is set up to screen only one married partner, the cost is $3,122,695. The hospital costs for the 990 cases of Tay-Sachs disease these individuals would produce over a thirty-year period in the United States is $34,650,000."[4] Another physician, apparently less interested or able to make such a precise audit has written: "Cost-benefit analyses have been made for the total prospective detection and monitoring of Tay-Sachs disease, cystic fibrosis (when prenatal detection becomes available for cystic fibrosis) and other disorders, and in most cases, the expenditures for hospitalization and medical care far exceed the cost of prenatal detection in properly selected risk populations, followed by selective abortion." Yet a third physician has calculated that the costs to the state of caring for children with Down's syndrome is more than three times that of detecting and aborting them. (These authors all acknowledge the additional nonsocietal "costs" of personal suffering, but insofar as they consider society, the costs are purely economic.)

There are many questions that can be raised about this approach. First, there are the questions about the accuracy of the calculations. Not all the costs have been reckoned. The aborted defective child will be "replaced" by a "normal" child. In keeping the ledger, the "costs" to society of his care and maintenance cannot be ignored—costs of educating him, or removing his wastes and pollutions, not to mention the "costs" in nonreplaceable natural resources that he consumes. Who is a greater drain on society's precious resources, the average inmate of a home for the retarded or the average graduate of Harvard College? I am not sure we know or can even find out. Then there are the costs of training the physician, and genetic counselors, equipping their laboratories, supporting their research, and sending them and us to conferences to worry about what they are doing. An accurate economic analysis seems to me to be impossible, even in principle. And even if it were possible, one could fall back on the words of the ordinary language philosopher, Andy Capp, who, when his wife said that she was getting really worried about the cost of living, replied: "Sweet'eart, name me one person who wants t'stop livin' on account of the cost."

A second defect of the economic analysis is that there are matters of social importance that are not reducible to financial costs, and others that may not be quantifiable at all. How does one quantitate the costs of real and potential social conflict, either between children and parents, or between the community and the "deviants" who refuse amniocentesis and continue to bear abnormal children? Can one measure the effect on racial tensions of attempting to screen for and prevent the birth of children homozygous (or heterozygous) for sickle-cell anemia? What numbers does one attach to any decreased willingness or ability to take care of the less fortunate, or to cope with

difficult problems? And what about the "costs" of rising expectations? Will we become increasingly dissatisfied with anything short of the "optimum baby"? How does one quantify anxiety? Humiliation? Guilt? Finally, might not the medical profession pay an unmeasurable price if genetic abortion and other revolutionary activities bring about changes in medical ethics and medical practice that lead to the further erosion of trust in the physician?

An appeal to social worthiness or usefulness is a less vulgar form of the standard of societal good. It is true that great social contributions are unlikely to be forthcoming from persons who suffer from most serious genetic diseases, especially since many of them die in childhood. Yet consider the following remarks of Pearl Buck (1968) on the subject of being a mother of a child retarded from phenylketonuria:

> My child's life has not been meaningless. She has indeed brought comfort and practical help to many people who are parents of retarded children or are themselves handicapped. True, she has done it through me, yet without her I would not have had the means of learning how to accept the inevitable sorrow, and how to make that acceptance useful to others. Would I be so heartless as to say that it has been worthwhile for my child to be born retarded? Certainly not, but I am saying that even though gravely retarded it has been worthwhile for her to have lived.
>
> It can be summed up, perhaps, by saying that in this world, where cruelty prevails in so many aspects of our life, I would not add the weight of choice to kill rather than to let live. A retarded child, a handicapped person, brings its own gift to life, even to the life of normal human beings. That gift is comprehended in the lessons of patience, understanding, and mercy, lessons which we all need to receive and to practice with one another, whatever we are.

The standard of potential social worthiness is little better in deciding about abortion in particular cases than is the standard of economic cost. To drive the point home, each of us might consider retrospectively whether he would have been willing to stand trial for his life while a fetus, pleading only his worth to society as he now can evaluate it. How many of us are not socially "defective" and with none of the excuses possible for a child with phenylketonuria? If there is to be human life at all, potential social worthiness cannot be its entitlement.

Finally, we should take note of the ambiguities in the very notion of societal good. Some use the term "society" to mean their own particular political community, others to mean the whole human race, and still others speak as if they mean both simultaneously, following that all-too-human belief that what is good for me and mine is good for mankind. Who knows what is genetically best for mankind, even with respect to Down's syndrome? I would submit that the genetic heritage of the human species is largely in the care of persons who do not live along the amniocentesis frontier. If we in the industrialized West wish to be really serious about the genetic future of the species, we would concentrate our attack on mutagenesis, and especially on our large contribution to the pool of environmental mutagens.

But even the more narrow use of society is ambiguous. Do we mean our "society" as it is today? Or do we mean our "society" as it ought to be? If the former, our standards will be ephemeral, for ours is a faddish "society." (By far the most worrisome feature of the changing attitudes on abortion is the suddenness with which they changed.) Any such socially determined standards are likely to provide too precarious a foundation for decisions about genetic abortion, let alone for our notions of human rights. If we mean the latter, then we have transcended the societal standard, since the "good society" is not to be found in "society" itself, nor is it likely to be discovered by taking a vote. In sum, societal good as a standard for justifying genetic abortion seems to be unsatisfactory. It is hard to define in general, difficult to apply clearly to particular cases, susceptible to overreaching and abuse (hence, very dangerous), and not sufficient unto itself if considerations of the good community are held to be automatically implied.

A second major alternative is the standard of parental or familial good. Here the argument of justification might run as follows. Parents have a right to determine, according to their own wishes and based upon their own notions of what is good for them, the qualitative as well as the quantitative character of their families. If they believe that the birth of a seriously deformed child will be the cause of great sorrow and suffering to themselves and to their other children and a drain on their time and resources, then they may ethically decide to prevent the birth of such a child, even by abortion.

This argument I would expect to be more attractive to most people than the argument appealing to the good of society. For one thing, we are more likely to trust a person's conception of what is good for him than his notion of what is good for society. Also, the number of persons involved is small, making it seem less impossible to weigh all the relevant factors in determining the good of the family. Most powerfully, one can see and appreciate the possible harm done to healthy children if the parents are obliged to devote most of their energies to caring for the afflicted child.

Yet there are ambiguities and difficulties perhaps as great as with the standard of societal good. In the first place, it is not entirely clear what would be good for the other children. In a strong family, the experience with a suffering and dying child might help the healthy siblings learn to face and cope with adversity. Some have even speculated that the lack of experience with death and serious illness in our affluent young people is an important element in their difficulty in trying to find a way of life and in responding patiently yet steadily to the serious problems of our society (Cassell, 1969). I suspect that one cannot generalize. In some children and in some families, experience with suffering may be strengthening, and in others, disabling. My point here is that the matter is uncertain, and that parents deciding on this basis are as likely as not to be mistaken.

The family or parental standard, like the societal standard, is unavoidably elastic because "suffering" does not come in discontinuous units, and because parental wishes and desires know no limits. Both are utterly subjective, relative, and notoriously subject to change. Some parents claim that they could not tolerate having to raise a child of the undesired sex; I know of one case where the woman in the delivery room, on being informed that her child was a son, told the physician that she did not even wish to see it and that he should get rid of it. We may judge her attitude to be pathological, but even pathological suffering is suffering. Would such suffering justify aborting her normal male fetus?

Or take the converse case of two parents, who

for their own very peculiar reasons, wish to have an abnormal child, say, a child who will suffer from the same disease as grandfather or a child whose arrested development would preclude the threat of adolescent rebellion and separation. Are these acceptable grounds for the abortion of "normals"?

Granted, such cases will be rare. But they serve to show the dangers inherent in talking about the parental right to determine, according to their wishes, the quality of their children. Indeed, the whole idea of parental rights with respect to children strikes me as problematic. It suggests that children are like property, that they exist for the parents. One need only look around to see some of the results of this notion of parenthood. The language of duties to children would be more in keeping with the heavy responsibility we bear in affirming the continuity of life with life and in trying to transmit what wisdom we have acquired to the next generation. Our children are not our children. Hopefully, reflection on these matters could lead to a greater appreciation of why it is people do and should have children. No better consequence can be hoped for from the advent of amniocentesis and other technologies for controlling human reproduction.

If one speaks of familial good in terms of parental duty, one could argue that parents have an obligation to do what they can to insure that their children are born healthy and sound. But this formulation transcends the limitation of parental wishes and desires. As in the case of the good society, the idea of "healthy and sound" requires an objective standard, a standard in reality. Hard as it may be to uncover it, this is what we are seeking. Nature as a standard is the third alternative.

The justification according to the natural standard might run like this. As a result of our knowledge of genetic diseases, we know that persons afflicted with certain diseases will never be capable of living the full life of a human being. Just as a no-necked giraffe could never live a giraffe's life, or a needleless porcupine would not attain true "porcupine-hood," so a child or fetus with Tay-Sachs disease or Down's syndrome, for example, will never be truly human. They will never be able to care for themselves, nor have they even the potential for developing the distinctively human capacities for thought or self-consciousness. Nature herself has aborted many similar cases, and has provided for the early death of many who happen to get born. There is no reason to keep them alive; instead, we should prevent their birth by contraception or sterilization if possible, and abortion if necessary.

The advantages of this approach are clear. The standards are objective and in the fetus itself, thus avoiding the relativity and ambiguity in societal and parental good. The standard can be easily generalized to cover all such cases and will be resistant to the shifting sands of public opinion.

This standard, I would suggest, is the one which most physicians and genetic counselors appeal to in their heart of hearts, no matter what they say or do about letting the parents choose. Why else would they have developed genetic counseling and amniocentesis? Indeed, the notions of disease, of abnormal, of defective, make no sense at all in the absence of a natural norm of health. This norm is the foundation of the art of the physician and of the inquiry of the health scientist. Yet, as Motulsky and others in this volume have pointed out, the standard is elusive. Ironically, we are gaining increasing power to manipulate and control our own nature at a time in which we are increasingly confused about what is normal, healthy, and fit.

Although possibly acceptable in principle, the natural standard runs into problems in application when attempts are made to fix the boundary between potentially human and potentially not human. Professor Lejeune (1970) has clearly demonstrated the difficulty, if not the impossibility, of setting clear molecular, cytological, or developmental signposts for this boundary. Attempts to induce signposts by considering the phenotypes of the worst cases is equally difficult. Which features would we take to be the most relevant in, say, Tay-Sachs disease, Lesch-Nyhan syndrome, Cri du chat, Down's syndrome? Certainly, severe mental retardation. But how "severe" is "severe"? As Abraham Lincoln and I argued earlier, mental retardation admits of degree. It too is relative. Moreover, it is not clear that certain other defects and deformities might not equally foreclose the possibility of a truly or fully human life. What about blindness or deafness? Quadriplegia? Aphasia? Several of these in combination? Not only does each kind of defect admit of a continuous scale of severity, but it also merges with other defects on a continuous scale of defectiveness. Where on this scale is the line to be drawn: after mental retardation? blindness? muscular dystrophy? cystic fibrosis? hemophilia? diabetes? galactosemia? Turner's syndrome? XYY? club foot? Moreover, the identical two continuous scales—kind and severity—are found also among the living. In fact, it is the natural standard which may be the most dangerous one in that it leads most directly to the idea that there are second-class human beings and subhuman human beings.

But the story is not complete. The very idea of nature is ambiguous. According to one view, the one I have been using, nature points to or implies a peak, a perfection. According to this view, human rights depend upon attaining the status of humanness. The fetus is only potential; it has no rights, according to this view. But all kinds of people fall short of the norm: children, idiots, some adults. This understanding of nature has been used to justify not only abortion and infanticide, but also slavery.

There is another notion of nature, less splendid, more humane and, though less able to sustain a notion of health, more acceptable to the findings of modern science. Animal nature is characterized by impulses of self-preservation and by the capacity to feel pleasure and to suffer pain. Man and other animals are alike on this understanding of nature. And the right to life is ascribed to all such self-preserving and suffering creatures. Yet on this understanding of nature, the fetus—even a defective fetus—is not potential, but actual. The right to life belongs to him. But for this reason, this understanding of nature does not provide and may even deny what it is we are seeking, namely a justification for genetic abortion, adequate unto itself, which does not simultaneously justify infanticide, homicide, and enslavement of the genetically abnormal.

There is a third understanding of nature, akin to the second, nature as sacrosanct, nature as created by a Creator. Indeed, to speak about this reminds us that there is a fourth possible standard for judgments about genetic abortion: the religious standard. I shall leave the discussion of this standard to those who are able to speak of it in better faith.

Now that I am at the end, the reader can better share my sense of frustration. I have failed to provide myself with a satisfactory intellectual and moral justification for the practice of genetic abortion. Perhaps others more able than I can supply one. Perhaps the pragmatists can persuade me that we should abandon the search for principled justification, that if we just trust people's situational decisions or their gut reactions, everything will turn out fine. Maybe they are right. But we should not forget the sage observation of Bertrand Russell: "Pragmatism is like a warm bath that heats up so imperceptibly that you don't know when to scream." I would add that before we submerge ourselves irrevocably in amniotic fluid, we take note of the connection to our own baths, into which we have started the hot water running.

Notes

1. This strikes me as by far the most important inference to be drawn from the fact that men in different times and cultures have answered the abortion question differently. Seen in this light, the differing and changing answers themselves suggest that it is a question not easily put under, at least not for very long.

2. Other ways include: one should not do violence to living or growing things; life is sacred; respect nature; fetal life has value; refrain from taking innocent life; protect and preserve life. As some have pointed out, the terms chosen are of different weight, and would require reasons of different weight to tip the balance in favor of abortion. My choice of the "rights" terminology is not meant to beg the questions of whether such rights really exist, or of where they come from. However, the notion of a "fetal right to life" presents only a little more difficulty in this regard than does the notion of a "human right to life," since the former does not depend on a claim that the human fetus is already "human." In my sense of the terms "right" and "life," we might even say that a dog or a fetal dog has a "right to life," and that it would be cruel and immoral for a man to go around performing abortions even on dogs for no good reason.

3. For a discussion of the possible biological rather than moral price of attempts to prevent the birth of defective children see Neel (1970) and Motulsky, Fraser, and Felsenstein (1971).

4. I assume this calculation ignores the possibilities of inflation, devaluation, and revolution.

References

Buck, P. S.   (1968). Foreword to *The Terrible Choice: The Abortion Dilemma*. New York, Bantam Books, pp. ix–xi.

Cassell, E.   (1969). "Death and the Physician," Commentary (June), pp. 73–79.

Lejeune, J.   (1970). *American Journal of Human Genetics*, 22, p. 121.

Lincoln, A.   (1854). In *The Collected Works of Abraham Lincoln*, R. P. Basler, editor. New Brunswick, New Jersey, Rutgers University Press, Vol. II, p. 222.

Motulsky, A. G., G. R. Fraser, and J. Felsenstein (1971). In Symposium on Intrauterine Diagnosis, D. Bergsma, editor. *Birth Defects: Original Article Series*, Vol. 7, No. 5.

Neel, J.   (1972). In *Early Diagnosis of Human Genetic Defects: Scientific and Ethical Considerations*, M. Harris, editor. Washington, D.C. U.S. Government Printing Office, pp. 366–380.

Ethical Issues in Biological Engineering

Martin P. Golding

I. Obligations to the Future

In the popular literature on biology and genetics—and undoubtedly in the technical literature, too—a frequent topic of discussion is whether man can consciously control the future of human evolution. It is pointed out that civilization has, in a sense, suspended the normal processes of natural selection, or at least that the form that the struggle for existence takes has been materially affected by human culture.[1] The interpretation of the current stage is not entirely clear. Is it a "new kind of biological evolution" or is it a "new state of evolution" in which the "psychosocial" aspects are paramount?[2] The topic is a heady one, full of deep philosophical significance. The issue that I shall now consider seems easy by comparison—what are our obligations toward the future?

The occasion for this question is plain. One ground on which a social program of biological engineering might be justified is that its goal is ethically mandatory, an obligation. The goal is that of maintaining (or enhancing) genetic quality. We must still consider what this goal (or set of goals) consists of. At this point, however, there is no need to go into the details. I am now concerned, rather, with a general question about social doctoring, of which biological engineering is only a kind, albeit an important kind. Put more precisely, though in quite general terms, the above question

may be formulated as a complex of three questions: (i) is there now an obligation to bring about any given situation in the future?; (ii) if there is such an obligation, on whom does it fall?; and, (iii) if there is such an obligation, what ought be done now to fulfill it? I shall concentrate on the first of these three. It is clearly the most important, although I would hardly go so far as to say that social programs of biological engineering are completely foreclosed if it is answered in the negative.

But even as now formulated, question (i) is unsatisfactory. "Future" is a vague term, and no headway can be made until we settle on the "future" that is the subject of concern. Purposive conduct is future-oriented; one does something now in order to bring about some condition at a later date. But this later date may vary from the next second on into eternity. I move towards the switch in order momentarily to turn on the light. A nation goes to war in order to make the world safe for democracy twenty years later. It would be easy to multiply examples. On the other hand, we accuse someone of short-sightedness. He acts in the present for the present, so to speak. And the "present" for which he acts might be a point five years from now, when that point should be—we think—ten or twenty or fifty years hence. What relevantly counts as the future in one context, counts as the present in another.

How do we fix the future for the problem-area

Reprinted by permission of the author and publisher from UCLA Law Review 15 (1968): 443–479. *Editor's Note: The footnotes and section numbers in this reading have been renumbered.*

that constitutes the topic of this paper? In order to get a foothold I must advert to the problem of genetic quality, although the following discussion has application, I believe, to any social program for which the dimensions of the future are the same. The outer boundary of this future is not easy to establish. It is that point at which a critical situation will obtain unless steps are taken in order to prevent it. The nearest I have come to a definite statement on this is contained in the following remarks of Sir Julian Huxley:

> [I]f we don't do something about controlling our genetic inheritance, we are going to degenerate. Without selection, bad mutations inevitably tend to accumulate; *in the long run, perhaps 5,000 to 10,000 years from now,* we [sic] shall certainly have to do something about it. . . . Most mutations are deleterious, but we now keep many of them going that would otherwise have died out. If this continues indefinitely . . . then the whole genetic capacity of man will be much weakened.[3]

I hasten to add that my reading of the literature suggests that the situation is somewhat more urgent. The inner boundary of this future would be set, I suppose, at that point at which a society begins seriously to suffer from the failure to maintain genetic integrity. I am, frankly, at loss to supply a date for this, especially since "seriously to suffer" is both vague and ambiguous (suffer in what respects?). In any case, it would seem that the "future" with which we are concerned is—in relation to programs of social action—what we ordinarily think of as the *remote* future. A social program of biological engineering would be planning for this remote future. We may therefore reformulate our original question as follows: Is there now an obligation to bring about any given situation in the remote future? Unfortunately, I cannot be more precise. (Obviously, I am not concerned with eugenic programs that might be aimed at our immediate descendants, but I shall say a few words about them later.)

This reformulation takes us back to . . . the communal context of social programs. . . . Sometimes a social program is initiated in one communal context in order to bring about an allegedly desirable situation in another communal context. We are thus raising a question about our moral relations to the community of the remote future. I submit that this relationship is far from clear, cer-

tainly less clear than our moral obligations to communities of the present.

I think it worthwhile to dwell a bit on this point. It appears that a social program may be justified on three grounds (singly or in combination): (1) self-interest, (2) an obligation to prevent an undesirable situation or promote a desirable one, and (3) humanitarian considerations. Frequently, these tend to converge.

To justify a policy on grounds of self-interest is not necessarily to condemn it to the realm of the immoral. Considerations of self-interest are always legitimate, even if they are not always overriding. Now when a social program is justified in this manner, the "self" which is involved is an extended self, so to speak. In the United States we are currently engaged in a number of programs of social welfare, and it is in our interest to be so engaged. The "self" encompasses a community of individuals. But as the "self" is thus extended, it becomes less plausible to view our concern with the communal welfare as "self-interested." This would be true whenever the "self" is extended so as to transcend spatial and temporal boundaries, where the "self" is enlarged to encompass wider and wider communities. If the individuals whose welfare is the object of the program are included in the "self" whose interest is being maximized, then the ground of the programs would be virtually indistinguishable from an obligation to promote the good of humanitarianism.

A social program may be justified by appeal to an obligation to promote a desirable situation or prevent an undesirable one—but, I take it, not a desirable or undesirable situation *simpliciter*. It must be desirable or undesirable *for some community*. I have elsewhere elaborated upon the importance of the notion of community in the development of a theory of human rights.[4] For our purposes we may note that the extension of rights is historically conditioned by two factors. Individuals and groups put forward *claims* to the goods of life, demand them as their right. In this way the content of a system of rights is increasingly expanded towards the inclusion of more of these goods. . . . Secondly, there is an increasing expansion of the "moral community," namely, those individuals and groups whose claims to the goods of life are entitled to recognition. The altruistic impulse breaks out of narrow confines towards a concern for the well-being of larger segments of mankind.

Of course, not every claim is recognized as conferring a right; not every claim is recognized as a claim upon me or a claim upon society, imposing an *obligation*. Some claims may be frivolous. Here a third factor enters the picture: *the social ideal*, a conception of the good life for man, which serves as the yardstick by which such claims are measured. In speaking of the good life I do not have in mind the ideal life of saints, which may be a personal ideal, but that kind of good life which is feasible for society at large. It must surely contain a material or economic component. . . . I am far from maintaining that a social ideal is subject to easy formulation; it is certainly not static. In any case, it is in reference to claims, the scope of the community, and the ideal that our social obligations are determined.

These three also play a role in humanitarianism. . . . At its heart humanitarianism is concern for the well-being of others. Viewed from the inside, humanitarianism is the desire that others should have the goods of life, or at least not suffer its pains. Men do have genuine other-regarding affections, which are not disguised forms of self-love. . . . There are, of course, significant differences among those "others" whose well-being motivates us, as will be evident to anyone who compares his concern for the well-being of his own child with his concern for the starving child in a far-off land. These differences derive from the kind of obligation one has for the other's welfare and the strength of the altruistic impulse. It would be just as much a mistake to conclude that humanitarianism involves no degree of obligation to the stranger, as it would be to conclude that the normal father-child relationship involves no altruistic impulse. . . . We do have an "obligation of benevolence, or humanity," as Bishop Butler called it, an obligation that extends out from the family to increasingly wider communities. The character of this obligation is determined by the kinds of moral relationships one has to these communities, or to put it in other terms, by one's membership in different kinds of community. The concept of community is, admittedly, obscure. The analysis of it is beyond the scope of this paper. Here I would point out that it is not a biological notion. It is ethical and metaphysical, if you will, a spiritual idea.

In considering the social programs that this country has undertaken in order to promote the welfare of other societies and nations, one can hardly deny that a good share of our motivation is self-interest in a narrow sense, *i.e.*, our national interest. But this is not the whole story, for we do also acknowledge an obligation toward other peoples. This obligation, of course, is not of the same order as the special obligation we have to promote the welfare of various individuals and groups in our own society, who are entitled to be recognized as part of our moral community. A crucial factor in the home situation . . . is an awareness of the *relevance* to them of our social ideal, and therefore a receptiveness to their claims to what we regard as the goods of life. Now the notion of "the relevance to X of a social ideal" is extremely complicated, and I am unable to give a full explication of it. (I suspect that it has both normative and descriptive components.) Undoubtedly, the condition of someone's life is an important, and perhaps the important, element in determining this relevance. And it would seem, in turn, that composition of a moral community is a partial function of the degree to which a social ideal has relevance for a set of individuals, given their conditions of life.

We may conclude, I think, that our obligation to engage in social programs for the peoples of distant lands has a problematical status. The more remote the conditions of their life from ours and the stranger they are, the less relevant does our social ideal become for them and the farther they get pushed towards the fringes of our moral community. It requires a great effort of mind to see in them the same humanity that we share with our next-door neighbors. I do not say this in order to justify the kinds of vicious colonialism that so-called advanced nations practice against the unadvanced. Rather, the issue is the justification of social policies for the betterment of life of the less advanced. The more remote the conditions of their life from ours and the stranger they are, the less do we know what to desire for them.[5] Of course, it does not follow that we have no obligations in respect of strange peoples in remote lands. What is exceedingly questionable, however, is the extent to which we should think of them as having claims to the goods of life as we conceive these goods. If I may be permitted to indulge in a bit of science fiction, the point I am making will, perhaps, become clearer. Suppose there are rational beings on other planets. They are bound to be very different from us and the conditions of their life would be very different from ours. Since they are rational I assume that we would have an obligation of truth-telling in respect of them, if we could communicate with them. But we would be at a loss to say whether we have any social obligation to secure for them what we consider the goods of life. I readily concede that the strange peoples of the earth are in a better case than Martians or Venusians.

In this respect our immediate descendants, though yet unborn, are better off than strange peoples. After all, we do know—or at least think we know—what to hope for our children. The conditions of their life will probably be much like ours and they will be much like us. Our social ideal has relevance for them and they—though unborn—are part of our moral community. They have claims upon us. If someone finds it difficult to think of having an obligation towards his unborn child, then he should find it difficult to think of having an obligation toward a community of humans (humanoids?) fifty generations hence. (I must confess to finding it odd when the same people who put biological engineering for the future on ethical grounds also defend abortion of a foetus on the ground that we have no obligation in respect of an unborn child.)

The conclusion to be drawn from the above discussion should be apparent. It is highly doubtful that we have an obligation to establish social programs that would secure a "good life" (prevent the undesirable, promote the desirable) for the community of the *remote* future. The conditions of life then are likely to be so different from anything we can now imagine that we do not know what to desire for them. Now this does not *prove* that we have no such obligation; but it does put a heavy burden of argument on anyone who comes forward with proposals regarding the remote future. We shall have to inquire further into whether a case can be made for biological engineering. In so doing we need to be sensitive to the probability that any effective program of biological engineering will itself alter the conditions of life. . . .

II. Positive Eugenics

In the next . . . sections I shall consider aspects of some possible programs of biological engineering. My discussion is confined, in the main, to their goal-component. Except for a few instances I pass no judgment on their desirability. I am concerned, rather, to bring to light issues that have to be settled in order for such judgments to be made. It goes without saying that I approach the topic with trepidation, as any layman must.

I begin with positive eugenics[6] because I find it simpler for me to handle. This type of biological engineering, according to Julian Huxley who is one of its leading exponents, "has a far larger scope and importance than negative [eugenics]. It is not concerned merely to prevent genetic deterioration, but aims to raise human capacity and performance to a new level." Moreover, according to Huxley, "negative eugenics is of minor evolutionary importance and the need for it will gradually be superseded by efficient measures of positive eugenics."[7]

Except for *Rassenhygiene*, I am not aware of any attempt to carry out a program of positive eugenics on a wide scale excluding animal stock-breeding. One of the reasons for this is the lack of clearly defined aims.[8] The clarification of these aims would necessarily have two facets. One involves specification of the traits that are to be enhanced, and the other would be a showing that their enhancement would truly be advantageous for the community for which they are to be enhanced. As far as I can tell, there is paltry attention given to the second. There is a tendency readily to assume that characteristics which we all take to be desirable, and whose absence we deplore, would not only be valuable under all conditions but also would be universally more valuable if they could be improved on. This may be true, but it needs to be supported by argument. Mere reference to the fact that culture can survive only if human beings possess the genetic equipment which is favorable for culture is not sufficient. To know only that culture has a genetic basis is not much more useful than knowing it has a solar basis. Perhaps it is asking for what no one could possibly supply, but it seems to me that what is required is the establishment of connections between genetic constitution and specifically characterized features of culture. However, it is generally accepted that "genes determine the possibility of culture but not its content."[9]

The first of the facets mentioned above has been more widely discussed. It is interesting to take note of the shift from the talk of races or strains, found in earlier eugenic literature, to talk of mental or social characteristics. Thus, Francis Galton, the coiner of the term "eugenics," states that the aim of eugenics is "to give to the more suitable races or strains of blood a better chance of prevailing speedily over the less suitable than they otherwise would have had."[10] Behind this way of speaking were, first, Galton's conviction "that the English propertied and governing classes were a repository of virtually all that is biologically precious in the English nation and possibly in mankind,"[11] and, second, an incorrect theory of heredity (blending inheritance). Even such a liberal-minded follower of Galton as the English philosopher F. C. S. Schiller lapses into this way of speaking. Consider, for example, his statement that "the reason why the symptoms of racial decay are not more pronounced is probably that European civilization is still living on its biological capital, on the qualities bred into the Nordic stock by the severest natural selection, while it was still barbarian, only 1500 years ago."[12]

With the rise and development of genetics such talk tends to disappear and is replaced with the notion of the production of the "ideal genotype." A strong elitist tone remains, however, with ideological overtones. This is illustrated in Hermann J. Muller's removing of Marx and Sun Yat Sen from his 1935 list of eminent men and his adding of Einstein and Lincoln.[13] If Muller is now sanguine about the prospects of positive eugenics, it seems that in 1932 he was prepared to jettison the whole affair. In a speech given before the Eugenics Society in New York, he said:

> Only the impending revolution in our economic system will bring us into a position where we can properly judge, from a truly social point of view, what characteristics are most worthy of a man. . . .
>
>   Thus [he concluded] it is up to us, if we want eugenics that functions, to work for it in the only way now practicable, by first turning our hand to help throw over the incubus of the old, outworn society.[14]

The ideological overtone is also to be found in a 1962 article by Julian Huxley, who would stress:

> . . . . the need for planning the environment in such a way as will promote our eugenic aims. By 1936, it was already clear that the net effect of present-day social policies could not be eugenic, and was in all probability dysgenic. But, as Muller has demonstrated, this was not

always so. In that long period of human history during which our evolving and expanding hominid ancestors lived in small and tightly knit groups competing for territorial and technological success, the social organization promoted selection for intelligent exploration of possibilities, devotion and co-operative altruism: the cultural and genetic systems reinforced each other. It was only much later, with the growth of bigger social units of highly organized civilization based on status and class differentials, that the two became antagonistic. . . .[15]

I do not wish to suggest that ideological perspectives are irrelevant to the choice of an ideal genotype; obviously they are not. But this is one reason why there is likely to be much disagreement over the choice. Furthermore, the moral to be drawn from Muller's changing of his list is that—assuming we could produce our ideal genotype of today—we might regret our choice in 25 years. And we still need assurance that the kind of culture we regard as desirable could in fact be maintained by our ideal genotype.[16]

In any case, if I correctly understand the exponents of positive eugenics, it is not an ideal genotype that they wish to produce, but an ideal phenotype. This would be in line with their insistence on planning the proper environment for the development of certain human capacities. Huxley explicitly maintains that eugenics needs a phenotypic approach, and goes so far as to criticize the "geneticism" of Medawar and Penrose in their purely scientific work.[17] While the phenotypic approach makes more sense to me, it is clear that it poses serious difficulties for biological engineering. It seems that there are few normal human characters that are governed by allelomorphs of a single gene (e.g., ability or inability to taste PTC). Most characteristics are brought about through the interplay of many different genes. Matters are complicated by the fact that so-called graded characters (e.g., stature), and certainly mental and social traits, depend on many genes and on environmental influences. Therefore, "any simple genetical analysis is ruled out."[18] I have the distinct impression that although many of the more enthusiastic exponents of biological engineering always say that a sharp heredity-environment dichotomy must be rejected, this amounts to lip-service.[19] The production of definite phenotypes by means of genic selection seems impossible.

"Few of us would have advocated preferential multiplication of Hitler's genes through germinal selection. Yet who can say that in a different cultural context Hitler might not have been one of the truly great leaders of men, or that Einstein might not have been a diabolical villain.[20]

It would be very misleading and unfair to Huxley and Muller, at least, to imply that they propose as a goal the production of an ideal phenotype. Judging from the criticisms frequently made of them, they do give this impression. But they are now quite explicit that there is no single type that they have in mind. What they seek is an increase in the relative number of individuals who possess such human excellences as altruism, a spirit of cooperativeness, fellow-feeling, imagination, a sense of discipline and duty, and intelligence.[21] Whether they intend that these should be produced only in combination, and not singly, is unclear to me; but if I am not mistaken they would support a relative increase in the number of persons who have any of these traits. Moreover, they would support an increase in the strength of any of these traits. The method they propose is artificial insemination by deliberately preferred donors. Muller goes on to add that the sperm of the chosen ones be stored for later use.[22]

This program raises a number of questions. (1) Are these characteristics hereditary? (2) If they are, and if it were technologically feasible to produce them, would it be desirable to do so? (3) What should be the institutional framework of such a program? I shall briefly take up each.

A detailed discussion of the first question would take me way out of my competence, so I shall only raise a few issues that seem to me to call for attention. With respect to all of the traits except intelligence, I know of no experimental studies that are designed to establish whether or not they are inherited. (It would be fascinating to have an experiment for testing the inheritability of vanity, to take something out of the scope of the above list.) Of course, one is always in a position to say that there *must* be a genetic basis for them. This would be to make the term "genetic basis" a panchreston that explains everything in general, but nothing in particular. In any case, it is not easy to see how such experiments are to be designed. One of the problems is conceptual. Consider altruism. What does the term refer to: a feeling? a motive? or a set of behavior patterns? Is it not the case that the

social meaning of altruism (as well as the other "social virtues") depends on the kinds of context that elicit altruistic feelings, motives, and behavior? The problem here is very much like one that besets those who argued that criminal tendencies are heritable. What constitutes a crime may vary from society to society and from legal system to legal system. Whatever it is that the altruistic donor might transmit to his progeny, it is hardly necessary that it should be exhibited as anything that would be recognized as altruism (or any of the other social virtues that would be involved.).[23] The following remark hits the nail on the head:

> Our distinguished geneticist [Muller] has suggested that fellowship, co-operation, moral courage and integrity, appreciation of nature and art, and aptness of expression and communication are desirable human traits. One must agree. But, since each of these qualities has meanings peculiar to its particular evolutionary stage and social type, he surely cannot mean they are genetically determined.[24]

The heritability of intelligence is a complicated topic. There have been numerous studies on it. Identical and non-identical twins have been researched, and there have been longitudinal family studies on mental retardation. Generations of school children have been I.Q.'d. I am quite prepared to admit that intelligence has a genetic basis: I take my own children as evidence. In a more serious vein, however, what seems to be established is that certain tendencies that fall within a wide range are inherited.[25] Studies of long-lasting eminent families do not permit the strengthening of this conclusion, for the unsuccessful branches are lost to history.[26] On the question of I.Q., the following seem to me to be words of wisdom:

> [T]here are two questions the geneticist may be asked. The first is: if for example individuals with higher I.Q.s breed more than those with lower (or vice versa) will the I.Q. of the population change, and at what rate? The second question is, if we were effectively to encourage such differential reproduction in favor of I.Q., what would be the consequent changes in characteristics other than I.Q.? The first of these is of course difficult enough to answer, witness the problem of interpreting the facts concerning correlations of I.Q. and family size. The second is at present impossible to answer for even if we were to suspect negative correlations between other

attributes we deem desirable and I.Q., establishment of the facts concerning the degree to which the correlations had genetic causes would be a difficult task indeed.[27]

It is sometimes suggested that mankind as a whole or at least a considerable segment of it may be evolving in the direction of less intelligence.[28] If true, this would be a reason for undertaking a particular kind of program of biological engineering. Although it may readily be conceded that heredity is a strong factor in intelligence (as is shown by studies on twins and foster children), a comparison of results of intelligence tests given to Scottish school children in 1932 and 1947 seems to indicate that this is not true.[29] In conclusion we may say that considerably more research needs to be done on the genetic basis of intelligence before we give the go-ahead to Professors Muller and Huxley. (It is not necessary for me to compound the problem by here taking up the questions of the definition of ''intelligence'' and the role of environmental influences.)

But suppose the heritability of the various mental and social characters could be established. Would it be desirable to enhance their occurrence if it could be accomplished? I need not repeat my previous points that turn upon the issue of whether this would be desirable *for* the community of the future. Here I wish to bring out other issues. Consider, for example, the sense of discipline and duty to which Huxley refers. Now, I would not go so far as David Hume who maintains that the various social virtues are approved of solely on grounds of their tendency to maximize utility (happiness).[30] Nevertheless, I strongly doubt that anyone would endorse the enhancement of a sense of discipline and duty under what he regards as an evil social system and in the presence of immoral values. Admittedly, we may have a kind of morbid admiration for the Nazi's sense of discipline and duty, but we would have gladly preferred its *dis*-enhancement. A similar line of argument applies to other of the social virtues. It would seem that their promotion would be undesirable unless we could also determine the conditions of life of the community of the future, including also its values. Secondly, it is doubtful that we would welcome an increase in the relative numbers of intelligent men unless altruists could be increased in the same proportions, otherwise the result may be a disadvantageously large number of

clever and crafty mean men. But what guarantee is there that selective eugenic insemination—if that is the method adopted—would work itself out in the desired manner? Finally, I submit that no one knows what would be the effects of an enhancement of the social virtues, although we all imagine that the world would be a happier place. It is quite conceivable, however, that the survival of culture is dependent upon a certain blend of altruism and self-interest for example, and that this would be upset by the program of biological engineering.

Assuming that these matters could be laid to rest, we still have the institutional framework of the social program to consider. This is an important matter, for institutional frameworks are not morally neutral. The construction of such frameworks is, as indicated previously, a complicated task; moreover frameworks must be adjusted to the techniques that are to be employed. Therefore, only a brief general discussion of a few points is possible here. One of these techniques, A.I.D. with preferred donors, has already been mentioned. Others include controlled mating and controlled breeding (by devices other than A.I.D.). It may some day be possible chemically to modify the phenotype by improving the genetic material, as is suggested by discoveries about the structure of D.N.A. Other possibilities that cannot now be foreseen may be in the offing.

The ethical issues relative to the institutional framework turn on: (a) the degree to which the use of these techniques would be dependent on voluntary adoption or coercive measures; and (b) the degree to which their utilization would be subject to democratic control, with safeguards against abuse. Obviously, no ethical assessment of any social program of biological engineering can be made until these points are straightened out.

Two of the leading exponents of the A.I.D. method of positive eugenics, Huxley and Muller, insist that adoption should be completely voluntary. In answering the objection that effective selection needs authoritarian methods, Huxley writes:

> For one thing, dogmatic tyranny in the modern world is becoming increasingly self-defeating: partly because it is dogmatic and therefore essentially unscientific, partly because it is tyrannical and therefore in the long run intolerable. But the chief point is that human improvement never works solely or even

mainly by such methods and is doing so less and less as man commits himself more thoroughly to the process of general self-education.[31]

This, I think, misses the point. The objector could perfectly well agree with everything just said. And he would stress that human improvement would not result from a program of positive eugenics because it needs authoritarian methods: rather than making better men, it would make men worse. It is no reply for Huxley to say that authoritarian methods wouldn't work.

Muller, if I understand him rightly, adds another point in support of voluntary adoption:

> If we are to preserve that self-determination which is an essential feature of human intelligence, success and happiness, our individual actions in the realm of genetics must be steps based upon our own personal judgments and inclinations. Although these decisions are all conditioned by the mores about us, these mores can be specifically shaped and channelized by our own distinctive personalities.[32]

This I interpret to imply that authoritarian methods would counteract the goal of the program, namely, the maximization of intelligence and the social virtues. If true, this is tantamount to the admission of the *environmental* factor in these characters, and raises again the question as to the degree to which they are genetically transmitted, if at all.

In the last analysis, the question of whether positive eugenics can be effective without authoritarian methods remains open. It is a straightforward question of fact, once the standard of effectiveness is specified. My personal opinion—for what it is worth—is that authoritarian methods would be required. Plato and the Spartans, who respectively supported controlled mating and breeding, were more realistic than their modern counterparts. (Plato supposed that married couples could be made to believe that their unions were based on voluntary choice.) I am not convinced by the instancing of the spread of voluntary birth control. But if authoritarian methods are required it is doubtful that the game is worth the candle. The argument that since assortive mating occurs anyway there can be nothing wrong with the complete coercive control of mating is hardly deserving of a reply.

In the absence of a detailed proposal for an institutional framework it is difficult to discuss the question of democratic control and safeguards against abuse. Suffice it to say that the benevolence of Professors Huxley and Muller is no guarantee against abuse by a state subject to changing ideals and tastes.[33]

In closing this section it is appropriate to call attention to the profound social consequences that programs of positive eugenics (by a currently contemplated technique) would have. It would be bound, for example, to alter the institution of the family. Now this institution is already undergoing change, but it is hardly clear what these changes are or whether they are changes for the better. Plainly, selection by "delegated parenthood runs counter to a deep-rooted sense of proprietary parenthood."[34] The adoption of this method is certain to have a profound impact on the conditions of life in the community of the future. I do not share Huxley's confidence that these changes are bound to be beneficent.[35]

I should add that my strong doubts about the desirability of a social program of positive eugenics do not necessarily bear upon the use of A.I.D. in individual cases. My general outlook is that we should maintain strict principles (against its use), but be flexible in practice. However, this is another matter.

III. Negative Eugenics[36]

Negative eugenics is a subject that the layman approaches with even greater trepidation. In addition to lacking a proper grounding in the technicalities of genetics, he faces the problem of "what to do when doctors disagree." For we do not find complete unanimity among experts on the necessity for certain types of social programs of negative eugenics or their effectiveness. The following discussion is guided by what seem to me the most persuasive arguments. . . . Most of the topics I shall discuss in this section are not in themselves ethical issues, but nevertheless bear upon the question of whether we ought to engage in programs of biological engineering that aim at the reduction of genetically caused defects. A number of the points that I have tried to make in the preceding sections are relevant here. But I shall not review them. They should be fairly obvious to the reader who has made it this far.

It is well known that various defects (both psychic and physical) are heritable. Indeed, for certain defects, the probability that a child born of a "defective" parent will also have such a defect can be calculated. The genetics of abnormality, in fact, is better known than the genetics of normality. The agents of transmission of these heritable defects are the genes. Some harmful genes are, of course, eliminated in each generation before their carriers have a chance to reproduce. War, famine, disease, etc., make a contribution in this regard, although they also eliminate "good" genes. In addition, a deleterious gene may be eliminated by virtue of its killing off its carrier. New defective genes, however, enter the gene pool by a process of mutation. Some of these are transmitted to future generations. The maintenance of biological efficiency for a species is dependent upon the operation of selective survival, the winnowing out of a large number of carriers of harmful genes before they have a chance to reproduce. The natural processes of selection are no longer operating with the degree that is required for the human species to maintain its efficiency in the long run (Huxley's 5,000 to 10,000 years). Medical technology, by prolonging the lives of defect carriers, enables the transmission of harmful genes; it has a "dysgenic" effect. The "load of mutations" thus increases in every generation. Some type of artificial selection for survival is needed, lest man commit biological suicide.[37]

The above paragraph is a condensed statement of the justification for a social program of biological engineering aimed at reducing the "unfit." I do not find it convincing, nor do many experts in the field. First, it is not clear that medicine *is* dysgenic in its effects. Secondly, it is not clear that any program of negative eugenics would be much help in dealing with the problem in any way that would be significant for the species. And thirdly, it is not clear that any such a program wouldn't do more harm than good. I shall present a condensed statement of the counter-considerations.

Whether medicine has dysgenic effects is a normative question, though not necessarily an ethical one. It is true that medicine protects certain genes from natural selection. But the harmfulness of a gene (or of any trait) is partially dependent, at the very least, on its environment.[38] We do not have the genetic capacity to synthesize certain vitamins. This cannot be thought of as a defect so long as we can get an adequate supply of vitamins in our food or in chemical compounds. Some genes which are "bad" in one environment are "good" in another (as is the case with certain genes that determine susceptibility to malaria and sickle-cell anemia). Moreover, and especially, if the harmful effects of a gene can be overcome by medical technology it is not clear that the situation can be described as dysgenic. "If, for instance, diabetes mellitus (known to involve a strong genetic predisposition) can be fully controlled by simple and universally available medication, then the predisposing genes do no harm and their spread in a population would do no harm."[39] We can expect further advances in medicine that not only will protect deleterious genes from natural selection, but also provide an environmental adjustment to the genetic system. Medical science might not be able to handle completely the effects of the harmful gene, but then neither would negative eugenics.

For many hereditary defects there are no known treatments. The negative eugenist proposes that these be reduced by eliminating as far as possible the harmful genes. The methods suggested are, usually, sterilization or controlled mating. No one seems prepared to opt for Spartanism, . . . Of the other two, sterilization would be the more efficient, and I shall confine myself to its prospects.

Even if a thoroughgoing program of sterilization of carriers of defective genes were adopted (and one of the difficulties here is that all of us probably carry a few harmful genes), its success would depend upon the type of gene involved. Dominant genes with complete penetration show up in every carrier, so that even if new ones arose by mutation, a program of sterilization would readily eliminate them. Huntington's chorea (a highly debilitating nervous disease) is due to such a gene. However, it usually appears too late for action to take place before reproduction. In any case such genes are rare. Moreover, for many of the most harmful dominant genes sterilization is not necessary, as they are self-eliminating. They kill or sterilize their carriers. Most new occurrences of such genes are due to mutation rather than inheritance, so that the complete elimination of such genes is impossible.

In the case of deleterious recessive genes, the prospects of sterilization are decidedly poor. The rarer the gene the more slowly does the elimination take place. It has been calculated that it would take sterilization about two hundred generations to reduce the proportion of albinos in the population to half the present frequency.[40] Most recessive harmful genes are rare, and they are carried more often in heterozygotes than in homozygotes. The elimination of these genes by sterilizing the visibly affected rare homozygotes would have a low rate of success.[41] Here we are supposing that sterilization would be employed against all persons visibly affected by a harmful gene. The success rate would be even lower if many such persons escape sterilization. I need not go into the ethical issues that a program of coercive sterilization occasions.[42]

Nothing that I have said above negates the desirability of a program of genetic counselling. Such a program is designed to aid the individual family in reducing the risks of personal tragedy. Nor does anything I have said necessarily rule out sterilization when these risks are high and the defect serious (*e.g.,* in the case of amaurotic idiocy). Undoubtedly, as genetics learns how to identify harmful genes in phenotypically normal persons, genetic counselling and education should be expanded. We do desire a full and satisfactory life for our children, and ought to avail ourselves of all the resources of biological science to realize it. But, as I have argued, this is quite different from programs that aim at promoting a desirable life for the community of the remote future. "It is, perhaps, not too selfish to say that posterity should be allowed to tackle its own problems and to hope that it may have better means for doing so than we have."[43]

Finally, it is not clear that a social program of negative eugenics wouldn't do more harm than good. This, of course, might depend upon the kind of defects that it would aim to eliminate. Nevertheless it is plain that "good" genes would be reduced in the process. A conflict could arise between the aims of positive and negative eugenics. Sweden has had a ban on the marriage of endogenous epileptics since 1757. This has been attacked by a Swedish geneticist not only on the grounds that the chances for an epileptic to have epileptic children are not very high, but also on the grounds "that many epileptics are highly intelligent and socially valuable members of their community, well fitted to bring up children, and that they may carry valuable genes whose transmission will be prevented by the existing law."[44]

I do not suppose that anyone will go so far as to maintain that society should insure itself a sup-

ply of defectives so as to provide occasions for altruism and self-sacrifice, which are classified among the highest virtues. Nevertheless, eugenics is certain to find itself in a dilemma in the cases of "a blind poet, a deaf musician, a consumptive novelist, and a hunchback physicist [who] have contributed so much to our intellectual heritage as to be classified as geniuses."[45] Secondly, and here I repeat myself, we do not know what the conditions of life in the remote future will be. It is difficult to imagine that certain severe defects will ever have a good side to them, yet we may be doing a great favor for the future if we preserve genetic diversity even on pain of allowing various defectives to transmit their genes to the future. There is something to be said for "genetic waste."[46]

IV. The Control of Biological Control[47]

In this section I wish to stress the need for mutual confidence between layman and biological scientist. A breakdown in confidence can only be detrimental to both parties. To secure this trust the layman, on his part, must keep himself informed as far as possible on scientific advance thereby to acquire an intelligent appreciation of the requirements of the developing discipline; and the scientist, on his part, must act with a sense of responsibility towards the community. Our technological civilization is dependent upon science, and this is a fact which the layman knows. He can never hope to master the specialized sciences; he can get a "feel" for them, at best. Inevitably, the layman, if he wishes to preserve this civilization, must have some measure of faith in the moral integrity of the scientist. And this faith will be impaired whenever the scientist fails to act responsibly in the layman's judgment. Plainly, this judgment ought to be grounded upon the intelligent appreciation of the science, and not on ignorance or caprice. The scientist on his side must both act and appear to act in a manner that justifies the layman's faith. He must therefore not only show a concern for the advancement of his discipline, but also for its bearing upon the communal good. Among other things this means that the scientist must allow for the possibility that the communal good might at times over-ride scientific advance. In order to act responsibly towards the community, the scientist must be conscientious. That is to say, he must attempt to judge his prospective conduct from an impartial perspective, and not merely as a scientist interested in advancing his discipline. He must pass moral judgments upon himself and be willing to let such judgments influence his conduct as a scientist. In this way the layman's trust in the scientist can be maintained.

It is in the field of biological engineering that we are likely to have a crisis of confidence. Control over the direction of mutation, which is possible now in a limited area, is bound to be extended. If it has not already been done, babies will be grown in test-tubes. The imagination is staggered by the possibilities—for evil as well as good. Both positive and negative eugenics, which are the products of benevolent if often misguided men (in my opinion), will be overtaken by *atypogenics*, the creation of the abnormal, the weird, and the bizarre. It is generally true that any new technique which is discovered is put to use. The strange world of the science fiction writer will become a reality.

There is much concern today over moral problems raised by experimental medicine.[48] These problems are occasioned by a shift in the traditional orientation of medicine, which is therapeutic and patient-centered. Rather than aiming at doing good for the patient, curing not merely the disease but the whole man, there is a trend towards viewing the patient as a subject or specimen for study and research. These problems, however, are likely to pale in the light of atypogenics, which *ab novo* will be able to create its subjects for research.

At this point a crisis in confidence could become real. There is a certain casuistry of the mind whereby men convince themselves that everything is permitted. This is a special danger when one has in view an apparently good end, such as the expansion of human knowledge. But even knowledge doesn't justify any and every act. If we should ever come to believe this we shall be in the death-throes of the struggle between man's creations and himself. This is the moral of the story of Dr. Frankenstein, a piece of fiction that will soon become fact.

Perhaps I am exaggerating. Nevertheless it does seem to me that some recent statements by a leading geneticist are hardly calculated to inspire the layman's confidence in the biological engineer. Professor Joshua Lederberg can "see nothing fundamentally different between vaccinating with a live virus and introducing new genetic information into an individual." Now presumably this need not frighten us so long as we understand that this might be old-fashioned negative eugenics using new techniques. But Professor Lederberg is also reported as saying that "an overzealous policing to keep people from doing seemingly bizarre genetic experiments would be as dangerous as forcing their use on society."[49] These remarks sound like a threat, a threat which is not likely to be well-taken by the layman. It is important, to say the least, that Professor Lederberg should clarify his position. Furthermore, it is important that geneticists at large should make their views explicit.

With all due respect for Professor Lederberg, I suggest that we are heading towards the day when policing of atypogenics will become necessary. Naturally, we should wish to avoid "overzealous" policing, and it can be avoided only if the geneticist maintains the confidence of the lay public. This he can do by showing his conscientiousness.

I would propose that control of atypogenics, and of genetic experimentation in general, be initially exercised by the discipline itself. Geneticists at large must become the conscience that passes judgment on the conduct of the individual researcher. This requires full *publicity* regarding prospective experiments and their results. Discussion should then take place over whether or how the work should proceed, a judgment on its permissibility should be rendered. *Primum non nocere*—first, do no harm—may serve as a guiding principle. Individuals who violate either the requirement of publicity or the sense of the discipline on permissibility, should be censured, and perhaps be subject to some kind of penalty. I do not know how to construct the institutional framework for the control of biological control, but I think we are approaching the day when its construction will become necessary. It is possible that the discipline of genetics will be unable to police itself and that legal sanctions will be necessary to deter what the public (in its ignorance, perhaps) regards as abuses. This, of course, is not a happy prospect. The legal control of biological engineering is itself liable to abuse in ways that are easily imagined, especially after our imagination has been stretched by the thought of atypogenics.

V. Concluding Remarks

As control is extended over the direction of mutation, the subjects of positive and negative eugenics will need re-thinking. In this paper I have argued, on the whole, against lending our assent to programs of these types. It may turn out, however, that we shall not have to make a choice between positive or negative eugenics, on the one hand, and the amelioration of failings and ills by more standard methods, on the other. The choice may be between eugenics and atypogenics. In any case, it would be sad if we had no choice in the matter at all. Many experts in the field assure us that atypogenics lies far in the future. Let us hope so. Meanwhile, we would do well to bear in mind the words of Benjamin Jowett, one of the Victorian commentators on Plato: "We know how human nature may be degraded; we do not know how by artificial means any improvement in the breed can be effected."[50]

Notes

1. *See* G. HARDIN, NATURE AND MAN'S FATE 219 (1961).

2. *See* Huxley, *The Emergence of Darwinism*, in 1 EVOLUTION AFTER DARWIN 1, 19–21.

3. Taken from a television broadcast and printed in 3 EVOLUTION AFTER DARWIN 61 (emphasis added).

4. Golding, *Towards a Theory of Human Rights* [THE MONIST 52 (1968), 521–549].

5. Sometimes, the better we get to know these peoples, the clearer we are on the irrelevance of our social ideal for them. Few of us today—and probably the fewer the better—feel an obligation to export Western culture to the corners of the earth.

6. *See* Batt, p. 529; Gorney, p. 294; Grad, pp. 486, 491 [UCLA LAW REVIEW 15 (1968)].

7. Huxley, *Eugenics in Evolutionary Perspective*, 54 EUGENICS REV. 123, 135 (1962).

8. *See* C. AUERBACH, THE SCIENCE OF GENETICS 97–99 (1961).

9. Dobzhansky, *Evolution at Work*, 127 SCIENCE 1091, 1097 (1958).

10. Quoted in L. DUNN & T. DOBZHANSKY, HEREDITY, RACE AND SOCIETY 9 (1946).

11. *Id.* at 8.

12. F. SCHILLER, EUGENICS AND POLITICS 92 (1926).

13. *See* Muller, [*The Guidance of Human Evolution*, EVOLUTION AFTER DARWIN 454 (S. Tax ed. 1960); noted by L. C. Dunn, *Cross-Currents in the History of Human Genetics*, 54 EUGENICS REV. 69 (1962), at 75].

14. Quoted in G. HARDIN, *supra* note [1], at 230.

15. Huxley, *supra* note [7], at 133.

16. *See* Dunn, *supra* note [13], at 75.

17. Huxley, *supra* note [7], at 132, 137.

18. C. AUERBACH, *supra* note [8], at 60.

19. I shall not list examples. The following comment is of interest: "Statements such as the 'Jukes-Kallikaks, "bad heredity" concept may have been too enthusiastically rejected by perfectionists,' and meaningless pronouncements such as 'Heredity controls intelligence more than twice as much as does environment in families that adopt one of a pair of white identical twins' add nothing but noise to our available information.

"These statements, derived from a paper presented by an American Nobel laureate, William Shockley, must be disturbing to any serious scientist, not because they reflect an uncongenial set of social attitudes, but because they revive an outmoded but ever recurring dichotomy between nature and nurture. Any contemporary mode of thought concerning behavior and genetics which continuously fails to appreciate the functional inseparability of gene complex and environment in the development of phenotype is scientifically worthless." Birch, *Bright Rats and Dull Rats*, 10 COLUM. U.F. 30 (1967).

20. Beadle, *Genes Culture, and Man*, COLUM. U.F. 12, 15–16 (1965).

21. *See* Huxley, *supra* note [7], at 133; Muller, *supra* note [13], at 440–45.

22. "Moreover, those who repeatedly proved their worth would surely be called upon to reappear age after age until the population in general had caught up with them." Muller, *supra* note [13], at 454.

23. I am unsure as to what generalizations are permissible from the study of animal ethology. (Lorenz, Tinbergen, etc.) Neither side of the dispute over the heritability of aggression convinces me, anyway. And when these arguments are extended to deal with the question whether "war is in our genes," I am even less convinced. One of the problems, as above, is the social meaning of aggression. If a layman may be allowed to express agreement with an expert, I would also endorse the following statement: "Perhaps the most ubiquitous difficulty in interpreting the data of behavioral genetics is that the genetics is sometimes sound but almost always the behavioral analysis is terribly poor." Birch, *supra* note [19], at 31.

24. Steward, in 3 EVOLUTION AFTER DARWIN 241.

25. *Cf.* Burt, *The Inheritance of Mental Ability*, 13 AM. PSYCHOLOGIST 1 (1958), who seems both properly cautious and over-enthusiastic in generalizing from his data.

26. *See, e.g.*, A. WAGNER, ENGLISH ANCESTRY (1961).

27. Thoday, *Causes and Functions of Genetic Variety*, 54 EUGENICS REV. 195 (1963).

28. *See* G. Simpson, This View of Life 277 (1964). I do not present the considerations that support this suggestion. Simpson implies that they are not conclusive, and the matter is in need of study. I fully agree that we should approach it with an unbiased mind.

29. *See* C. Auerbach, *supra* note [8], at 149–52. Perhaps I am only betraying my own ignorance, but if intelligence *is* declining, we may ask when this decline began. It seems to me ludicrous that there should be a significantly higher proportion of stupid individuals in the world today than there was in the time of Caesar.

30. An Inquiry Concerning the Principals of Morals §§ II–III (Hendel ed. 1957).

31. Huxley, *supra* note [7], at 138.

32. Muller, *supra* note [13], at 460.

33. *See* Dunn, *supra* note [13], at 75.

34. Huxley, *supra* note [7], at 139.

35. *Cf.* Matthews, *Eugenics and the Family*, 53 Eugenics Rev. 193 (1962). Matthews is a moderate proponent of eugenics.

36. *See* Gorney, p. 293; Grad, p. 487 [UCLA Law Review, 15 (1968)].

37. *See* Gorney, p. 306 [UCLA Law Review, 15 (1968)].

38. *See* Thoday, *supra* note [27], at 198.

39. G. Simpson, *supra* note [28], at 279. *See also* C. Auerbach, *supra* note [8], at 95.

40. L. Dunn & T. Dobzhansky, *supra* note [10], at 87–92.

41. *See* C. Auerbach, *supra* note |8|, at 86–91.

42. Huxley, if I understand him correctly, supports a program of *voluntary* sterilization. *See* Huxley, *supra* note [7], at 135. I think it utopian to suppose that such a program would be very effective.

43. L. Dunn & T. Dobzhansky, *supra* note [10], at 93–94.

44. C. Auerbach, *supra* note |8|, at 94; *see* Gorney, p. 308; Grad, p. 492 [UCLA Law Review, 15 (1968)].

45. Steward, *Evolutionary Principles and Social Types*, in 2 Evolution after Darwin 169.

46. *See* G. Hardin, *supra* note [1], ch. 13. *See also* Thoday, *supra* note [27], at 199.

47. *See generally* Burger, p. 436 [UCLA Law Review, 15 (1968)].

48. *See* Beecher, *Ethics and Clinical Research*, 274 N. Eng. J. Med. 1354 (1966); Freund, *Ethical Problems in Human Experimentation*, 273 N. Eng. J. Med. 687 (1965); Stumpf, *Some Moral Dimensions of Medicine*, 64 Annals Internal Med. 460 (1966); *Informed Consent in Drug Research*, Columbia Journal of Law and Social Problems, Oct. 24, 1966, at 4–8.

49. Report of a symposium on genetics and development held at Columbia University. N.Y. Times, Oct. 22, 1967, at 67, col. 1.

50. I Works of Plato 246 (B. Jowett transl. 1937).

Inquiring into Inquiry

Robert L. Sinsheimer

For what specific purposes might we wish to limit inquiry? Do we wish to curb only the means or even the ends of inquiry? Let me advance some suggestions.

One is the preservation of human dignity. We should not do experiments that involuntarily make of *man* a means rather than an end. The ethics of human experimentation are, I think, now rather well accepted, even though it must be recognized that such restraints blunt pure inquiry.

Another reason to limit at least the means of inquiry is the avoidance of involuntary physical or biological hazard. As might be expected, the level of hazard which demands restraint will be arguable. We have already one instance of such limita-tion in the—not universally accepted—ban on atmospheric nuclear testing. The field of recombinant DNA research has an analogous potential for widespread, inadvertent danger from the leak-out of possibly toxic organisms. It is a danger difficult to quantitate, so that the limited precautions already proposed are certain to be the subject of continued controversy.

Another reason to limit inquiry may be the sheer cost of a research project. This issue introduces a new perspective—the ends of the research. By introducing the element of cost one asks if the primary consequence of the inquiry, that is, the knowledge to be gained, is worth the expenditure of talent, time, and resources. Deci-

Reprinted with permission of the author and the publisher from Hastings Center Report, 6 *(August 1976): 18.* © *Institute of Society, Ethics and the Life Sciences, 360 Broadway, Hastings-on-Hudson,N.Y. 10706.*

sions about the allocation of resources are usually, and properly, left to the political sphere. However, scientists are also citizens and despite our enthusiasms we should endeavor to be at least dimly aware of the realities of competing concerns.

Progressing ever deeper into controversy, one may extend inquiry into the ends of inquiry and question whether, in particular instances, we want to know the answer in every case. Given the nature of man and of human society, are the secondary consequences of such knowedge, on balance, likely to be beneficial? Here it may be that the highest wisdom is to recognize that we are not wise enough to know what we do not want to know, and thus to leave the ends of inquiry unrestrained. Indeed, I expect there are only a few instances where prudence would be in order. But the set may not be null. Let me give four selected illustrations of research whose likely consequences would seem to me to be major and at this time in our society to be of appreciably less advantage than harm.

Should we attempt to contact presumed "extraterrestrial intelligences"? I wonder if the authors of such experiments have ever considered the impact upon the human spirit if it should develop that there are other forms of life, to whom we are, for instance, as the chimpanzee is to us. Once it were realized someone already knew the answers to our questions, it seems to me, the impact upon science itself would be especially devastating. We know from our own history the shattering impact more advanced civilizations have upon the less advanced. In my view the human race has to make it on its own, for our own self-respect.

Research upon improved, easier, simpler, cheaper methods of isotope separation? Result: slightly cheaper power, far easier bombs. Is that, on balance, in anyone's best interest?

Research upon a simple means for predetermination of the sex of children? Result: some boon to animal husbandry, boys or girls upon parental request, and the potential for a major imbalance in the human sex ratio. Is this disruption of a balance already provided by nature really a desirable advance?

Indiscriminate research upon the aging process? What is the long-range purpose? The purpose of cancer research is clear: the eradication of cancer. Is the purpose of aging research the eradication of aging? None would quarrel with research to relieve the infirmities of old age. But the section, "Purpose of Legislation," in the House Committee statement accompanying the Research on Aging Act of 1974, states that, "This Institute (the National Institute of Aging) will provide a natural focus for the research necessary to achieve the great goal of keeping our people as young as possible as long as possible." Is this, on balance, a desirable goal?

The very success of science has ended its pleasant isolation. The impact of science and the increasing coupling of science to human affairs do encumber us with new responsibilities. Yet at the same time we do not wish to shackle inquiry with the bonds of responsibility. Somehow we need to find a way to be doubly responsible, both to mainkind and to science, as one of man's finest creations. That will not be easy.

When May Research Be Stopped?

Carl Cohen

The uses and possible misuses of recombinant DNA are so threatening, some believe, that research into that technology should now be stopped. But reasons good enough to justify prohibition of research in this sphere must, in fairness, apply equally to other spheres, if threats of similar gravity arise there.

I ask, therefore: What are the alternative prin-

ciples that, if adopted, might reasonably justify prohibition of research in a given sphere? Which of these alternative principles should be rejected, and which accepted in some form or part? And to the extent that any one of these principles is acceptable, what bearing does it have upon continued research with recombinant DNA?

My answers to these questions rest upon two

Reprinted by permission from the New England Journal of Medicine 296, *no. 21, (1976): 1203–1210.*
Editor's Note: Footnotes in this reading have been renumbered.

fundamental propositions, very generally agreed upon. First: freedom of inquiry is a value of such profound importance that it must not be abridged without the most compelling reasons. This proposition, true generally, carries great weight in a society holding liberty as a paramount ideal; it carries extraordinary weight in universities and research institutions committed explicitly to the enlargement of knowledge. Second: some research undertakings should properly be restricted. Everyone may not agree upon particular cases, but it will be agreed that a rational commitment to freedom of inquiry does not protect every research enterprise in every circumstance.

The task is to characterize the enterprises and circumstances in which prohibition may prove defensible or even obligatory.

Alternative Principles of Prohibition

To justify prohibition, some would present a practical syllogism in this form: Major premise: research having certain identifiable features (p, q, r . . .) may (or must) be stopped. Minor premise: this research (in recombinant DNA, or in nuclear fission, or . . .) has precisely those features. Hence, this research may (or must) be stopped. My first objective is to formulate alternative, plausible major premises of such syllogisms.

Principles of prohibition must pertain either to the product or to the process of the research in question. The line between the two may be hard to draw, but under one or the other can be listed all the general principles that seem remotely tenable.

Set A: By-product (#1–#3)

1. Research should not be permitted when it aims at (or is likely to result in) the discovery of knowledge that is wrong for human beings to possess.

2. Research should not be permitted when it aims at (or is likely to result in) the discovery of knowledge that is not wise to place in human hands.

   2a. When there is any probability that the knowledge developed will be used with very injurious consequences.

   2b. When there is moderate probability that the knowledge developed will be used with very injurious consequences.

   2c. When there is high probability that the knowledge developed will be used with very injurious consequences.

3. Research should not be permitted when it aims specifically at the development or perfection of instruments for killing or injuring human beings.

Set B: By-process (#4–#6)

4. Research should not be permitted when it is not conducted openly, for all to examine the ongoing process and results.

5. Research should not be permitted when its continuation is unfair, either to the subjects of the experimentation or to those otherwise involved in the research. Research is unfair when, through coercion or deceit, or in some other way, the rights of those involved are not respected.

6. Research should not be permitted when its conduct (as distinct from its product) presents risks so great as clearly to outweigh the benefits reasonably anticipated. Risks here must be understood to include all hazards that that process of inquiry entails, of which there are two large categories: risks of "misfire" (i.e., achieving results different from and more dangerous than those sought) and risks of "accident" (i.e., unforeseen mishap during the process).

   6a. When the risks are essentially to persons involved in the research:

   (6a1) the subjects of experimentation;

   (6a2) the researchers and their associates.

   6b. Where the risks are essentially to others than those involved in the research.

These exhaust the alternative principles that are at all reasonable, or arguably tenable, for the prohibition of research. Phrasing (and the degree of specificity) may vary, but every plausible candidate, I contend, will fall under one or another of the six kinds distinguished.

As an illustration: Robert Sinsheimer, professor of biophysics at the California Institute of Technology and an acute critic of recombinant DNA research, has suggested some possible answers to the question, "For what specific purposes might we wish to limit inquiry?" He proposes, or at least entertains, several candidates.[1]

(a) To preserve human dignity. "We should not do experiments that involuntarily make of man a means rather than an end."[1] But, of course, human subjects in medical experiments are means. Sinsheimer surely intends to emphasize, with Kant, that one must not treat human beings as means only, but also as ends—for which reason research committees do rigorously insist that their participation be truly voluntary and informed. This is but a more elaborate statement of principle (5), above, demanding fairness.

(b) To avoid "involuntary physical or biological hazard."[1] Sinsheimer recognizes, of course, that one cannot avoid all such hazards. He wants us all to be very sensitive to the level of danger. This is but another formulation, less precise, of principle (6), above, addressing the balance of risk and benefit.

(c) Cost. "[One] asks if the primary consequences of the inquiry, that is, the knowledge to be gained, is worth the expenditures of talent, time and resources."[1] But refusing to support research is one thing, prohibiting it is another. When the research enterprise involves heavy expense, one is right to insist that the worth of the knowledge to be gained be very carefully estimated. Protecting free inquiry does not entail irrationality in the expenditure of resources. And it is true that institutional refusal to fund a research project often has the effect of blocking that project in that context. Many research activities, however (work with recombinant DNA technology being one important example), do not require very large investments of institutional or governmental funds. Although one may conclude, therefore, that for some projects the object does not justify the expenditure, it is essential to see that cost cannot serve as grounds for prohibition. Some research is simply not worth doing, but reasons for not troubling to do certain things ourselves must not be taken as reasons for keeping other persons from doing them.

Some principles, very different from those stated above, are procedural, requiring special machinery for the approval of research protocols in certain areas. Approval (some say) must be given by the appropriate bodies, with appropriate membership, deliberating with appropriate care. Others say that the decision to permit research of certain kinds may be made only by some larger community (city or state) through some demo-cratic voting procedure. Such regulation, although awkward, is being tried in some quarters. But, even when feasible and fitting, those procedural requirements are not germane here. One seeks to discover reasons that may serve to deny approval. Whatever the decision-making machinery, the individual users of that machinery need grounds for concluding yea or nay. These grounds—not the system of their application—are what I am concerned with here.

Finally, I note that the six alternative principles are not mutually exclusive; one could rationally hold (say) both (3) [on killing], and some variant of (6) [risks over benefits]. They may overlap, relying upon the same feature of a given inquiry—for example, what is objectionable under (4) [openness] may also be objectionable under (5) [unfairness].

It remains to determine which (if any) of these principles should be adopted, and which (if any) apply to the sphere of recombinant DNA research, and to identify the restrictions (if any) that properly follow therefrom.

The Six Principles Reconsidered

What follows is a critical appraisal of the six alternative principles listed above. The conclusions reached unavoidably rely upon some personal judgments, but are put forward for general agreement.

Principles Based upon the Product of Research (#1–#3)

(1) "Research should not be permitted when it aims at (or is likely to result in) the discovery of knowledge that is wrong for human beings to possess."

This principle should be rejected utterly. There is no body of knowledge, or item of knowledge, that is intrinsically wrong to possess. The conviction that there are forbidden precincts, that there is an intellectual sanctum sanctorum into which all entry is sinful, must rely upon some claim of special revelation, or some other nonrational restriction that has no rightful authority to limit inquiry in a university or research institution.

Principles of privacy, it is true, may render certain sorts of knowledge about individuals not suitable for public scrutiny. But there is a vast difference between the claim that some knowledge is not properly public and the claim that some knowledge is intrinsically unfit for human acquisition. Individuals are free, of course, to limit themselves if they honestly hold beliefs of the latter sort. The search here, however, is not for principles that some persons may cling to but for the principles research institutions ought to defend.

Note that this principle, (1), is widely attractive. Much of the anxiety that attends DNA research, I submit, flows from vague, unformulated doubts about whether this probe into "the code of life itself" might not be a form of human presumption, a playing of God. One is understandably awed by the cumulative powers of human intelligence; those powers can be (and often have been) misused. But fear of that misuse does not give rational warrant for closing the avenues of exploration. If one did believe that there are domains in which human knowing is taboo, molecular genetics might indeed be one of them. Inquiry into nuclear fusion or celestial exploration might then be equally taboo, as might be the study of theories of relativity, or the development of contraceptive technics. The penetration of every intellectual frontier threatens deeply held convictions. Every striking advance in human prowess frightens many, horrifies some and appears to a few as the profane invasion of the holy of holies. The difficulty lies not in discriminating between the real holy of holies and those only mistakenly supposed; it lies in the unwarranted assumption that there are any spheres of knowledge to which ingress is forbidden. This first principle is wholly untenable; a fortiori it is not tenable as applied to the biochemistry of genetics.

(2) "Research should not be permitted when it aims at (or is likely to result in) the discovery of knowledge that is not wise to place in human hands."

Of this principle I distinguish three varieties, depending on the degree of probability with which great injury may be anticipated as a result of the possession of that knowledge. Of course, there will be argument about what constitutes great injury, about how such probabilities are to be calculated or estimated, and about what the probabilities are in a particular case. But supposing rough agreement is reached on these matters, the rightness (or wrongness) of the principle here formulated remains to be determined, and is of profound importance.

Principle (2a) [that prohibition of research is justified when there is any probability of very injurious consequences] may be rejected categorically; it verges on the absurd. On that principle one ought not rise from bed.

Principle (2b) [that prohibition of research is justified when there is moderate probability of very injurious consequences] must be more seriously considered—but it too deserves rejection in the end. It is true, of course, that the results of inquiry will often be such that there is some moderate likelihood that their use will prove very injurious, even disastrous. But the ubiquity of such possibilities renders (2b) [as it does (2a)] so sweeping as to entail the cessation of a great deal of the research—both in biologic and in physical sciences—best calculated to improve the human condition.

Nevertheless, serious thinkers have urged the adoption of some such principle. Two especially—one a historian, and the other a biophysicist—deserve response.

Shaw Livermore, professor of history at the University of Michigan, in concluding that his university should not proceed with the development of recombinant DNA technology, argues as follows:[2]

(i) Research on recombinant DNA promises the development of a special, elemental capability: that of overcoming the natural genetic barriers that separate the species, and (ultimately) of uniting genetic components of different species to produce new forms of life.

(ii) This capability would be so great, so overwhelming, as to exceed the capacity of society to direct and control it.

Therefore, (iii) success in this research "will bring with it a train of awesome and possibly disastrous consequences,"[2]

and (iv) decisions demanded by this technology may well have effects that are "unintended but irreversible."[2]

Livermore suggests, in effect, that scientists here are like the Sorcerer's Apprentice, conjuring into existence what they do not fully understand and none of them can control. Although appealing, the argument fails upon careful test. Consider its elements in reverse order.

(iv) That decisions regarding DNA will sometimes have unintended and irreversible effects is surely true, but not very weighty. That is precisely the case for every important human enterprise in research and development—it leaves the world in an irreversibly different condition from that in which it was before, and has consequences that could not have been foreseen, and therefore could not have been intended. Many of the discoveries that have proved the greatest boons to mankind have arisen from basic research in ways that were—when that research was first pursued—wholly unforeseen and unintended. That some consequences (bad and good) of any major inquiry will be irreversible and unintended is evident, and cannot reasonably be taken as grounds for the prohibition of inquiry.

(iii) But the consequences of this inquiry may be awesome—possibly disastrous. Awesomeness, again, may be for good as well as evil. One should bear in mind, in weighing arguments like these, that recombinant DNA technology also opens possibilities for monumental improvements in the human condition. Both sides must be weighed. But it is the "possibly disastrous" results that are the nub of this complaint—a complaint that cuts either not at all or entirely too well. There are no grounds for supposing that the likelihood of disaster is greater in this arena than in other research arenas that one would not seriously think of foreclosing. There is "moderate probability," I suppose, that the results of research into nuclear fusion will one day be put to malevolent uses—but one would not on this ground seriously suggest a prohibition of inquiry into the ways in which the nuclei of atoms may combine. In any sphere knowledge may be put to devilish use; that is a poor reason for prohibiting its acquisition.

(ii) It is suggested that the acquisition of certain awesome capabilities be barred because the capacity to direct them, once acquired, is lacking. But do we lack that power? The supposition is very doubtful. Many reflective historians and philosophers would insist that we have the capacity for the direction and control of the products of research. Whether we will sharpen such capacities as finely as we ought remains to be seen. Recent self-imposed restraints, followed by extended public deliberation, precisely in this sphere of recombinant DNA, strongly suggest that the capacity to control does exist and is being applied. Some present uncertainty about the outcome of this application surely does not justify the cessation of the inquiry. And even if only the potential for wise

control is now present, the realization of that potential can be stimulated and encouraged only with the advance of the inquiry in question. Professor Livermore, although reflectively, gives up hope for Dame Reason; I judge that one is ill advised to join him in despair.

(i) His anxieties—and indeed most arguments of this variety—stem largely from the "elemental" nature of the capabilities in view. But there is confusion hidden in the slippage between fears arising from the alleged probabilities of disaster (probabilities not ever established) and fears arising from the allegedly special, extraordinary properties of the knowledge to be discovered. The implicit suggestion that the knowledge sought is too godlike for human frailty gives seeming (but unjustifiable) plausibility to the claim that its acquisition will bring catastrophe. Once it is clearly seen that knowledge is not to be feared, that it may prove valuable everywhere, risky anywhere, and intrinsically improper nowhere, it will also be seen that the specialness of the discoveries in view, though in some ways real, ceases to serve as any ground for prohibition. Research in genetics, as in every science, moves ever onward; inquiry into the controlled manipulation of genetic macromolecules is a natural and inevitable phase of that advance. Fears that human beings are incapable of dealing with the products of their own intelligence are as much and as little justified on every other research continuum as on this one.

A differing effort to provide a tenable variant of this principle, (2b) is made by Sinsheimer. He writes:

> [One] may extend inquiry into the ends of inquiry and question whether, in particular instances, we want to know the answer in every case. Given the nature of man and of human society, are the secondary consequences of such knowledge, on balance, likely to be beneficial? Here it may be that the highest wisdom is to recognize that we are not wise enough to know what we do not want to know, and thus to leave the ends of inquiry unrestrained. Indeed, I expect there are only a few instances where prudence would be in order. But the set may not be null.[1]

What does this say? Sinsheimer is guarded, tentative, unsure. From his questions and modalities emerge at last his suggestion of four actual spheres in which—because the secondary consequences of knowledge are not likely, on balance, to prove beneficial—he seriously believes that inquiry might appropriately be restricted.

(i) "Should we attempt to contact presumed 'extraterrestrial intelligences'?" Sinsheimer believes that "the impact upon the human spirit" if it should develop that there are vastly superior forms of life, and the impact of that knowledge upon science itself would be "devastating."[1]

(ii) "Research upon improved, easier, simpler, cheaper methods of isotope separation?" Sinsheimer doubts whether such research is in man's best interest, yielding "slightly cheaper power, far easier bombs."[1]

(iii) "Research upon a simple means for the predetermination of the sex of children?" Sinsheimer appears to believe that the resultant potential for "a major imbalance in the human sex ratio" shows advances here to be undesirable.[1]

(iv) "Indiscriminate research upon the aging process?" Sinsheimer appears to believe that the stated goal accompanying legislation to advance such research, "keeping our people as young as possible, as long as possible," is not, on balance, desirable.[1]

It is hard to know what to make of these suggestions. They are very cautiously put, half in interrogative form. But (whatever Sinsheimer believes or may find desirable), if such speculations are treated as arguments for the principle of restriction here involved, they fail utterly. Two observations will suffice.

First. The most that such apprehensions could establish—supposing that everyone shared them—is that it might be that certain inquiries will not prove beneficial on balance. Of course that may be. What follows? Precisely that argument has been presented (with greater force than in most of Professor Sinsheimer's instances) against every scientific advance: against Galileo, against Darwin, against Freud. Such obstinacy (it was urged that good men not even look through Galileo's "infernal glass") is now considered indefensible. It is not an iota more defensible now than it was then. It was entirely correct for the opponents of these seminal thinkers to insist that inquiry of the kinds that they opposed might not prove beneficial in the end. What does that tell about the principle invoked? If, now, the same principle is used not merely to discourage but to prohibit research—in recombinant DNA, for

example—one will operate under strictures of essentially the same character as those that persuaded so many rational men to condemn the teaching of the Copernican hypothesis.

Second. The illustrations given by Professor Sinsheimer of the applicability of his principle, his pleas for "prudence," where ignorance seems to him more desirable than knowledge, are self-convicting. If principle (2b) when applied means—as it appears to for him—that researches into the aging process, into nuclear power, into extraterrestrial contact and so on are to be blocked or restricted because of what may transpire if they are successful, the upshot of the argument is revealed. He helps one to see the extreme consequences forced upon everyone, unacceptable to most, if the principle of restriction that he has put forward is taken seriously.

Finally respecting (2b), one variety of great injury that some foresee (unlike catastrophic decisions having unintended impact) deserves remark. It is the gradual deterioration of human culture resulting from ever more extended subjection to technical control. As technology comes to pervade culture (some contend), human values must retreat—even wither. So we can defend our most humane interests only by disarming the technologists. Well, the probability of this feared outcome is very difficult to estimate. Its likelihood, in my judgment, though not trivial, is not great. To prohibit research on such grounds would be intolerably repressive. On this interpretation of disaster, too, the principle would cut against technological advance in every sphere, not that of molecular genetics alone.

For principle (2c) [that research be prohibited when the probability of its very injurious consequences is high or very high] the case is different. Were we to believe that in a given case, the prohibition of that specific inquiry would be, I judge, at least arguable. In such circumstances—the only persuasive candidate I can think of is research into nuclear explosives—the alleged probability would have to be explored, documented, established as fully as resources would then permit. Even here potentiality for benefit would also need to be weighed. Recognizing that rational men may ultimately differ in the resolution of such cases, one must allow that for some research ventures the probability of disastrous use of the products might be so high as to justify prohibition.

Again, two observations respecting (2c). First. Our rational commitment to freedom of inquiry is such that, in judging any claim of highly probable disaster, the burden of proof clearly rests upon those who would prohibit on that basis. They must present a convincing account of what concrete disasters are envisaged, what the methods are for determining the probability of such outcomes, and how those methods establish the high probability of the catastrophe pictured. The burden here is not light, nor ought it to be. Scientific inquiry should not be blocked simply upon the presentation by critics of a parade of imagined horribles of unspecified nature and doubtful likelihood.

Secondly, principle (2c) does not, in any case, apply to research with recombinant DNA. There is some probability (it may be supposed) that, after years of further development, the products of such research might be put to malevolent use—as instruments of war (although better, more convenient killers are already at hand) or in the realization of some (now far-fetched but then realizable) brave new world. There is some probability of that, one must grant. But that probability, on the best evidence now available, is slight; at its gravest interpretation, which very few would accept, that probability is no more than moderate. A high probability it is not. Hence in this sphere principle (2c) does not apply.

I conclude that principle (2) is generally inapplicable in most of its forms, and that in none of its forms may it properly serve to prohibit any research in the biochemistry of genetics now contemplated.

(3) "Research should not be permitted when it aims specifically at the development or perfection of instruments for killing or injuring human beings."

This is a reasonable principle for both persons and institutions; it is now accepted and applied by some universities. There are times, circumstances and some institutions to which it might not properly apply.

Although this principle may serve as major premise in a practical syllogism forbidding some kinds of research in some contexts, it cannot serve in a syllogism forbidding recombinant DNA research in any context at present. Research now contemplated with recombinant DNA does not faintly resemble the "munitions" development that would be the target of such a principle. If such an aim were proposed, or even seriously entertained, this principle might, indeed, be called into play. Under present and foreseeable circumstances, however, principle (3) simply has no bearing on the problem at hand.

I conclude that no tenable principle for the prohibition of research based upon its product can now serve to restrict research into recombinant DNA.

Principles Based upon the Process of Research (#4–#6)

(4) "Research should not be permitted when it is not conducted openly, for all to examine the ongoing process and results."

This attractive principle is of a kind very different from the others so far reviewed. Rightly understood, it presents not a limitation upon research but the statement of an ideal—one that we all properly share and promote. The realization of this ideal cannot and should not be taken as an inviolable condition for the conduct of the inquiry. It simply is not that. National security, proprietary interests (of firms or individuals) justly acquired, or other special concerns may render full openness an impractical ideal in many circumstances, certainly not justifying the cessation of all research whose conduct falls short of that ideal.

Openness—both in the research process and for the results of research—is an ideal widely and genuinely honored. Some universities do not permit in their precincts (or are inhospitable toward) research so classified as to restrict access to its results. But complete openness of the research process is very deliberately not applied as a necessary condition by universities, governmental institutions or private enterprises. If it were to be so applied, a great deal of research in progress would have to be discontinued. Much research that is planned would not (under such restriction) go forward. One would not seriously wish to insist upon this discontinuation and blockage. I conclude that the publicity principle is not even remotely acceptable as a basis for prohibition. Since it cannot serve for prohibition generally, it cannot serve so for research in recombinant DNA unless this inquiry can be shown to be specially prone to the evils of secrecy. That cannot be shown. There is no reason to believe that review of the research process in this field, and timely publication of its results, will fail to meet normal standards of the scientific community.

In fact, the circumstances surrounding DNA research lead to the very opposite conclusion. The nature, location and conditions of recombinant DNA research have been subject to a publicity surpassing that in any other comparable scientific sphere. Largely as a result of initiatives taken by the scientific community itself, public scrutiny in this area has been intense, and the researchers' standards of openness have been, and are sure to continue to be, much higher than normal. Therefore, even if the demand for openness in the process were an appropriate ground for restricting some inquiries in some contexts, it could not serve to restrict, in this context, inquiry using recombinant DNA.

(5) "Research should not be permitted when its continuation is unfair, either to the subjects of the experimentation or to those otherwise involved in the research."

This principle is sound; research whose process does substantial injustice ought not to be pursued, no matter its kind. Often disregarded in the past, this principle is now generally accepted, and is applied concretely to research activities in which unfairness can become a problem. To this end, all experiments proposing to put human subjects at risk—in any way, and to any degree, even the slightest—must be screened by a specially organized human-subjects review committee (HSRC), one kind of institutional review board. No such research may go forward without the explicit approval of an HSRC—and this restriction applies fully to any work with DNA that proposes to put human subjects at risk in any way.

Restrictions for the protection of human subjects being already in force, they need no special restatement for a specific sphere of inquiry. Experiments with recombinant DNA involving human beings have not yet been proposed. If they become a real possibility, and are proposed, the task of the HSRC screening that enterprise may be a delicate one. One will surely agree, in any case, that fairness (noncoercion, full information and so on) toward proposed subjects must be a condition for the continuation of that investigation.

Fairness to other researchers—respect for the present state of the work of others, full information to all investigators involved about what is in view and what is at risk—is also a demand reason-

ably made. But it, like openness, is a principle for the guidance of conduct, not the restriction of it. It cannot serve for the prohibition of research of a given kind.

Principle (5), I conclude, although important and sound, has no special application to research in recombinant DNA. So far as it does have institutional applicability, its application must be (and is) general, screening out research protocols in every sphere that fail to measure up to the requirements of justice. But measuring up to this standard is not a function of the subject matter of the research.

(6) "Research should not be permitted when the conduct of such research (as distinct from its product) presents risks (either of misfire or of accident) so great as clearly to outweigh the benefits reasonably anticipated." A misfire might be, for example, the creation, through DNA recombination, of an organism with unintended pathogenic capacity against which ordinary antibiotics proved ineffective. An accident might be, for example, the undetected escape, from a laboratory thought to be sealed, of a micro-organism giving rise to contagion.

This principle also is sound and applicable. Bringing it to bear upon DNA research, however, is complicated, and the outcome of that application is uncertain. Just here lie the major technical problems that have been and remain the focus of much scientific debate. The problem of containing the recombined DNA, either by physical retention within the laboratory or by weakening the host organism so as to render it not viable outside the laboratory, has been the major topic in controversy over what is unreasonably risky and what is not. Only in the light of the present state of effectiveness of containment measures can risks be rationally estimated. Hence the emergence of guidelines (laid down by the National Institutes of Health) for containment, and for permissible risks given known levels of effective containment. Hence, too, the need to reassess what is reasonably safe to do in the light of existing technical capacities to contain—especially since the capacity to contain biologically, by "disarming the bug," is being steadily improved. Recombined DNA molecules do create special dangers, which do, rightly, require special attention to the conditions and precautions under which specific research activities are carried on.

Still, the principle accepted here, that risks must be minimized, and never allowed to exceed the reasonably anticipated benefits, is one of general application. It applies to all research in medicine, in physics, in biology, in aeronautics, and so on. It has a bearing upon DNA research, to be sure—but only to the extent that the risks encountered in a specific experimental project within that domain appear to equal or to outweigh the anticipated benefits of that project.

Critical here are the risks to persons other than those involved in the research (6b): the people in the street who may be endangered by accident or misfire. Risks to experimental subjects (6a1) must be screened by human-subjects review committees [described above under (5)] designed precisely for that purpose. Risks to researchers themselves or to others formally involved in the research project (6a2) may be grouped for present purposes with risks to outsiders. It is for this combined group that the key question arises.

That key question, now heatedly argued, is this: Are the risks of recombined DNA, whether of misfire or of accident, of such enormity and such probability as to justify prohibition of further research in that sphere?

The first thing to notice about this question is that although here framed in the singular, it must in fact be asked about a host of very different research proposals. Estimating risk-benefit balance for some proposed investigation is often a vexing task. But it should be emphasized that the decisions called for in this family of cases are not, in principle, different from those we are commonly obliged to make when data are incomplete, the time-frame long, the object risky but promising. In this family of cases, as elsewhere, we will do the best we can.

Some contend that in this sphere of research, unlike others, the general sum of anticipated risks, taking into consideration both their degree of seriousness and their probability, outweighs the general sum of anticipated benefits, their value and likelihood similarly weighed. Therefore (they conclude) the proper estimate of risk-benefit balance calls for cessation now of all further research in this sphere.

This argument is unsound. Consider:

First, the key premise is false; it makes a stronger claim than the evidence supports. Granting that the present state of knowledge is short, all indications are that, if one weighed, as on a balance scale, the expected goods in view, multiplied by the likelihood of their probability, the result would be very different from that supposed by this argument. Everyone will allow that there are dangers, some not yet fully known, but the most careful and sophisticated discussions of these dangers, taking severity and probability into account, do not begin to show that they outweigh, or even approach, the sum of advantages likely to accrue from such research over the long term.[3]

The fact remains that some future proposals for investigation in molecular genetics, because of the special risks entailed in the process (and with full consideration of the nature and probability of the benefits in view) may, after thoughtful deliberation, then be rejected by the research institution. Clearly, such rejections, if they transpire, will require the continuing activity of an institutional review board, on the model of a human-subjects review committee, but with a differing focus. Rejection on the grounds of excessive risk is a step that must not be taken lightly, but it probably will be taken in some cases.

Since general prohibition is not in order, and approval for individual proposals must be given on a case-by-case basis, it is appropriate that such continuing review bodies set the conditions for the permissible pursuit of the risky inquiry proposed. Here lies the operative force of the general conviction that, whatever the level of risks found tolerable, there must be a commensurate level of precaution. Only through a process of ongoing review will it be possible to adjust restriction to enterprise rationally. Only through such deliberation can improvements in the effectiveness of containment (both physical and biologic) be weighed, as well as any special likelihood of misfire that the specific nature of the investigation at hand may present.

Finally, it is the singularity of this sphere of research, the uniqueness of its risks and promises, that is so specially provocative. That singularity must be taken account of, but should not be overplayed. Special attentions are rightly given, on a continuing basis, to proposals for experimentation with recombinant DNA, all agree. But it has been my aim to show that the form of the questions to be answered is not essentially different in this domain of scientific research from that in any other. There is a temptation to treat the recombination of DNA as fundamentally different just because of the character of the knowledge aimed at. But if I am right about the first set of principles entertained(#1–#3) pertaining to the product of research, this temptation should not be yielded to.

In summary, for the general prohibition of scientific research in any sphere, the only arguments that might suffice require premises vastly stronger than any now available or likely soon to be available. There is no valid practical syllogism, having true premises, whose conclusion is that research into recombinant DNA should be stopped. Of proposed arguments to this end it may be fairly said either that the major premise (the principle of prohibition) is false, or when true principles are provided, that the minor premise (specifying recombinant DNA research as defective in the ways indicated) is very far from established.

Notes

1. Sinsheimer, R. Inquiring into inquiry. Hastings Cent Rep 6(4):18, 1976.

2. Livermore, S. Statement of dissent, Report of the University Committee to Recommend Policy for the Molecular Genetics and Oncology Program, Office of the Vice President for Research, University of Michigan, Ann Arbor, March, 1976. Appendix B1, pp 46–47.

3. A number of bodies, with members both in the sciences and in the humanities, have deliberated long and carefully upon the likely balance of risk and benefit, over long term and short, of recombinant DNA research. Perhaps the two most thorough and probing studies are the Report of the Working Party on the Experimental Manipulation of the Genetic Composition of Micro-Organisms. Presented to Parliament by the Secretary of State for Education and Science, London, January, 1975 (this document is widely known as the Ashby Report, after the Chairman of the Working Party, Lord Eric Ashby), and the report of the University Committee to Recommend Policy for the Molecular Genetics and Oncology Program, presented to the vice-president for research at the University of Michigan, Ann Arbor, March, 1976 (attached to this document, widely known as the Report of Committee B, is a dissent and a reply to the dissent). Subsequently appeared a critique of the Report of Committee B, a response to that critique by Committee B, and a separate endorsement of the Committee's original report, all presented to the Regents of the University of Michigan.

Decision Scenario 1

Sara Straus was frightened. She sat in the counselor's office with her hands folded in her lap, trying to look calm.

"Mrs. Straus," the counselor said, "I have the results back on your AFP test. I'm sorry to tell you that the level of alpha protein in your blood is quite high."

"What does that mean?" Mrs. Straus asked.

"It means," said the counselor, "that your chances of having a baby with what we call neural tube defect are quite high. Your child might be born with an open spine or with part of its brain missing."

"Oh, my God. Is there anything I can do?"

The counselor shook her head. "If you mean can you do anything to make the baby normal, the answer is no. This test is about 90 percent accurate. The only reasonable course is to have an abortion and begin another child when you feel ready."

"But I don't believe in abortion," said Mrs. Straus.

"There's no way we can force you to have one. But according to the law if you have been informed of the chances of such a defect and do not have an abortion, then you and your husband must accept full financial responsibility for the care of the defective child."

"How much would that cost?"

"Probably around fifty thousand dollars a year."

"We can't afford that," said Mrs. Straus. "Nobody could afford to pay money like that."

"I'm just telling you the law," said the counselor.

"What if we have the child and then can't pay?"

"The law requires that you and your husband declare yourselves bankrupt. The child will then be placed in a public institution, and a fixed percentage of your future earnings will go to pay for its upkeep. Even after its death you must continue to pay until the accumulated costs to the state have been repaid."

"That's unfair," said Mrs. Straus. "We're being forced to go against what we think is right."

The facts about the AFP test are correct. But of course, there is no such law at this time. Should there be such a law?

Is it ever right to force people to act in ways that they consider to be morally wrong?

Should genetic screening programs be voluntary and advisory or should they be backed up by laws that aim at protecting society by requiring that individuals act in certain ways as the results of the screening?

What objections to involuntary screening are presented by Murray?

Would those in Rawls's original position be likely to favor compulsory screening laws?

Decision Scenario 2

"I'm sorry I wasn't able to bring you better news," Dr. Valery Mendez said. "I hope our first consultation helped prepare you for it."

Timothy Schwartz shook his head. "We gambled and lost," he said. "We can't say we didn't know what we were doing."

"That doesn't make it much easier," Judith Schwartz said. "When you said we were both Tay-Sachs carriers, I thought, 'Well, it won't happen to us.' But I was wrong."

"The odds were in our favor," Mr. Schwartz said. "I still think we did the right thing."

"Maybe we shouldn't even have had ourselves tested," Mrs. Schwartz said. "Then we wouldn't even know we've got a problem."

"But we'd have one anyway," her husband said. "Ignorance is bliss only when it's folly to be wise. Now we at least know what we're up against."

"What about this new test?" Mrs. Schwartz asked. "Can we really trust the results?"

"I'm afraid so," said Dr. Mendez. "The fetal cells taken during amniocentesis were cultured, and the chromosome study showed that the child you're carrying will have Tay-Sachs."

"What do you recommend?" Mr. Schwartz asked.

"It's not for me to recommend. I can give you some information—tell you the options—but you've got to make your own decision."

"Is abortion the only solution?" Mrs. Schwartz asked.

"If you call it a solution," Mr. Schwartz said.

"The disease is almost invariably fatal," Dr. Mendez said. "And there is really no effective treatment for it. A lot of people think there may be in the future, but that doesn't help right now."

"So what does it involve?" Mr. Schwartz asked.

"At first your child will seem quite normal, but that's only because it takes time for a particular chemical to build up in the brain. After the first year or so, the child will start to show signs of deterioration. He'll start losing his sight. Then as brain damage progresses, he'll lose control over his muscles, and eventually he will die."

"And we just have to stand by and watch that happen?" Mrs. Schwartz asked.

"Nothing can be done to stop it," Dr. Mendez said. "It's a terrible and sad disease."

"We certainly do want to have a child," Mr. Schwartz said. "But we don't want to have one that is going to suffer all his life. I don't think I could stand that."

Are there good utilitarian reasons for believing that the Schwartzes would be justified in choosing abortion in these circumstances?

How might a Kantian argue that it is their moral duty to the fetus as a potential person to choose abortion?

How persuasive is Kass's argument that genetic abortion constitutes a threat to the principle that each person is of equal worth?

Kass contends that none of the three standards he examines can allow us to justify selective abortion. State and evaluate his arguments.

Is this the sort of case in which Murray would consider ignorance to be bliss?

Decision Scenario 3

When Carla Lambrodi was thirty-eight years old she became pregnant for the first time. She was thirty-nine when her son Peter was born. Immediately after his birth, Peter was diagnosed as suffering from Down's syndrome.

Carla and her husband Thomas were both distraught that the child they had been hoping for and planning for should be so sadly abnormal. They had done everything that they knew to do to ensure that the baby would be healthy. Carla had gone to Doctor's Medical Center for regular checkups, had done the exercises prescribed for her, and had followed the diet she had been given.

"We knew I was older than most mothers," she said. "But I thought that the doctors would help me and advise me and that everything would be all right."

"We talked about abortion if anything went wrong," Thomas said. "We didn't like the idea, but we were both prepared to accept it. We didn't want an abnormal child. We didn't think it would be fair to us, and we didn't want to bring a child into the world that was doomed to suffer the way that Peter is."

The Lambrodi's were particularly upset and angry when they learned that Carla's physicians at the medical center had failed to tell her about the possibility of amniocentesis. Because of her age, the chance of Carla's having a child with Down's syndrome was significantly greater than the risk run by younger women. The test would have determined whether the fetus she was carrying had the genetic defect that causes the syndrome.

The Lambrodi's decided to sue Doctor's Medical Center for damages. They claimed that it was the duty of the physicians at the medical center to inform Carla Lambrodi of the risk that her child would be defective and to inform her about the possibility and advantages of amniocentesis.

The lawyers for the medical center argued that medical standards did not require physicians to inform their patients about the possibility of prenatal tests.

"Physicians exercise their judgment in dealing with patients," the lawyers argued. "They may decide that patients should have certain tests, but they have no duty to tell patients about the tests. It is the physicians who have the responsibility of caring for patients, and within the limits of the standards of good medical practice, the decision about what to tell patients is up to the physicians themselves."

Evaluate the argument formulated by the medical center lawyers.

If Kass is correct in his belief that there are no compelling considerations that justify selective abortion, then can it be right for a physician to inform a patient about a test that might have the effect of encouraging her to seek an abortion?

How might a rule utilitarian defend a physician's decision not to inform a patient about the possibility of prenatal genetic tests?

Is it compatible with the natural law view to hold both that abortion is wrong for genetic reasons and that a physician has a duty to inform patients about prenatal tests?

On what grounds might a Kantian argue that a physician has such a duty?

Decision Scenario 4

"The concept behind the bill is very simple, Senator," said Mrs. Laude. "We want to improve the human race, and we know exactly how to do it. The principles of genetics can be used to guide changes in the population."

"You mean," said the Senator, "you can make people smarter?"

"Not as individuals. But we can increase the level of intelligence in the society. We can do this by seeing to it that intelligent people have more children than the less intelligent. Over time, the statistical balance will shift towards intelligence."

"And does your draft of the bill make that possible?"

"By a system of financial incentives and disincentives," said Mrs. Laude. "Those above a certain level of intelligence will be offered a yearly stipend to pay part of the expenses for each of their children. Those below that level will receive nothing, and, having to bear the full cost themselves, they are likely to limit the number of children they have. We will also make use of genetic counseling programs to encourage or discourage children, whatever is appropriate in each case."

"These genetic counseling programs will be government run and supported?" the Senator asked.

"That's right. The law will require that everyone be screened and classified before his or her fifteenth birthday."

"Is intelligence all that you'll screen for?"

"It's the only positive trait we will try to increase. We will also screen against genetic diseases, like Tay-Sachs and sickle-cell anemia."

"This will be very controversial, you know," said the Senator.

"We know," Mrs. Laude said. "It will take a person of courage to introduce such a bill into the Senate. But we think it's the most important piece of legislation imaginable. The improvement of our society and of the whole human race will be the end result."

> *What problems and dangers are inherent in Mrs. Laude's proposal for a program of positive and negative eugenics?*
>
> *What can be said in defense of such a program?*
>
> *Would a utilitarian be likely to favor such a program?*
>
> *Could such a program be defended as compatible with Rawl's principles of justice?*
>
> *What arguments against any such program does Golding present?*

Decision Scenario 5

"Here's the theory," said Dr. Larry Torland. "Homocystinuria is produced because cystahionine synthetase is not available to catalyze the condensation of homocystine to form cystahionine."

"Another inborn error of metabolism," Cynthia Pruett said. "What are the clinical signs?"

"Renal hypertension, arterial thrombosis, myocardial infarction, and stroke are some of the outcomes. Usually there are skeletal abnormalities, variable mental retardation, progressive arterial thrombosis, and mental confusion that's easily confused with schizophrenia if you don't know what you're looking at. And of course there's a lot of homocystine excrete in the urine."

"Okay," Cynthia said. "Now get back to the theory."

"The enzyme we're talking about is produced in several places. In the kidney, the liver, and the brain primarily. Now one possibility is that it's not produced because there is a missing precursor. If that's the case, there's not much we can do."

"But there's another possibility?"

"Right. It may be that we're dealing with a missing or dysfunctioning gene the way we are in PKU or Tay-Sachs. So if we could get some cells in place that manufacture chystahionine sythetase, get them to multiply, they might produce enough CS to do some good."

"I assume there's no good therapy for this disease."

"None. It can be treated symptomatically by medical means, but there's no way to really bring it under control."

"So what are you going to try to do?" Cynthia asked.

"I've got a cell line already that will produce CS. It's one I developed from mouse tumor cells. I want to inject some into the kidney of a patient and just see if we can get some CS production."

"You're not going to use whole cells, are you?"

"Of course not," Larry said. "Just the DNA. I'm going to try for transformation."

"Do you have any animal data?" Cynthia asked.

"Not yet. I'm going to do a large-scale trial if I get a grant. But right now, I'm just going to go on the basis of the likelihood that the procedure might do some good."

"I think you're making a big mistake," Cynthia said.

On what grounds might one disapprove of the proposed therapy?

What sort of information, might we demand, should be available before the direct use of recombinant DNA as a part of therapy can be considered legitimate?

If the therapy is not likely to do any harm and if it holds the promise of doing some good and if the patient is fully informed, then what reason can there be for not employing the therapy?

What advantages are there to having review boards or committees decide when a proposed therapy can be employed? Are there any disadvantages?

Decision Scenario 6

"The trick," said Martin Anders, "is to make use of the virus as part of our production system."

"How's that?" Hilda Presti asked.

"The DNA of the virus contains a segment of DNA that we've introduced into it. When the virus attacks a bacterial cell, it injects its DNA into the cell. The viral DNA takes over the cell machinery enough to get the cell to make copies of the viral DNA and get it to synthesize the proteins that the DNA directs."

"That means then that if the proteins are something that are useful—like insulin—then you've got a chemical factory working under your control."

"That's the idea," said Anders. "We should be able to harness the powers of millions of bacteria to make what we want."

"Isn't that dangerous, though?" Presti asked.

"What do you mean?"

"Don't viruses also sometimes carry DNA segments that make the bacteria they infect resistant to antibiotics?"

"It's true," Anders nodded. "Sometimes they do. But we would be careful to select our viruses very carefully."

"Can you really be that careful? Isn't it possible that the viruses you use could start an epidemic of something like cholera, one that we wouldn't be able to control because antibiotics would be useless?"

"It could happen. I don't deny it. But the point is, the potential gains far outweigh the risks."

"Gains of what sort?" Presti asked.

"Two kinds," said Anders. "The gain in knowledge. We will learn a great deal about the biochemical mechanisms that regulate life processes. This knowledge may be applicable to humans. For example, we might someday be able to turn on the genes that direct the developmental processes so that we can regenerate lost or diseased organs. Second, there are more immediate gains, such as having a cheap source of biochemical products such as insulin. There really is no limit to what we might be able to do in the future."

"I'm afraid that one of the things that we might be able to do is to wipe out the human race," Presti said. "I think such research should be stopped."

One of the potential dangers of genetic engineering is mentioned here. What are some others?

Can the principles of utilitarianism be used to justify laws against conducting certain kinds of research?

Should moral principles ever be used to regulate research?

Is it possible to conduct research in a wholly "value-free" fashion?

What considerations mentioned by Sinsheimer might be used to support the claim that research of the sort described above should be prohibited?

Evaluate Cohen's critique of the arguments against research involving genetic engineering.

8

REPRODUCTIVE CONTROL:
IN VITRO FERTILIZATION,
ARTIFICIAL INSEMINATION, AND
STERILIZATION

CASE PRESENTATION
Louise Brown

Under other circumstances, the birth announcement might have been perfectly ordinary, the sort that appear in newspapers every day: *Born to John and Lesley Brown: a baby girl, Louise, 5 lbs. 12 ozs., 11:47 p.m., July 25, 1978, Oldham General Hospital (Oldham, England).*

But the birth of Louise Brown was far from being an ordinary event, and the announcement of its occurrence appeared in headlines throughout the world. For the first time in history, a child was born who was conceived outside the mother's body under controlled laboratory conditions.

Louise Brown was the world's first "test-tube baby."

For John and Lesley Brown, the birth of Louise was a truly marvelous event. "She's so small, so beautiful, so perfect," her mother told a reporter. "It was like a dream. I couldn't believe it," her father said.

The joy of the Browns was understandable, for, from the time of their marriage in 1969, they had both very much wanted to have a child. Then they discovered that Mrs. Brown was unable to conceive because of blocked fallopian tubes—the ova would not descend so fertilization could not occur. In 1970, she underwent an operation in an attempt to correct the condition, but the procedure was unsuccessful.

The Browns decided they would adopt a child, since they couldn't have one of their own. After two years on a waiting list, they gave up that plan. But the idea of having their own child was rekindled when a nurse familiar with the work of embryologist Robert Edwards and gynecologist Patrick Steptoe referred the Browns to them.

For the previous twelve years, Steptoe and Edwards had been working on the medical and biochemical techniques required for embryo transfer. Steptoe developed techniques for removing a ripened ovum from a woman's ovaries, then reimplanting it in the uterus after it has been fertilized. Edwards improved the chemical solutions needed to keep ova functioning and healthy outside the body and perfected a method of external fertilization with sperm.

Using their techniques, Steptoe and Edwards had successfully produced a pregnancy in one of their patients in 1975, but it had resulted in a miscarriage. They continued to refine their procedures and were confident that their techniques could produce a normal pregnancy that would result in a healthy baby.

They considered Lesley Brown an excellent candidate for an embryo transfer. She was in excellent general health, at thirty-one she was not too old for pregnancy, and she was highly fertile. In 1976, Steptoe did an exploratory operation and found that Mrs. Brown's fallopian tubes were not functional and could not be surgically repaired. He removed them so that he would have clear access to the ovaries.

In November of 1977, Mrs. Brown was given injections of a hormone to increase the maturation rate of her egg cells. Then in a small private hospital in Oldham, Dr. Steptoe performed a minor surgical procedure. Using a laparoscope—a tube with a built-in eyepiece and light source that is inserted through a tiny slit in the abdomen—to guide him he extracted an ovum with a suction needle from a ripened follicle.

The ovum was then placed in a small glass vessel containing biochemical nutrients and sperm that had been secured from John Brown. Once the egg was fertilized, it was transferred to another nutrient solution. More than fifty hours later, the ovum had reached the eight-cell stage of division. Guided by their previous experience and research, Steptoe and Edwards had decided that it was at this stage that an ovum should be returned to the womb. Although in normal human development, the ovum has divided to produce sixty-four or more cells before it completes its descent down the fallopian tube and becomes attached to the uterine wall, they had learned that attachment is possible at an earlier stage. The stupendous difficulties in creating and maintaining the proper biochemical environment for a multiplying cell made it reasonable to reduce the time outside the body as much as possible.

Mrs. Brown had been given another series of hormone injections to prepare her uterus. Two and a half days after the ovum was removed, a fertilized egg—an embryo—was reimplanted. Using a laparoscope and a hollow plastic tube (a cannula), Dr. Steptoe introduced the small sphere of cells into Mrs. Brown's uterus. It successfully attached itself to the uterine wall.

Mrs. Brown's pregnancy proceeded normally, but because of the special nature of her case, seven weeks before the baby was due, she entered the Oldham Hospital maternity ward so that she could be continuously monitored. About a week before the birth was expected, the baby was delivered by caesarean section. Mrs. Brown had developed toxemia, a condition associated with high blood pressure that can lead to stillbirth.

The baby was normal, and all concerned were jubilant. "The last time I saw the baby it was just eight cells in a test tube," Dr. Edwards said. "It was beautiful then, and it's still beautiful now." After the delivery, Dr. Steptoe said, "She came out crying her head off, a beautiful normal baby."

Mr. Brown almost missed the great event, because no one on the hospital staff had bothered to tell him that his wife was scheduled for the operation. Only when he had been gone for about two hours and called back to talk to his wife did he find out what was about to happen.

He rushed back and waited anxiously until a nurse came out and told him, "You're the father of a wonderful little girl." As he later told a reporter, "Almost before I knew it, there I was holding our daughter in my arms."

Like many ordinary fathers, he ran down the halls of the hospital telling people he passed, "It's a girl! I've got a baby daughter."

To calm down, he went outside and stood in the rain. It was there that a reporter from a London newspaper captured Mr. Brown's view of the event. "The man who deserves all the praise is Mr. Steptoe," he said. "What a man to be able to do such a wonderful thing."

Introduction

"Oh, brave new world that has such people in it!" exclaims Miranda in Shakespeare's *The Tempest*.

It is a phrase from this line that provided Aldous Huxley with the title for his dystopian novel *Brave New World*. A dystopia is the opposite of a utopia, and the future society depicted by Huxley is one which we are invited to view with shock and disapproval.

In this society, "pregnancy" is a dirty word, sex is purely recreational, and children are produced according to explicit genetic standards in the artificial wombs of state "hatcheries." Furthermore, an individual's genetic endowment determines the social position and obligations that he or she has within the society. Of course, everyone is conditioned to believe that the role he finds himself in is the best one to have.

In significant ways, that future is now. The new and still developing medical technologies of human reproduction have now reached a stage in which the technical innovations imagined by Huxley in 1932 to make such a society possible are well within the limits of feasibility.

We have no state hatcheries and no artificial uteruses. But we do have sperm banks and surrogate mothers. We have it within our power to remove an ovum from a woman's body, fertilize it, then return it so that it may develop into a child. By relatively simple surgical procedures, we can end forever the reproductive potentialities of otherwise fertile men or women.

The new technology associated with human reproduction is so powerful that it differs only in degree from that of Huxley's dystopian world. What we have yet to do is to employ the technology as part of a deliberate social policy to restructure our world along the lines imagined by Huxley.

Yet the potentiality is there. Perhaps more than anything else, it is the bleak vision of such a mechanistic and dehumanized future that has motivated much of the criticism of current reproductive technology. The "brave new world" of

Huxley is one in which traditional values associated with reproduction and family life, values based on individual autonomy, have been replaced by values of a purely social kind. In such a society, it is the good of the society or of the species, not the good of individuals, that is the touchstone of justification.

The possible loss of personal values is a legitimate and serious concern. The technologies of human reproduction are sometimes viewed as machines that may be employed to pave the road leading to a world of bleakness and loss. Yet it is important to remember that those same technologies also promise to enhance the lives of those presently living and to prevent potential suffering and despair.

Some women who are unable to bear children may now find it possible to do so through the use of in vitro fertilization techniques. Artificial insemination offers a means of impregnation when biological dysfunction makes the normal means impossible. Further, those women who would be at risk from becoming pregnant may now be protected by choosing surgical sterilization.

These are all potentialities that have become actualities; in vitro fertilization, artificial insemination, and sterilization are all procedures currently being performed. In the view of some, these procedures merely mark a beginning, and the possibilities inherent in reproductive technology still remain relatively unrealized. If we wish, we can employ the technology to change the very fabric and pattern of our society.

Should we do that? Or will the use of the technology necessarily promote the development of a dystopia? One way of thinking about these general questions is to turn once more to Huxley.

It is frequently overlooked that in 1962 Huxley published a utopian novel. Like the society in *Brave New World*, Huxley's ideal society also relies upon the principles of science, but in the ideal society they are used to promote autonomy and personal development.

Island portrays a society on the island of Pala that for over a hundred years has developed itself in accordance with the principles of reason and science. Living is communal, sexual repression is nonexistent, children are cared for by both their biological parents and other adults, drugs are used to enhance perceptual awareness, and social obligations are assigned on the basis of personal interest and ability.

More to the present point, the society makes use of reproductive technology to achieve its ends. It practices contraception, eugenics, and artificial insemination. Negative eugenics to eliminate genetic diseases is considered only rational. But more than this, by the use of "DF" and "AI" (Deep Freeze and Artificial Insemination), sperm from donors with superior genetic endowments is available for the use of couples who wish to improve their chances of having a child with special talents or with higher than usual intelligence.

Huxley's ideal society is not above criticism, even from those who are sympathetic toward the values he endorses. Yet *Brave New World* is such a powerful cautionary tale of what might happen if science were pressed into the service of repressive political goals that it makes it difficult to imagine other possible futures in which some of the same technology plays a more benign role. Since *Island* is an attempt to present such an alternate future, in thinking about the possibilities inherent in reproductive technology, fairness demands that we also consider Palinese society and not restrict our attention to the world of soma and state hatcheries.

In Vitro Fertilization

The birth of Louise Brown (see the Case Presentation) in 1978 was treated as a major media event. Photographs, television coverage, interviews, and news stories presented the world with minute details of the lives of the people involved and with close accounts of the technical procedures that had led to Louise's conception.

Despite the unprecedented character of the event, few people seemed surprised by it. The idea of a "test-tube baby" was one already familiar from fiction and folklore. The medieval alchemist was thought capable of generating life within his retorts, and hundreds of science fiction stories depicted a future in which the creation of life within the laboratory was an ordinary occurrence. In some ways, then, the birth of Louise Brown was seen as merely a matter of science and medicine catching up with imagination. (Indeed, they didn't quite catch up, for the "test tube" contained sperm and an egg, not just a mixture of chemicals.)

Although it is doubtful whether the public appreciated the magnitude of the achievement that resulted in the birth of Louise Brown, it was one of considerable significance. The first embryo transfer was performed in rabbits in 1890, but it was not until the role of hormones in reproduction, the nutritional requirements of developing cells, and the reproductive process itself were better understood that it became possible to consider seriously the idea of fertilizing an egg outside the mother's body and then returning it for ordinary development.

"In vitro" is a Latin phrase that means "in glass," and in embryology, it is used in contrast with "in utero" or "in the uterus." Ordinary human fertilization takes place in utero (strictly speaking, in the fallopian tubes) when a sperm cell unites with an ovum. In vitro fertilization, then, is fertilization that is artificially performed outside the woman's body—in a test tube, so to speak.

The ovum that produced Louise Brown was fertilized in vitro. But the entire process involved *embryo transfer*. That is, an ovum had to be taken from her mother's body, then after it was fertilized and had become an embryo, it was returned for in utero development.

Robert Edwards and Patrick Steptoe were the individuals responsible for developing and performing the techniques of in vitro fertilization and embryo transfer that led to the birth of Louise Brown. Basically, they followed a four-step process that has now become almost standard.

1. The patient is given a reproductive hormone in order to cause ova to ripen. A few hours before ovulation can be expected to occur, a small incision is made in the abdomen just below the navel. A laparoscope (an instrument with a built-in lens and light source) is inserted through the incision, and the ovaries are examined directly. When mature eggs are found that are about to break free from the thin walls of the ovarian follicle, the walls are punctured

and the contents are removed by a vacuum aspirator (a hollow suction needle). Several eggs may be removed.

2. The eggs are transferred to a nutrient solution that is biochemically similar to that found in the fallopian tubes. Sperm is then added to the solution. As soon as a single sperm cell penetrates the ovum, the ovum is fertilized.

3. The fertilized egg is transferred to another nutrient solution where, after about a day, it begins to undergo cell division. When the ovum reaches the eight-cell stage, it is ready to be returned to the uterus. The patient is given injections of hormones to prepare her uterus to receive the fertilized egg.

4. The small ball of cells is placed in the uterus through the cervix (the opening that leads to the vagina) by means of a hollow plastic tube called a cannula. The fertilized egg continues to divide, and somewhere between the thirty-two- and sixty-four-cell stage, it attaches itself to the uterine wall.

If the attachment is successful, from this point on, development should proceed as though fertilization had taken place in the ordinary fashion.

On December 28, 1981, Elizabeth Jordan Carr was born at Norfolk General Hospital, Norfolk, Virginia. She has the distinction of being the first baby conceived in vitro born in the United States. Like Louise Brown, she also weighed five pounds, twelve ounces, was born ahead of schedule and was perfectly healthy.

At present, at least fifteen babies have been born in this manner. Except for Elizabeth Carr, the births all took place in England or Australia. So far, more than a hundred women have become pregnant through the in vitro procedure, and the number can be expected to increase greatly in the future.

A number of American clinics (the first opened in Norfolk) are making use of the procedure in dealing with selected childless couples. The rate of success has not yet been great. The procedure involves a high level of skill on the part of the physician, and a great number of factors are involved.

However, most observers believe that as physicians gain in experience and as we acquire a better understanding of the relevant factors, the in vitro procedure will become a standard and quite commonplace treatment for infertility.

By virtue of being first, Louise Brown continues to be a symbol of what it is possible to achieve by the procedures pioneered by Steptoe and Edwards. But in the future it is likely that she will quietly take her place among the ranks of literally hundreds of others whose conception occurred in a glass bottle.

Benefits

Obviously, the processes involved in in vitro fertilization and embryo transfer are complicated and require a great amount of skill and knowledge. An obvious question to ask about the whole procedure is, what is to be gained by it? That is, what are the benefits of such a technically difficult and expensive medical procedure?

The most direct and perhaps the most persuasive answer is that in vitro fertilization makes it possible for many couples to conceive children who would not otherwise be able to do so. It is estimated that as much as 45 percent of all cases of female infertility is caused by abnormal or obstructed fallopian tubes. In such cases, although normal ova are produced, they cannot move down the tubes to be fertilized. In some cases, tissue blocking the tubes may be removed or the tubes may be reconstructed. In other cases, however, the tubes may be absent or impossible to repair. This means that the only way in which the woman can expect to have a child of her own is by means of in vitro fertilization.

At present, the in vitro fertilization procedures developed by Steptoe and Edwards produce pregnancies in only about 1 percent of the cases treated. Additional research, however, is very likely to increase the percentage of successful pregnancies and births. Thus, for many couples who once had no hope of having a child, there promises to be a realistic possibility of becoming parents.

Second, and quite ironically, research into improving in vitro fertilization and embryo transfer may lead to better and more effective contraceptives. This almost paradoxical result is due to the fact that the sort of knowledge required to make fertilization and reimplantation of the embryo successful is also knowledge that can be employed to prevent pregnancy. For example, a knowledge of the biochemical mechanism by which a sperm penetrates an ovum and renders the ovum impenetrable to all other sperm cells can be turned in the direction either of promoting fertilization or of preventing it. Similarly, understanding how the embryo attaches itself to the wall of the uterus may lead to methods for either decreasing or increasing the likelihood of an embryo's becoming attached.

Third, research with animals using the techniques of in vitro fertilization and embryo transfer can be employed to determine the ways in which various environmental toxins and drugs affect the developing fetus. At present, research groups are exposing fertilized monkey ova to chemicals, then reimplanting them. The aim is to discover the means by which specific chemicals alter development and result in defective offspring.

Such information is of obvious value. If we are to be successful in eliminating or reducing human birth defects that are caused by chemical agents, then we must know what the chemicals do. Only in such ways can safe levels of exposure be determined and steps taken to avoid or prevent the presence of environmental toxins and harmful ingredients in drugs.

These are just three of the more direct advantages associated with in vitro fertilization. Other possibilities inherent in the procedure might make up a substantial list. Here are merely two of them.

Gene repair.   The way in which the genetic code contained in the DNA of a fertilized egg directs the development of the egg into a baby is far from being understood. Nonetheless, fragments of the total picture are now emerging. The technology of recombinant DNA (see the Case Presentation of Chapter 7) has made it possible to isolate single genes and to identify their products. It is a long way from this stage to being able, for example, to outline all of the steps by which the heart develops. Yet such work is promising enough to fuel the hope that we shall eventually understand the way in which DNA controls the entire developmental process.

This kind of detailed knowledge might make it possible to locate defects in genes that, when uncorrected, lead to faulty development of the fetus. At present, to avoid the birth of a child with birth defects associated with damaged or missing genes, abortion is the only recourse.

Additional knowledge might allow faulty genes to be replaced or repaired. Thus, developmental failures like Down's syndrome and spinal bifida or heritable genetic defects like Tay-Sachs disease might be treated at the level of the genes. An entirely new chapter of fetal medicine would then be opened.

Surrogate mothers. This is perhaps the most dramatic possibility opened up by in vitro fertilization and embryo transfer. It has already been demonstrated in animal experiments that embryos from one female can be removed and transferred to another female to undergo the process of development and birth. Thus a cow that is considered genetically superior (in terms of milk production or resistance to disease, for example) can be artificially inseminated, then as many as sixteen embryos can be removed. Afterwards, the embryos can be implanted in the uteruses of less valuable cows. In this way, a desirable strain of cattle can be developed much more quickly than by ordinary breeding techniques.

Although a few people have advocated using "genetically superior" women as a source of ova and "less superior" women as surrogate mothers, it is highly unlikely that such a program will ever be endorsed by society. (See the Introduction to Chapter 7 for the difficulties in determining genetic "superiority.")

Nevertheless, the basic procedure might well be employed with human beings. A woman with an abnormal uterus who is not capable of a normal pregnancy might contribute an ovum that, after being fertilized in vitro, is implanted in the uterus of a second woman whose uterus has been prepared to receive it. The "host" or surrogate mother then carries the baby to term.

Surrogate mothers of a certain kind are already a fact of contemporary life. At least two cases have received widespread news coverage. In one of them, an unmarried woman who had never been pregnant agreed to be artificially inseminated, then give up the resulting child to a couple that was incapable of having a child of their own. In the other case, a woman was paid ten thousand dollars to bear a child for another childless couple.

These cases involve artificial insemination, rather than in vitro fertilization and embryo transfer. But the practice of employing a surrogate mother has already become established to a limited degree. Furthermore, the wives of the couples using the services of a surrogate mother were themselves unable to bear children. However, it is only a short step from being unable to bear children to being *unwilling* to bear children, though physically able.

Thus, it is easy to imagine that some women might choose to free themselves from the rigors of pregnancy by hiring a surrogate mother. The employer would be the source of the ovum, which would then be fertilized in vitro and implanted as an embryo in the uterus of the surrogate. Women who could afford to do so could have their own natural children without ever having to be pregnant.

An additional possibility is what has been called "prenatal adoption." A woman unable to ovulate normally, but otherwise capable of pregnancy, might choose to "adopt" an embryo carried by another woman. The embryo would be transferred to the first woman's uterus (after preparation by appropriate hormone injections), and there it would develop into a child. This procedure is not one that has been performed yet.

The possibilities inherent in in vitro fertilization and embryo transfer that have been mentioned here as sources of immediate or future benefits are all ones considered to be quite realistic by most researchers. By contrast, although it is possible to imagine such a thing, the development of "baby factories" or "hatcheries" similar to those described in *Brave New World* are technologically unlikely, judged in terms of current science and medicine. Machines would have to serve the function now served by the uterus, and designing such machines would require knowing enough about the needs of the developing fetus to reproduce that function. At the present, it is not possible even to state all the problems that would have to be solved.

Difficulties

This is not the place to discuss the ethical and social issues connected with the possibilities of in vitro fertilization mentioned above. There are aspects of the procedure itself and the current way in which it is being employed that some people find troublesome. Very briefly, we shall consider just five.

1. The ova that are removed for fertilization are not all used. Although they may all be mixed with sperm and several may be fertilized, only a single fertilized ovum is selected for implantation. The others are simply discarded.

For those who believe that human life begins at the moment of conception, the destruction of fertilized ova may be viewed as tantamount to abortion. Thus, for some people, the destruction may be regarded as destroying innocent human life.

Others, who are not prepared to ascribe the status of being a person to a fertilized ovum, may still be troubled by its pointless destruction. They may believe that its potentiality to develop, under certain conditions, into a human being at least requires that it be treated with concern and respect. Those who subscribe to such a view might well argue that the only legitimate form of in vitro fertilization is one in which the effort is made to fertilize only a single ovum. A failure in fertilization would then be similar to the failure that occurs naturally, and what would be eliminated would be the necessity of destroying fertilized eggs that cannot be implanted.

2. At present, when human in vitro fertilization is a wholly new procedure, it is impossible to assess the risks to the fetus and to the person it may become. A fetus that is conceived from an ovum that is removed to an alien environment and sustained by a nutrient solution that may not contain some necessary ingredients for development may well be at much greater risk than a fetus conceived in the ordinary way. Not only may the child be more likely to suffer defects evident at birth, but it may suffer some defects that will not show up until years later. (Mrs. Brown is rumored to have signed an agreement stating that she would submit to an abortion if there were signs that the fetus she was carrying was not developing normally.)

3. In vitro fertilization may encourage the development of eugenic ideas about improving the species. Rather than having children of their own, would-be parents might be motivated to seek out ova (and sperm) from people who

possess physical and intellectual characteristics that are particularly admired. Thus, even without an organized plan of social eugenics (see Chapter 7), individuals might be tempted to follow their own eugenic notions.

4. Similarly, would-be parents might be inclined to exercise the potential for control over the sex of their offspring. Only males contain both an X and a Y chromosome, and their presence is detectable in the cells of the developing embryo. Determination of the sex of the embryo would allow the potential parents to decide whether they wish to have a male or female child. Consequently, a potential human being (the developing fetus) might be destroyed for what is basically a trivial reason.

5. In vitro fertilization is likely to promote a social climate in which having children becomes severed from the family. The procedure places emphasis on the mechanics of fertilization and, in doing so, minimizes the significance of the shared love and commitments of the parents of a child conceived by normal intercourse. Furthermore, the procedure offers the opportunity for an unmarried woman to have a child without having anything at all to do with the biological father of the child.

Obviously, these difficulties are not ones likely to be considered equally serious by everyone. Those who do not believe that life begins at conception will hardly be troubled by the discarding of unimplanted embryos. Additional research and experience will no doubt reduce whatever risks there may be to a fetus conceived in vitro. Sex choice is possible now by the use of amniocentesis so is not a problem unique to in vitro fertilization, and the same is true of the implementation of eugenic ideas. Finally, whether in vitro procedures actually lead to a weakening of the values associated with the family is partly an empirical question that only additional use of the method will show. Even if childbearing does become severed from current family structure, it still must be shown that this is itself something of which we ought to disapprove. It is clearly not impossible that alternative social structures for childbearing and childrearing might be superior to ones currently dominant in western culture.

Artificial Insemination

In 1909, an unusual letter appeared in the professional journal *Medical World*. A. D. Hard, the author of the letter, claimed that when he was a student at Jefferson Medical College in Philadelphia, a wealthy businessman and his wife consulted a physician on the faculty about their inability to conceive a child.

A detailed examination of each of the people showed that the man was incapable of producing sperm. The case was presented for discussion in a class of which Hard was a member. According to Hard, the class suggested that semen should be taken from the "best-looking member of the class" and used to inseminate the wife.

The letter claimed that this was done while the woman was anesthetized and that neither the husband nor the wife were told about the process. The patient became pregnant and give birth to a son. The husband was then told how the pregnancy was produced, and, although he was pleased with the result, he asked that his wife not be informed.

The event described by Hard took place in 1884, and there is reason to believe that Hard was "the best-looking member of the class."

The Philadelphia case is generally acknowledged to be the first recorded instance of artificial insemination of donor sperm in a human patient. However, the process of artificial insemination itself has a much longer history. Arab horsemen in the fourteenth century apparently inseminated mares with semen-soaked sponges, and in the eighteenth century the Italian physiologist Spallansani documented experiments in which he fertilized dogs, reptiles, and frogs.

The first recorded case of the artificial insemination of a human being occurred in 1790, when the English physician John Hunter used semen obtained from a husband to inseminate his wife. Sporadic uses of the technique continued to occur in England, France, and the United States, and during the early part of the present century, they became more and more frequent. At present, probably more than two thousand children a year are born in this country who were conceived by artificial insemination.

Artificial insemination has become generally recognized as a legitimate medical procedure. The process is employed by hospitals, fertility clinics, and physicians who specialize in problems involving conception. Before looking at some of the ethical and legal issues involved in artificial insemination, it is useful to consider some relevant factual information about the process.

The Artificial Insemination Procedure

Artificial insemination is a relatively simple procedure. It is initiated one or two days before the woman's body temperature indicates that ovulation is about to take place. It is then repeated one or two more times until her body temperature shows that ovulation is completed. Typically, three inseminations are performed during a monthly cycle.

In the insemination, the patient is usually placed in a position so that her hips are raised. A semen specimen, collected earlier through masturbation or taken from a sperm bank, is placed in a syringe attached to a narrow tube or catheter. The catheter is gently inserted into the cervical canal and the semen is slowly injected into the uterus. The patient then stays in her position for fifteen or twenty minutes to increase the chances that the sperm will fertilize an ovum.

The overall success rate of artificial insemination is about 85 percent. Success on the first attempt is quite rare, and the highest rate occurs in the third month. In unusual cases, efforts may be made every month for as long as six months or a year. Such efforts are continued, however, only when a detailed examination shows that the woman is not suffering from some unrecognized problem preventing her from becoming pregnant.

When sperm taken from donors is used, the rate of congenital abnormalities is a little lower than that for the general population. There seems to be no evidence to support the fear that manipulating the sperm causes any harm. (Many physicians prefer to employ fresh, rather than frozen, sperm to minimize the amount of environmental change the sperm is subjected to. Other physicians claim that frozen sperm is to be preferred, for it provides a means of screening out defective cells or chromosome abnormalities.)

Reasons for Seeking Artificial Insemination

Artificial insemination may be sought for a variety of reasons. When a couple is involved, the reasons are almost always associated with physiological or physical factors that make it impossible for the couple to conceive a child in the usual sexual way.

About 15 percent of all married couples are infertile, and 40 percent of those cases are due to factors involving the male. In some instances, the male may be unable to produce any sperm at all (a condition called asospermia) or the number of sperm the male produces may be too low to make impregnation of the female likely (a condition called oligospermia). In other cases, adequate numbers of sperm cells may be produced, but they may not function normally. They may not be sufficiently motile to make their way past the vaginal canal and through the opening to the uterus. Hence, their chances of reaching and penetrating an ovum are slight. Finally, the male may suffer from a neurological condition that makes ejaculation impossible or from a disease (such as diabetes) which renders him impotent.

If the female cannot ovulate or if her fallopian tubes are blocked so that ova cannot descend, then artificial insemination can accomplish nothing. (See the section above on in vitro fertilization.) Yet there are factors affecting the female that artificial insemination can be helpful in overcoming. For example, if the female has a vaginal environment that is biochemically inhospitable to sperm, then artificial insemination may be successful. Because the sperm need not pass through the vagina, they have a better chance of surviving. Also, if the female has a small cervix (the opening to the uterus) or if her uterus is in an abnormal position, then artificial insemination may be used to deliver the sperm to an advantageous position for fertilization, a position they otherwise might not reach.

A couple might also seek artificial insemination for genetic reasons. Both may be carriers of a recessive gene for a genetic disorder (Tay-Sachs disease, for example) or the male may be the carrier of a dominant gene for a genetic disorder (Huntington's chorea, for example). In either case, the couple may not want to run the statistical risk of their child being born with a genetic disease. To avoid the possibility, they may choose to make use of artificial insemination with sperm secured from a donor.

The traditional recipient of artificial insemination is a married woman who, in consultation with her husband, has decided to have a child. Some physiological or physical difficulty in conceiving leads them to turn to artificial insemination.

But the traditional recipient is no longer the only recipient. Those seeking to have the procedure performed now include single women who wish to have a child but do not wish to have it fathered in the usual fashion. Some estimates place the number of such women at 150 a year. The percentages of such inseminations may increase in the future if the notion of being a single parent continues to be met with acceptance or approval within our society. The increase may be quite rapid if the attitudes of physicians, in particular, change. At present, single women who wish to become mothers are likely to be discouraged, and some physicians will not accept them as candidates for artificial insemination.

Types of Artificial Insemination

Artificial insemination can be divided into types in accordance with the source of the sperm employed in the procedure.

Artificial insemination (homologous) uses sperm obtained from the male partner. The name of the process is usually abbreviated as AIH, and the H is frequently taken to stand for "husband." While it is true that the male of a couple is most frequently the woman's husband, legal marriage is not necessary for AIH. The male need only be, in some sense, the functional equivalent of a husband.

Artificial insemination (heterologous) uses sperm from a sperm donor. For this reason, the process is usually referred to by the abbreviation AID. The use of semen obtained from a donor is the most frequent of AI procedures, and it is the one that gives rise to most of the social and legal issues surrounding the practice.

Artificial insemination (confused) employs a mixture of sperm from the male partner and sperm obtained from a donor. CAI, as it is commonly called, has no particular biological advantage, but it does offer a couple a degree of psychological support. Because they cannot be sure that it was not sperm from the male partner that resulted in conception, they may be more inclined to accept the child as the product of their union. The role of the third-party sperm donor is thus psychologically minimized.

Sperm Donors

Sperm donors are typically selected from medical-student and hospital-staff volunteers. An effort is made to employ as donors people in excellent health with a high level of intellectual ability. Their family histories are reviewed to reduce the possibility of transmitting a genetic disorder, and their blood type is checked to determine its compatibility with that of the AID recipient.

Such general physical features of the donor as body type, hair and eye color, and complexion are matched in a rough way with those of the potential parents. To be a donor, an individual must also be known to be fertile. This means that he must already be a biological parent or that he must fall within the normal range in several semen analyses.

Donors are typically paid for their services. What is more, their identity is kept secret from the recipient and her husband. A coding system is ordinarily used both to preserve the anonymity of the donor and to ensure that the same donor is used in all inseminations.

Sperm contributed by a donor might be employed in an insemination within one to three hours after the semen is obtained. As mentioned earlier, some physicians prefer to use freshly obtained sperm in the procedure. But sperm may also be maintained in a frozen condition and, after being restored to the proper temperature, used in the same way as fresh sperm. Sperm banks are no more than freezers containing racks of coded plastic tubes holding donated sperm.

The semen stored in sperm banks is not necessarily that of anonymous donors. For a variety of reasons, individuals may wish to have their sperm preserved and pay a fee to a sperm-bank operator for this service. For example, a man planning a vasectomy (see the section on sterilization below) or one expecting to become sterile because of a progressive disease may store his sperm in the event that he may later want to father a child.

Issues in Artificial Insemination

Artificial insemination presents a great variety of moral, legal, and social issues. The truth is, most of those issues have not been addressed in a thorough fashion. Legal scholars have explored some of the consequences that AI has for traditional legal doctrines of paternity, legitimacy, and inheritance. They have also made recommendations for formulating new laws (or reformulating old ones) to take into account the reality of the practice of AI.

Others who have written about AI have mostly focused on its potential for altering the relationship between husbands and wives and for producing undesirable social changes. Many of the objections to in vitro fertilization have also been offered to artificial insemination. For example, it has been argued that AI will take the love out of sexual procreation and make it a purely mechanical process, that AI will promote the practice of eugenics and so denigrate the worth of babies that fall short of some ideal, and that AI is just another step down the road toward the society of *Brave New World*.

While such issues are of great importance, they have usually been discussed in such a general fashion that specific ethical questions about the use of artificial insemination as a medical procedure have rarely been raised. As a result, those questions have not been subjected to the dialectical process of argument and criticism that is important in helping us arrive at reasoned opinions.

Some of the issues that need close attention from philosophers concern individual rights and responsibilities. This is not the place for a discussion of such issues, but at least a few of them ought to be mentioned to indicate the sort of intellectual work that needs to be done. For example, does a man who has served as a sperm donor have any special moral responsibilities? He certainly must have some responsibilities. For example, it would be wrong for him to lie about any genetic diseases in his family history. But does he have any responsibilities to the child that is produced by AI employing his sperm? If donating sperm is no different from donating blood, then perhaps he does not. But is such a comparison apt?

Can a child born as a result of AI legitimately demand to know the name of his biological father? We need not assume that mere curiosity might motivate such a request. Someone might need to know his family background in order to determine how likely it is that a potential child might have a genetic disorder. After all, it is unreasonable to assume that a donor is fully informed about his own biological background. Perhaps the current practice of maintaining the anonymity of sperm donors is not one that can stand critical scrutiny.

Should a woman be allowed to order sperm donated by someone who approximates her concept of an ideal person? Should she be able to request a donor from a certain ethnic group, with particular eye and hair color, certain minimum or maximum height, physical attractiveness, with evidence of intelligence, and so on? At present, the physician who performs the procedure also makes the choice of the donor. But why should the physician be granted the right to make the selection? One might argue that allowing the physician to exercise such a power violates the autonomy of the AI recipient.

A number of other ethical questions are easily raised about AI: Does any woman (married or single, or any age) have the right to demand AI? Can a wife justifiably refuse AI when her husband wishes her to receive it? Can a wife decide to receive AID, even if her husband is opposed?

Other questions concerning the proper procedures to follow in the practice of AI are also of considerable significance. For example, how thoroughly must sperm donors be screened for genetic defects? What standards of quality must sperm as a biological material be required to satisfy? What physical, educational, or general social traits (if any) should individual donors possess? Should records be maintained and shared through an established network to prevent the marriage or mating of individuals born from AID with the same biological father?

At present, these questions have been answered only by individual physicians or clinics, if at all. There are no general medical or legal policies that govern the practice of AI. Even if present practices are adequate, most people would agree that there is a need to develop uniform policies to regulate AI.

Obviously, we have touched upon only a few of the ethical and social issues that the practice of artificial insemination generates. Indeed, at the moment, it is not wholly clear even what the more significant issues may be. In this area of medical ethics, in particular, philosophers still have a great deal of work to do.

Sterilization

A person is *sterile* when he or she is biologically incapable of reproduction, either because of an inability to produce or supply sex cells (gametes) or because of a more general physiological condition.

Sterility may be the natural result of a variety of causes. In women, for example, undeveloped fallopian tubes may make it impossible for ova to descend to be fertilized. In men, viral diseases such as mumps may impair the capacity of the testes to produce sperm.

Sterility may also be an incidental result of a medical or surgical procedure required for the treatment of an illness. Radiation therapy, for example, may lead to sterility in both men and women. Or the treatment of certain kinds of cancer may require the removal of the ovaries, thus destroying a woman's ability to produce ova.

Finally, sterility may be produced deliberately by surgical intervention. That is, surgery may be performed with the sole aim of rendering the patient incapable of biological reproduction. The most common procedure employed with men is *vasectomy*. This involves the surgical removal of a segment of the vas deferens, the tube that transfers sperm cells to the ejaculatory duct. Although ejaculation remains unimpaired, the ejaculate will no longer contain sperm cells. The surgery involved is relatively minor.

The most frequent sterilization procedure used with women is *tubal ligation.* A surgical incision is made in the abdominal wall to gain access to the fallopian tubes. Then the tubes are simply tied off so that the ova produced by the ovaries cannot descend to the uterus. The surgery has more risk associated with it than does vasectomy, but it is considered a relatively simple and safe procedure.

The next most common means of female sterilization is *total hysterectomy.* In this procedure, the entire uterus (womb) is removed. After an ovum is fertilized by a sperm cell, during the ordinary course of development, the embryo attaches itself to the wall of the uterus. Thus, removal of the uterus makes it impossible for a woman to have children. (There must be good medical reasons to remove the ovaries when a hysterectomy is performed, for their excision leads to hormonal disturbances. Removing the ovaries just for the purpose of sterilization is not considered good medical practice.) A hysterectomy is regarded as a major surgical procedure, and it involves a much greater risk to the patient than tubal ligation.

Voluntary Sterilization

Some people choose sterilization voluntarily as a method of contraception. Since it is almost totally reliable as a means of birth control, those who are certain that they want to surrender their option to have children may select sterilization for this reason.

The preferred procedures for contraceptive sterilization are vasectomy and tubal ligation. Although the consequences of both can sometimes be reversed surgically (less often with vasectomy), the results are more reasonably thought of as permanent.

Except for those who accept a natural law view of sexual reproduction, voluntary sterilization as a contraceptive measure has not been *in itself* the source of major ethical or social controversy. However, in connection with questions about coercion and individual rights under publicly funded welfare and medical assistance programs, voluntary sterilization has been at the center of a political and ethical storm.

In 1973, it was called to public attention that a clinic in Alabama had sterilized a number of girls under circumstances that suggested either a misunderstanding of what was involved or lack of proper consent. Two of the girls, Minni Relf (age fourteen) and Mary Alice Relf (twelve) were the daughters of Lonni Relf, a poor black man from Montgomery. Mr. Relf was called to testify at a federal hearing in Washington. "I didn't want it done," he told the committee.

Partly as a result of the hearing, federal regulations were issued in 1974 to attempt to guarantee that sterilization would always be voluntary. Despite the regulations, studies by both an independent consumer group and the federal General Accounting Office showed that abuses were not only continuing, but actually seemed to be increasing.

In particular, vulnerable groups such as Indian and Hispanic women, poor blacks, minors, and women just recovering from pregnancy were found to be the targets of a disproportionately large number of sterilizations of doubtful legitimacy. Furthermore, those who agreed to sterilization were often subjected to full hysterectomies, rather than the simpler and safer procedure of tubal ligation. The reason for selecting the more complicated and dangerous procedure seemed to have more to do with the surgeon's desire for challenge than with any legitimate medical reason.

When asked why he chose to perform a hysterectomy to sterilize a patient, one surgeon is reported to have replied: "It's more of a challenge. You know, a well-trained chimpanzee can do a tubal ligation. . . . [A hysterectomy] is good training."

In 1977, the federal government reaffirmed its regulations governing sterilization and proposed to cut off funds to clinics and hospitals if there was evidence that the rules were not being followed. The regulations require that a person be given a "fair" explanation of the sterilization procedure, that the benefits and risks be pointed out, and that the irreversible character of the procedure be made clear. The person must also be informed orally before the question of consent is raised that a refusal to accept sterilization will not be used as a basis for denying welfare benefits. The same information must also appear on a consent form, and a seventy-two-hour waiting period is required between the time the consent form is signed and the surgery is performed.

In addition, in keeping with the 1974 regulations, federal funds cannot be used to sterilize anyone under the age of twenty-one or anyone who is not mentally competent. A federal district court injunction extended these same restrictions to sterilization under state laws.

The federal regulations are clearly aimed at protecting the welfare of those groups that are most vulnerable to pressures to consent to sterilization—the poor, minors, and the mentally incompetent. However, critics of the regulations maintain that they are so strict that they actually deny to women who are dependent on public assistance for their medical care the right to make a decision about their own bodies. While women with money can ordinarily arrange for sterilization without question or delays, purely as a result of their own decision, poor women must have their decisions subjected to a government policy and its requirements. Thus, according to the critics, the regulations are no more than a case of unjustifiable paternalism.

Opponents of the regulations object particularly to the mandatory waiting period. They point out that it prevents a woman from being sterilized at the end of a pregnancy while still in the hospital. If she chooses sterilization surgery, she must say that she does, then return to the hospital at additional public and private cost, and once more undergo the risk of anesthesia. Consequently, poor women are more subject to government interference in their private lives than are women with adequate financial resources.

Even the requirement that minors be considered ineligible for sterilization paid for by federal funds is not acceptable to critics of the regulations. They contend that age is not itself an indicator of maturity. In their view, it should be left up to the patient's physician to determine whether she adequately understands the nature and consequences of sterilization—even if the patient is a minor. Like any other medical or surgical procedure, informed consent should be required, and it is the job of the physician to make certain this condition is met. If it is not, then the physician ought to be held liable.

Both defenders and critics of the regulations agree that the sterilization of the mentally incompetent poses special problems.

Involuntary Sterilization and the Mentally Incompetent

Starting at the beginning of this century, a complicated network of federal, state, and even city laws and regulations governing sterilization has developed. Many of the laws were inspired by the eugenics movement of the 1920s and 1930s and were intended to "improve" the human race by preventing the "mentally and morally defective" from reproducing.

The most influential court decision from this period was the 1927 Supreme Court ruling in *Buck* v. *Bell*. Carrie Buck was (in the language of the time) a "feeble-minded" white patient at an institution in Virginia. She was the daughter of a feeble-minded woman confined to the same institution, and she herself was the mother of an illegitimate feeble-minded child.

According to a Virginia law, whenever the superintendent of a state institution considered it in the best interest of the patient and society, a patient "afflicted with hereditary forms of insanity and imbecility" might be considered a candidate for sterilization. A hearing was then held by a special board, and if the board ruled in favor of sterilization, then the patient or her representative might appeal to the courts. Otherwise, the sterilization would take place.

An appeal all the way to the Supreme Court was made on behalf of Carrie Buck, and Justice Oliver Wendell Holmes wrote the majority opinion upholding the Virginia law:

> We have seen more than once that the public welfare may call upon the best citizens for their lives. It would be strange if it could not call upon those who already sap the strength of the state for these lesser sacrifices . . . in order to prevent our being swamped with incompetence. It is better for all the world if, instead of waiting to execute degenerate offspring for crime, or to let them starve for their imbecility, society can prevent those who are manifestly unfit from continuing their kind . . . Three generations of imbeciles are enough.

The Holmes opinion relied on an analogy with laws requiring vaccination. The implicit view was that if we can require vaccination in order to protect the society from the spread of infectious diseases, then we can require sterilization to protect society from the spread of feeble-mindedness.

Holmes's opinion and the sterilization laws themselves rest on assumptions about the nature of mental retardation and mental illness that we now recognize to be both simplistic and fundamentally in error. Mental deficiency varies greatly in severity and can have many causes, many of which are quite unknown. Although some forms of mental impairment involve an indirect genetic component, the most common forms do not. Furthermore, there is no evidence at all to show a causal connection between mental deficiency and crime. So far as "hereditary forms of insanity" are concerned, there is good evidence to show that schizophrenia involves a genetic factor, but the evidence is not conclusive. In addition, the pattern of heritability is not as simple as that assumed in the nineteenth and early twentieth centuries.

The sterilization laws and the Supreme Court decision are an outstanding example of how common beliefs and prejudices can do a great deal of social damage when they are used as a substitute for reliable scientific knowledge. To some extent, we are continuing to pay today for the complacent ignorance of an earlier time.

Some twenty-seven states still have so-called involuntary sterilization laws. Yet medical, legal, and public attitudes toward sterilizing the mentally deficient have undergone a radical change. Today no responsible person advocates the compulsory sterilization of the mentally incompetent. However, most of those who do not oppose sterilization in principle also believe that people who are mentally impaired ought to have the same right to sterilization as those of normal intelligence.

The basic moral and social difficulty consists in providing access to sterilization for the mentally deficient, while protecting them from coercion. The federal regulations discussed earlier forbid the sterilization of minors and those incapable of giving informed consent.

Most professionals who work with the mentally handicapped tend to support these restrictions. At present, there are some five million mentally deficient people in the United States. Most of them can care for themselves and many hold jobs and have families. There are, however, about three hundred thousand people who are profoundly retarded and require care and supervision.

It is this last group that presents the most difficulty for any policy about sterilization. If they are incapable of giving informed consent, then under the government regulations, they cannot receive sterilization surgery. This has led some people to object that in attempting to protect the mentally deficient, the restrictions deny them a right open to others. Furthermore, the restrictions implicitly force the families of such people to bear all the responsibility for the retarded person's sexual conduct and any resulting pregnancies or births. Families are thus deprived of a means of dealing with the problems that they face.

This is essentially the view taken by three groups of parents in Hartford, Connecticut who decided to fight a legal battle to have their daughters sterilized. The girls are aged twelve, thirteen, and fifteen; all are blind and severely retarded, and one is deaf.

A hospital in Hartford refused to allow sterilization surgery to be performed, even though the parents requested it and physicians who were consulted agreed that the surgery would be beneficial to the girls. The parents tried several other private hospitals in the area, but they also refused the sterilization request.

The federal regulations do not apply to patients whose expenses are privately paid. Nevertheless, the lawsuits based on the regulations have had a general effect on the medical community and made hospitals and physicians reluctant to perform sterilizations in cases in which consent is at issue. Because the children in the Hartford case were not institutionalized, relevant state laws were not applicable to them either. As a result, the hospitals in Hartford moved in the direction of legal and social pressure and refused to allow the sterilizations.

A court has yet to decide the outcome of the suit by the Hartford parents. But the case itself dramatically reveals the difficulty of finding a satisfactory way of protecting mentally defective people, while allowing actions to be taken in their interest.

Ethical Theories and Reproductive Control

One of the themes of Mary Shelley's famous novel *Frankenstein* is that it is both wrong and dangerous to tamper with the natural forces of life. It is wrong because it disturbs the natural order of things, and it is dangerous because it unleashes forces beyond human control. The "monster" that is animated by Dr. Victor Frankenstein stands as a warning and reproach to all who seek to impose their will on the world through the powers of scientific technology.

The fundamental ethical question about the technology of human reproductive control is whether it ought to be employed at all. Is it simply wrong for us to use our knowledge of human biology to exercise power over the processes of human reproduction?

The natural law view, as represented by currently accepted doctrines of the Roman Catholic Church, suggests that all three of the techniques for controlling human reproduction that we have discussed here are fundamentally wrong.

Children may ordinarily be expected as a result of sexual union within marriage. However, if no measures are wrongfully taken to frustrate the possibility of their birth (contraception, for example), then a married couple has no obligation to attempt to conceive children by means such as artificial insemination or in vitro fertilization.

Indeed, those processes themselves are inherently objectionable. Artificial insemination requires male masturbation, which is prima facie wrong, since it is an act that can be considered to be unnatural, given the natural end of sex. Furthermore, AI, even when semen from the husband is used, tends to destroy the values inherent in the married state. It makes conception a mechanical act.

In vitro fertilization is open to the same objections. In addition, the process itself involves the destruction of fertilized ova. On the view that human conception takes place at the moment of fertilization, this means that the discarding of unimplanted embryos amounts to the destruction of human life.

Sterilization, whether voluntary or not, is also inherently wrong, for it involves defeating the natural purpose of the reproductive organs. Furthermore, according to the principle of totality, we have a natural duty to preserve the integrity of our bodies. This means that any procedure that involves "mutilation" or the destruction of the capacity of an organ to function properly is morally wrong. Thus, vasectomies and tubal ligations are both ruled out. (Of course, if sterilization is the unintended consequence of a surgical procedure required to save the patient's life, then it is not wrong. We have a natural duty to preserve our lives, and the principle of double effect justifies such unintended sterilizations.)

On the utilitarian view, no reproductive technology is in itself objectionable. The question that has to be answered is whether the use of any particular procedure, in general or in a certain case, is likely to lead to more good than not. In general, it is reasonable to believe that a utilitarian would be likely to approve of the three sorts of procedures we have discussed here.

However, it is worth mentioning that a rule utilitarian might well oppose any or all of the procedures. If there is strong evidence to support the view that the use of reproductive technology will lead to a society in which the welfare of its members will not be served, then a rule utilitarian would be on firm ground in arguing that reproductive technology ought to be abandoned.

According to Ross's ethical theory, we have prima facie duties of beneficence. That is, we have an obligation to assist others in bettering their lives. This suggests that the use of reproductive technology may be justified as a means to promote the well-being of others. For example, if a couple desires to have a child but is unable to conceive one, then either in vitro fertilization procedures or artificial insemination might be employed to help them satisfy their shared desire.

Similarly, if someone wishes to be sterilized for the purpose of contraception, then there seems to be no reason why he or she should not be. Of course, there is also a prima facie duty to avoid causing anyone harm. This means that we have an obligation to make certain that a candidate for voluntary sterilization understands the nature and consequences of the procedure. In effect, informed consent is required. Thus, in cases where consent may be in question, sterilization may not be legitimate.

Is the involuntary sterilization of the mentally incompetent ever right on Ross's view? One could argue that it sometimes is. If a person is unable to care for herself, then it may be that we have a duty to promote her interest by removing the possibility that she will be burdened by a child. It may be that by performing a sterilization procedure we are doing her no harm and are, in fact, acting beneficently.

Kantian principles do not seem to supply grounds for objecting either to in vitro fertilization or to artificial insemination as inherently wrong. However, the maxim involved in each action must always be one that satisfies the categorical imperative. Consequently, some instances of in vitro fertilization and artificial insemination would no doubt be morally wrong.

It is not clear whether Kantian principles would make the involuntary sterilization of the mentally retarded an unethical procedure. One could argue that sterilization without consent would violate the autonomy of the person. The act might provide benefits for the person's family or for society, but this would offer no legitimate justification. We would be treating the person as a means to satisfy the wishes of others and not as an end in herself.

However, in contrast, one might argue that in dealing with a severely retarded person who is incapable of giving meaningful consent, we have a duty to treat the person in a way that acknowledges her intrinsic worth. This may mean doing for her what she would do for herself if she were rational and seeking her own welfare. Thus, sterilization might be justifiable if it is done for her sake only.

The technology of reproduction is a reality of ordinary life. So far it has made our society into neither a dystopia nor a utopia. It is just one set of tools among the many others that science and medicine have forged.

Yet the tools are powerful ones, and we should beware of allowing familiarity to produce indifference. The moral and social issues raised by reproductive technology are just as real as the technology. So far we have not treated some of them with the seriousness that they deserve.

The Selections

Before the birth of Louise Brown, Paul Ramsey vigorously argued against the moral legitimacy of in vitro fertilization. In his view, it was more a kind of experimentation than a form of therapy. One of Ramsey's major objections was that the procedure subjected the potential child to unknown risks. In "Manufacturing Our Offspring," Ramsey continues to maintain that, despite the apparent good health of Louise Brown, the procedure is unacceptable. The earlier trials in fertilization are not justified by successful results, and the risk of injury to the unborn still remains.

Ramsey is also much concerned about the future developments that may follow in vitro fertilization. Its very success, he fears, will encourage more experimentation and even more radical changes in human reproduction—the creation of chimeras (formed by joining cells from humans and animals), sex-choice procedures, and the development of artificial wombs. The great risk, for Ramsey, is that human procreation will lose its humanity and become a form of mechanical reproduction—that Huxley's hatcheries will become a reality.

John A. Robertson deals directly with the two basic issues raised by Ramsey. First, Robertson points out, our society will not necessarily move toward the sort of dehumanized reproduction feared by Ramsey. How far we wish to go with any biomedical technology is a decision we must make, and it is quite possible that we might wish to accept in vitro conception but reject the establishment of hatcheries.

Second, Robertson does not see the problems associated with risks to the potential child as sufficiently compelling to forbid the in vitro procedure. If one has no objection to abortion in general, then the higher risk of spontaneous abortion is not a persuasive reason. Moreover, now that the procedure has been demonstrated to be relatively safe, there are no good utilitarian grounds for rejecting it.

The general deontological principle that it is wrong to impose a burden to benefit others without the consent of the burdened might seem to make in vitro fertilization prima facie wrong. Knowingly risking a deformed birth to benefit the desires of the parents for a child might be thought to violate the right of the child. But, Robertson claims, this position is misconceived. At the time of conception, there was no child with rights to be violated. We cannot respect a person's rights by refraining from an action that prevents his existence.

Robertson's general view is that it is proper for the state both to regulate in vitro procedures to minimize the frequency of abnormal births and to encourage couples to seek other alternatives. However, banning in vitro techniques totally would not be justified.

In the selection "Artificial Insemination: The Legal Position Today," Walter Wadlington reviews the history of court decisions on issues involving AI. Wadlington himself presents no argument in this selection, but the reasoning behind the court decisions is mentioned in his account. What is particularly worth noticing are the specific issues in contention, for these are issues that have moral as well as legal dimensions. Questions that arise concern AI and adultery, legitimacy, paternity, parental responsibilities and rights, and the duties of the physician who performs an AI procedure. These are questions with substantial philosophical content that deserve close attention.

In the last selection, George J. Annas lists three possible positions that courts can take with respect to the sterilization of the mentally retarded: to refuse approval where consent is not possible, to approve when sterilization is in the best interest of the individual, and to take a "*Quinlan*-type" approach and leave the decision in the hands of the individual's family and physician. Annas reviews the New Jersey case of Lee Ann Grady, in which the state Supreme Court, the same court that made the *Quinlan* decision, took the second approach. Most important, Annas presents the kind of evidence the court considered relevant to establish that sterilization is indeed in the best interest of the individual. Annas suggests that this approach is one that avoids the drawbacks of total prohibition and also provides protection for the person concerned.

Manufacturing Our Offspring: Weighing the Risks

Paul Ramsey

Pope Pius XII once warned against reducing the cohabitation of married persons to the transmission of germ life. This would, he said, "convert the domestic hearth, sanctuary of the family, into nothing more than a biological laboratory" (*Acta Apostolicae Sedis* 43:850 [1951]). That quaint language was spoken about artificial insemination. The Pontiff feared the nemesis of humanity under the fluorescent light of laboratories. He warned of this in 1951—eons ago!

For more than a decade, medical teams have been racing to bring to birth a baby fertilized in a laboratory. The British team of Steptoe and Edwards is the winner. "Brown" is an ordinary name; the father is a railway worker, the mother a Lancashire housewife. Baby Louise Brown is not so ordinary. On the advice of the gynecologist Patrick C. Steptoe an agent has been hired, supposedly to protect the Browns from undue pressure and to guarantee the newborn Brown a good start in life. To the fluorescent light of the laboratory has been added the media spotlight.

The Possibility of Damage

The first question to be raised concerns damage to the new Brown from these procedures in their entirety. In a 1974 scientific article the other member of the winning team, Robert G. Edwards, a physiologist at Cambridge University, asserted,

Reprinted with permission of the author and The Hastings Center from Hastings Center Report, *8 (October 1978): 7–9.* © *Institute of Society, Ethics and the Life Sciences, 360 Broadway, Hastings-on-Hudson, NY 10706.*

"if there is no undue risk of deformity additional to those of natural conception, and publicity is avoided, the children should grow up and develop normally and be no more misfits than other children born today after some form of medical help" (R. G. Edwards, "Fertilization of Human Eggs in Vitro: Morals, Ethics and the Law," *The Quarterly Review of Biology*, 49:1 [March 1974], 3-26). Here Edwards raised two points: how we were to estimate "undue" additional risks of deformity (and whether *any* such risks should be imposed) and the psychological damage that may result if publicity is not avoided.

On the first point, Edwards argues for fifteen pages that there is no risk of deformity from the procedure. I understand why the risks are very low. The developing life (the blastocyst, not yet called the embryo) that is manipulated is a cluster of cleaving cells. These cells have "totipotency." As yet none is on its way to become, say, blood, or has "clicked-off" its potency for becoming, say, a liver cell or a bone. At this point in human development the individual (like an earthworm) can renew itself even if momentarily injured. After differentiation into various tissues and organs, the embryo and fetus is more vulnerable to irreversible damage; for example, from thalidomide taken by the mother during pregnancy.

However small, there is still risk of induced injury. The question of "undue" additional risk remains at the heart of the moral question whether human genesis should ever have been attempted in this way. Having carefully built the case for no undue risk in his article, Edwards then spends four pages warning all participants in this procedure that they are liable to "wrongful life" suits for tort compensation. As defendants, all the participants would have to prove that any damage did not result from manipulating the blastocyst. (Among the parties liable, and to be warned, is the "semen donor," not only the husband—which shows that the procedure is not intended to be used only to the good end of overcoming a married women's oviduct blockage.)

I was stunned by this contradiction in a single article by an eminent scientist because heretofore I had supposed that only theologians were reputed to "fudge" in their arguments. In any case, the knowledge that one may induce injury, though not predictable, cannot be excluded. This seems to me to be significant in a conclusive moral argument against the experiments that have gone on

for more than a decade. Moreover, if the new Brown is normal as announced, this will prove only that this kind of human genesis is now and for the future not to be condemned for this reason. Such success will not show that all the past trials at irremovable possible risk (including baby Brown's) were for that period of time excusable.

I once expressed the "macabre 'hope'" that the first child conceived by laboratory fertilization would prove to be a bad result—and that it be well advertised, not hidden from view. That might halt the practice! Edwards missed my irony, failing to note that I also said: "I do not actually believe that the good to some from public revulsion in such an event would justify the impairment of that child. But then for the same reasons, neither is the manipulation of embryos a procedure that can possibly be morally justified"—even if the result happens to be a Mahalia Jackson. (Paul Ramsey, "Shall We 'Reproduce?'," *Journal of the American Medical Association*, 220:11 [June 12, 1972], 1482). A small risk of grave induced injury is still a morally unacceptable risk.

The Damage of Publicity

Concerning the second source of possible grave damage—publicity—I do not know whether or why Edwards changed his mind. Perhaps there was only a breakdown of communication between him and Steptoe who advised that Louise Brown be capitalized from birth. One can speculate, however, as follows concerning the dilemma the winning team faced. They needed to prove their accomplishment to the scientific community and to the world at large. A British doctor had announced previously that there were one or more babies already born in Europe by this procedure. He offered no proof, and was disbelieved. Nobody wins a Nobel prize for science that way.

If the Steptoe-Edwards team wanted both to advance science and/or their scientific reputations and to protect the next Brown from damaging publicity, they should have tried to create a new "institution" for doing both. The British Medical Association could have been asked to appoint a monitor who could now certify the team's achievement while at the same time avoiding publicity focused upon the subjects (the Browns) with whom the scientist-physician have achieved their success.

In the absence of this anticipatory solution,

there was no other recourse than to try to control the publicity and to enable Louise Brown to garner the revenues. This baby will be hailed or stigmatized all her life as the first laboratory-fertilized progeny to be birthed in all human history. Think of the enormity of that reputation! If this child is not physically or psychologically damaged from its beginning, socio-psychological ruin seems invited. If she is the world's best tennis player or if she becomes a juvenile delinquent, the outcome will be explained or excused by her unique genesis. Mahalia Jackson had a more obscure and normal passage into maturity. So also did the parents Brown, and Drs. Steptoe and Edwards. What now have they visited upon this child?

We are told that this sort of "assisted pregnancy" is a "far cry" from Aldous Huxley's pharmacological, genetic, and womb-free paradise. This is true for the moment. Women with fallopian tube blockage now will be able with their husbands to have children. That is all.

Doris Del Zio* says that she only wanted a child, although the press begins to report or insinuate that Doris and John Del Zio now say that they might have been the "first." Destructive prevention of that notoriety could also be cause for damage claims in our commercial civilization. Clearly, however, Doris's egg and John's sperm and the cultured blastocyst (if such it was) belonged to them and to no one else. On the other hand a physician is not a patient's plumber. He has professional standards, and is held to them by review committees.

Still there is more to be said about medical and public policy than that a woman's infertility can be "cured." This medical technology is another "long step for mankind" toward Aldous Huxley's "Brave New World." Host "mothers" with wombs-for-hire are immediately possible. Nothing technically limits the fertilization to the husband's sperm. We already have sperm banks. Egg banks will be next. People will be able to go to either to select. Bearing the child can be arranged by contract and financial payment. The consequences to come from opening of the human uterus to medical technological control are not likely to contribute to the emancipation of women.

There is still more. We are not limited to human progeny growing their own natural genetic endowments. We are not limited to the child Lesley Brown has or Doris Del Zio wanted. Gene splicing soon can be done before the blastocyst or embryo is transferred to the womb of the woman— any woman. "The procedures," Edwards and David Sharpe wrote in a 1971 scientific article, "open the way to further work on human embryos in the laboratory" (R. G. Edwards and D. J. Sharpe, "Social Values and Research in Human Embryology." *Nature* 231 [May 14, 1971] 87–91).

The authors do not mean only benign attempts to correct genetic defects. They also mention cloning and the creation of "chimeras" by importing cells from other blastocysts (perhaps from other species). These creations also need women to carry them through pregnancy. Noting that the first principle of medical ethics—Do no harm— permits the alleviation of infertility, and that this "has been stretched to cover destruction of fetuses with hereditary defects," Edwards and Sharpe ask rhetorically whether the first principle of medical ethics can be stretched to justify "the more remote techniques of modifying embryos"?

Even more ominous is the announced claim that scientists have the "right" to "exercise their professional activities to the limit that is tolerable by society . . . as lay attitudes struggle to catch up with what scientists can do." Publics must be "helped to keep pace." In short, science does not operate within the ethics of a wider human community. It is a scientific ethic, or whatever can be done, that should shape our public philosophy. Let laggards beware.

True, in his 1974 article, Edwards stated that there is "hardly any point in making chimeras until some clinical advantage can be shown to accrue from the method." But he also speaks of "sexing blastocysts" before transfer. His remedy for the problems this remedy will lead to is: "Imbalance of the sexes could probably be prevented by recording the sex of newborn children, and adjusting the choice open to parents." Scientist-kings will manage everything. His only reservation is that the use of "surrogate mothers" should be avoided at the present time until more is known about the inter-

*Background Note: In 1972 Dr. W. J. Sweeney told Doris Del Zio about the possibility of in vitro fertilization. Del Zio requested the procedure, and Dr. Sweeney and Dr. Landrum Shettles removed ova and fertilized them with sperm from Del Zio's husband John. The procedure was halted by Dr. Shettles's superior, Dr. Raymond Vande Wiele, on the grounds that it had not been approved by the Columbia University-Presbyterian Hospital human experimentation committee. The Del Zios sued Vande Wiele and the institutions involved and in 1974 were awarded damages in a jury trial.

locking psychological relationships among the parties. Edwards does not say how we can acquire such knowledge without (on his own terms) doing an unethical experimentation now in order to find out whether we ought to do it or not.

Finally, the human womb is a halfway technology. It is replaceable by more "perfect" artifices. Given recent advances in newborn intensive care units, only about twenty-two weeks remain to be conquered in which the human female must necessarily participate in procreation. Then "reproduction" can replace procreation, and we will come to Huxley's Hatcheries. His was a vision of society in which everyone was quite happy. The way there is also a happy one, and we go along that way always motivated by good ends, such as the relief of women's infertility.

For all the motherhood intended at present, the truth is that as C. S. Lewis wrote in *The Abolition of Man*: "the regenerate science . . ., would not do even to minerals and vegetables what modern science threatens to do to man himself" (New York: Macmillan, 1947, p. 49).

Readers may wish to perform the following experiment on themselves. Turn off the tube. Don't pick up the newspaper for two days. Instead, read *That Hideous Strength*, the third book in C. S. Lewis's science fiction trilogy (New York: MacMillan, 1946). The final assault upon humanity is gathering in Edgestow, a fictional British college town. The forces of technology, limited no more by the Christian ages, are trying to combine with pre-Christian forces, represented by Merlin the Magician whose body is buried on the Bracton College grounds. Only the philologist Ransom can save humankind from the powers of the present age concentrated in the National Institute of Coordinated Experiments (acronym NICE).

It is NICE that the Browns have a wonderful baby. Lewis need not have thought of his fictional college, Bracton. Cambridge University is NICE too. To give couples a baby sexed to their desires will be NICE. Every other step taken will certainly be NICE. Finally, *Brave New World* is entirely NICE. For everyone is happy. Only there is no poetry there. Nor will a baby ever be a surprise.

In Vitro Conception and Harm to the Unborn

John A. Robertson

The recent birth of Louise Brown raises the question of whether society ought to permit willing couples and doctors to use in vitro fertilization to overcome infertility. Although no law currently prohibits use of in vitro fertilization as a treatment for infertility, DHEW regulations prohibit institutions receiving federal research funds for conducting research involving implantation of human ova, unless the Ethics Advisory Board determines its "ethical acceptability." While further study is needed, ethical questions about this research seem less salient now that the technique has apparently produced a healthy baby.

Two justifications have been asserted for restricting in vitro conception as a means to relieve infertility. It is said that extra-utero conception, though not in itself harmful, might move us to-

ward total artificial manipulation of reproduction, ending in Huxley's dehumanized hatcheries, where babies are "decanted" from bottles with predetermined characteristics. The problem of technologizing natural processes, however, is not unique to reproductive advances; it arises with most new biomedical capabilities, and appears no more a ground for restriction here than elsewhere. The slope may not be as slippery as feared—we can employ in vitro conception without also producing clones in artificial wombs. Moreover, practices antithetical to our values might, when they finally occur, be acceptable to future generations with very different value systems from our own.

The second justification asserts that relieving infertility through in vitro conception is morally impermissible because of the greater risk that the

Reprinted with permission of the author and the publisher from Hastings Center Report, 8 (October 1978): 13–14. © Institute of Society, Ethics and the Life Sciences, 360 Broadway, Hastings-on Hudson, N.Y. 10706.

implanted cells will abort or produce defective children. In my view, this argument does not withstand scrutiny, and is therefore not a sufficient moral or legal ground for banning the procedure, though it would justify regulation to minimize the frequency of such outcomes.

This argument could be viewed as a plea for distributive justice for the aborted fetuses and deformed children resulting from these procedures. They bear significant burdens, without consent, in order to confer the benefits of parenthood on childless couples who cannot otherwise conceive. Generally, heavy burdens may not be imposed without consent or overriding justification. But consent is absent, and though relief of infertility is a worthy goal, it is insufficient to justify the suffering of aborted fetuses and deformed children. Treating them justly means that we must treat them as we treat other nonconsenting, incompetent persons, and must prohibit the use of procedures that harm them.

As a claim for distributive justice for aborted fetuses, the argument seems plainly insufficient, unless one believes that abortion is generally wrong. If one believes that pregnant women should have wide discretion to decide whether to abort, then the higher risk of spontaneous or induced abortion from in vitro conception techniques is not a sufficient reason for banning them. Public policy currently grants the pregnant woman autonomy over the abortion decision. She may override the interests of the fetus, at least until viability, for any reason she chooses. The state can no more stop women from conceiving because they might abort and hence harm fetal interests, than it can stop abortion altogether. Given the current state of the law, a higher risk that fetuses conceived ex utero will abort should not preclude infertile women from conceiving by the only means available to them.

Prevention of Harm to Offspring

Prevention of harm to a deformed offspring, however, seems a more persuasive argument, for parents free to abort fetuses may not harm children. The parents, it is said, are a direct cause of the deformed child's suffering, because they choose to conceive in a manner that risks producing a deformed child. On utilitarian grounds these burdens cannot be justified, because the suffering of the child who lacks capacity for normal develop-

ment and interaction is so much greater than the suffering of a couple who must remain barren.

The utilitarian argument seemed especially compelling while in vitro techniques remained experimental and the risk of deformity appeared great. If the magnitude and probability of deformity lessen as more babies are born, this argument loses force. As the teratogenic effects of the procedure decrease and prenatal detection of defective fetuses increases, the resulting satisfaction to parents made fertile may well outweigh the suffering of infants born deformed from in vitro conception.

But opposition to in vitro conception because of harm to offspring rests more on a deontological or rights position than on a utilitarian calculus of burdens and benefits. On Kantian principles of respect for persons, the imposition of burdens without consent to benefit others is prima facie wrong, even if net utility is increased. Knowingly risking a deformed birth violates the right of the child, for it imposes harm without its consent, whether or not others are greatly benefited.

Both the utilitarian and rights position seem misconceived, however, for it is unclear how the deformed child has been harmed. At the time of the in vitro conception, there was no child with rights that could be violated. The parents have not caused a child who would otherwise be normal to be born defective, for there is no child to be harmed aside from the very act creating the risk of harm. The act creating the risk of injury also brings about the very being that is said to be injured. But for that act, the child would never have existed at all. From the child's perspective, the only alternative to the action that allegedly violates his right not to be harmed is even less desirable, for it means no existence at all. One does not respect a person's rights by refraining from an activity that prevents his existence altogether.

It is difficult to escape the conclusion, shared by the courts in "wrongful life" cases, that a non-normal child has no cause of action against persons causing the abnormality if the alternative to their action is no life at all. On this view, human existence, however imperfect, is, in most cases to the individual involved, preferable to nonexistence. Children deformed as a result of in vitro techniques at least are alive, and, unless their lives are full of incessant pain, they are better off than if they were never conceived at all. The couple's choice of procreative technique thus does not violate the child's rights, and should not be banned on that ground. Indeed, under *Roe* v. *Wade*, such concern would not amount to the compelling state interest necessary to justify interference with procreative choice.

An opposite conclusion would, in other situations, lead to results that clearly do violate the rights of deformed persons. If it is better that such children not be born at all, rather than be born with less than full capacities, then it follows that once born, such persons would be better off dead than alive. Killing them would then be morally justified (or obligatory) as a means to promote their interests, for life in their condition is said to justify preventing their birth altogether. Most of us would recoil in horror at such a practice. Rather than serving their interests, killing deformed persons to save them from the suffering of a life with handicaps would, except in the rare case of irremediable suffering, be an intolerable violation of their rights, which the criminal law would punish.

This conclusion would also lead to intolerable results in the case of a couple who are heterozygote carriers of a genetic defect not diagnosable prenatally and who knowingly decide to take the one-in-four risk of conceiving a deformed child; in the case of a thirty-eight-year-old woman who rejects prenatal diagnosis for Down's syndrome because she is morally opposed to abortion; and in the case of the pregnant woman exposed to rubella who also refuses to have an abortion. Have they violated any right of the child who is born deformed, when the only alternative would have been no child at all? Does the risk of deformity justify depriving them of the chance to procreate? The logic of the argument against in vitro conception necessarily encompasses these cases as well. If the state may ban in vitro conception to prevent possible harm to resulting offspring, it may also require sterilization, amniocentesis, or abortion to prevent deformed births in other situations. Yet procreative autonomy in those other situations seems essential. No morally relevant ground distinguishes in vitro conception.

Opposition to in vitro conception because of possible harm to the offspring may stem in part from a perception that couples resorting to in vitro techniques callously sacrifice the interests of potential offspring in order to improve their own lot. But children born deformed from such procedures do not suffer alone. A couple plagued by infertility will also suffer greatly if in vitro conception yields a deformed birth. They have every incentive to minimize that possibility, for the burden on them is also great. As the risk of serious deformity increases, infertile couples will be reluctant to use these procedures. A choice to take that risk might involve love for the desired child as much as self-interest.

In any event, the state may regulate in vitro conception to minimize the frequency of abnormal births, even though it may not ban in vitro techniques altogether. Doctors who perform these procedures without informed consent, without a high degree of skill, or without exhausting other medical options, can be made legally liable. The state may encourage alternative methods of satisfying desires for parenthood, or choose not to fund the research necessary to make in vitro procedures more widely available. But it should not ban the use by willing, informed parties as a last resort to overcome infertility due to oviduct blockage, on the ground that a defective child may suffer who would not exist at all but for use of that technique.

Artificial Insemination: The Legal Position Today

Walter Wadlington

AI and the Courts

Most of the legal profession today is either in ignorance or in hiding concerning artificial insemination. Until recently a handful of British Commonwealth decisions and a few trial court cases, not always officially reported, were the only sources available upon which to construct a legal framework for the process. In the past several

Reprinted from "Artificial Insemination: The Dangers of a Poorly Kept Secret," Northwestern University Law Review, 64, no. 6 (January-February 1970): 785–793. *Editor's note: The footnotes in this selection have been renumbered.*

years more cases have been the subject of formally reported decisions, including one from the California Supreme Court.

To the extent that any consensus is appearing, the general rule seems to be that, in the absence of a conclusive presumption of legitimacy of a child born during wedlock, the AID child is illegitimate. It also seems, however, that judicial effort is made to encourage or enforce his support by a consenting husband/nonfather. Whether AID will be considered to be adultery in some circumstances is not as clear. Thus far we have little to aid us in our speculation on how the courts will view the responsibility of the AID practitioner, or the third party donor of semen, when eventually faced with an action calling for such a determination.

Three reported Commonwealth decisions illustrate the confused judicial tone which exists in the absence of legislation. *Orford* v. *Orford,*[1] the earliest of the triumvirate, reached the Supreme Court of Ontario in 1921. The wife, who lived in England, brought suit for alimony against the husband, who lived in Canada. The couple had not consummated their marriage by sexual intercourse before their separation. The husband, upon discovering that the wife had given birth to a child, asserted her adultery in bar of an alimony award. The wife asserted that the child had been conceived through AID. After both a factual finding that the wife had engaged in adultery "in the ordinary way" at some time during the separation, and a statement that the wife's story about having gone through the process was "not to be believed," the court still felt constrained to discuss the legal effects of artificial insemination. In these *obiter* remarks, it was concluded that AID under such circumstances would have amounted to adultery because the "essence" of that offense is not so much the joinder of sexual organs as it is "the voluntary surrender . . . of the reproductive powers or faculties" by the wife to someone other than her husband.[2]

In 1948 an English court in *L.* v. *L.*[3] faced a case bearing strong resemblance to our opening hypothetical illustration. After seven years of marriage, the wife sought an annulment on the ground that her husband either was impotent or had wilfully refused to consummate the marriage. Although he had at first refused to seek psychological counsel, he later had agreed to do so; at the same time the couple sought to have a child through AIH. The latter endeavor was the more successful, and the couple who had never copulated with each other nevertheless produced a child.

The court's opinion seems to reveal that the husband's problems were largely (if not wholly) psychic. He admitted that there had been no intercourse, but denied that there had been willful refusal on his part. Under these circumstances, the court annulled the marriage, even though it meant that the child would be illegitimate.[4] The court rejected the husband's contention of an estoppel on the wife's part, pointing out that the wife had "not misled her husband to do anything on the faith of her acquiescence in an abnormal marriage."[5] By way of consolation to the husband, it was pointed out that "he has the privilege of having a child by the woman he loved, and, apparently, still loves, which is no small privilege to a man."[6]

in Scotland, it was held in 1949 that AID would not be considered adultery. Proof of conception in this manner could, therefore, be used to rebut the obvious inference which would otherwise be drawn from the fact of childbirth following a long period of the husband's non-acess.[7] The fairly detailed explanation of the medical technique involved was of considerable importance in the court's reasoning. Lord Wheatley pointed out that a woman alone in her room could impregnate herself with a third party's semen through the use of a syringe. He then stated that "Unilateral adultery is possible, as in the case of a married man who ravishes a woman not his wife, but self-adultery is a conception as yet unknown to the law."[8]

The jurisprudence in our own country has been equally varied. The courts have seemingly been no less willing to discuss the problems of AID whether necessary to the actual decision or not. This was first evident in a 1948 New York case, *Strnad* v. *Strnad,*[9] involving the question of a husband's visitation rights to a child born through AID. After confirming previously awarded custody rights, the court ostensibly declined opinion as to the propriety of the AID process generally, and as to the specific property rights which might later come into issue in this particular situation. The court, however, added that "the child has been potentially adopted or semi-adopted" by the consenting husband.[10] The court failed to mention that adoption is a wholly statutory proceeding, and that there is no established concept of semi-adoption. The court did not clarify matters by adding that the child should logically and realistically be considered in the same position as a child who is born out of wedlock, but legitimated by the subsequent marriage of the parents.

Probably the most widely mentioned of the unreported trial court cases[11] has been the 1954 Illinois decision of *Doornbos* v. *Doornbos*.[12] There the court, in a declaratory proceeding, indicated that a child produced through AI would be considered illegitimate, and the act itself considered adulterous on the part of the wife so inseminated. The court added that AID seemed to raise no serious legal problems. That much publicized case was followed quietly by a New York decision in 1958 which refused to allow a mother to cut off parental rights of her divorced husband by asserting the AID conception of the child.[13] The child previously had been designated as that of the couple, both in a support agreement executed by them, and in a bilateral Nevada divorce decree entitled to full faith and credit. The court indicated some impatience with the mother for having tried to raise the AID issue in the later proceeding.[14]

In 1963 the New York Supreme Court finally met the question of legitimacy of an AID child in a head-on encounter. In *Gursky* v. *Gursky*,[15] as in the previously discussed English case of *L.* v. *L.*,[16] a wife was granted an annulment because of her husband's impotence. Like the parties in our hypothetical case, the couple, before annulment, had consented to AID for the wife and a child had been born. In contrast with the approach in *Strnad*,[17] the court this time noted that there was no means for effecting an adoption in New York except as provided by statute, and that there was no basis for asserting that consent to AI met the statutory requirements. The court further acknowledge the "deeply imbedded" concept in our law "that a child who is begotten through a father who is not the mother's husband is illegitimate."[18] The court, however, did find that the conduct and declarations of the husband implied a promise on his part to support any child born through the AID process; this promise was held to be legally enforceable either by virtue of an implied contract or through the doctrine of equitable estoppel.[19] At that point the court stopped, with the specific notation that it was not passing on any other personal rights (including property rights) between the child and the mother's husband.

Latest in this collection of judicial and gene-alogical nightmares was *People* v. *Sorenson*,[20] a California criminal prosecution of a father for failure to provide support for a child born to his wife through consensual AID before she had divorced him.[21] The birth certificate had designated the husband as father, despite the fact that he was sterile. The decree of divorce, entered several years later, did not order immediate child support, but reserved the right to have support added at a later time. When the mother applied for public assistance during an illness, the district attorney sought support from the ostensible father. His refusal to contribute resulted in the prosecution.

In reinstating a lower court conviction which had been vacated by the appellate court,[22] the California Supreme Court, in bank, held that regardless of the AID conception the accused, who had consented to the process, would be considered the "lawful father" of the child for purposes of the penal provision. As the court noted, their specific review of the effect of AID probably was unnecessary in view of the California rule that "the issue of a wife cohabiting with her husband, who is not impotent, is conclusively presumed to be legitimate."[23] The end result of their further response has been amendment of both the Penal Code[24] and Civil Code[25] provisions to conform to the holding of the court as to parental support duties. It is also significant that the California court, in reasoning quite similar to that of Lord Wheatley in the *MacLennan* case, pronounced that AID logically could not be considered adultery.[26]

A case which must not be overlooked in this early chapter of the legal history of artificial insemination is *Zepeda* v. *Zepeda*,[27] decided by the appellate court of Illinoi in 1963. Widely celebrated as seeking to establish an "action or wrongful life,"[28] it involved a child's action against his putative father for having caused him to be born with the serious legal and social impediment of illegitimacy. The court noted that substantial hardships still accrued to one of illegitimate birth in Illinois despite recent legislative attempts toward amelioration. Although it then characterized the father's action as a tort against the child, the court refused to allow recovery because of the staggering potential effects which this could have.[29]

One possible troublemaker which bothered the court considerably was the practice of artificial insemination.[30] Since that time, a New York court has used the reasoning of the *Zepeda* opinion to allow recovery of damages by a defective child in a somewhat different factual situation. Although this decision was reversed on appeal,[31] the theory is continually being advanced[32] and there are signs that it may be on the threshold of at least partial acceptance.[33] From the standpoint of the AID child who is declared illegitimate, such a breakthrough could be of particular significance as a means of effectively reaching both the physician and the donor.

Some Cases Still to Be Seen

There are a number of possible actions or situations which might lead to litigation, which as yet have not surfaced among the reported decisions. One such action is a paternity suit against the donor of the semen. The signing of consent forms by all parties prior to the artificial insemination would not necessarily preclude such an action inasmuch as the child, whose rights will be at issue, has not then been conceived. It seems doubtful that a mother could consent in advance to a waiver of any paternity action her unborn child ultimately might have.[34] It is unlikely, however, that such action will reach the courts very often under present medical practice both because of the anonymity of the donor in most cases (outside New York City, at least) and because the child himself probably will never learn that he was conceived through AID.[35] These, however, are factual rather than legal obstacles. That such cases as *Gursky*[36] and *Orford*[37] have been decided should bear warning that cases which squarely present the AID issue can reach the courts. It is most likely that the donor will be held to be the legal parent in such cases inasmuch as he is, after all, the biological parent. In support of this conclusion, one can cite such cases as the "splash pregnancy," where the biological father in a non-AID framework was considered to be the legal father, even though he had not experienced intercourse with the mother.[38]

Another potential action would be a malpractice suit against the physician. This could arise in several ways. One of the most obvious would be the use of semen from a clearly defective or diseased donor. Another could arise from the failure to pay attention to such a matter as incompatible Rh typing, resulting in erythroblastosis fetalis.[39] Taking this one short step further, we can also imagine a malpractice action by an AID child who is determined to be illegitimate on the basis of exclusionary blood groupings between himself and his mother's husband. Under the present circumstances, which amply warn the physician of the legal consequences which may result, it would seem that he should be careful to guard against this possibility. Of course, if the lack of paternity is proved through some other evidence (*e.g.*, the husband's sterility, or non-access) the physician would be less likely to be held for malpractice.

It is also possible that a donor could assert some rights with regard to a child born through use of his semen. The likelihood of such an action in practice seems slim at this time for the same reasons already outlined with regard to the child's action against the donor. In addition, usually the donor has consciously and calculatedly entered the situation with the understanding, acknowledged in writing, that his role will remain secret. The current increasingly legal concern, however, for the rights of an unwed father who has sired a child through copulation[40] could be considered as having equal effect with regard to the AID donor-father. The question then arises: if neither the mother nor the mother's husband wishes to maintain the child, should the biological father be allowed to assert his rights to him for purposes such as legitimating him, adopting him, or obtaining custody?

Notes

1. 58 D.L.R. 251 (1921).
2. Id. at 258. The court added: "Sexual intercourse is adulterous because in the case of the woman it involves the possibility of introducing into the family of the husband a false strain of blood. Any act on the part of the wife which does that would, therefore, be adulterous." Id.
3. [1949] 1 All E.R. 141 (1948).
4. English law had never provided for the legitimation of children of void or voidable marriages. Most American jurisdictions long ago enacted provisions to the effect that the children of void or voidable marriages will be deemed legitimate. . . . Seemingly the child born through AIH would fit within such coverage because biologically he is the child of both parents.
5. One question which also might be posed in some jurisdictions is whether the voidable marriage has been "ratified." If it is in fact possible to ratify a marriage with an impotent spouse, it seems

difficult to conjure up any better case for ratification than having a child through AIH.

6. [1949] 1 All E.R. 141, 145 (1948). Although concern for the feelings of husband and wife occupy more of the discussion, mention also is made of the child's interests: "The future holds better augury for the child, I think, if I grant the decree than if he is brought up by an embittered mother who may be tied for life to a marriage that has never been a real marriage, and which, only through the unnatural aid of science, has produced the fruit of a real marriage." Id. at 146.

7. *MacLennan* v. *MacLennan.* [1958] Sess. Cas. 105.

8. Id. at 114.

9. 190 Misc. 786, 78 N.Y.S.2d 390 (Sup. Ct. 1948).

10. Id. at 787, 78 N.Y.S.2d at 391.

11. No attempt has been made by the author to catalogue the various trial level decision dealing with this problem. At least one other beside *Doornbos* which has been frequently noted, however, is *Hoch* v. *Hoch*, a 1945 decision in the Circuit Court of Cook County, Illinois, in which it was indicated that AID did not constitute adultery for the purpose of obtaining a divorce.

12. 23 U.S.L.W. 2308 (Super. Ct., Cook County, Ill., Dec. 13, 1954).

13. *People* v. *Dennett*, 15 Misc. 2d 260, 184 N.Y.S.2d 178 (Sup. Ct. 1958).

14. Id. at 265, 184 N.Y.S.2d at 184.

15. 39 Misc. 2d 1083, 242 N.Y.S.2d 406 (Sup. Ct. 1963), noted at 64 *Colum. L. Rev.* 376 (1964).

16. [1949] 1 All E.R. 141.

17. 190 Misc. 786, 78 N.Y.S.2d 390 (Sup. Ct. 1948.)

18. 39 Misc. 2d 1083, 1085, 242 N.Y.S.2d 406, 408 (Sup. Ct. 1963.)

19. The court stated: "The 'consent' was in its terms a request to the physician to conduct the artificial insemination for the express purpose of providing a child for the mutual happiness of the parties. There is nothing in the record to indicate that the wife would have undergone artificial insemination in the absence of the husband's consent. Hence it is reasonable to presume that she was induced so to act and thus changed her position in reliance on the husband's express wishes." Id. at 1089, 242 N.Y.S.2d at 411-12.

20. 66 *Cal. Rptr.* 7, 437 P.2d 495 (1968).

21. He was prosecuted under §270 of the California Penal Code of 1955 which provides for punishment of the father of either a legitimate or illegitimate child for willful failure to render necessary support.

22. *People* v. *Sorensen*, 62 Cal. Rptr. 462 (Ct. App. 1967).

23. Cal. Evid. Code §621 (West 1966).

24. Following the *Sorenson* decision, an additional paragraph was added to Penal Code §270 in 1968, providing: "The husband of a woman who bears a child as the result of artificial insemination shall be considered the father of that child for the purposes of this section, if he consented in writing to the artificial insemination." Cal. Pen. Code §270 (West 1968).

25. 7 Cal. Leg. Serv. ch. 1615, §2 at 3174 (West 1969).

26. While Lord Wheatley's remarks, quoted in the text accompanying note [8] supra, presented the picture of the woman inseminating herself while alone in her room, the court in *Sorenson* adds that "to consider it an act of adultery with the donor, who at the time of insemination may be a thousand miles away or may even be dead is . . . absurd." *People* v. *Sorenson*, 66 Cal. Rptr. 7, 13, 437 P.2d 495, 501 (1968). As to whether the doctor is the adulterer, the court raises the usual question as to how this would be handled if one used a female doctor.

27. 41 Ill. App. 2d 240, 190 N.E.2d 849 (1963), cert. denied, 379 U.S. 945 (1964).

28. This unfortunate, ethically inconsistent characterization of the action comes from the court's own opinion: "Recognition of the plaintiff's claim means creation of a new tort: A cause of action for wrongful life." See *Zepeda* v. *Zepeda*, 41 Ill. App. 2d 240, 262, 190 N.E.2d 849, 858 (1963), *cert. denied*, 379 U.S. 945 (1964).

29. The court took the view that basically the problem was inseparable from a larger consideration of illegitimacy. They pointed out: "Although the legal questions unfolded are new, the problem is not; the social conditions producing the problem have existed since the advent of man." Id. at 263, 190 N.E.2d at 859. In closing they stated: "The interest of society is so involved, the action needed to redress the tort could be so far-reaching, that the policy of the State should be declared by the representatives of the People [referring specifically to the legislature]." Id.

30. As pointed out already, discussion of the potential effects of AID seems almost irresistible to many courts when it seems possible to work it into an opinion. In *Zepeda* the court pointed out the possibility in the future of "public sperm banks" and "sperm injections like present day blood transfusions." Id. at 261, 190 N.E.2d at 859.

31. See *Williams* v. *State*, 46 Misc. 2d 824, 260 N.Y.S.2d 953 (Ct. Cl. 1965), reversed in *Williams* v. *State*, 18 N.Y.2d 481, 276 N.Y.S.2d 885 (1966).

32. See, e.g., *Pinkney* v. *Pinkney* 198 So. 2d 52 (Fla. Ct. App. 1967). A variation sometimes referred to

as "the right not to be born" was involved in *Gleitman* v. *Cosgrove*, 49 N.J. 22, 227 A.2d 689 (1967). This suit was brought in the form of a malpractice action by a husband, wife, and child against a physician for not advising a pregnant mother with rubella that her child was likely to be defective. The court did not allow recovery. It should be noted that abortion was not legally permitted in the particular state under such circumstances, though the court indicated that the child's action would not have been affected had it been possible. In the light of recent abortion law reform dealing with this particular medical indication, it seems probable that such a case is likely to come up elsewhere with a better prognosis for recovery regardless of the New Jersey court's views.

For more general discussion of *Zepeda* and its progeny see Note, Compensation for the Harmful Effects of Illegitimacy, 66 *Colum. L. Rev.* 127 (1966); Note, Liability To Bastard For Negligence Resulting In His Conception, 18 *Stan. L. Rev.* 530 (1966).

33. See *Custodio* v. *Bauer*, 251 Cal. App. 303, 59 Cal. Rptr. 463 (Ct. App. 1967). This case involved an action against two physicians for negligent performance of sterilization on a wife, after which she gave birth to a tenth child. Although the action is by the child's parents, the opinion indicates a willingness to at least consider the effect of the birth of an unwanted child into a family. Id. at 319, 59 Cal. Rptr. at 477. *Cf. In Re*

Guardianship of C., 98 N.J. Super. 474, 237 A2d 652, 659 (1967).

34. *Cf. Berry* v. *Chaplin*, 169 P.2d 442, 445, 446 (Ct. App. Cal. 1946).

35. In adoption the practice of revealing to a child that he is in fact the biological offspring of some other couple is widely prevalent. In cases of artificial insemination, however, this does not seem to be the case at all. The fact that the child is usually born to a married woman living with her husband, and the steps taken to insure that the identity of the semen donor remains unknown are all part of the process of anonymity.

36. 39 Misc. 2d 1083, 242 N.Y.S.2d 406 (Sup. Ct. 1963).

37. 58 D.L.R. 251 (1921).

38. *T. v. M.*, 100 N.J. Super. 530, 242 A.2d 670 (Ch. 1968).

39. Erythroblastosis fetolis is a hemolytic disease of the fetus. As already explained, one of the indications for AID is to avoid such a result through the mating of married couples with such an incompatibility.

40. See, e.g., *In Re* Adoption of Krueger, 104 Ariz. 26, 448 P.2d 82 (1968); *Mixon* v. *Mize*, 198 So. 2d 373 (Ct. App. Fla. 1967); *In re* Mark T., 8 Mich. App. 122, 154 N.W.2d 27 (1967); *In re* Brennan, 270 Minn. 455, 134 N.W.2d 126 (1965); *In re* Guardianship of C., 98 N.J. Super. 474, 237 A.2d 652 (1967).

Sterilization of the Mentally Retarded: a Decision for the Courts

George J. Annas

In the most notorious case involving sterilization of a mentally retarded person, the United States Supreme Court upheld a Virginia statute that was the basis for sterilizing Carrie Buck, a "feeble-minded eighteen-year-old" who was "the daughter of a feeble-minded mother and the mother of an illegitimate feeble-minded child." Oliver Wendell Holmes, speaking for the Court, argued:

It is better for all the world, if instead of waiting to execute degenerate offspring for crime, or let them starve for their imbecility,

society can prevent those who are manifestly unfit from continuing their kind. . . . Three generations of imbeciles are enough (*Buck* v. *Bell*, 274 U.S. 200[1927]).

After an orgy of eugenic sterilizations, the pendulum has swung back to the point where this opinion represents neither good law nor good genetics. On the way, in 1942, the same Supreme Court concluded in a different context that the right to procreate was a basic constitutional right. Sterilization "forever deprived" an individual of

Reprinted with permission of the author and the publisher from Hastings Center Report, 11 *(August 1981), 18–19. © Institute of Society, Ethics and the Life Sciences, 360 Broadway, Hastings-on-Hudson, N.Y. 10706.*

this right, which is "fundamental to the very existence and survival of the race" (*Skinner* v. *Oklahoma*, 316 U.S. 535 [1942]).

At least three approaches are now possible. One—the majority approach—is for courts in states that have no specific statutes authorizing sterilization simply to declare that it cannot be done on individuals who cannot personally consent to it. Another is for courts individually to evaluate cases in which sterilization of a mentally retarded individual is contemplated, and to authorize it only if it is in the person's "best interests." And the third is for courts to adopt a "*Quinlan*-type approach" by defining the test to be applied in making a decision to sterilize and permitting the family of the incompetent and their physician (with or without the help of a review committee) to make the decision without resort to the courts. (See George J. Annas, "In re Quinlan: Legal Comfort for Doctors," *Hastings Center Report*, June 1976, pp. 29–31.)

If any court could be expected to take a *Quinlan* approach it would be the New Jersey Supreme Court, the same court that wrote the *Quinlan* decision. Thus it will undoubtedly surprise some *Quinlan* enthusiasts that this court opted for the second choice, requiring a court to decide if an incompetent may be sterilized.

The Case of Lee Ann Grady

The case that brought the issue to the New Jersey Supreme Court involved Lee Ann Grady, a nineteen-year-old with Down's syndrome. She is the oldest of three children, lives at home with them and her parents, and has never been institutionalized. Her IQ is in the "upper 20s to upper 30s range." She can converse, count to some extent, and recognize letters of the alphabet. She can dress and bathe herself. Her life expectancy and physical maturation are normal; however, her mental deficiency has prevented the normal emotional and social development of sexuality. If she becomes pregnant, she will not understand her condition, and she will not be capable of caring for a baby alone.

Because of her sexual development, her parents have provided her with birth control pills for the past four years, although there is no evidence that she has ever engaged in sexual activity or has any interest in it. At the age of twenty she will leave her special class in the public school system.

Her parents would like to have her placed in a sheltered work group, and eventually in a group home for retarded adults so that she can begin a more independent life and have a place to live after they die. They believe that dependable and continuous contraception is a prerequisite to this change; and they and their doctor sought to have her sterilized, using a tubal ligation, at the Morristown Memorial Hospital. The hospital refused without court approval, and a lawsuit followed. (*In the Matter of Lee Ann Grady*, 426 A. 2d 467 [N.J., 1981]).

The Appeal

The lower court granted the parents' application; and the public advocate and attorney general, both invited to appear by the trial judge, appealed. The appeals court begins its analysis by recognizing that "sterilization [destroys] an important part of a person's social and biological identity"; and rejects any notion that it might assign fewer rights to the mentally retarded than to other citizens. The court declines to classify the proposed sterilization as either voluntary (since she could not understand the problem or the proposed solution) or compulsory (since no one is actually objecting to the procedure on her behalf). Instead it defines a new category: a procedure "lacking personal consent because of a legal disability."

Following closely the logic of the *Quinlan* case, the court concludes that the right to prevent contraception through sterilization is one of the privacy rights protected by the U.S. Constitution, and declines to discard it for the mentally retarded "solely on the basis that [their] condition prevents conscious exercise of the choice." As in *Quinlan*, this court sees its task as fashioning a way to preserve the right of choice for incompetent persons. Unlike *Quinlan*, however, the court refuses to permit the person's parents and a court-appointed guardian to make the decision. Instead it insists that only the court can make this decision for an incompetent. The reasons for this departure from *Quinlan* are instructive.

The court gives two reasons for distinguishing this case from *Quinlan*. First, it sees the alternatives in *Quinlan* as "much more clear cut": indefinite life in a coma versus natural death. It believes such a choice is "not conducive to detached evaluation and resolution by the person exercising it in behalf of the patient," but that the decision relies more "on instinct than reasoned calculation." Second, there was no history of abuse in *Quinlan*-type decisions. In contrast, many choices are open to Lee Ann Grady; and there is a history of horrible abuses in this area.

The court notes that similar decisions in adoption and child custody cases are routinely made by the courts, and holds that, under its inherent *parens patriae* power, the courts have the authority to protect incompetents who cannot protect themselves because of an innate legal disability. This power has been applied in medical cases, including authorizations to treat children over the parents' objection, kidney and bone marrow transplant cases, and in the *Quinlan* case itself.

The court understands that its decision is *not* Lee Ann's, but

> . . . it is a genuine choice . . . designed to further the same interests she might pursue had she the ability to decide herself. We believe that having the choice made in her behalf produces a more just and compassionate result than leaving Lee Ann with no way of exercising a constitutional right. *Our Court should accept the responsibility of providing her with a choice* to compensate for her inability to exercise personally an important constitutional right. (Emphasis supplied.)

Standards for Decision

Having decided that a court is a proper decision maker, the appeals court considered the standards and procedures to be employed. The court stops short of requiring a showing of "strict necessity," but does enunciate very strict criteria that must be met before sterilization can be authorized. The Court must appoint a guardian *ad litem* to represent the interests of the ward, and "should receive" independent medical and psychological evaluations by qualified professionals. The trial judge must personally meet with the individual before concluding that the person lacks capacity to make a decision about sterilization and that the incapacity is unlikely to change. This incapacity must be proven by clear and convincing evidence. Finally, the court must be persuaded, also by clear and convincing evidence, that the sterilization is in the person's *best interests*. In making this determination, the court must consider the

- Possibility of pregnancy;

- Possibility of physical and mental harm from pregnancy and from sterilization;
- Likelihood of sexual activity;
- Inability of the person to understand contraception;
- Feasibility of a less drastic means of contraception;
- Possibility of postponing sterilization;
- Ability of the person to care for a child, or the possibility of marriage at a future date with ability of the couple to care for the child;
- Evidence of relevant medical advances;
- Demonstration that the proponents of sterilization are seeking it in good faith for the primary concern of the person and not their own or the public's convenience.

This list is not meant to be inclusive, and "the ultimate criterion is the best interests of the incompetent person." Because the trial court did not apply the stringent "clear and convincing" standard of proof (it used the more traditional "preponderance of evidence" standard) to the best interests conclusion, the case was remanded for further proceedings.

Protecting Individual Rights

The court finds a new substantive right—the right to sterilization—and seeks to protect incompetents from its arbitrary use by demanding strict due process protection. This is far superior to a blanket prohibition of sterilization, and much more protective of individual rights than permitting families to make this decision on their own. The basis on which *Quinlan* is distinguished is instructive. It supports the notion that a terminally ill patient in a chronic vegetative state has suffered a form of "death" and therefore has no good options. Since the only two choices for such a patient are both so bleak, the court thinks that "instinct" rather than logic must be called upon to make this choice. If the court's words are taken seriously, New Jersey courts might be inclined to require a court decision in cases like *Saikewicz*, where the choices are much more complex, since an individual presumably has a greater interest in preserving life than in preserving an ability to procreate.

The second distinction from *Quinlan*, the history of abuse, seems to indicate that should abuses in other areas of medical care for incompetents come to light, courts will step in to protect this class of persons. If *Quinlan* was read by some as a judicial retreat from protecting incompetent individuals, the New Jersey courts have clearly signaled that this "retreat" was made under very specific circumstances from which we cannot generalize.

If a structural problem exists with the decision, it is in the role of the guardian *ad litem*. The court defines the guardian's role as "representing the interests of his ward." This seems inappropriate for a proceeding in which the judge, not the guardian, will make the judgment as to whether the sterilization is in the person's best interests. Since the petitioners will always be arguing in favor of the sterilization, it would make more sense if the guardian *ad litem* were required to present all of the arguments against sterilization to the best of his ability. As Professor Charles Baron of Boston College Law School has argued, "Without advocates on both sides of the issue to develop

the record, the court is too likely to face mental set and path-of-least-resistance pitfalls. . . . [A] general pattern will seem to emerge from the evidence; an accustomed label is waiting for the case, and without awaiting further proofs, this label is promptly assigned to it." (Charles Baron, "Voluntary Sterilization of the Mentally Retarded" in Aubrey Milunsky, George J. Annas, editors, *Genetics and the Law*, New York: Plenum, 1976, pp. 273–74.)

The New Jersey model is as good as anything that exists, but it stands almost alone in the country. Since most courts will not act without them, statutes should be enacted in each state to prohibit sterilization of the mentally retarded and other incompetent individuals except when a court finds, after an adversary hearing, that the sterilization is in the best interests of the individual. Such a procedure permits sterilization in cases where a compelling case can be made, and protects potential victims from sterilization abuse for the benefit of others.

Decision Scenario 1

"I'm sorry we can't help you," Patricia Spring said. "But what you want is simply against our policy."

Charles Blendon and Carla Neuman didn't try to hide their disappointment. The San Diego Reproductive Clinic had been their last hope. They very badly wanted to have a child but Carla's fallopian tubes had been surgically removed as part of a successful effort to treat precancerous growths.

"In fact," Patricia Spring said, "you don't meet at least two of our criteria."

"We can afford to pay," Charles Blendon said.

"That's not it. First of all, Carla is thirty-eight, and we set thirty-five as the upper limit. And second, you two are not married, and we require that the donor and the patient be husband and wife."

"Who makes those rules?" Carla Neuman asked. "It seems to me that if we want to have a child, then that's our business and nobody else's."

"The Clinic makes the rules," Patricia Spring said. "You see, there is some greater risk of birth defects in women who are over the age of thirty-five. There are sound medical reasons for our criteria."

"But what if we're willing to take the risk?" Charles Blendon asked.

"You can't take a risk that is likely to affect an unborn child."

But I'm willing to have tests," Carla Neuman said. "And neither of us is against abortion. If there is something wrong with the fetus, then I'll have an abortion."

"And just what sort of medical basis is there for the marriage requirement?" Charles Blendon asked. "It seems to me that the Clinic is just imposing its own moral standards on Carla and me."

"Look," Patricia Spring said, "I know you're both upset and disappointed. I sympathize with you. But the Clinic operates in a community, and our criteria reflect both good medical judgment and the standards of the community."

"Does the Clinic receive any public money," Carla Neuman asked.

"We have some research grants."

"Then it seems to me that we have grounds for a suit," Carla said. "The Clinic is discriminating against us because we aren't married, and it's denying us the right to take a risk we're willing to take."

"I can only tell you what our criteria are," Patricia Spring said. "I can't arrange for you to be accepted as a patient here, and there's nothing you or I can do about it."

"That remains to be seen," Charles Blendon said.

> *In Robertson's view, is the Clinic justified in setting an age limit on the women it will accept as patients? If so, why?*
>
> *How might a rule utilitarian justify the Clinic's requirement that a couple be married in order for the woman to be accepted as a patient?*
>
> *Does the fact that the Clinic receives public funds provide any reason to believe that its services should be open to everyone?*
>
> *On what grounds might Ramsey object to the very existence of such a clinic?*

Decision Scenario 2

In a television program in January of 1982, Dr. Robert Edwards outlined a plan to freeze embryos for later use. If the embryos could be stored in this way and then unfrozen without any damage to chromosomes, then an embryo transplant could be delayed until the potential mother had reached the most favorable time in her menstrual cycle.

Furthermore, according to Dr. Edwards, embryos that are not needed by the ovum donor might be implanted in women who are unable to ovulate. Such women would then be able to carry the developing fetus to term and so become mothers, something they otherwise would not be able to do.

A representative of Life, a British anti-abortion organization, criticized the plan outlined by Dr. Edwards. Nuala Scarisbrick said that the idea "raises horrendous legal and moral implications."

Dr. Michael Thomas, the chairman of the British Medical Association's ethics committee, said that Dr. Edwards's plan was a case of "medical technology running ahead of morality." He requested that Dr. Edwards and his collaborator Dr. Patrick Steptoe stop their experiments until his committee could review their work.

> *What are the ethical issues raised by such experiments?*

Assuming that Dr. Edwards's plan could be put into effect immediately, what ethical problems does it prevent?

Is there any justification for stopping the experiment? If so, on what grounds might they be stopped?

Is there any point in having an ethics committee review the experiments?

Decision Scenario 3

Dr. Charles Davis quickly scanned the data sheet on his desk then looked at the woman seated across from him. Her name was Nancy Callahan. She was twenty-five years old and worked as a print conservator at an art museum.

"I see that you aren't married," Dr. Davis said.

"That's right," Nancy Callahan said. "That's basically the reason I'm here." When Dr. Davis looked puzzled, she added, "I still want to have a child."

Dr. Davis nodded and thought for a moment. Nancy Callahan was the first unmarried person to come to the Bayside Fertility Clinic to request AID. As the legal owner and operator of the Clinic, as well as the Chief of Medical Services, Dr. Davis was the one ultimately responsible for the Clinic's policies.

"I hope you understand that I have to ask you some personal questions," Dr. Davis said.

"Of course."

"You're not engaged or planning to get married?"

"No. At least not at the moment. I don't want to rule out the possibility that I will want to get married someday."

"Don't you know anybody you would want to have a child with in the ordinary sexual way?"

"I might be able to find someone," Nancy Callahan said. "But you see, I don't want to get involved with anybody right now. I'm ready to be a mother, but I'm not ready to get into the kind of situation that having a child in what you call 'the ordinary sexual way' would require."

"I see."

"I hope you do. This is something I really want to do. I think I'll be a good mother. I want a child very much, and I can afford to support one."

"It's just somewhat unusual," Dr. Davis said."

"But it's not illegal, is it?"

"No," Dr. Davis said. "It's not illegal."

"So what's the problem? I'm healthy. I'm financially sound and mentally stable, and I'm both able and eager to accept the responsibility of being a mother."

"It's just that at the moment the policy of our clinic requires that patients be married and that both husbands and wives agree to the insemination procedure."

"But there's nothing magical about a policy," Nancy Callahan said. "It can be changed for good reasons, can't it?"

"Perhaps so," said Dr. Davis.

What utilitarian arguments can be advanced in favor of the policy mentioned by Dr. Davis?

Does the natural law view support such a policy? (See the discussion of the natural law theory of ethics in the introductory chapter.)

Could it be argued on the basis of Ross's ethical theory that Dr. Davis has a prima facie duty to provide Ms. Callahan with the service that she requests?

Might a Kantian argue that respect for Ms. Callahan's autonomy as a rational being would make it morally wrong to deny her the service she requests, while providing it to a married woman?

Decision Scenario 4

"My husband and I have talked over the matter in great detail," Marge Gower said. "We don't care about the sex of the child, but we know exactly the kinds of features we want to try for."

"Mrs. Gower," Dr. Louise Singh said. "You've got to understand that we're not running a mail-order catalog business for babies."

"I'm not trying to order a *baby*. I just want to tell you what I'm looking for in a sperm donor. I want somebody who is at least six feet tall, muscular—not fat—has light-colored hair and is very good looking. Also, I want some proof that he has a good sense of humor and is intelligent. He has to have at least a college degree. I'll leave all the rest to you. I mean, things about health."

"Thank you," said Dr. Singh. "But I really don't think I can go along with that."

"I don't see why not. If I were going to have a child in the usual way and I were deliberately going to get pregnant, I would certainly choose somebody like I described."

"But you aren't doing it in the usual way. You're going to be using donor semen."

"But who is going to choose the donor? You are, aren't you?"

"I plan to. I'll select somebody from our list of applicants who resembles you and your husband in a general way."

"I don't see why you should have that kind of power," Mrs. Gower said. "It's going to be my baby. I think I have the right to say what the father should be like."

"That's against Reproductive Medicine's policy."

"Well, that's too bad. Just tell me who to talk to to get the policy changed. I'm going to have a baby like my husband and I want. As long as I have to have artificial insemination, I want to get the most good out of it."

On what grounds might a utilitarian support the claim that Dr. Singh ought to be wholly responsible for choosing the sperm donor?

On what grounds might a utilitarian support the claim that Mrs. Gower and her husband ought to be able to select the features that a sperm donor should have?

Would it be better for the potential recipient of artificial insemination if the sperm donor were known personally to her and her husband? What are some of the problems caused by anonymity mentioned by Wadlington?

Might the choice of a sperm donor by the physician be regarded as an unacceptable form of paternalism? (See the discussion of paternalism in Chapter 4.)

Consider the issue involved here from the standpoint of the potential sperm donor. Should a sperm donor have some control over the use of his sperm in artificial insemination? Mrs. Gower argues that since the child will be hers, she should be the one who specifies what traits the donor should have. Since, biologically speaking, the child will equally be the offspring of the sperm donor, should he be able to specify the traits the sperm recipient should have?

Decision Scenario 5

"Now Ms. Ralston, I don't know if you fully realize the consequences of tubal ligation," Dr. Swabey said.

"I'm perfectly aware of them," Teri Ralston said. "It means that ova will no longer come down the fallopian tubes and be available for fertilization. It means that I will never get pregnant, and I believe the operation is best thought of as irreversible."

Dr. Swabey was somewhat taken aback. The young woman seated in his office seemed intelligent and well informed. However, he was almost certain that what she wanted would be a big mistake.

"That's all quite right," he said. "But now here you are, twenty-eight years old, coming to me and asking to be sterilized. You may think that's what you want, that may *be* what you want. But that's what you want right now. You may change your mind next week or next year. You may meet a man you want to have children with, and you won't be able to have any. You'll be sorry you ever chose this path."

Teri Ralston shook her head. "I'm not likely to change my mind. I know I never want to have children. It just doesn't fit into my life style."

"That's what you say now, but I'm talking about the future."

"That's what I say now, and that's what I'll say later," Teri Ralston insisted. "You see, Dr. Swabey, I'm an active feminist. You would probably consider me a radical. I've been one for over ten years, and I know what I want to do with my life. I don't want to have children—ever—and I don't want to run the risk of getting pregnant. I don't believe in abortions unless they are absolutely necessary, and I want to do what I can to see that one isn't ever necessary in my case."

"I suppose I understand your views," Dr. Swabey said. "But I never sterilize a woman as young as you are, unless there are medical indications of the need to do so."

"What do you mean?"

"Well, say, if you were the carrier of a genetic disease, then I would agree to sterilize you."

"But you won't do it just on the basis of my own ideas about my life."

"No, I won't."

Is there any reason to believe that Teri Ralston's decision to be sterilized is anything but voluntary?

Is there any reason to believe that Dr. Swabey is violating Ms. Ralston's individual autonomy in refusing to perform a sterilization procedure?

On what grounds might a rule utilitarian argue in favor of the position taken by Dr. Swabey?

On what grounds might a defender of the natural law theory object to Teri Ralston's decision?

Decision Scenario 6

Louise Tredle was twenty-years-old and retarded. Her IQ measured less than thirty on the WAIS, and she had difficulty understanding even very simple concepts.

Louise Tredle was also a mother. Her child was four years old. Both he and Louise lived with Louise's widowed mother. The child's father was unknown.

Mrs. Tredle never felt it was safe to leave Louise and the child by themselves. Louise could be trusted to perform routine chores, but she simply was not able to protect either herself or the child from the hazards of ordinary life. Because of this, Mrs. Tredle couldn't take a job outside the home. She was forced to operate the household on the money she got from social security and from payments made by state and federal welfare agencies.

When Mrs. Tredle found out that Louise had started stopping in at a neighborhood bar on her way back from the grocery store, Mrs. Tredle became fearful. Louise was sexually naive, and her intelligence level made her easy to take advantage of. Mrs. Tredle was very much afraid that Louise would become pregnant again. For Mrs. Tredle, abortion was out of the question, and she didn't know if she would be able to take care of another child.

Mrs. Tredle decided that she would have to try to get Louise sterilized. Only then would there be full protection for Louise and the rest of the family. Dr. Feldman, the physician who had arranged for Louise to be declared legally incompetent, also arranged for Mrs. Tredle to talk to someone in a community legal services organization. After Mrs. Tredle explained the situation, Mr. Olson, one of the agency's lawyers, took the necessary steps to set up a court hearing.

Mrs. Tredle testified at the court hearing. She explained her fears and tried to make the judge see that she was just not able to take responsibility for Louise and her child and, perhaps, another child. She explained the difficulty of watching Louise all the time and trying to make sure she didn't become sexually involved with anyone.

Mr. Olson arranged for a psychiatrist to examine Louise, and the psychiatrist testified that Louise was indeed of subnormal intelligence and unable to function in an ordinary responsible way. Louise herself was questioned by the court. She responded to questions about how she liked being a mother by saying that she liked it very much and that she loved her child. When she was asked if she knew what sterilization was, she said that she knew it meant she wouldn't be able to have children. She also said that she didn't want that to happen to her.

To Mrs. Tredle's surprise, the judge ruled against her request. In the court's opinion, Louise's wish not to lose the capacity to have children outweighed all other considerations. The court refused to approve sterilization.

> *What sort of evidence should be considered to show that sterilization is in the best interest of the individual? (See the discussion by Annas.)*

> *Would a Quinlan-type approach to the decision be more likely to emphasize considerations other than the best interest of the person?*

> *According to Rawls, what features must a paternalistic action have to justify it as legitimate? Does the fact that Mrs. Tredle will gain benefits from having Louise sterilized necessarily mean that such an action cannot be justified?*

> *Would a utilitarian consider Louise's mental limitations and Mrs. Tredle's situation and wishes relevant to deciding whether a decision to sterilize Louise would be justified?*

> *Does the fact that Louise knows that sterilization means she won't be capable of having more children show that she is sufficiently informed to make her wish not to lose that capacity equivalent to a refusal to give consent?*

Part IV
RESOURCES

9
COMPETITION AND ALLOCATION

CASE PRESENTATION
Selection Committee

In 1966 Brattle, Texas, proper had a population of about ten thousand people. In Brattle County there were twenty thousand more people who lived on isolated farms deep within the pine forests, or in crossroads towns with a filling station, a feed store, one or two white, frame churches, and maybe twenty or twenty-five houses.

Brattle was the marketing town and county seat, the place all the farmers, their wives, and children went to on Saturday afternoon. It was also the medical center because it had the only hospitals in the county. One of them, Conklin Clinic, was hardly more than a group of doctor's offices. But Crane Memorial Hospital was quite a different sort of place. Occupying a relatively new three-story brick building in downtown Brattle, the hospital offered new equipment, a well-trained staff, and high quality medical care.

This was mostly due to the efforts of Dr. J. B. Crane, Jr. The hospital was dedicated to the memory of his father, a man who practiced medicine in Brattle County for almost fifty years. Before Crane became a memorial hospital, it was Crane Clinic. But J. B. Crane, Jr., after returning from the Johns Hopkins Medical School, was determined to expand the clinic and transform it into a modern hospital. The need was there, and private investors were easy to find. Only a year after his father's death, Dr. Crane was able to offer Brattle County a genuine hospital.

It was only natural that when the County Commissioner decided that Brattle County should have a dialysis machine, he would turn to Dr. Crane's hospital. The machine was bought with county funds, but Crane Memorial Hospital would operate it under a contract agreement. The hospital was guaranteed against loss by the county, but the hospital was also not permitted to make a profit on dialysis. Furthermore, although access to the machine was not restricted to county residents, residents were to be given priority.

Dr. Crane was not pleased with this stipulation. "I don't like to have medical decisions influenced by political considerations," he told the Commissioner. "If a guy comes in and needs dialysis, I don't want to tell him that he can't have it because somebody else who doesn't need it as much is on the machine and that person is a county resident."

"I don't know what to tell you," the Commissioner said. "It was county tax money that paid for the machine, and the County Council decided that the people who supplied the money ought to get top priority."

"What about the kind of case that I mentioned?" Dr. Crane asked. "What about somebody who could wait for dialysis who is a resident as opposed to somebody who needs it immediately who's not a resident?"

"We'll just leave that sort of case to your discretion," the Commissioner said. "People around here have confidence in you and your doctors. If you say they can wait, then they can wait. I know you won't let them down. Of course if somebody died while some outsider was on the machine. . . . Well, that would be embarrassing for all of us, I guess."

Dr. Crane was pleased to have the dialysis machine in his hospital. Not only was it the only one in Brattle County, none of the neighboring counties had one either. Only the big hospitals in places like Dallas, Houston, and San Antonio had the machines. It put Crane Memorial up in the top rank.

Dr. Crane was totally unprepared for the problem when it came. He hadn't known there were so many people with chronic renal disease in Brattle County. But when news spread that there was a kidney machine available at Crane Memorial Hospital, twenty-three people applied for the dialysis program. Some were Dr. Crane's own patients or patients of his associates on the hospital staff. But a number of them were ones referred to the hospital by other physicians in Brattle and surrounding towns. Two of them were from neighboring Lopez County.

Working at a maximum, the machine could accommodate fourteen patients. But the staff decided that maximum operation would be likely to lead to dangerous equipment malfunctions and breakdowns. They settled on ten as the number of patients that should be admitted to the program.

Dr. Crane and his staff interviewed each of the program's applicants, reviewed their medical history, and got a thorough medical workup on each. They persuaded two of the patients to continue to commute to Houston, where they were already in dialysis. In four cases, renal disease had already progressed to the point that the staff decided that the patients could not benefit sufficiently from the program to make them good medical risks. In one other case, a patient suffering intestinal cancer and in generally poor health was rejected as a candidate. Two people were not in genuine need of dialysis but could be best treated by a program of medication.

That left fourteen candidates for the ten positions. Thirteen were from Brattle County and one from Lopez County.

"This is not a medical problem," Dr. Crane told the Commissioner. "And I'm not going to take the responsibility of deciding which people to condemn to death and which to give an extra chance at life."

"What do you want me to do?" the Commissioner asked. "I wouldn't object if you made the decision. I mean, you wouldn't have to tell everybody about it. You could just decide."

"That's something I won't do," Dr. Crane said. "All of this has to be open and aboveboard. It's got to be fair. If I decide, then everybody will think I am favoring my own patients or just taking the people who can pay the most money."

"I see what you mean. If I appoint a selection committee, will you serve on it?"

"I will. So long as my vote is the same as everybody else's."

"That's what I'll do then," the Commissioner said.

The Brattle County Renal Dialysis Selection Committee was appointed and operating within the week. In addition to Dr. Crane, it was made up of three people chosen by the Commissioner. Amy Langford, a Brattle housewife in her middle fifties whose husband owned the largest automobile and truck agency in Brattle County, was one member. Reverend David Johnson was another member. He was the only black on the committee and the pastor of the largest predominantly black church in Brattle. The last member was Jacob Sims, owner of a hardware store in the nearby town of Silsbee. He was the only member of the committee not from the town of Brattle.

"Now I'm inclined to favor this fellow," said Mr. Sims at the Selection Committee's first meeting. "He's twenty-four years old, he's married and has a child two years old."

"You're talking about James Nelson?" Mrs. Langford asked. "I had some trouble with him. I've heard that he used to drink a lot before he got sick, and from the looks of his record he's had a hard time keeping a job."

"That's hard to say," said Reverend Johnson. "He works as a pulp-wood hauler, and people who do that change jobs a lot. You just have to go where the work is."

"That's right," said Mr. Sims. "One thing, though. I can't find any indication of his church membership. He says he's a Methodist, but I don't see where he's told us what his church is."

"I don't either," said Mrs. Langford. "And he's not a member of the Mason's or the Lion's Club or any other sort of civic group. I wouldn't say he's made much of a contribution to this community."

"That's right," said Reverend Johnson. "But let's don't forget that he's got a wife and baby depending on him. That child is going to need a father."

"I think he is a good psychological candidate," said Dr. Crane. "That is, I think if he starts the program he'll stick to it. I've talked with his wife, and I know she'll encourage him."

"We should notice that he's a high school dropout," Mrs. Langford said. "I don't think we can ever expect him to make much of a contribution to this town or to the county."

"Do you want to vote on this case?" asked Mr. Sims, the chairman of the committee.

"Let's talk about all of them, then go back and vote," Reverend Johnson suggested.

Everyone around the table nodded in agreement. The files were arranged by date of application, and Mr. Sims picked up the next one from the stack in front of him.

"Alva Algers," he said. "He's a fifty-three-year-old lawyer with three grown children. His wife is still alive, and he's still married to her. He's Secretary of the Layman's Board of the Brattle Episcopal Church, a member of the Rotary Club and the Elk's. He used to be a scoutmaster."

"From the practical point of view," said Dr. Crane, "he would be a good candidate. He's intelligent and educated and understands what's involved in dialysis."

"I think he's definitely the sort of person we want to help," said Mrs. Langford. "He's the kind of person that makes this a better town. I'm definitely in favor of him."

"I am too," said Reverend Johnson. "Even if he does go to the wrong church."

"I'm not so sure," said Mr. Sims. "I don't think fifty-three is old—I'd better not, because I'm fifty-two myself. Still, his children are grown, he's led a good life. I'm not sure I wouldn't give the edge to some younger fellow."

"How can you say that," Mrs. Langford said. "He's got a lot of good years left. He's a person of good character who might still do a lot for other people. He's not like that Nelson, who's not going to do any good for anybody except himself."

"I guess I'm not convinced that lawyers and members of the Rotary Club do a lot more good for the community than drivers of pulp-wood trucks," Mr. Sims said.

"Perhaps we ought to go on to the next candidate," Reverend Johnson said.

"We have Mrs. Holly Holton, a forty-three-year-old housewife from Mineral Springs," Mr. Sim said.

"That's in Lopez County, isn't it?" Mrs. Langford asked. "I think we can just reject her right off. She didn't pay the taxes that bought the machine, and our county doesn't have any responsibility for her."

"That's right," said Reverend Johnson.

Mr. Sims agreed and Dr. Crane raised no objection.

"Now," said Mr. Sims, "here's Alton Conway. I believe he's our only black candidate."

"I know him well," said Reverend Johnson. "He owns a dry cleaning business, and people in the black community think very highly of him."

"I'm in favor of him," Mrs. Langford said. "He's a married man and seems quite settled and respectable."

"I wouldn't want us to take him just because he's black," Reverend Johnson said. "But I think he's got a lot in his favor."

"Well," said Mr. Sims, "unless Dr. Crane wants to add anything, let's go on to Nora Bainridge. She's a thirty-year-old divorced woman whose eight-year-old boy lives with his father over in Louisiana. She's a waitress at the Pep Cafe."

"She is a very vital woman," said Dr. Crane. "She's had a lot of trouble in her life, but I think she's a real fighter."

"I don't believe she's much of a churchgoer," said Reverend Johnson. "At least she doesn't give us a pastor's name."

"That's right," said Mrs. Langford. "And I just wonder what kind of morals a woman like her has. I mean, being divorced and working as a waitress and all."

"I don't believe we're trying to award sainthood here," said Mr. Sims.

"But surely moral character is relevant," said Mrs. Langford.

"I don't know anything against her moral character," said Mr. Sims. "Do you?"

"I'm only guessing," said Mrs. Langford. "But I wouldn't say that a woman of her background and apparent character is somebody we ought to give top priority to."

"I don't want to be the one to cast the first stone," said Reverend Johnson. "But I wouldn't put her at the top of our list either."

"I think we had better be careful not to discriminate against people who are poor and uneducated," said Dr. Crane.

"I agree," said Mrs. Langford. "But surely we have to take account of a person's worth."

"Can you tell us how we can measure a person's worth?" asked Mr. Sims.

"I believe I can," Mrs. Langford said. "Does the person have a steady job? Is he or she somebody we would be proud to know? Is he a churchgoer? Does he or she do things for other people? We can see what kind of education the person has had, and consider whether he is somebody we would like to have around."

"I guess that's some of it all right," said Mr. Sims. "But I don't like to rely on things like education, money, and public service. A lot of people just haven't had a decent chance in this world. Maybe they were born poor or have had a lot of bad luck. I'm beginning to think that we ought to make our choices just by drawing lots."

"I can't approve of that," said Reverend Johnson. "That seems like a form of gambling to me. We ought to choose the good over the wicked, reward those who have led a virtuous life."

"I agree," Mrs. Langford said. "Choosing by drawing straws or something like that would mean we are just too cowardly to make the decisions. We would be shirking our responsibility. Clearly, some people are more deserving than others, and we ought to have the courage to say so."

"All right," said Mr. Sims. "I guess we'd better get on with it then. Simon Gootz is a forty-eight-year-old baker. He's got a wife and four children. Owns his own bakery—probably all of us have been there. He's Jewish."

"I'm not sure he's the sort of person who can stick to the required diet and go through the dialysis program," Dr. Crane said.

"I'll bet his wife and children would be a good incentive," said Mrs. Langford.

"There's not a Jewish church in town," said Reverend Johnson. "So of course we can't expect him to be a regular churchgoer."

"He's an immigrant," said Mr. Sims. "I don't believe he has any education to speak of, but he did start that bakery and build it up from nothing. I think that says a lot about his character."

"I think we can agree he's a good candidate," said Mrs. Langford.

"Let's just take one more before we break for dinner," Mr. Sims said. "Rebecca Scarborough. She's a sixty-three-year-old widow. Her children are all grown and living somewhere else."

"She's my patient," Dr. Crane said. "She's a tough and resourceful old woman. I believe she can follow orders and stand up to the rigors of the program, and her health in general is good."

Reverend Johnson said, "I just wonder if we shouldn't put a lady like her pretty far down on our list. She's lived a long life already, and she hasn't got anybody depending on her."

"I'm against that," Mrs. Langford said. "Everybody knows Mrs. Scarborough. Her family has been in this town for ages. She's one of our most substantial citizens. People would be scandalized if we didn't select her."

"Of course I'm not from Brattle," said Mr. Sims. "And maybe that's an advantage here, because I don't see that she's got much in her favor except being from an old family."

"I think that's worth something," said Mrs. Langford.

"I'm not sure it's enough, though," said Reverend Johnson.

After dinner at the Crane Memorial Hospital cafeteria, the Selection Committee met again to discuss the seven remaining candidates. It was past ten o'clock before their final decisions were made. James Nelson, the pulp-wood truck driver, Holly Holton, the housewife from Mineral Springs, and Nora Bainridge, the waitress, were all rejected as candidates. Mrs. Scarborough was rejected also. The lawyer, Alva Algers, the dry cleaner, Alton Conway, and the baker, Simon Gootz, were selected to participate in the dialysis program. Others selected were a retired secondary school teacher, an assembly-line worker at the Rigid Box Company, a Brattle County Sheriff's Department patrolman, and a twenty-seven-year-old woman file clerk in the office of the Texas Western Insurance Company.

Dr. Crane was glad that the choices were made so that the program could begin operation. But he was not pleased with the selection method and resolved to talk to his own staff and with the County Commissioner about devising some other kind of selection procedure.

Without giving any reasons, Mr. Sims sent a letter to the County Commissioner resigning from the Renal Dialysis Selection Committee.

Mrs. Langford and Reverend Johnson also sent letters to the Commissioner. They thanked him for appointing them to the Committee and indicated their willingness to continue to serve.

CASE PRESENTATION
Policy Decision

Jake Hanna (as we will call him) stood by the admitting desk in the emergency room of Commerce County Hospital and couldn't believe what was happening. It was like being trapped in a nightmare.

Less than ten miles away, his wife Christine lay in a recovery room at Valley View Hospital. She had just given birth to their first child and was still groggy from the anesthesia.

Martha, as they had already decided to name their daughter before her birth, had been premature. She was almost six weeks early, and both Jake and Chris had been surprised when Chris began to experience labor pains. At first they didn't know what the pains were, then they decided that to be safe, they had better get Chris to the hospital Chris's obstetrician had told them to go to. They were lucky to have gotten to Valley View in time, because the birth was a difficult one and Chris had needed help and reassurance.

In another respect, they hadn't been so lucky. Valley View was a small private hospital with restricted facilities. It had an emergency room, but no intensive care or neonatal units.

And Martha needed help. She was small and underdeveloped. Her heart sounds were weak and slightly irregular, she was having difficulty breathing, and her blood chemistry was unbalanced and showed inadequate kidney function. If she was to have a good chance at living, she needed special treatment and continuous monitoring.

"You need to get her into a special facility," Dr. Birk told Jake. "We're doing all we can for her here, but that's not very much. We aren't even set up to do dialysis. We simply don't have the equipment or the personnel to provide her with the kind of care she needs."

"Where could she go?" Jake asked.

"Commerce County Hospital—it's the only place in the area with a neonatal setup."

"Can you make the arrangements?"

"I'm sorry, I can't. They won't take referrals anymore. Somebody on their staff has to do the admitting. I think they're trying to cut back on their program."

"Can I get her in?"

"I'm not sure," Dr. Birk said. "but she needs to be there. They may take her as a walk-in. So you're going to have to go in person and take the baby with you. Do you have a friend or family member here?"

"Chris's mother is with her. But isn't it dangerous to move the baby?"

"Not really. She's in a stable condition, and if you take her you'll save a lot of time. She needs help as fast as she can get it."

With Martha wrapped in a grey hospital blanket and held by Chris's mother, Jake drove the ten miles to Commerce County Hospital and double-parked at the emergency entrance. He literally ran through the wide doors.

He explained to the clerk at the admitting desk that Dr. Birk had said that the baby needed to be in a neonatal unit at once. The clerk said that he had no authority to make that kind of admission and told Jake to sit down while he paged Dr. Donna Chavez, the director of the unit.

The wait seemed interminable to Jake, but in less than ten minutes Dr. Chavez appeared in the emergency room. Jake walked over to her, and while they stood by the admitting desk with a dozen people waiting for their names to be called, he explained the problem once again.

When Jake had finished, Dr. Chavez shook her head. "We can't admit the child," she said. "I'm sorry, but we just can't do it."

"Why not?" Jake asked. "Don't you have room or something?"

"That's not the problem. We actually have enough space."

"Then what is it?"

"This is going to be hard for you to understand," Dr. Chavez said. "But the hospital has adopted a new policy. At no time can we have more than twenty patients in the neonatal unit, and that's the number we have now. The problem is with costs."

"But I'm willing to pay, and I have insurance."

"It's not particular costs, Mr. Hanna. It's the cost of the whole unit, and Commerce has just decided to cut back on its size. That's why they've imposed a twenty-infant limit."

"But what about my child?" Jake asked. "She needs help, and she needs it right now."

"I'm very, very sorry," Dr. Chavez said. "If the decision were mine alone, I would admit her at once. But as things are, I simply have to follow the hospital's policy guidelines."

"So you refuse to take her?"

"I must. I don't have any real choice in the matter."

"What am I supposed to do? Just let her die?"

"I suggest you take the child back to Valley View. They will do everything they can, and with luck things will work out for her. I certainly hope so."

Jake thought he had never had a nightmare as bad as this. He had never before felt so helpless, so powerless. There was no way he could force them to admit Martha, and there was nothing he could do for her himself. It surprised him that he didn't feel particularly angry at Dr. Chavez or at the hospital. He was simply too numb to feel much of anything.

Jake said nothing more to Dr. Chavez. He went out to the car and drove back to Valley View. Mrs. Williams cried all the way back, and Jake wished that he could.

Inside the emergency room at Valley View, a nurse took the baby from Mrs. Williams. They took Martha to a small treatment room and gave her oxygen to help her breathing.

Jake and Mrs. Williams sat in the waiting area. They agreed that there was no need to tell Chris anything yet. She was asleep and no purpose would be served by waking her.

Three hours later, a doctor Jake had never seen before came to tell him that Martha was dead.

Note: This case is a fictional account that is based on a real incident. For an actual case that parallels the fictional one in some respects, see the St. Louis *Post-Dispatch*, 5 July 1981, p. 14A, for the story about the policy at Tampa General Hospital.

INTRODUCTION

The story of Robin Cook's novel *Coma* takes place in a large Boston hospital at the present time. What sets the novel apart from dozens of others with similar settings and characters is the fact that the plot hinges on the operations of a large-scale blackmarket in transplant organs. For enormous fees, the criminals running the operation will supply corneas, kidneys, or hearts to those who can pay the price.

Cook claims that the inspiration for his novel came from an advertisement in a California newspaper. The anonymous ad offered to sell for five thousand dollars any organ that a reader wanted to buy. Thus, Cook's novel seems to be rooted firmly in the world we know today and not just a leap into the speculative realms of science fiction.

Organ transplants have attracted a considerable amount of attention in the last few years. Not only are transplants dramatic, often offering last-minute salvation from an almost certain death, but the very possibility of organ transplants is bright with promise. We can easily imagine a future in which any injured or diseased organ can be replaced almost as easily as the parts on a car. Yet the present state of biomedical technology makes this more a distant dream than a current reality.

If blood is considered to be an organ, it is the only organ that can currently be "transplanted" in a relatively unproblematic way. Corneas, skin grafts, and bone segments have the next best records of success, although kidney transplants have become successful enough to justify their widespread use. Heart transplants, by contrast, continue to be uncertain and highly controversial procedures. The basic problem with organ transplants is the phenomenon of tissue rejection by the immune system. Alien proteins trigger the body's defensive mechanisms. For this reason, the proteins in the transplanted tissues must be matched as carefully as possible with those of the recipient, and then powerful immunosuppressive drugs have to be used in an effort to allow the host body to accommodate itself to the foreign tissue. These drugs leave the body open to infections that it could normally cope with without much difficulty. Even "successful" kidney transplants are not wholly satisfactory as a general medical procedure because about half of the recipients die within two years of the transplant.

Despite the imperfections of organ transplants, the need for organs (kidneys in particular) is always greater than the supply. (The blackmarket operations in Cook's novel may not be wholly unrealistic.) In such a situation, where scarcity and need conflict, it is frequently necessary to decide who among the candidates for a transplant will receive an available organ. Relatively objective considerations such as the "goodness" of tissue matching may rule out some candidates. But it does happen that choices have to be made.

Who should make such choices? Should they be made by a physician, following his or her own intuitions? Should they be made by a committee or board? If so, who should be on the committee? Should a patient have a representative to speak for his or her interest—someone to "make a case" for receiving the transplant organ?

Should the decision be made in accordance with a set of explicit criteria? If so, then what criteria are appropriate? Are matters such as age, race, sex, and place of residence irrelevant? Should the character and accomplishments of the candidates be given any weight? Should people be judged by their estimated "worth to the community"? Should the fact that someone is a parent be given any weight?

These are just some of the questions that are relevant to the general issue of deciding how to allocate medical goods in situations in which the available supply is surpassed by a present need. Transplant organs are just an example of one type of goods. In the future, with the improvement of transplant technology, the allocation of organs will no doubt become an even more frequent problem than it is at present. It is, of course, already a morally serious problem.

It was not organ transplants that first called public attention to the issue of resource allocation. This occurred most dramatically in the early 1960s when the Artificial Kidney Center in Seattle, Washington initiated an effective large-scale treatment program for people with renal diseases. Normal kidneys filter from the blood waste products that have accumulated as a result of ordinary cellular metabolism—salt, urea, creatinine, potassium, uric acid, and other substances. These waste products are sent from the kidneys to the bladder, where they are then secreted as urine. Kidney failure, which can result from one of a number of diseases, allows waste products to build up in the blood. This can cause high blood pressure and even heart failure, tissue edema (swelling), and muscular seizure. If unremedied, the condition results in death.

When renal failure occurs, hemodialysis is a way of cleansing the blood of waste products by passing it through a cellophanelike tube immersed in a chemical bath. The impurities in the blood pass through the membrane and into the chemical bath by osmosis, and the purified blood is then returned to the patient's body.

At the beginning of the Seattle program, there were many more candidates for dialysis than there were units ("kidney machines") to accommodate them. As a response to this situation, the Kidney Center set up a committee to select those patients who would receive treatment. (See the Case Presentation for an account of how such a committee might work.) In effect, the committee was offering to some a better chance for life than they would have without access to dialysis equipment.

As other centers and hospitals established renal units, they faced the same painful decision that Seattle did. Almost always there were many more patients needing hemodialysis than there was equipment available to treat them. It was partly in response to this situation that Section 299–1 of Public Law 92–603 was passed by Congress in 1972. Those that require hemodialysis or kidney transplants are now eligible for Medicare payments that cover as much as 80 percent of the costs involved.

At present more than twenty-three thousand patients are now receiving dialysis supported by Medicare. Present costs are over three hundred million dollars a year. By the 1980s it is expected that about fifty thousand people will be in federally supported dialysis programs, at a cost of over a billion dollars a year.

Quite apart from the cost, which is much higher than originally expected, dialysis continues to present moral difficulties. Resources are still finite so that at a given time more patients may both need and want dialysis than can be accommodated. Hence the need to make choices among patients is still present. It brings with it all the problems that we mentioned above.

In addition, because more dialysis equipment is available and is financially available to virtually everyone, physicians face a serious difficulty. Even if a physician believes that a patient is not likely to gain benefits from dialysis to an extent to justify the expense, should he recommend the patient for dialysis anyway? Not to do so may mean almost certain death for the patient in the near future, yet the social cost (measured in terms of the cost of equipment and its operation, hospital facilities, and the time of physicians, nurses, and technicians) may be immense. It can be as much as seventy-five to one hundred thousand dollars a year for a single person.

It is important to notice that dialysis does not solve all the problems for patients with terminal kidney diseases. Although time spent on the machine varies, some patients spend five hours, three days a week, attached to the machine. Medical and psychological problems are typical even when the process works at its most efficient. Prolonged dialysis can produce neurological disorders, severe headaches, gastrointestinal bleeding, and bone diseases. Psychological and physical stress is always present, and particularly before dialysis treatments, severe depression is common. A 1971 study showed that 5 percent of dialysis patients take their own lives, and a number of others simply drop out of treatment programs and allow themselves to die. For these reasons, strong motivation, psychological stability, age, and a generally sound physical condition are factors considered important in deciding whether to admit a person to dialysis.

The characteristics required to make someone a "successful" dialysis patient are to some extent "middle-class virtues." A patient must not only be motivated to save his life, but he must also understand the need for the dialysis, be capable of adhering to a strict diet, show up for scheduled dialysis sessions, and so on. As a consequence, where decisions about whether to admit a patient to dialysis are based on estimates of the likelihood of the patient's doing what is required, members of the white middle class have a definite edge over others. Selection criteria that are apparently objective may actually involve hidden class or racial bias.

The problems of transplants and dialysis are ones that involve decisions that affect individuals in a direct and immediate way—either a person is accepted into a dialysis program or he is not. As we will see in the next chapter, there are a number of broader social issues connected with providing and distributing medical resources. But our concern here is with the sort of decision making that involves the welfare of particular people in specific situations. The situations are ones in which there is not enough of what is needed to go around. The basic question, of course, is who shall get it and who shall go without?

Earlier, in connection with transplants, we mentioned some of the more specific questions that have to be asked. The questions generally fall into two categories: Who shall decide? and What criteria or standards should be employed in making the decision? These are appropriate questions whether the medical resources we are talking about are transplant organs, dialysis machines, drugs, hospital beds, operating rooms, medical the.apy, physician's time, or whatever. Any commodity or service that can be in short supply relative to the need for it raises the issue of legitimate distribution.

Ethical Theories and the Allocation of Medical Resources

An analogy that is frequently used in the discussion of the distribution of limited medical resources compares such a situation to the plight of a group of people adrift in a lifeboat. If some of the group are sacrificed, then the others will have a much better chance of surviving. But who should be sacrificed?

One answer to this question is that no one should be. Simply by virtue of being human, each person in the lifeboat has an equal worth. An action that involved sacrificing anyone for the good of the others in the boat would not be morally defensible. This suggests that the only right course of action would be simply to do nothing.

This point of view is one that may be regarded as compatible with Kant's ethical principles. Because each individual may be considered to have inherent value, considerations such as talent, intelligence, age, social worth, and so on are morally irrelevant. Accordingly, there seems to be no grounds for distinguishing those who are to be sacrificed from those who may be saved. In the medical context, this would mean that when there are not enough goods and services to go around, then no one should receive them.

This is not a result that is dictated by Kant's principles, however. One might also argue that just because every person is equal to every other in dignity and worth does not require the sacrifice of all. A random procedure—such as drawing straws—might be used to determine who is to have an increased chance of survival. In such a case, each person is being treated as having equal value, and the person who loses might be regarded as exercising his autonomy by sacrificing himself or herself. The maxim underlying the sacrifice would, apparently, be one that would meet the test of the categorical imperative. Any rational person might be expected to sacrifice himself in such a situation and under the conditions in which the decision was made. In the case of medical resources, a random procedure would seem to be a morally legitimate procedure.

The natural law view and Ross's would seem to support a similar line of argument. Although we all have a duty, on these views, to preserve our lives, this does not mean that we do not sometimes have to risk them. Just such a risk might be involved in agreeing to abide by the outcome of a random procedure to decide who will be sacrificed and who saved.

Utilitarianism does not dictate a specific answer to the question of who, if anyone, should be saved. It does differ radically in one respect, however, from those moral views that ascribe an intrinsic value to each human life. The principle of utility suggests that we ought to take into account the consequences of sacrificing some people rather than others. Who, for example, is more likely to make a contribution to the general welfare of the society, an accountant or a nurse? This approach opens the way to considering the "social worth" of people and makes morally relevant such characteristics as education, occupation, age, record of accomplishment, and so on.

To take this approach would require working out a set of criteria that would assign value to various properties of people. Those to be sacrificed would be those whose point total put them at the low end of the ranking. Here, then, a typical "calculus of utilities" would be relied on to solve the decision problem. Decisions about the allocation of medical resources would follow exactly the same pattern.

This approach is not one required by the principle of utility, however. Someone might argue that a policy formulated along those lines would have so many harmful social consequences that some other solution would be preferable. Thus, a utilitarian might argue that a better policy would be one based on some random process. In connection with medical goods and services, a "first come, first served" approach might be superior. (This, at least, is a possible option for rule utilitarianism. It could be argued that an act utilitarian would be forced to adopt the first approach.)

Rawls's principles of justice seem clearly to rule out distributing medical resources on the grounds of "social worth." Where special benefits are to be obtained, those benefits must be of value to all and open to all. It is compatible with Rawls's view, of course, that there should be no special medical resources. But if there are and they must be distributed under conditions of scarcity, then some genuinely fair procedure, such as random selection, must be the procedure used.

No ethical theory that we have considered gives a straightforward answer to the question of who shall make the selection. Where a procedure is random or "first come, first served," the decision-making process requires only establishing the right kind of social arrangements to implement the policy. Only when social worth must be judged and considered as a relevant factor in decision making does the procedure assume importance. (This is assuming that medical decisions about appropriateness have already been made, decisions that establish a class of candidates for the limited resources.)

A utilitarian answer as to who shall make the allocation decision might be that the decision should be made by those who are in a good position to judge the likelihood of an individual's contributing to the welfare of the society as a whole. Since physicians are not uniquely qualified to make such judgments, decisions by an individual physician or a committee of physicians would not be the best approach. A better one would probably be a committee composed of a variety of people representative of the society.

There are many more questions of a moral kind connected with the allocation of scarce resources than we have mentioned here. We have not, for example, considered whether an individual should be allowed to make a case for receiving resources. Nor have we examined any of the problems with employing specific criteria for selection for treatment (such as requiring that a person be a resident of a certain community or state). We have, however, touched upon enough of the basic issues that it should be easy to see how other appropriate questions might be asked.

The Selections

Nicholas Rescher in his essay makes a useful distinction between two kinds of criteria: criteria of inclusion (for the selection of candidates) and criteria of comparison (for selection of recipients). Rescher argues that three areas need to be considered in establishing a class of candidates: (1) constituency (Is the person a member of the community the institution is designed to serve?); (2) progress of science (Can new knowledge be gained from the case?); and (3) success (Is the treatment of the person likely to be effective?).

Five factors, Rescher claims, ought to be considered in deciding upon recipients of the goods or services: (1) the likelihood of successful treatment compared with others in the group; (2) the life-expectancy of the person; (3) the person's family role; (4) the potential of the person in making future contributions; and (5) the person's record of services or contributions.

Rescher argues that it is necessary to have a rational selection system, but he admits that the exact manner in which a system takes into account relevant factors cannot be fixed and exact. In his view, which is basically a utilitarian one, an acceptable selection system might be one that makes use of point ratings of the factors mentioned above. This would establish a smaller group, but as a final step, he suggests, the best procedure might well be to make use of a chance factor (such as a lottery) to choose recipients.

Childress's essay is explicitly critical of the utilitarian approach that would make "social worth" the source of selection criteria. Such criteria, Childress argues, lead us to value only the person who is a conformist. What is more, they have the effect of reducing people to their social roles. Childress favors some sort of random selection procedure ("first come, first served," or a lottery). Only an approach of this kind, he argues, preserves an individual's "personal and transcendent dignity, which on the utilitarian approach would be submerged in his social role and function." Also, Childress suggests, the random approach contributes to the preservation of such values as the maintenance of trust between patient and physician.

It can be argued that Childress is wrong to identify the utilitarian approach with the use of criteria based on social roles. As we mentioned earlier, it seems possible for rule utilitarianism to endorse the random approach advocated by Childress, although for very different reasons. Yet Childress's criticisms do hit at the utilitarian solutions recommended by Rescher.

In "Human Organs and the Open Market," Clifton Perry addresses another aspect of the problem of distributing scarce medical resources. Perry is not so much interested in criteria for selection under conditions of scarcity as in reducing the scarcity. His focus is on transplant organs.

In the view of some, the relative scarcity of transplant organs such as kidneys, corneas, and pituitary glands is due primarily to the fact that the availability of the organs is almost wholly dependent on individual donations. Exactly why a policy for securing organs that is based on donation has not been effective is probably due to a number of practical considerations. For example, many people are quite uncertain about how to arrange to donate their organs, mechanisms for retrieving organs from those who have signed donor cards have not been well worked out, and it is often difficult to get the permission of a bereaved family to remove an organ for transplant from a recently dead family member.

Perry points out that, in addition to donation, two other approaches to securing organs have been generally favored: automatically "harvesting" or salvaging needed organs after death and trading organs. The idea of selling organs has met with very little acceptance. Although donation is frequently taken as the morally ideal policy, as a matter of fact, Perry claims, the values that we associate with it can also be shown to be present in the other approaches.

Perry's fundamental argument is that a careful consideration of all four approaches shows that a social policy based on selling transplant organs might be the best one. Not only could it be more effective in making needed organs available, but it could also satisfy such moral restraints and social goals as saving lives, assisting survivors, protecting the autonomy of the living, and preserving the integrity of the dead.

The Allocation of Exotic Medical Lifesaving Therapy

Nicholas Rescher

I. The Problem

Technological progress has in recent years transformed the limits of the possible in medical therapy. However, the elevated state of sophistication of modern medical technology has brought the economists' classic problem of scarcity in its wake as an unfortunate side product. The enormously sophisticated and complex equipment and the highly trained teams of experts requisite for its utilization are scarce resources in relation to potential demand. The administrators of the great medical institutions that preside over these scarce resources thus come to be faced increasingly with the awesome choice: *Whose life to save?*

A (somewhat hypothetical) paradigm example of this problem may be sketched within the following set of definitive assumptions: We suppose that persons in some particular medically morbid condition are "mortally afflicted": It is virtually certain that they will die within a short time period (say ninety days). We assume that some very complex course of treatment (e.g., a heart transplant) represents a substantial probability of life prolongation for persons in this mortally afflicted condition. We assume that the facilities available in terms of human resources, mechanical instrumentalities, and requisite materials (e.g., hearts in the case of a heart transplant) make it possible to give a certain treatment—this "exotic (medical) lifesaving therapy," or ELT for short—to a certain, relatively small number of people. And finally we assume that a substantially greater pool of people in the mortally afflicted condition is at hand. The problem then may be formulated as follows: How is one to select within the pool of afflicted patients the ones to be given the ELT treatment in question; how to select those "whose lives are to be saved"?

Faced with many candidates for an ELT process that can be made available to only a few, doctors and medical administrators confront the decision of who is to be given a chance at survival and who is, in effect, to be condemned to die.

As has already been implied, the "heroic" variety of spare-part surgery can pretty well be assimilated to this paradigm. One can foresee the time when heart transplantation, for example, will have become pretty much a routine medical procedure, albeit on a very limited basis, since a cardiac surgeon with the technical competence to transplant hearts can operate at best a rather small number of times each week and the elaborate facilities for such operations will most probably exist on a modest scale. Moreover, in "spare-part" surgery there is always the problem of availability of the "spare parts" themselves. A report in one British newspaper gives the following picture: "Of the 150,000 who die of heart disease each year [in the U.K.], Mr. Donald Longmore, research surgeon at the National Heart Hospital [in London] estimated that 22,000 might be eligible for heart surgery. Another 30,000 would need heart and lung transplants. But there are probably only between 7,000 and 14,000 potential donors a year."[1] Envisaging this situation in which at the very most something like one in four heart-malfunction victims can be saved, we clearly confront a problem in ELT allocation.

A perhaps even more drastic case in point is afforded by long-term haemodialysis, an ongoing process by which a complex device—an "artificial kidney machine"—is used periodically in cases of chronic renal failure to substitute for a nonfunctional kidney in "cleaning" potential poisons from the blood. Only a few major institutions have chronic haemodialysis units, whose complex op-

Reprinted from Ethics 79 (April 1969), *by permission of The University of Chicago Press and the author.* © 1979 by The University of Chicago Press.

eration is an extremely expensive proposition. For the present and foreseeable future the situation is that "the number of places available for chronic haemodialysis is hopelessly inadequate."[2]

The traditional medical ethos has insulated the physician against facing the very existence of this problem. When swearing the Hippocratic Oath, he commits himself to work for the benefit of the sick in "whatsoever house I enter."[3] In taking this stance, the physician substantially renounces the explicit choice of saving certain lives rather than others. Of course, doctors have always in fact had to face such choices on the battlefield or in times of disaster, but there the issue had to be resolved hurriedly, under pressure, and in circumstances in which the very nature of the case effectively precluded calm deliberation by the decision maker as well as criticism by others. In sharp contrast, however, cases of the type we have postulated in the present discussion arise predictably, and represent choices to be made deliberately and "in cold blood."

It is, to begin with, appropriate to remark that this problem is not fundamentally a medical problem. For when there are sufficiently many afflicted candidates for ELT then—so we may assume—there will also be more than enough for whom the purely medical grounds for ELT allocation are decisively strong in any individual case, and just about equally strong throughout the group. But in this circumstance a selection of some afflicted patients over and against others cannot *ex hypothesi* be made on the basis of purely medical considerations.

The selection problem, as we have said, is in substantial measure not a medical one. It is a problem *for* medical men, which must somehow be solved by them, but that does not make it a medical issue—any more than the problem of hospital building is a medical issue. As a problem it belongs to the category of philosophical problems—specifically a problem of moral philosophy or ethics. Structurally, it bears a substantial kinship with those issues in this field that revolve about the notorious whom-to-save-on-the-lifeboat and whom-to-throw-to-the-wolves-pursuing-the-sled questions. But whereas questions of this just-indicated sort are artificial, hypothetical, and far-fetched, the ELT issue poses a *genuine* policy question for the responsible administrators in medical

institutions, indeed a question that threatens to become commonplace in the foreseeable future.

Now what the medical administrator needs to have, and what the philosopher is presumably *ex officio* in a position to help in providing, is a body of *rational guidelines* for making choices in these literally life-or-death situations. This is an issue in which many interested parties have a substantial stake, including the responsible decision maker who wants to satisfy his conscience that he is acting in a reasonable way. Moreover, the family and associates of the man who is turned away—to say nothing of the man himself—have the right to an acceptable explanation. And indeed even the general public wants to know that what is being done is fitting and proper. All of these interested parties are entitled to insist that a reasonable code of operating principles provides a defensible rationale for making the life-and-death choices involved in ELT.

II. The Two Types of Criteria

Two distinguishable types of criteria are bound up in the issue of making ELT choices. We shall call these *Criteria of Inclusion* and *Criteria of Comparison*, respectively. The distinction at issue here requires some explanation. We can think of the selection as being made by a two-stage process: (1) the selection from among all possible candidates (by a suitable screening process) of a group to be taken under serious consideration as candidates for therapy, and then (2) the actual singling out, within this group, of the particular individuals to whom therapy is to be given. Thus the first process narrows down the range of comparative choices by eliminating *en bloc* whole categories of potential candidates. The second process calls for a more refined, case-by-case comparison of those candidates that remain. By means of the first set of criteria one forms a selection group; by means of the second set, an actual selection is made within this group.

Thus what we shall call a "selection system" for the choice of patients to receive therapy of the ELT type will consist of criteria of these two kinds. Such a system will be acceptable only when the reasonableness of its component criteria can be established.

III. Essential Features of an Acceptable ELT Selection System

To qualify as reasonable, an ELT selection must meet two important "regulative" requirements: it must be *simple* enough to be readily intelligible, and it must be *plausible*, that is, patently reasonable in a way that can be apprehended easily and without involving ramified subtleties. Those medical administrators responsible for ELT choices must follow a modus operandi that virtually all the people involved can readily understand to be acceptable (at a reasonable level of generality, at any rate). Appearances are critically important here. It is not enough that the choice be made in a *justifiable* way; it must be possible for people—*plain* people—to "see" (i.e., understand without elaborate teaching or indoctrination) that *it is justified*, insofar as any mode of procedure can be justified in cases of this sort.

One "constitutive" requirement is obviously an essential feature of a reasonable selection system: all of its component criteria—those of inclusion and those of comparison alike—must be reasonable in the sense of being *rationally defensible*. The ramifications of this requirement call for detailed consideration. But one of its aspects should be noted without further ado: it must be *fair*—it must treat relevantly like cases alike, leaving no room for "influence" or favoritism, etc.

IV. The Basic Screening Stage: Criteria of Inclusion (and Exclusion)

Three sorts of considerations are prominent among the plausible criteria of inclusion/exclusion at the basic screening stage: the constituency factor, the progress-of-science factor, and the prospect-of-success factor.

A. The Constituency Factor

It is a "fact of life" that ELT can be available only in the institutional setting of a hospital or medical institute or the like. Such institutions generally have normal clientele boundaries. A veterans' hospital will not concern itself primarily with treating nonveterans, a children's hospital cannot be expected to accommodate the "senior citizen," an army hospital can regard college professors as outside its sphere. Sometimes the boundaries are geographic—a state hospital may admit only residents of a certain state. (There are, of course, indefensible constituency principles—say race or religion, party membership, or ability to pay; and there are cases of borderline legitimacy, e.g., sex.[4]) A medical institution is justified in considering for ELT only persons within its own constituency, provided this constituency is constituted upon a defensible basis. Thus the haemodialysis selection committee in Seattle "agreed to consider only those applications who were residents of the state of Washington. . . . They justified this stand on the grounds that since the basic research . . . had been done at . . . a state-supported institution—the people whose taxes had paid for the research should be its first beneficiaries."[5]

While thus insisting that constituency considerations represent a valid and legitimate factor in ELT selection, I do feel there is much to be said for minimizing their role in life-or-death cases. Indeed a refusal to recognize them at all is a significant part of medical tradition, going back to the very oath of Hippocrates. They represent a departure from the ideal arising with the institutionalization of medicine, moving it away from its original status as an art practiced by an individual practitioner.

B. The Progress-of-Science Factor

The needs of medical research can provide a second valid principle of inclusion. The research interests of the medical staff in relation to the specific nature of the cases at issue is a significant consideration. It may be important for the progress of medical science—and thus of potential benefit to many persons in the future—to determine how effective the ELT at issue is with diabetics or persons over sixty or with a negative RH factor. Considerations of this sort represent another type of legitimate factor in ELT selection.

A very definitely *borderline* case under this head would revolve around the question of a patient's willingness to pay, not in monetary terms, but in offering himself as an experimental subject, say by contracting to return at designated times for a series of tests substantially unrelated to his own health, but yielding data of importance to medical knowledge in general.

C. The Prospect-of-Success Factor

It may be that while the ELT at issue is not without *some* effectiveness in general, it has been established to be highly effective only with patients in certain specific categories (e.g., females under forty of a specific blood type). This difference in effectiveness—in the absolute or in the probability of success—is (we assume) so marked as to constitute virtually a difference in kind rather than in degree. In this case, it would be perfectly legitimate to adopt the general rule of making the ELT at issue available only or primarily to persons in this substantial-promise-of-success category. (It is on grounds of this sort that young children and persons over fifty are generally ruled out as candidates for haemodialysis.)

We have maintained that the three factors of constituency, progress of science, and prospect of success represent legitimate criteria of inclusion for ELT selection. But it remains to examine the considerations which legitimate them. The legitimating factors are in the final analysis practical or pragmatic in nature. From the practical angle it is advantageous—indeed to some extent necessary—that the arrangements governing medical institutions should embody certain constituency principles. It makes good pragmatic and utilitarian sense that progress-of-science considerations should be operative here. And, finally, the practical aspect is reinforced by a whole host of other considerations—including moral ones—in supporting the prospect-of-success criterion. The workings of each of these factors are of course conditioned by the ever-present element of limited availability. They are operative only in this context, that is, prospect of success is a legitimate consideration at all only because we are dealing with a situation of scarcity.

V. The Final Selection Stage: Criteria of Selection

Five sorts of elements must, as we see it, figure primarily among the plausible criteria of selection that are to be brought to bear in further screening the group constituted after application of the criteria of inclusion: the relative-likelihood-of-success factor, the life-expectancy factor, the family role factor, the potential-contributions factor, and the services-rendered factor. The first two represent the *biomedical* aspect, the second three the *social* aspect.

A. The Relative-Likelihood-of-Success Factor

It is clear that the relative likelihood of success is a legitimate and appropriate factor in making a selection within the group of qualified patients that are to receive ELT. This is obviously one of the considerations that must count very significantly in a reasonable selection procedure.

The present criterion is of course closely related to item *C* of the preceding section. There we were concerned with prospect-of-success considerations categorically and *en bloc*. Here at present they come into play in a particularized case-by-case comparison among individuals. If the therapy at issue is not a once-and-for-all proposition and requires ongoing treatment, cognate considerations must be brought in. Thus, for example, in the case of a chronic ELT procedure such as haemodialysis it would clearly make sense to give priority to patients with a potentially reversible condition (who would thus need treatment for only a fraction of their remaining lives).

B. The Life-Expectancy Factor

Even if the ELT is "successful" in the patient's case he may, considering his age and/or other aspects of his general medical condition, look forward to only a very short probable future life. This is obviously another factor that must be taken into account.

C. The Family Role Factor

A person's life is a thing of importance not only to himself but to others—friends, associates, neighbors, colleagues, etc. But his (or her) relationship to his immediate family is a thing of unique intimacy and significance. The nature of his relationship to his wife, children, and parents, and the issue of their financial and psychological dependence upon him, are obviously matters that deserve to be given weight in the ELT selection process. Other things being anything like equal, the mother of minor children must take priority over the middle-aged bachelor.

D. The Potential Future-Contributions Factor (Prospective Service)

In "choosing to save" one life rather than another, "the society," through the mediation of the particular medical institution in question—which should certainly look upon itself as a trustee for the social interest—is clearly warranted in considering the likely pattern of future *services to be rendered* by the patient (adequate recovery assumed), considering his age, talent, training, and past record of performance. In its allocations of ELT, society "invests" a scarce resource in one person as against another and is thus entitled to look to the probable prospective "return" on its investment.

It may well be that a thoroughly egalitarian society is reluctant to put someone's social contribution into the scale in situations of the sort at issue. One popular article states that "the most difficult standard would be the candidate's value to society," and goes on to quote someone who said: "You can't just pick a brilliant painter over a laborer. The average citizen would be quickly eliminated."[6] But what if it were not a brilliant painter but a brilliant surgeon or medical researcher that was at issue? One wonders if the author of the *obiter dictum* that one "can't just pick" would still feel equally sure of his ground. In any case, the fact that the standard is difficult to apply is certainly no reason for not attempting to apply it. The problem of ELT selection is inevitably burdened with difficult standards.

Some might feel that in assessing a patient's value to society one should ask not only who if permitted to continue living can make the greatest contribution to society in some creative or constructive way, but also who by dying would leave behind the greatest burden on society in assuming the discharge of their residual responsibilities.[7] Certainly the philosophical utilitarian would give equal weight to both these considerations. Just here is where I would part ways with orthodox utilitarianism. For—though this is not the place to do so—I should be prepared to argue that a civilized society has an obligation to promote the furtherance of positive achievements in cultural and related areas even if this means the assumption of certain added burdens.[8]

E. The Past Services-Rendered Factor (Retrospective Service)

A person's services to another person or group have always been taken to constitute a valid basis for a claim upon this person or group—of course a moral and not necessarily a legal claim. Society's obligation for the recognition and reward

of services rendered—an obligation whose discharge is also very possibly conducive to self-interest in the long run—is thus another factor to be taken into account. This should be viewed as a morally necessary correlative of the previously considered factor of *prospective* service. It would be morally indefensible of society in effect to say: "Never mind about services you rendered yesterday—it is only the services to be rendered tomorrow that will count with us today." We live in very future-oriented times, constantly preoccupied in a distinctly utilitarian way with future satisfactions. And this disinclines us to give much recognition to past services. But parity considerations of the sort just adduced indicate that such recognition should be given *on grounds of equity.* No doubt a justification for giving weight to services rendered can also be attempted along utilitarian lines. ("The reward of past services rendered spurs people on to greater future efforts and is thus socially advantageous in the long-run future.") In saying that past services should be counted "on grounds of equity"—rather than "on grounds of utility"—I take the view that even if this utilitarian defense could somehow be shown to be fallacious, I should still be prepared to maintain the propriety of taking services rendered into account. The position does not rest on a utilitarian basis and so would not collapse with the removal of such a basis.[9]

As we have said, these five factors fall into three groups: the biomedical factors A and B, the familial factor C, and the social factors D and E. With items A and B the need for a detailed analysis of the medical considerations comes to the fore. The age of the patient, his medical history, his physical and psychological condition, his specific disease, etc., will all need to be taken into exact account. These biomedical factors represent technical issues: they call for the physicians' expert judgment and the medical statisticians' hard data. And they are ethically uncontroversial factors—their legitimacy and appropriateness are evident from the very nature of the case.

Greater problems arise with the familial and social factors. They involve intangibles that are difficult to judge. How is one to develop subcriteria for weighing the relative social contributions of (say) an architect or a librarian or a mother of

young children? And they involve highly problematic issues. (For example, should good moral
character be rated a plus and bad a minus in judging services rendered?) And there is something
strikingly unpleasant in grappling with issues of
this sort for people brought up in times greatly
inclined towards maxims of the type "Judge not!"
and "Live and let live!" All the same, in the situation that concerns us here such distasteful problems must be faced, since a failure to choose to
save some is tantamount to sentencing all. Unpleasant choices are intrinsic to the problem of ELT
selection; they are of the very essence of the
matter.[10]

But is reference to all these factors indeed inevitable? The justification for taking account of the
medical factors is pretty obvious. But why should
the social aspect of services rendered and to be
rendered be taken into account at all? The answer
is that they must be taken into account not from
the *medical* but from the *ethical* point of view. Despite disagreement on many fundamental issues,
moral philosophers of the present day are pretty
well in consensus that the justification of human
actions is to be sought largely and primarily—if
not exclusively—in the principles of utility and of
justice.[11] But utility requires reference of services to
be rendered and justice calls for a recognition of
services that have been rendered. Moral considerations would thus demand recognition of these
two factors. (This, of course, still leaves open the
question of whether the point of view provides a
valid basis of action: Why base one's actions upon
moral principles?—or, to put it bluntly—Why be
moral? The present paper is, however, hardly the
place to grapple with so fundamental an issue,
which has been canvassed in the literature of
philosophical ethics since Plato.)

VI. More than Medical Issues Are Involved

An active controversy has of late sprung up in
medical circles over the question of whether non-
physician laymen should be given a role in ELT
selection (in the specific context of chronic
haemodialysis). One physician writes: "I think
that the assessment of the candidates should be
made by a senior doctor on the [dialysis] unit, but I
am sure that it would be helpful to him—both in
sharing responsibility and in avoiding personal
pressure—if a small unnamed group of people
[presumably including laymen] officially made the
final decision. I visualize the doctor bringing the
data to the group, explaining the points in relation
to each case, and obtaining their approval of his
order of priority."[12]

Essentially this procedure of a selection committee of laymen has for some years been in use
in one of the most publicized chronic dialysis
units, that of the Swedish Hospital of Seattle,
Washington.[13] Many physicians are apparently reluctant to see the choice of allocation of medical
therapy pass out of strictly medical hands. Thus in
a recent symposium on the "Selection of Patients
for Haemodialysis,"[14] Dr. Ralph Shakman writes:
"Who is to implement the selection? In my opinion
it must ultimately be the responsibility of the consultants in charge of the renal units . . . I can see
no reason for delegating this responsibility to lay
persons. Surely the latter would be better
employed if they could be persuaded to devote
their time and energy to raise more and more
money for us to spend on our patients."[15] Other
contributors to this symposium strike much the
same note. Dr. F. M. Parsons writes: "In an attempt to overcome . . . difficulties in selection
some have advocated introducing certain specified
lay people into the discussions. Is it wise? I doubt
whether a committee of this type can adjudicate as
satisfactorily as two medical colleagues, particularly as successful therapy involves close cooperation between doctor and patient."[16] And Dr. M. A.
Wilson writes in the same symposium: "The
suggestion has been made that lay panels should
select individuals for dialysis from among a group
who are medically suitable. Though this would relieve the doctor-in-charge of a heavy load of responsibility, it would place the burden on those
who have no personal knowledge and have to
base their judgments on medical or social reports. I
do not believe this would result in better decisions
for the group or improve the doctor-patient relationship in individual cases."[17]

But no amount of flag waving about the doctor's facing up to his responsibility—or prostra-
tions before the idol of the doctor-patient relationship and reluctance to admit laymen into the
sacred precincts of the conference chambers of

medical consultations—can obscure the essential fact that ELT selection is not a wholly medical problem. When there are more than enough places in an ELT program to accommodate all who need it, then it will clearly be a medical question to decide who does have the need and which among these would successfully respond. But when an admitted gross insufficiency of places exists, when there are ten or fifty or one hundred highly eligible candidates for each place in the program, then it is unrealistic to take the view that purely medical criteria can furnish a sufficient basis for selection. The question of ELT selection becomes serious as a phenomenon of scale—because, as more candidates present themselves, strictly medical factors are increasingly less adequate as a selection criterion precisely because by numerical category-crowding there will be more and more cases whose "status is much the same" so far as purely medical considerations go.

The ELT selection problem clearly poses issues that transcend the medical sphere because—in the nature of the case—many residual issues remain to be dealt with once *all* of the medical questions have been faced. Because of this there is good reason why laymen as well as physicians should be involved in the selection process. Once the medical considerations have been brought to bear, fundamental social issues remain to be resolved. The instrumentalities of ELT have been created through the social investment of scarce resources, and the interests of the society deserve to play a role in their utilization. As representatives of their social interests, lay opinions should function to complement and supplement medical views once the proper arena of medical considerations is left behind.[18] Those physicians who have urged the presence of lay members on selection panels can, from this point of view, be recognized as having seen the issue in proper perspective.

One physician has argued against lay representation on selection panels for haemodialysis as follows: "If the doctor advises dialysis and the lay panel refuses, the patient will regard this as a death sentence passed by an anonymous court from which he has no right of appeal."[19] But this drawback is not specific to the use of a lay panel. Rather, it is a feature inherent in every *selection* procedure, regardless of whether the selection is done by the head doctor of the unit, by a panel of physicians, etc. No matter who does the selecting among patients recommended for dialysis, the feelings of the patient who has been rejected (and knows it) can be expected to be much the same, provided that he recognizes the actual nature of the choice (and is not deceived by the possibly convenient but ultimately poisonous fiction that because the selection was made by physicians it was made entirely on medical grounds).

In summary, then, the question of ELT selection would appear to be one that is in its very nature heavily laden with issues of medical research, practice, and administration. But it will not be a question that can be resolved on solely medical grounds. Strictly social issues of justice and utility will invariably arise in this area—questions going outside the medical area in whose resolution medical laymen can and should play a substantial role.

VII. The Inherent Imperfection (Non-Optimality) of Any Selection System

Our discussion to this point of the design of a selection system for ELT has left a gap that is a very fundamental and serious omission. We have argued that five factors must be taken into substantial and explicit account:

A. *Relative likelihood of success* Is the chance of the treatment's being "successful" to be rated as high, good, average, etc.?[20]

B. *Expectancy of future life* Assuming the "success" of the treatment, how much longer does the patient stand a good chance (75 per cent or better) of living—considering his age and general condition?

C. *Family role* To what extent does the patient have responsibilities to others in his immediate family?

D. *Social contributions rendered* Are the patient's past services to his society outstanding, substantial, average, etc.?

E. *Social contributions to be rendered* Considering his age, talents, training, and past record of performance, is there a substantial probability that the patient will—*adequate recovery being assured*—render in the future services to his society that can be characterized as outstanding, substantial, average, etc.?

This list is clearly insufficient for the construction of a reasonable selection system, since that would require not only *that these factors be taken into account* (somehow or other), but—going beyond this—would specify *a specific set of procedures for taking account of them*. The specific procedures that would constitute such a system would have to take account of the interrelationship of these factors (e.g., B and E), and to set out exact guidelines as to the relevant weight that is to be given to each of them. This is something our discussion has not as yet considered.

In fact, I should want to maintain that there is no such thing here as a single rationally superior selection system. The position of affairs seems to me to be something like this: (1) It is necessary (for reasons already canvassed) to *have* a system, and to have a system that is rationally defensible, and (2) to be rationally defensible, this system must take the factors A–E into substantial and explicit account. But (3) the exact manner in which a rationally defensible system takes account of these factors cannot be fixed in any one specific way on the basis of general considerations. Any of the variety of ways that give A–E "their due" will be acceptable and viable. One cannot hope to find within this range of workable systems some one that is *optimal* in relation to the alternatives. There is no one system that does "the (uniquely) best"—only a variety of systems that do "as well as one can expect to do" in cases of this sort.

The situation is structurally very much akin to that of rules of partition of an estate among the relations of a decedent. It is important *that there be* such rules. And it is reasonable that spouse, children, parents, siblings, etc., be taken account of in these rules. But the question of the exact method of division—say that when the decedent has neither living spouse nor living children then his estate is to be divided, dividing 60 per cent between parents, 40 per cent between siblings versus dividing 90 per cent between parents, 10 per cent between siblings—cannot be settled on the basis of any general abstract considerations of reasonableness. Within broad limits, a *variety* of resolutions are all perfectly acceptable—so that no one procedure can justifiably be regarded as "the

(uniquely) best" because it is superior to all others.[21]

VIII. A Possible Basis for a Reasonable Selection System

Having said that there is no such thing as *the optimal* selection system for ELT, I want now to sketch out the broad features of what I would regard as *one acceptable* system.

The basis for the system would be a point rating. The scoring here at issue would give roughly equal weight to the medical considerations (A and B) in comparison with the extramedical considerations (C = family role, D = services rendered, and E = services to be rendered), also giving roughly equal weight to the three items involved here (C, D, and E). The result of such a scoring procedure would provide the essential *starting point* of our ELT selection mechanism. I deliberately say "starting point" because it seems to me that one should not follow the results of this scoring in an *automatic* way. I would propose that the actual selection should only be guided but not actually be dictated by this scoring procedure, along lines now to be explained.

IX. The Desirability of Introducing an Element of Chance

The detailed procedure I would propose—not of course as optimal (for reasons we have seen), but as eminently acceptable—would combine the scoring procedure just discussed with an element of chance. The resulting selection system would function as follows:

1. First the criteria of inclusion of Section IV above would be applied to constitute a *first phase selection group*—which (we shall suppose) is substantially larger than the number *n* of persons who can actually be accommodated with ELT.

2. Next the criteria of selection of Section V are brought to bear via a scoring procedure of the type described in Section VIII. On this basis a *second phase selection group* is constituted which is only *somewhat* larger—say by a third or a half—than the critical number *n* at issue.

3. If this second phase selection group is relatively homogeneous as regards rating by the scoring procedure—that is, if there are no really major disparities within this group (as would be likely if the initial group was significantly larger than n)—then the final selection is made by *random* selection of n persons from within this group.

This introduction of the element of chance—in what could be dramatized as a "lottery of life and death"—must be justified. The fact is that such a procedure would bring with it three substantial advantages.

First, as we have argued above (in Section VII), any acceptable selection system is inherently non-optimal. The introduction of the element of chance prevents the results that life-and-death choices are made by the automatic application of an admittedly imperfect selection method.

Second, a recourse to chance would doubtless make matters easier for the rejected patient and those who have a specific interest in him. It would surely be quite hard for them to accept his exclusion by relatively mechanical application of objective criteria in whose implementation subjective judgment is involved. But the circumstances of life have conditioned us to accept the workings of chance and to tolerate the element of luck (good or bad): human life is an inherently contingent process. Nobody, after all, has an absolute right to ELT—but most of us would feel that we have "every bit as much right" to it as anyone else in significantly similar circumstances. The introduction of the element of chance assures a like handling of like cases over the widest possible area that seems reasonable in the circumstances.

Third (and perhaps least), such a recourse to random selection does much to relieve the administrators of the selection system of the awesome burden of ultimate and absolute responsibility.

These three considerations would seem to build up a substantial case for introducing the element of chance into the mechanism of the system for ELT selection in a way limited and circumscribed by other weightier considerations, along some such lines as those set forth above.[22]

It should be recognized that this injection of *man-made* chance supplements the element of *natural* chance that is present inevitably and in any

case (apart from the role of chance in singling out certain persons as victims for the affliction at issue). As F. M. Parsons has observed: "any vacancies [in an ELT program—specifically haemodialysis] will be filled immediately by the first suitable patients, even though their claims for therapy may subsequently prove less than those of other patients refused later."[23] Life is a chancy business and even the most rational of human arrangements can cover this over to a very limited extent at best.

Notes

1. Christine Doyle, "Spare-Part Heart Surgeons Worried by Their Success," *Observer*, May 12, 1968.

2. J. D. N. Nabarro, "Selection of Patients for Haemodialysis," *British Medical Journal* (March 11, 1967), p. 623. Although several thousand patients die in the U.K. each year from renal failure—there are about thirty new cases per million of population—only 10 per cent of these can for the foreseeable future be accommodated with chronic haemodialysis. Kidney transplantation—itself a very tricky procedure—cannot make a more than minor contribution here. As this article goes to press, I learn that patients can be maintained in home dialysis at an operating cost about half that of maintaining them in a hospital dialysis unit (roughly an $8,000 minimum). In the United States, around 7,000 patients with terminal uremia who could benefit from haemodialysis evolve yearly. As of mid-1968, some 1,000 of these can be accommodated in existing hospital units. By June 1967, a world-wide total of some 120 patients were in treatment by home dialysis. (Data from a forthcoming paper, "Home Dialysis," by C. M. Conty and H. V. Murdaugh. See also R. A. Baillod *et al.*, "Overnight Haemodialysis in the Home," *Proceedings of the European Dialysis and Transplant Association*, VI [1965], 99 ff.)

3. For the Hippocratic Oath see *Hippocrates: Works* (Loeb ed.; London, 1959), I, p. 298.

4. Another example of borderline legitimacy is posed by an endowment "with strings attached," e.g., "In accepting this legacy the hospital agrees to admit and provide all needed treatment for any direct descendant of myself, its founder."

5. Shana Alexander, "They Decide Who Lives, Who Dies," *Life*, LIII (November 9, 1962), 102–25 (see p. 107).

6. Lawrence Lader, "Who Has the Right To Live?" *Good Housekeeping* (January 1968), p. 144.

7. This approach could thus be continued to embrace the previous factor, that of family role, the preceding item (C).

8. Moreover a doctrinaire utilitarian would presumably be willing to withdraw a continuing mode of ELT such as haemodialysis from a patient to make room for a more promising candidate who came to view at a later stage and who could not otherwise be accommodated. I should be unwilling to adopt this course, partly on grounds of utility (with a view to the demoralization of insecurity), partly on the non-utilitarian ground that a "moral commitment" has been made and must be honored.

9. Of course the difficult question remains of the relative weight that should be given to prospective and retrospective service in cases where these factors conflict. There is good reason to treat them on a par.

10. This in the symposium on "Selection of Patients for Haemodialysis," *British Medical Journal* (March 11, 1967), pp. 622–24. F. M. Parsons writes: "But other forms of selecting patients [distinct from first come, first served] are suspect in my view if they imply evaluation of man by man. What criteria could be used? Who could justify a claim that the life of a mayor would be more valuable than that of the humblest citizen of his borough? Whatever we may think as individuals none of us is indispensable." But having just set out this hard-line view he immediately backs away from it: "On the other hand, to assume that there was little to choose between Alexander Fleming and Adolf Hitler . . . would be nonsense, and we should be naive if we were to pretend that we could not be influenced by their achievements and characters if we had to choose between the two of them. Whether we like it or not we cannot escape the fact that this kind of selection for long-term haemodialysis will be required until very large sums of money become available for equipment and services [so that *everyone* who needs treatment can be accommodated]."

11. The relative fundamentality of these principles is, however, a substantially disputed issue.

12. J. D. N. Nabarro, *op. cit.*, p. 622.

13. See Shana Alexander, *op. cit.*

14. *British Medical Journal* (March 11, 1967), pp. 622–24.

15. *Ibid.*, p. 624. Another contributor writes in the same symposium, "The selection of the few [to receive haemodialysis] is proving very difficult—a true 'Doctor's Dilemma'—for almost everybody would agree that this must be a medical decision, preferably reached by consultation among colleagues" (Dr. F. M. Parsons, *ibid.*, p. 623).

16. "The Selection of Patients for Haemodialysis," *op. cit.* (n. 10 above), p. 623.

17. Dr. Wilson's article concludes with the perplexing suggestion—wildly beside the point given the structure of the situation at issue—that "the final decision will be made by the patient." But this contention is only marginally more ludicrous than Parsons's contention that in selecting patients for haemodialysis "gainful employment in a well chosen occupation is necessary to achieve the best results" since "only the minority wish to live on charity" (*ibid.*).

18. To say this is of course not to deny that such questions of applied medical ethics will invariably involve a host of medical considerations—it is only to insist that extra-medical considerations will also invariably be at issue.

19. M. A. Wilson, "Selection of Patients for Haemodialysis," *op. cit.*, p. 624.

20. In the case of an ongoing treatment involving complex procedure and dietary and other mode-of-life restrictions—and chronic haemodialysis definitely falls into this category—the patient's psychological makeup, his willpower to "stick with it" in the face of substantial discouragements—will obviously also be a substantial factor here. The man who gives up, takes not his life alone, but (figuratively speaking) also that of the person he replaced in the treatment schedule.

21. To say that acceptable solutions can range over broad limits is *not* to say that there are no limits at all. It is an obviously intriguing and fundamental problem to raise the question of the factors that set these limits. This complex issue cannot be dealt with adequately here. Suffice it to say that considerations regarding precedent and people's expectations, factor of social utility, and matters of fairness and sense of justice all come into play.

22. One writer has mooted the suggestion that: "Perhaps the right thing to do, difficult as it may be to accept, is to select [for haemodialysis] from among the medical and psychologically qualified patients on a strictly random basis" (S. Gorovitz, "Ethics and the Allocation of Medical Resources," *Medical Research Engineering*, V [1966], p. 7). Out-right random selection would, however, seem indefensible because of its refusal to give weight to considerations which, under the circumstances, *deserve* to be given weight. The proposed procedure of superimposing a certain degree of randomness upon the rational-choice criteria would seem to combine the advantages of the two without importing the worst defects of either.

23. "Selection of Patients for Haemodialysis," *op. cit.*, p. 623. The question of whether a patient for chronic treatment should ever be terminated from the program (say if he contracts cancer) poses a variety of difficult ethical problems with which we need not at present concern ourselves. But it does seem plausible to take the (somewhat anti-utilitarian) view that a patient should not be terminated simply because a "better qualified" patient comes along later on. It would seem that a quasi-contractual relationship has been created through established expectations and reciprocal understandings, and that the situation is in this regard akin to that of the man who, having undertaken to sell his house to one buyer, cannot afterward unilaterally undo this arrangement to sell it to a higher bidder who "needs it worse" (thus maximizing the over-all utility).

24. I acknowledge with thanks the help of Miss Hazel Johnson, Reference Librarian at the University of Pittsburgh Library, in connection with the bibliography.

Bibliography[24]

S. Alexander. "They Decide Who Lives, Who Dies," *Life*, LIII (November 9, 1962), 102–25.

C. Doyle. "Spare-Part Heart Surgeons Worried by Their Success," *Observer* (London), May 12, 1968.

J. Fletcher. *Morals and Medicine*. London, 1955.

S. Gorovitz. "Ethics and the Allocation of Medical Resources," *Medical Research Engineering*, V (1966), 5–7.

L. Lader. "Who Has the Right To Live?" *Good Housekeeping* (January, 1968), pp. 85 and 144–50.

J. D. N. Nabarro, F. M. Parsons, R. Shakman, and M. A. Wilson. "Selection of Patients for Haemodialysis," *British Medical Journal* (March 11, 1967), pp. 622–24.

H. M. Schmeck, Jr. "Panel Holds Life-or-Death Vote in Allotting of Artificial Kidney," *New York Times*, May 6, 1962, pp. 1, 83.

G. E. W. Wolstenholme and M. O'Connor (eds.). *Ethics in Medical Progress*. London, 1966.

Who Shall Live When Not All Can Live?

James F. Childress

Who shall live when not all can live? Although this question has been urgently forced upon us by the dramatic use of artificial internal organs and organ transplantations, it is hardly new. George Bernard Shaw dealt with it in "The Doctor's Dilemma":

> *Sir Patrick.* Well, Mr. Savior of Lives: which is it to be? that honest decent man Blenkinsop, or that rotten blackguard of an artist, eh?
> *Ridgeon.* It's not an easy case to judge, is it? Blenkinsop's an honest decent man; but is he any use? Dubedat's a rotten blackguard; but he's a genuine source of pretty and pleasant and good things.
> *Sir Patrick.* What will he be a source of for that poor innocent wife of his, when she finds him out?
> *Ridgeon.* That's true. Her life will be a hell.
> *Sir Patrick.* And tell me this. Suppose you had this choice put before you: either to go through life and find all the pictures bad but all the men and women good, or go through life and find all the pictures good and all the men and women rotten. Which would you choose?[1]

A significant example of the distribution of scarce medical resources is seen in the use of penicillin shortly after its discovery. Military officers had to determine which soldiers would be treated—those with venereal disease or those wounded in combat.[2] In many respects such decisions have become routine in medical circles. Day after day physicians and others make judgments and decisions "about allocations of medical care to various segments of our population, to various types of hospitalized patients, and to specific individuals,"[3] for example, whether mental illness or cancer will receive the higher proportion of available funds. Nevertheless, the dramatic forms of "Scarce Life-Saving Medical Resources" (hereafter abbreviated as SLMR) such as hemodialysis and kidney and heart transplants have compelled us to examine the moral questions that have been con-

Reprinted with the permission of the publisher from Soundings, An Interdisciplinary Journal 53, no. 4 (Winter 1970). *Editor's Note: The footnotes in this reading have been renumbered.*

cealed in many routine decisions. I do not attempt in this paper to show how a resolution of SLMR cases can help us in the more routine ones which do not involve a conflict of life with life. Rather I develop an argument for a particular method of determining who shall live when not all can live. No conclusions are implied about criteria and procedures for determining who shall receive medical resources that are not directly related to the preservation of life (e.g. corneal transplants) or about standards for allocating money and time for studying and treating certain diseases.

Just as current SLMR decisions are not totally discontinuous with other medical decisions, so we must ask whether some other cases might, at least by analogy, help us develop the needed criteria and procedures. Some have looked at the principles at work in our responses to abortion, euthanasia, and artificial insemination.[4] Usually they have concluded that these cases do not cast light on the selection of patients for artificial and transplanted organs. The reason is evident: in abortion, euthanasia, and artificial insemination, there is no conflict of life with life for limited but indispensable resources (with the possible exception of therapeutic abortion). In current SLMR decisions, such a conflict is inescapable, and it makes them so morally perplexing and fascinating. If analogous cases are to be found, I think that we shall locate them in moral conflict situations.

Analogous Conflict Situations

An especially interesting and pertinent one is *U.S. v. Holmes*.[5] In 1841 an American ship, the *William Brown*, which was near Newfoundland on a trip from Liverpool to Philadelphia, struck an iceberg. The crew and half the passengers were able to escape in the two available vessels. One of these, a longboat, carrying too many passengers and leaking seriously, began to founder in the turbulent sea after about twenty-four hours. In a desperate attempt to keep it from sinking, the crew threw overboard fourteen men. Two sisters of one of the men either jumped overboard to join their brother in death or instructed the crew to throw them over. The criteria for determining who should live were "not to part man and wife, and not to throw over any women." Several hours later the others were rescued. Returning to Philadelphia, most of the crew disappeared, but one, Holmes, who had acted upon orders from the

mate, was indicted, tried, and convicted on the charge of "unlawful homicide."

We are interested in this case from a moral rather than a legal standpoint, and there are several possible responses to and judgments about it. Without attempting to be exhaustive I shall sketch a few of these. The judge contended that lots should have been cast, for in such conflict situations, there is no other procedure "so consonant both to humanity and to justice." Counsel for Holmes, on the other hand, maintained that the "sailors adopted the only principle of selection which was possible in an emergency like theirs, —a principle more humane than lots."

Another version of selection might extend and systematize the maxims of the sailors in the direction of "utility"; those are saved who will contribute to the greatest good for the greatest number. Yet another possible option is defended by Edmond Cahn in *The Moral Decision*. He argues that in this case we encounter the "morals of the last day." By this phrase he indicates that an apocalyptic crisis renders totally irrelevant the normal differences between individuals. He continues:

> In a strait of this extremity, all men are reduced—or raised, as one may choose to denominate it—to members of the genus, mere congeners and nothing else. Truly and literally, all were "in the same boat," and thus none could be saved separately from the others. I am driven to conclude that otherwise—that is, if none sacrifice themselves of free will to spare the others—they must all wait and die together. For where all have become congeners, pure and simple, no one can save himself by killing another.[6]

Cahn's answer to the question "who shall live when not all can live" is "none" unless the voluntary sacrifice by some persons permits it.

Few would deny the importance of Cahn's approach although many, including this writer, would suggest that it is relevant mainly as an affirmation of an elevated and, indeed, heroic or saintly morality which one hopes would find expression in the voluntary actions of many persons trapped in "borderline" situations involving a conflict of life with life. It is a maximal demand which some moral principles impose on the individual in the recognition that self-preservation is not a good which is to be defended at all costs. The absence of this saintly or heroic morality should not mean, however, that everyone perishes. Without making survival an absolute value and without justifying all means to achieve it, we can maintain that simply letting everyone die is irresponsible. This charge can be supported from several different standpoints, including society at large as well as the individuals involved. Among a group of self-interested individuals, none of whom volunteers to relinquish his life, there may be better and worse ways of determining who shall survive. One task of social ethics, whether religious or philosophical, is to propose relatively just institutional arrangements within which self-interested and biased men can live. The question then becomes: which set of arrangements—which criteria and procedures of selection—is most satisfactory in view of the human condition (man's limited altruism and inclination to seek his own good) and the conflicting values that are to be realized?

There are several significant differences between the *Holmes* and SLMR cases, a major one being that the former involves *direct* killing of another person, while the latter involves only *permitting* a person to die when it is not possible to save all. Furthermore, in extreme situations such as Holmes, the restraints of civilization have been stripped away and something approximating a state of nature prevails, in which life is "solitary, poor, nasty, brutish and short." The state of nature does not mean that moral standards are irrelevant and that might should prevail, but it does suggest that much of the matrix which normally supports morality has been removed. Also, the necessary but unfortunate decisions about who shall live and die are made by men who are existentially and personally involved in the outcome. Their survival too is at stake. Even though the institutional role of sailors seems to require greater sacrificial actions, there is obviously no assurance that they will adequately assess the number of sailors required to man the vessel or that they will impartially and objectively weigh the common good at stake. As the judge insisted in his defense of casting lots in the *Holmes* case: "In no other than this [casting lots] or some like way are those having equal rights put upon an equal footing, and in no other way is it possible to guard against partiality and oppression, violence, and conflict." This difference should not be exaggerated since self-interest, professional pride, and the like obviously affect the outcome of many medical decisions. Nor

do the remaining differences cancel *Holmes'* instructiveness.

Criteria of Selection for SLMR

Which set of arrangements should be adopted for SLMR? Two questions are involved: Which standards and criteria should be used? and, Who should make the decision? The first question is basic, since the debate about implementation, e.g. whether by a lay committee or physician, makes little progress until the criteria are determined.

We need two sets of criteria which will be applied at two different stages in the selection of recipients of SLMR. First, medical criteria should be used to exclude those who are not "medically acceptable." Second, from this group of "medically acceptable" applicants, the final selection can be made. Occasionally in current American medical practice, the first stage is omitted, but such an omission is unwarranted. Ethical and social responsibility would seem to require distributing these SLMR only to those who have some reasonable prospect of responding to the treatment. Furthermore, in transplants such medical tests as tissue and blood typing are necessary, although they are hardly fully developed.

"Medical acceptability" is not as easily determined as many non-physicians assume since there is considerable debate in medical circles about the relevant factors (e.g., age and complicating diseases). Although ethicists can contribute little or nothing to this debate, two proposals may be in order. First, "medical acceptability" should be used only to determine the group from which the final selection will be made, and the attempt to establish fine degrees of prospective response to treatment should be avoided. Medical criteria, then, would exclude some applicants but would not serve as a basis of comparison between those who pass the first stage. For example, if two applicants for dialysis were medically acceptable, the physicians would *not* choose the one with the *better* medical prospects. Final selection would be made on other grounds. Second, psychological and environmental factors should be kept to an absolute minimum and should be considered only when they are without doubt critically related to medical acceptability (e.g., the inability to cope with the requirements of dialysis which might lead to suicide).

The most significant moral questions emerge when we turn to the final selection. Once the pool of medically acceptable applicants has been defined and still the number is larger than the resources, what other criteria should be used? How should the final selection be made? First, I shall examine some of the difficulties that stem from efforts to make the final selection in terms of social value; these difficulties raise serious doubts about the feasibility and justifiability of the utilitarian approach. Then I shall consider the possible justification for random selection or chance.

Occasionally criteria of social worth focus on past contributions but most often they are primarily future-oriented. The patient's potential and probable contribution to the society is stressed, although this obviously cannot be abstracted from his present web of relationships (e.g., dependents) and occupational activities (e.g., nuclear physicist). Indeed, the magnitude of his contribution to society (as an abstraction) is measured in terms of these social roles, relations, and functions. Enough has already been said to suggest the tremendous range of factors that affect social value or worth.[7] Here we encounter the first major difficulty of this approach: How do we determine the relevant criteria of social value?

How does one quantify and compare the needs of the spirit (e.g., education, art, religion), political life, economic activity, technological development? Joseph Fletcher suggests that "some day we may learn how to 'quantify' or 'mathematicate' to 'computerize' the value problem in selection, in the same careful and thorough way that diagnosis has been."[8] I am not convinced that we can ever quantify values, or that we should attempt to do so. But even if the various social and human needs, in principle, could be quantified, how do we determine how much weight we will give to each one? Which will have priority in case of conflict? Or even more basically, in the light of which values and principles do we recognize social "needs"?

One possible way of determining the values which should be emphasized in selection has been proposed by Leo Shatin.[9] He insists that our medical decisions about allocating resources are already based on an unconscious scale of values (usually dominated by material worth). Since there is really no way of escaping this, we should be self-conscious and critical about it. How should we proceed? He recommends that we discover the values that most people in our society hold and then use them as criteria for distributing SLMR. These values can be discovered by attitude or opinion surveys. Presumably if fifty-one percent in this testing period put a greater premium on military needs than technological development, military men would have a greater claim on our SLMR than experimental researchers. But valuations of what is significant change, and the student revolutionary who was denied SLMR in 1970 might be celebrated in 1990 as the greatest American hero since George Washington.

Shatin presumably is seeking criteria that could be applied nationally, but at the present, regional and local as well as individual prejudices tincture the criteria of social value that are used in selection. Nowhere is this more evident than in the deliberations and decisions of the anonymous selection committee of the Seattle Artificial Kidney Center where such factors as church membership and Scout leadership have been deemed significant for determining who shall live.[10] As two critics conclude after examining these criteria and procedures, they rule out "creative nonconformists, who rub the bourgeoisie the wrong way but who historically have contributed so much to the making of America. The Pacific Northwest is no place for a Henry David Thoreau with bad kidneys."[11]

Closely connected to this first problem of determining social values is a second one. Not only is it difficult if not impossible to reach agreement on social values, but it is also rarely easy to predict what our needs will be in a few years and what the consequences of present actions will be. Furthermore it is difficult to predict which persons will fulfill their potential function in society. Admissions committees in colleges and universities experience the frustrations of predicting realization of potential. For these reasons, as someone has indicated, God might be a utilitarian, but we cannot be. We simply lack the capacity to predict very accurately the consequences which we then must evaluate. Our incapacity is never more evident than when we think in societal terms.

Other difficulties make us even less confident that such an approach to SLMR is advisable. Many critics raise the spectre of abuse, but this should not be overemphasized. The fundamental difficulty appears on another level: the utilitarian approach would in effect reduce the person to his social role, relations, and functions. Ultimately it dulls and perhaps even eliminates the sense of the person's transcendence, his dignity as a person which cannot be reduced to his past or future contribution to society. It is not at all clear that we are willing to live with these implications of utilitarian selection. Wilhelm Kolff, who invented the artificial kidney, has asked: "Do we really subscribe to the principle that social standing should determine selection? Do we allow patients to be treated with dialysis only when they are married, go to church, have children, have a job, a good income and give to the Community Chest?"[12]

The German theologian Helmut Thielicke contends that any search for "objective criteria" for selection is already a capitulation to the utilitarian point of view which violates man's dignity.[13] The solution is not to let all die, but to recognize that SLMR cases are "borderline situations" which inevitably involve guilt. The agent, however, can have courage and freedom (which, for Thielicke, come from justification by faith) and can

> go head anyway and seek for criteria for deciding the question of life or death in the matter of the artificial kidney. Since these criteria are . . . questionable, necessarily alien to the meaning of human existence, the decision to which they lead can be little more than that arrived at by casting lots.[14]

The resulting criteria, he suggests, will probably be very similar to those already employed in American medical practice.

He is most concerned to preserve a certain *attitude* or *disposition* in SLMR—the sense of guilt which arises when man's dignity is violated. With this sense of guilt, the agent remains "sound and healthy where it really counts."[15] Thielicke uses man's dignity only as a judgmental, critical, and negative standard. It only tells us how all selection criteria and procedures (and even the refusal to act) implicate us in the ambiguity of the human condition and its metaphysical guilt. This approach is consistent with his view of the task of theological ethics: "to teach us how to understand and endure—not "solve"—the borderline situation."[16] But ethics, I would contend, can help us discern the factors and norms in whose light relative, discriminate judgments can be made. Even if all actions in SLMR should involve guilt, some may preserve human dignity to a greater extent than others. Thielicke recognizes that a decision

based on any criteria is "little more than that arrived at by casting lots." But perhaps selection by chance would come the closest to embodying the moral and nonmoral values that we are trying to maintain (including a sense of man's dignity).

The Values of Random Selection

My proposal is that we use some form of randomness or chance (either natural, such as "first come, first served," or artificial, such as a lottery) to determine who shall be saved. Many reject randomness as a surrender to non-rationality when responsible and rational judgments can and must be made. Edmond Cahn criticizes "Holmes' judge" who recommended the casting of lots because, as Cahn puts it, "the crisis involves stakes too high for gambling and responsibilities too deep for destiny."[17] Similarly, other critics see randomness as a surrender to "non-human" forces which necessarily vitiates human values (e.g., it is important to have persons rather than impersonal forces determining who shall live). Sometimes they are identified with the outcome of the process (e.g., the features such as creativity and fullness of being which make human life what it is are to be considered and respected in the decision). Regarding the former, it must be admitted that the use of chance seems cold and impersonal. But presumably the defenders of utilitarian criteria in SLMR want to make their application as objective and impersonal as possible so that subjective bias does not determine who shall live.

Such criticism, however, ignores the moral and nonmoral values which might be supported by selection by randomness or chance. A more important criticism is that the procedure that I develop draws the relevant moral context too narrowly. That context, so the argument might run, includes the society and its future and not merely the individual with his illness and claim upon SLMR. But my contention is that the values and principles at work in the narrower context may well take precedence over those operative in the broader context both because of their weight and significance and because of the weaknesses of selection in terms of social worth. As Paul Freund rightly insists, "The more nearly total is the estimate to be made of an individual, and the more nearly the consequence determines life and death, the more unfit the judgment becomes for human reckoning. . . . Randomness as a moral principle deserves serious study."[18] Serious study would, I think point toward its implementation in certain conflict situations, primarily because it preserves a significant degree of *personal dignity by providing equality* of opportunity. Thus it cannot be dismissed as a "non-rational" and "non-human" procedure without an inquiry into the reasons, including human values, which might justify it. Paul Ramsey stresses this point about the *Holmes* case:

> Instead of fixing our attention upon "gambling" as the solution—with all the frivolous and often corrupt associations the word raises in our minds—we should think rather of equality of opportunity as the ethical substance of the relations of those individuals to one another that might have been guarded and expressed by casting lots.[19]

The individual's personal and transcendent dignity, which on the utilitarian approach would be submerged in his social role and function, can be protected and witnessed to by a recognition of his equal right to be saved. Such a right is best preserved by procedures which establish equality of opportunity. Thus selection by chance more closely approximates the requirements established by human dignity than does utilitarian calculation. It is not infallibly just, but it is preferable to the alternatives of letting all die or saving only those who have the greatest social responsibilities and potential contribution.

This argument can be extended by examining values other than individual dignity and equality of opportunity. Another basic value in the medical sphere is the relationship of trust between physician and patient. Which selection criteria are most in accord with this relationship of trust? Which will maintain, extend, and deepen it? My contention is that selection by randomness or chance is preferable from this standpoint too.

Trust, which is inextricably bound to respect for human dignity, is an attitude of expectation about another. It is not simply the expectation that another will act toward him in certain ways— which will respect him as a person. As Charles Fried writes:

> Although trust has to do with reliance on a disposition of another person, it is reliance on a disposition of a special sort: the disposition to act morally, to deal fairly with others, to live up to One's undertakings, and so on. Thus to

trust another is first of all to expect him to accept the principle of morality in his dealings with you, to respect your status as a person, your personality.[20]

This trust cannot be preserved in life-and-death situations when a person expects decisions about him to be made in terms of his social worth, for such decisions violate his status as a person. An applicant rejected on grounds of inadequacy in social value or virtue would have reason for feeling that his "trust" had been betrayed. Indeed, the sense that one is being viewed not as an end in himself but as a means in medical progress or the achievement of a greater social good is incompatible with attitudes and relationships of trust. We recognize this in the billboard which was erected after the first heart transplants: "Drive Carefully. Christiaan Barnard Is Watching You." The relationship of trust between the physician and patient is not only an instrumental value in the sense of being an important factor in the patient's treatment. It is also to be endorsed because of its intrinsic worth as a relationship.

Thus the related values of individual dignity and trust are best maintained in selection by chance. But other factors also buttress the argument for this approach. Which criteria and procedures would men agree upon? We have to suppose a hypothetical situation in which several men are going to determine for themselves and their families the criteria and procedures by which they would want to be admitted to and excluded from SLMR if the need arose.[21] We need to assume two restrictions and then ask which set of criteria and procedures would be chosen as the most rational and, indeed, the fairest. The restrictions are these: (1) That men are *self-interested*. They are interested in their own welfare (and that of members of their families), and this, of course, includes survival. Basically, they are not motivated by altruism. (2) Furthermore, they are ignorant of their own talents, abilities, potential, and probable contribution to the social good. They do not know how they would fare in a competitive situation, e.g., the competition for SLMR in terms of social contribution. Under these conditions which institution would be chosen—letting all die, utilitarian selection, or the use of chance? Which would seem the most rational? the fairest? By which set of criteria would they want to be included in or excluded from the list of those who will be saved? The rational choice in this setting (assuming self-interest and ignorance of one's competitive success) would be random selection or chance since this alone provides equality of opportunity. A possible response is that one would prefer to take a "risk" and therefore choose the utilitarian approach. But I think not, especially since I added that the participants in this hypothetical situation are choosing for their children as well as for themselves; random selection or chance could be more easily justified to the children. It would make more sense for men who are self-interested but uncertain about their relative contribution to society to elect a set of criteria which would build in equality of opportunity. They would consider selection by chance as relatively just and fair.

An important psychological point supplements earlier arguments for using chance or random selection. The psychological stress and strain among those who are rejected would be greater if the rejection is based on insufficient social worth than if it is based on chance. Obviously stress and strain cannot be eliminated in these borderline situations, but they would almost certainly be increased by the opprobrium of being judged relatively "unfit" by society's agents using society's values. Nicholas Rescher makes this point very effectively:

> . . . a recourse to chance would doubtless make matters easier for the rejected patient and those who have a specific interest in him. It would surely be quite hard for them to accept his exclusion by relatively mechanical application of objective criteria in whose implementation subjective judgment is involved. But the circumstances of life have conditioned us to accept the workings of chance and to tolerate the element of luck (good or bad): human life is an inherently contingent process. Nobody, after all, has an absolute right to ELT [Exotic Lifesaving Therapy]—but most of us would feel that we have "every bit as much right" to it as anyone else in significantly similar circumstances.[22]

Although it is seldom recognized as such, selection by chance is already in operation in practically every dialysis unit. I am not aware of any unit which removed some of its patients from kidney machines in order to make room for later applicants who are better qualified in terms of social worth. Furthermore, very few people would recommend it. Indeed, few would even consider

removing a person from a kidney machine on the grounds that a person better qualified *medically* had just applied. In a discussion of the treatment of chronic renal failure by dialysis at the University of Virginia Hospital Renal Unit from November 15, 1965 to November 15, 1966, Dr. Harry Abram writes: "Thirteen patients sought treatment but were not considered because the program had reached its limit of nine patients."[23] Thus, in practice and theory, natural chance is accepted at least within certain limits.

My proposal is that we extend this principle (first come, first served) to determine who among the medically acceptable patients shall live or that we utilize artificial chance such as a lottery or randomness. "First come, first served" would be more feasible than a lottery since the applicants make their claims over a period of time rather than as a group at one time. This procedure would be in accord with at least one principle in our present practices and with our sense of individual dignity, trust, and fairness. Its significance in relation to these values can be underlined by asking how the decision can be justified to the rejected applicant. Of course, one easy way of avoiding this task is to maintain the traditional cloak of secrecy, which works to a great extent because patients are often not aware that they are being considered for SLMR in addition to the usual treatment. But whether public justification is instituted or not is not the significant question; it is rather what reasons for rejection would be most acceptable to the unsuccessful applicant. My contention is that rejection can be accepted more readily if equality of opportunity, fairness, and trust are preserved, and that they are best preserved by selection by randomness or chance.

This proposal has yet another advantage since it would eliminate the need for a committee to examine applicants in terms of their social value. This onerous responsibility can be avoided.

Finally, there is a possible indirect consequence of widespread use of random selection which is interesting to ponder, although I do *not* adduce it as a good reason for adopting random selection. It can be argued, as Professor Mason Willrich of the University of Virginia Law School has suggested, that SLMR cases would practically disappear if these scarce resources were distributed randomly rather than on social worth grounds. Scarcity would no longer be a problem because the holders of economic and political power would make certain that they would not be excluded by a random selection procedure; hence they would help to redirect public priorities or establish private funding so that life-saving medical treatment would be widely and perhaps universally available.

In the framework that I have delineated, are the decrees of chance to be taken without exception? If we recognize exceptions, would we not open Pandora's box again just after we had succeeded in getting it closed? The direction of my argument has been against any exceptions, and I would defend this as the proper way to go. But let me indicate one possible way of admitting exceptions while at the same time circumscribing them so narrowly that they would be very rare indeed.

An obvious advantage of the utilitarian approach is that occasionally circumstances arise which make it necessary to say that one man is practically indispensable for a society in view of a particular set of problems it faces (e.g., the President when the nation is waging a war for survival). Certainly the argument to this point has stressed that the burden of proof would fall on those who think that the social danger in this instance is so great that they simply cannot abide by the outcome of a lottery or a first come, first served policy. Also, the reason must be negative rather than positive; that is, we depart from chance in this instance not because we want to take advantage of this person's potential contribution to the improvement of our society, but because his immediate loss would possibly (even probably) be disastrous (again, the President in a grave national emergency). Finally, social value (in the negative sense) should be used as a standard of exception in dialysis, for example, only if it would provide a reason strong enough to warrant removing another person from a kidney machine if all machines were taken. Assuming this strong reluctance to remove anyone once the commitment has been made to him, we would be willing to put this patient ahead of another applicant for a vacant machine only if we would be willing (in circumstances in which all machines are being used) to vacate a machine by removing someone from it. These restrictions would make an exception almost impossible.

While I do not recommend this procedure of recognizing exceptions, I think that one can de-

fend it while accepting my general thesis about selection by randomness or chance. If it is used, a lay committee (perhaps advisory, perhaps even stronger) would be called upon to deal with the alleged exceptions since the doctors or others would in effect be appealing the outcome of chance (either natural or artificial). This lay committee would determine whether this patient was so indispensable at this time and place that he had to be saved even by sacrificing the values preserved by random selection. It would make it quite clear that exception is warranted, if at all, only as the "lesser of two evils." Such a defense would be recognized only rarely, if ever, primarily because chance and randomness preserve so many important moral and nonmoral values in SLMR cases.

Notes

1. George Bernard Shaw, *The Doctor's Dilemma* (New York, 1941), pp. 132–133.

2. Henry K. Beecher, "Scarce Resources and Medical Advancement," *Daedalus* (Spring 1969), pp. 279–280.

3. Leo Shatin, "Medical Care and the Social Worth of a Man," *American Journal of Orthopsychiatry*, 36 (1967), 97.

4. Harry S. Abram and Walter Wadlington, "Selection of Patients for Artificial and Transplanted Organs," *Annals of Internal Medicine*, 69 (September 1968), 615–620.5.

5. *United States v. Holmes* Fed Cas. 360 (C.C.E.D. Pa 1842). All references are to the text of the trial as reprinted in Philip E. Davis, ed. *Moral Duty and Legal Responsibility: A Philosophical-Legal Casebook* (New York, 1966), pp. 102–118.

6. *The Moral Decision* (Bloomington, Ind., 1955) p. 71.

7. I am excluding from consideration the question of the ability to pay because most of the people involved have to secure funds from other sources, public or private, anyway.

8. Joseph Fletcher, "Donor Nephrectomies and Moral Responsibility," *Journal of the American Medical Women's Association*, 23 (Dec. 1968), p. 1090.

9. Leo Shatin, *op. cit.*, pp. 96–101.

10. For a discussion of the Seattle selection committee, see Shana Alexander, "They Decide Who Lives, Who Dies," *Life*, 53 (Nov. 9, 1962), 102. For an examination of general selection practices in dialysis see "Scarce Medical Resources," *Columbia Law Review* 69:620 (1969) and Harry S. Abram and Walter Wadlington, op. cit.

11. David Sanders and Jesse Dukeminier, Jr., "Medical Advance and Legal Lag: Hemodialysis and Kidney Transplantation," *UCLA Law Review* 15:367 (1968) 378.

12. "Letters and Comments," *Annals of Internal Medicine*, 61 (Aug. 1964), 360. Dr. G. E. Schreiner contends that "if you really believe in the right of society to make decisions on medical availability on these criteria you should be logical and say that when a man stops going to church or is divorced or loses his job, he ought to be removed from the programme and somebody else who fulfills these criteria substituted. Obviously no one faces up to this logical consequence." (G. E. W. Wolstenholme and Maeve O'Connor, ed. *Ethics in Medical Progress: With Special Reference to Transplantation,* A Ciba Foundation Symposium [Boston, 1966], p. 127.)

13. Helmut Thielicke, "The Doctor as Judge of Who Shall Live and Who Shall Die," *Who Shall Live?* ed. by Kenneth Vaux (Philadelphia, 1970), p. 172.

14. Ibid., pp. 173–174.

15. Ibid., p. 173.

16. Thielicke, *Theological Ethics*, Vol. I, *Foundations* (Philadelphia, 1966), p. 602.

17. Cahn, op. cit., p. 71.

18. Paul Freund, "Introduction," *Daedalus* (Spring 1969), xiii.

19. Paul Ramsey, *Nine Modern Moralists* (Englewood Cliffs, N.J., 1961), p. 245.

20. Charles Fried, "Privacy," In *Law, Reason, and Justice,* ed. by Graham Hughes (New York, 1969), p. 52.

21. My argument is greatly dependent on John Rawls's version of justice as fairness, which is a reinterpretation of social contract theory. Rawls, however, would probably not apply his ideas to "borderline situations." See "Distributive Justice: Some Addenda," Natural Law Forum, 13 (1968), 53. For Rawls's general theory, see "Justice as Fairness," Philosophy, Politics and Society (Second Series), ed. by Peter Laslett and W. G. Runciman (Oxford, 1962), pp. 132–157 and his other essays on aspects of this topic.

22. Nicholas Rescher, "The Allocation of Exotic Medical Lifesaving Therapy," *Ethics* 79 (1969): 173–180.

23. Harry S. Abram, M.D., "The Psychiatrist, the Treatment of Chronic Renal Failure, and the Prolongation of Life: II" *American Journal of Psychiatry* 126:157–167 (1969), 158.

Human Organs and the Open Market

Clifton Perry

Because of the principle that commercial profit cannot be obtained as a result of the possession of a dead body, it is never seriously argued that a social policy should be framed which allows for the selling of cadaver or neomort organs for medical purposes, for example, transplantation or experimentation. Generally it is maintained that organs ideally should be given by the deceased premortem or given by the family of the deceased, barring any prior objection by the deceased.[1] A not uncommon but as yet somewhat less popular approach to the procurement of medically needed organs is the alternative policy of harvesting or salvaging organs. Rather than the socially accepted medical routine of not taking organs unless explicitly allowed, the harvesting or salvaging approach would allow, as a matter of general practice, the taking of organs unless explicitly denied

such access by the deceased prior to demise or by the family, barring any previous counter by the deceased.[2] There is in addition a third policy whereby the trading of organs allows for the procurement of credits, again barring opposition by the appropriate family members. Under the trading system, medically needed organs would be exchanged in a manner not unlike that exemplified by the blood-bank system.[3]

Although troubled by various problems, the three approaches for organ procurement are always seen as preferable to any policy which advocates the selling of cadaver or neomort organs. Consequently, it shall be the intent of this essay to note those considerations which militate acceptance of the three traditional approaches concerning the medical acquisition of human organs as well as to suggest a manner by which the selling of

Reprinted from Ethics *91 (October 1980): 63-71. Copyright © 1980 by The University of Chicago.*

human organs might circumvent these problems. In the course of the argument an attempt also will be made to negotiate successfully the problems which uniquely concern the selling of human organs as a policy for organ acquistion.

I

The need for human organs for transplant, for example, the cornea, the human kidney, etc., is already well known. More than once it has been noted that over eight thousand people in the United States who die from renal failure might have been saved by a kidney transplant. Transplants would reduce the number of kidney-related deaths in the United States by almost 15–20 percent.[4] The situation for other human parts, for example, arteries, eyes, skin, etc., is no less notable. Including the heart, it has been estimated that from one cadaver or neomort perhaps seventeen separate items might be obtained.[5] Yet, given the number of lives which might have been saved, and the long waiting list for other human parts which relate to the quality of human life, for example, the cornea, it appears obvious that the giving of cadaver or neomort organs is pragmatically insufficient for the task for which it was intended, namely, the relief of needless human suffering and death.

It is in virtue of this consideration that the argument for the harvesting of organs gains its basic appeal. If we routinely took needed organs, the rate of human suffering and death would decrease dramatically. All the advantages of the giving of organs may be duplicated by a policy of salvaging. For instance, it has been noted that, *pace* Ramsey, the virtue of generosity of donors might still be manifested in the giving of human organs for purposes of research. Such research organs would generally not be salvaged, thus allowing for premortem and family donation.[6] Any disadvantage, moreover, noted with salvaging will be found in a giving policy. For example, the routine salvaging of organs is interrupted only under conditions of responsible party denial. This denial unfortunately occurs during a period of extreme family grief, for example, at the time of the patient's death. The untimely encounter, however, between the family and the medical establishment occurs also in the case of donating organs. In order to satisfy transplant needs the medical establish-

ment must attempt, during the period of family grief, to obtain the family's approval to take the deceased patient's organs. In either event, the untimely confrontation between the bereaved family and the medical establishment occurs.[7]

If the above arguments are correct, the salvaging and the giving policies are on equal footing as regards their efficacy in providing the necessary organs for sustaining human life and reducing human suffering. Both policies make allowances for generosity, and where the policy of giving equals the salvaging policy in efficiency of supplying necessary organs, it duplicates the salvaging policy's fault of untimely family-medical confrontation. Where the giving policy circumvents the confrontation problem, it runs the risk of being unable to supply the necessary organs. If, therefore, the policy of giving organs has been justified upon those grounds mentioned above, and the policy of salvaging is no worse and perhaps even better, the policy of salvaging should be implemented.

It has been argued that a society in which the populace regularly gave organs in sufficient number to guarantee no unnecessary loss of life or needless suffering would be, in some sense, better than one in which the requisite numbers of organs could be supplied only through periodic or continual harvesting.[8] In such a situation, it could be argued, the giving policy would be comparably better than the salvaging policy in that both policies supplied the requisite number of organs, but only the giving policy eliminated the painful encounter between the family and the medical establishment. It is quite true that such a situation does not obtain, and the problems concerning fair organ distribution have arisen within a society where the populace, of its own volition, has failed to meet the constant need for human organs, even though it is within its physical power to do so.[9] However, if a situation obtained whereby the general populace did give in sufficient number to decrease human suffering and death, it is likely that salvaging would also be allowed in sufficient number to achieve the same end. The sole reason for the painful encounter between the family and the medical establishment would, in either case, be eliminated. Again, both policies appear to be on a par, and in fact, between the notions of giving or salvaging organs, one can make no unequivocal judgment regarding the humanity of either policy.

Nevertheless, does not the routine salvaging of human organs say something about the social attitudes of the public involved in such a system? Allegedly, the salvaging of body parts entails that the said parts be treated as property owned by the state.[10] The implication of salvaging, then, is that it demeans the intrinsic value of humanity, besides allowing unnecessary encroachment of the state within family affairs. Besides the fact that the notion of the equation of dead bodies with humanity is suspect, it has also been countered that state encroachment is not necessarily bad, and in this situation might even be quite beneficial.[11] It is, nonetheless, not clear that a policy of salvaging organs represents an encroachment of the state any more than would a policy of giving. It would seem that, if the salvaging procedure were such that the family was powerless to deny access to the organs, then we would definitely possess a clear case of state encroachment. But with the policy of harvesting organs the family does have the final word by either tacit consent or active denial. No medical procedure is performed or not performed upon the cadaver without the family's silent approval or active denial. This situation is, at least with respect to the state, no different from a policy of giving organs. If, therefore, a state were to enact a bill which allowed for the giving of human organs and such a state-entered policy usurped private interests no more than a similar policy of harvesting, then the harvesting policy would allow for state encroachment only if the giving policy would.

Thus it may be maintained that both policies for the acquisition of human organs are equal with respect to the dignity of human life and death. The equalization of the two policies has been demonstrated by noting that the policy of harvesting has none of the militating disadvantages formerly thought to accrue to it. The policy of harvesting has, moreover, all of the advantages of an effective policy of giving. A policy for the procurement of human organs which is based upon the exchange of monetary credit might be similarly justified.

II

First it might be noted that a selling policy for obtaining cadaver or neomort organs does not fall short of the previously mentioned policies with respect to those issues discussed above.[12] It is not, for instance, maintained that a policy of selling represents another example of state encroachment. Indeed, if state involvement were to occur at all, it would have to be to reverse the self-stultifying effects of the unbridled capitalistic treatment of human organs. Such state involvement, for the most part, is designed to protect the consumer from unfair and unjust treatment by avaricious individuals. Otherwise such a system, considered independently of abuse through perfidy, appears the paradigm of individualistic interaction.

Even should state-initiated consumer protection occur, it would be to eliminate unscrupulous behavior in the appropriate personal interactions. As such, state encroachment would be beneficial rather than detrimental. Such state encroachment, furthermore, would be of a type similar to that noted in the policies of giving and harvesting in that the family is not powerless to deny medical access to the required organs. As with the harvesting or the giving of organs, the selling policy would place the family's or the premortem's wishes concerning the disposition of the organs ahead of the state's needs.

It might, of course, be argued that a policy of selling human organs appears somewhat less humane than its two counterparts. The free acquisition of human organs, whether explicitly given in a giving policy or implicitly given as in a salvaging policy, seems infinitely more humane than a policy whereby needed human organs are placed upon the open market. But it is unclear why the exchange of monetary considerations lessens the humanity of a given enterprise. It is quite true that the impetus for the relinquishment of the human organs may be due to the expectation of monetary return rather than to thoughts of the benefits likely to accrue to the recipient. Nevertheless, not only might thoughts of recipient benefit along with thought of personal aggrandizement motivate the premortem donor or family of such, but a system whose sole orientation is the lessening of human suffering and the diminishing of needless human death is, regardless of individual impetus, oriented toward very humane goals. We do not, after all, think the medical profession any less humanely oriented because there are physicians who receive a staggering income and continue their medical practice because of that income.

Does such a policy, however, allow for the much needed opportunity for personal generosity? Without embellishment, it might be suggested that of all the policies advocated regarding the procurement of cadaver or neomort organs, none allows for personal generosity to the degree allowed by the policy of selling. As with other policies, not only may one allow the requested organs to be taken for purposes of lessening pain, saving lives, or experimentation, but, unlike the other policies, one may also deny the financial return for the organs. The two previously considered policies can satisfy the first mentioned opportunity for generosity, but only a selling policy can satisfy both.

The efficiency of the selling policy in producing the much needed organs is not dissimilar to the efficiency of the policies of giving organs and of harvesting. There are, in other words, two approaches to the selling of organs which compare favorably with the previously considered policies for organ acquisition. The first approach places the burden, or perhaps the opportunity, of the sale upon the individual or individuals responsible. Much like the policy of giving, it would be assumed that the needed organs were not for sale unless a permission-to-sell form had been signed. Unfortunately, neither the giving nor the selling policy may be completely successful in satisfying the needs of the medically ill (although the latter may be more efficient) unless there is a somewhat aggressive approach made by the medical profession to persuade the responsible party to sell the required organs. Thus both policies may require the unfortunate family–medical-profession encounter, if needs are to be satisfied.

The unfortunate and untimely encounter is, as in the case of harvesting organs, duplicated in the second approach to selling, that is, passive selling. Passive selling places the responsibility for not selling upon those who are responsible for the organs. If there is no pre- or postmortem denial of sale, the cadaver or neomort organs are taken to be "for sale," and the responsible living party is reimbursed. The passive selling policy, like the harvesting policy, has a good chance of satisfying the needs of those persons who might be helped or saved by transplants but, unlike the harvesting policy, it brings monetary advantage to those who accede to the sale. Both policies, however, place the burden of denying the sale upon those individuals for whom the present circumstances make such behavior prodigiously difficult.

As argued above, it would appear that any advantage enjoyed by the effective giving of organs is equally enjoyed by the harvesting of organs. Likewise, any disadvantage suffered by the harvesting of organs is suffered equally by the effective giving of organs. Moreover, the equalization of the same advantages and disadvantages appears duplicated between the two policies when monetary reimbursement is added; for example, the giving of organs becomes the active selling of such while the harvesting of organs becomes the passive selling of such. Therefore, if the above is correct, the four approaches to organ acquisition appear equal with respect to those problems which affect all of the policies. There is, nevertheless, at least one major problem connected with the selling of organs which is irrelevant to the nonselling policies. The selling of cadaver or neomort organs transgresses the accepted principle that no individual is entitled to claim ownership of a dead body for commercial profit.[13]

III

Is a policy of selling cadaver or neomort organs an instance of commercial profit being gained through ownership of a dead body? It is not obvious that an affirmative answer must be forthcoming. Does the centuries-old principle forbidding the ownership of a dead body for commercial reasons have anything whatsoever to do with profit? It seems obvious that ownership is not absolutely forbidden, as the system of trading organs might properly be so characterized. If, that is, "commercial" is not equated with "selling for a profit," and if the general policy of trading organs advocated by Ramsey[14] is acceptable, then ownership of a dead body or parts thereof for commercial but nonprofit purposes would likewise be acceptable. Not all such trade situations, however, need be assumed to be unprofitable. For instance, it might be construed as gaining profit to exchange a kidney for a cornea or a heart for bone marrow, regardless of the precise worth attached to each type of organ. It might, in other words, be extremely difficult to assign a precise quantity of worth to particular organs and to avoid making a profit by the sorts of exchanges noted above. Consider also an exchange of dissimilar organs during a period when, because of a particular situation, there occurs a greater demand for the one organ without a similar increase in demand for the other. Such lack of parity of worth might also be created by advancements in medical technology with respect to the same organs. It might, for example, be taken as an exchange which precipitated profit when one party traded a kidney when kidney transplants were considered the most efficacious means of renal rejuvenation, but a loss to the party who received a kidney when technological advancements rendered kidney transplants the least efficacious form of rejuvenation. In such a purely nonprofit context, profit may be extracted when the empirical circumstances are such that dissimilar organs are exchanged, or when the organs are exchanged during periods of great technological advancement. Nevertheless, under "normal" circumstances the commercial exchange or trade of organs may obviate reference to profit.

Might a similar comment be made concerning the selling of organs? Under normal conditions of exchange, might profit be eliminated in such a way as to allow money to be considered germane to the exchange? It is not, after all, the case that profit necessarily entails reference to money, nor is it the case that money necessarily entails reference to profit. So long as the commercial exchange—be it exchange of organs for organs or organs for money—does not involve a profit enjoyed by one party over the other, the antiprofit principle anent organ acquisition has not been violated.

The advantage of selling over trading organs is that the problems created by the possible trade of dissimilar organs would be largely eliminated. Since there would obtain, in the case of selling only, numerical value placed upon organs, differences in organ value could be compensated for by appropriate reimbursement. This would allow someone in need of a kidney to exchange the numerical equivalent of a dissimilar organ plus or minus the compensating sum. Moreover, a decrease or increase in demand for various organs, either because of significant advances in medical technology or because of a change in physical conditions, might be counterbalanced by previously assigned monetary values which, although not impervious to considerations of exchange conditions, are less volatile than the conditions themselves. If the above is correct, the policy of selling might be

more successful than that of trading, in those untoward circumstances which lend themselves to profit making in exchange situations.

However, there is one problem which, it is argued, is unique to the selling of organs. If such a policy were initiated, only the opulent would be in a position to afford them. What would the poor do in a situation where a cornea transplant were needed, let alone a heart transplant? This problem, however, would seem to affect similarly a trading policy. If a poor family has failed, because of lack of desire or opportunity, to donate a needed organ and now one of its members finds him or herself in vital need of such an organ, does the family "owe" the medical establishment an organ, or does the family "pay" for the organ? Under a trading policy, a family in such a position cannot simply be given, gratis, a needed organ. Consequently, it would seem that either only those families who have given may receive, or that those families who have received but who have failed to donate in some sense "owe," either directly or, what is more likely, indirectly, those who have donated. In either event, similar to a policy of selling, a policy of trading would institute a procedure whereby only those who give may receive; all others will incur a debt which must be paid in some fashion.

However, the problem of the high cost of needed organs might actually be circumvented in a selling situation. This might be accomplished by including the cost of the organ within the cost of surgery, both of which costs might be covered by the appropriate social agency or medical insurance company. This need not be an exorbitant addition if the price of buying remained the same as the price of selling and if both were nominal, thus eliminating the possibility of unfair advantage or profit being secured by any party. One would, consequently, not get rich selling cadaver or neomort organs, nor would one have to be rich in order to procure one.

As presented above, it would appear that any advantages of a policy of trading organs may be duplicated by a policy of selling organs, and, in addition, the latter policy may be implemented so as to circumvent those problems usually associated with the former policy. Moreover, any policy which allowed for the selling of cadaver or neomort organs might be seen as equal in all respects to either an effective giving policy or a salvaging policy, except that it had the added advantage of nominally rewarding the responsible parties. Thus the policy of reimbursement might be separated from its sinister image which has, through the ages, represented the selling of cadavers as the nadir of human rapacity. The selling policy, as outlined above, is rather a representation of a social attitude of gratefulness for the organs without which needless suffering and death would continue.

IV

It might, therefore, be suggested that a policy allowing for the selling of organs need not necessarily violate the age-old tradition of disallowing for the procurement of commercial profit by ownership of a dead body or parts thereof. Furthermore, such a policy might satisfy the following "moral restraints" and "social goals":[15] (1) provision for a fitting removal of the body from society; (2) protection of the integrity of the corpse; (3) protection of the bodily integrity and autonomy of the living; (4) saving of lives; (5) lack of interference with other social objectives; and (6) assistance for the bereaved survivors.

Indeed it might be suggested that if any policy might satisfy all six requirements, a selling policy could. This is not to suggest that other policies would fail with respect to such requirements. However, not only is a selling or reimbursing policy not to be dismissed a priori, but, with particular reference to the assistance for the bereaved survivors, such a policy may be more efficacious than other alternatives.

Notes

1. Paul Ramsey, *The Patient as Person* (New Haven, Conn.: Yale University Press, 1970), chap. 5.
2. David Sanders and Jesse Dukeminier, "Medical Advance and Legal Lag: Hemodialysis and Kidney Transplant," *UCLA Law Review* 15 (1968): 357–413, esp. p. 402.
3. Ramsey.
4. Robert Veatch, *Death, Dying and the Biological Revolution* (New Haven, Conn.: Yale University Press, 1976).
5. Willard Gaylin, "Harvesting the Dead," *Harper's Magazine* (1974), pp. 23–30; Albert Jonsen, "The Totally Implantable Artificial Heart," *Hastings Center Report* 3 (1973): 1–4; Ramsey.
6. James Muyskens, "An Alternative Policy for Obtaining Cadaver Organs for Transplantation," *Philosophy and Public Affairs* 8 (1978):88–99.
7. Ibid.
8. Ramsey.
9. Ibid.
10. Veatch.
11. Muyskens.
12. Perhaps only because the argued disadvantages appear sufficient for dismissal.
13. Muyskens.
14. Ramsey.
15. Muyskens.

Decision Scenario 1

"What do you mean you don't know who he is?" asked Dr. Bridewell, the head of the Oakbrook Hospital Renal Unit.

"He was unconscious when the police brought him to the ER. We started the IV, stopped his bleeding, and patched him up. But he still hasn't recovered consciousness. The police think it was a hit-and-run driver." Dr. Kathy McDowell spoke in a precise, matter-of-fact voice. Dr. Bridewell always frightened her, but she was determined not to show it.

"He didn't have any identification?"

"That's right. They think that either the driver robbed him or somebody else who came along did. Anyway, he was wearing jeans and a sweatshirt, nothing that gives any clue as to his background. There is one thing we do know definitely."

"What's that?" asked Dr. Bridewell.

"Both of his kidneys were hopelessly damaged, but his general physical condition is good. We think he's a good candidate for a transplant."

"Then you know we've got a guy whose brain waves we're waiting to flatten out?"

"Dr. Liebsbaum told me."

"He ought to keep his mouth shut," Dr. Bridewell said. "Oh, don't take that seriously. I'm just upset because this faces us with a big problem. We're only going to have one kidney to transplant. The other one's shot."

"That's all we want," said McDowell.

Bridewell ignored her. "You did a tissue check?" he asked.

"It's close enough."

"Too bad. What I mean is that I've got another candidate. Now we have to decide which of the two gets the kidney."

"Who's the other candidate?"

"A Mrs. Benson. She's a woman in her early sixties who's active in local affairs. She was on the school board. Her husband's a rich lawyer, and both of them move in high social circles. She does a lot of work now with a foundation that's supposed to help minority children in school. She also happens to be a pretty good candidate physically for a transplant."

"So you'll choose her over my patient?" McDowell felt herself getting angry.

"I didn't say that. How old is this guy?"

"I would estimate that he's in his early or middle thirties. He seems to be in good physical condition."

"But we don't know anything about him," said Dr. Bridewell. "He might just be a drifter passing through town. He's probably not a member of the community that this hospital is supposed to serve, the one that pays bills and makes donations."

"Not that we know of," Dr. McDowell admitted. "But he might be. He might be a person of great value. Maybe he's even a physician."

"But we don't know for sure, do we?" said Dr. Bridewell.

Suppose you are Dr. Bridewell and have to decide between the unknown man and Mrs. Benson. On what grounds might you make your decision?

How might the criteria offered by Rescher or Childress be employed?

Would Kant consider both people to have a claim on the available kidney?

Are Rawls's principles of any help in formulating a policy that might help resolve problems of this sort?

In what way, if any, is Perry's proposal relevant?

Decision Scenario 2

"It will be at least two weeks before that melts," Miller said. He stood at the top of the trail looking down into the snow-blocked canyon.

"There's no way to go around?" Jennifer Martin asked. Backpacking up the steep mountain trail had been a grand adventure until the spring snowslide had isolated their little group. Now things were awful. Carl had lost his footing and tumbled down a steep slope, breaking a rib and ripping open his left side. Then Alice had gotten sick and was running a high fever. Doug Miller thought it might be pneumonia. Both Carl and Alice lay in their sleeping bags on the floor of the drafty line shack at the top of the trail.

"That's the only way in or out," Miller said. "And the snow is too loose and filled with pockets to support anybody. At least we have enough food."

"But we really need to do something for Carl and Alice," said Jennifer. "I didn't want to say this where they could hear me, but without treatment both of them have a good chance of dying."

"I thought you brought enough supplies for treatment. We all thought it was wonderful to have our own doctor along."

"Both need antibiotic therapy," Jennifer said. "Infection is the great risk in each case. And I just don't have enough antibiotics to treat both of them. One maybe."

"We can't do that," Miller said. "Can't you just split what there is between them."

"Yes, but that would probably do little good. With antibiotics you've got to kill all the bugs to keep the infection under control. Partial treatment is like trying to put out a house fire with a cup of water."

"So partial treatment of both might not help either?"

"It would help some but probably not enough," Jennifer said.

"Then it seems to me that we shouldn't treat either of them. That's the only fair thing to do."

"Then both will probably die."

"Are you willing to make the decision?" Miller asked. "Are you willing to say, 'I'm going to treat you, but I'm not going to treat the other person'?"

"I don't want to do that. And I don't want to give partial treatment either. I want to be able to save at least one of them."

"How are you going to choose?" asked Miller. "I think Carl is a nicer person than Alice, but Alice is a chemist, and society would probably regard her as more valuable. After all, Carl is just an unsuccessful poet and a bookstore clerk."

"Maybe we should explain the situation to them," Jennifer said. "Maybe one of them will volunteer to let the other use all of the antibiotics."

"I think that's cruel," Miller said. "I'll go back to my original suggestion that we don't give either of them any drugs."

What do you consider to be the right thing to do in this situation? Justify your decision.

What might a utilitarian argue?

Should Alice and Carl be consulted? If so, does the categorical imperative require that each agree to give up his or her claim to the antibiotics for the sake of the other?

Does the duty to preserve one's life (in Kant's theory or natural law) require that Carl and Alice demand the antibiotics for themselves?

What light (if any) does a case such as this throw on the question of establishing a policy for allocating scarce resources?

Decision Scenario 3

Valdez Regional Hospital is the primary medical facility for the residents of Valdez County, Arizona. Its intensive care unit is the only one available in the entire county, and the closest comparable unit is eighty-five miles away in Somora County.

The Valdez ICU is a twelve-bed facility and, from the statistical point of view, it is generally adequate to serve the needs of its patient population. That is, the cost of adding extra equipment and staff to increase the size of the facility is much greater than its actual use would justify.

Valdez's ICU policy, which is similar to policies of hospitals everywhere, requires that the staff make the effort to keep at least one of the twelve beds free for use in a genuine emergency.

On a bright, clear afternoon one day after Christmas, sixty-eight-year-old Harry Aveni was brought to the emergency room of Valdez after he had collapsed on the patio of his house. Mr. Aveni had been brought to the emergency room twice before. Both were episodes of congestive heart failure, and this third occasion was no different. Mr. Aveni had broken his diet during the holidays and consumed an unaccustomed amount of salt.

Mr. Aveni responded well to emergency treatment. The fluid surrounding his heart was withdrawn, a glycoside medication was administered, and his condition seemed to stabilize. Then that evening, there was a sudden onset of fibrillation—his heart started beating erratically. Again, Mr. Aveni responded well to treatment, and after emergency defibrillation, his condition again stabilized.

"He needs to be put into the ICU," Dr. Ellen Gracian said. "We can't care for him sufficiently on the wards, because he's got to have constant monitoring."

"I don't think Dr. Franklin is going to want to admit him," the nurse said. "There's only one bed left."

Dr. Gracian immediately left the floor and went to the ICU director's office. She explained what she wanted and waited while he seemed to be thinking it over.

"I don't think I can admit him," Dr. Franklin said. "Here we have an elderly gentleman who has now gone through three episodes of congestive failure and also seems to have something wrong to cause the fibrillation. He didn't stick to his diet, and in general his days are likely to be in the rather small numbers."

"But if he doesn't have intensive care, the numbers may be even smaller," Dr. Gracian said.

"That's no doubt true. But as things are, we've got eleven people who need to stay right where they are for God knows how long, and we've got just one bed at our disposal."

"But that's all I need, just one bed."

"I understand that," said Dr. Franklin. "But let's suppose we install your patient in the ICU and fifteen minutes after we put him there an eighteen-year-old accident victim is brought in. She's going to have to have emergency treatment, then close and constant monitoring, or she's likely to die."

"But you don't know that somebody like that is going to come in," Dr. Gracian said. "And Mr Aveni is here right now and is in need right now."

"I'm sorry," said Dr. Franklin. "But the chances are very good that somebody is going to need that bed, somebody we can do more for than we can do for your patient. Somebody who's got a better chance to live a longer and more normal life."

"I see," Dr Gracian said. "But I thought we were in the business of savings lives."

"We are. But we can't save them all, and that's where the problems come in."

What argument can be made from the point of view of an actutilitarian to support Dr. Franklin's decision?

Would a Kantian approve or disapprove of the decision?

Would a selection procedure of the sort favored by Childress secure a bed in the ICU for Mr. Aveni?

Would any of the criteria presented by Rescher lead to the selection of Mr. Aveni over an eighteen-year-old accident victim?

Decision Scenario 4

The microsurgical team at Benton Public Hospital consisted of twenty-three people. Five were surgeons, three were anesthesiologists, three were internists, two were radiologists, and the remaining members were various sorts of nurses and technicians.

Early Tuesday afternoon on a date late in March, the members of the team that had to be sterile were scrubbing while the others were preparing to start operating on Mr. Hammond Cox. Mr. Cox was a fifty-nine-year-old, unmarried black man who worked as a janitor in a large apartment building. While performing his duties, Mr. Cox had caught his hand in the mechanism of a commercial trash compactor. The bones of his wrist had been crushed and the blood vessels severed.

The head of the team, Dr. Herbert Lagorio, believed that it was possible to restore at least partial functioning to Mr. Cox's hand. Otherwise, the hand would have to be amputated.

Mr. Cox had been drunk when the accident happened. When the police ambulance brought him to the emergency room, he was still so drunk that a decision was made to delay surgery for almost an hour to give him a chance to burn up some of the alcohol he had consumed. As it was, administering anesthesia to Mr. Cox would incur a greater than average risk. Furthermore, blood tests had shown that Mr. Cox already suffered from some degree of liver damage. In both short- and long-range terms, Mr. Cox was not a terribly good surgical risk.

Dr. Lagorio was already scrubbed when Dr. Carol Levine, a resident in emergency medicine, had him paged.

"This had better be important," he told her. "I've got a guy prepped and waiting."

"I know you do," Dr. Levine said. "But there's something you ought to know about before you start."

"Tell me quick."

"They just brought in a thirty-five-year-old white female with a totally severed right hand. She's a biology professor at Columbia and was working late in her lab when some maniac looking for drugs came in and attacked her with a cleaver."

"What shape is the hand in?"

"Excellent. The campus cops were there within minutes, and there was ice in the lab. One of the cops had the good sense to put the hand in a plastic bag and bring it with her."

"Is she in good general health?"

"It seems excellent," Dr. Levine said.

"This is a real problem."

"You can't do two cases at once?

"No way. We need everybody we've got to do one."

"How about sending her someplace else?"

"No place else is set up to do what has to be done," Dr. Lagorio said.

"So what are you going to do?"

"That's what I've got to decide," Dr. Lagorio said.

Does a "first-come, first-served" criterion like that defended by Childress require that Mr. Cox receive the surgery?

Does a "social-value" criterion require that the biology professor receive the surgery?

Can the chance of a successful outcome in each case be used as a criterion without violating the notion that all people are of equal inherent worth?

In your view, who should have the potential benefits of the surgery? Give reasons to support your view.

Decision Scenario 5

"Your baby's pituitary gland is not fully developed," Dr. Robert Amatin said.

Clarissa Austin nodded to show that she understood that at least something was wrong with her child. She had already made up her mind to do whatever she had to do to see to it that her baby was all right.

"That means he's not getting enough of a hormone—a chemical—produced there," Dr. Amatin went on. "He won't undergo the normal course of development without that chemical."

"Can you give it to him?"

Dr. Amatin avoided answering the question directly. "A transplant is the best hope," he said. "If we can surgically remove the malformed pituitary and attach a new one, then the baby has a very good chance of being normal."

"I'll be happy to give my permission, if that's what you're waiting for," Clarissa said.

"It's not that simple," Dr. Amatin said. He looked uncomfortable. "It really comes down to a matter of money."

"I don't have much money," Clarissa said. "You know my bills are being paid by Medicaid."

"I know that, and the government won't pay for transplant organs."

"How much does it cost?"

"I've got a family right now that says it wants five thousand dollars for the pituitary of their baby. She just died this morning."

"I can't get money like that," Clarissa said.

"I can ask them to come up and talk to you. Maybe they would take less or maybe you could work out some kind of deferred payment with them."

"What if I can't?"

Dr. Amatin shook his head. "I can't arrange for a transplant without an organ, and I suspect they will just try to find somebody else to sell it to."

"That don't seem fair," Clarissa said. "Just because I haven't got the money, my little baby is going to have to be some kind of cripple and maybe die."

If organs are sold on the open market, is such a situation possible?

What does Perry suggest might be done to avoid difficulties such as the one described?

Is Ms. Austin correct in saying that it would be unfair for her child not to have the organ because she cannot afford to pay the asking price? After all, surely it is not unfair for her child not to have, say, a silver drinking cup because she cannot afford to pay the asking price.

Is selling organs on the open market necessarily incompatible with Rawls's principles of justice?

Do such situations prove that the present policy of relying on donated organs is a superior one?

10
THE CLAIM TO HEALTH CARE

CASE PRESENTATION
The Crisis in American Health Care

A crisis exists in a social institution when there are factors present that tend to destroy the institution or render it ineffective in achieving its goals. Two major factors have led some observers to say that the American health care system is in a state of crisis: the increasing cost to the society of health care, and the failure to deliver health care to those who need it at prices they can afford. Let us examine each of these factors briefly and then turn to some solutions that have been offered.

Cost of Health Care

After defense, health care is the most expensive item in the federal budget, and the average American must work one month a year to pay for medical insurance, physicians' bills, and the cost of hospitalization.

Despite recent efforts to contain the costs of health care, they continue to rise at a rate greater than the increase in consumer prices. In 1981, the overall price index rose at a rate of 9.4 percent, while overall medical costs rose by 12.5 percent. This was the largest increase since 1935, the year the government began to collect such statistics.

Hospital costs, more than any other factor, are responsible for the increasing expense of health care. In the first nine months of 1979, hospital expenditures rose 13.4 percent. In 1980, the increase was 17 percent, and in 1981, it was 18.8 percent.

Various explanations have been given for the spiraling costs of health care. Stanley Hwang suggests that one factor is the lack of financial accountability from those responsible for operating the health-care system. Most Americans are covered by employee group insurance that pays physicians and hospitals on a fee-for-service basis. This system serves to hide the cost of medical care from the consumer. Because the consumer gets a relatively unlimited amount of medical services for a fixed premium and because the premium itself is hidden in the form of direct and indirect payroll deductions, the consumer has no incentive to avoid unnecessary or quite expensive medical services. Doctors and hospitals have no incentive to trim costs because the consumer is not concerned about the cost, and insurers respond to rising costs by increasing premiums. In such a situation, no one believes it is necessary to worry about cost.

Others, such as Bernard Winter, lay most of the blame on the greed for profit on the part of physicians, hospitals, drug companies, construction companies, equipment manufacturers, and all others who are involved in the gigantic "medical industry." Winter mentions as relevant such considerations as these:

> The Hill-Burton Act of 1946 provided federal funds to encourage the building of "non-profit" hospitals. Because of the money to be made from the construction and operation of the hospitals, there was a great amount of overbuilding. On a given day about 100,000 hospital beds are empty in the United States. It costs $20,000 a year to maintain an empty bed so $2 billion a year is spent on unneeded facilities.

> Studies show that as much as one-third of hospital stays are unnecessary. This adds $5 billion to health care.

> The United States has 780 open-heart surgery facilities. They cost $380 billion to build and several million dollars a year to maintain. Yet 11 percent are not used even once a year.

> "Medicaid Mills" operated by physicians add millions to health care costs, while at the same time providing poor medical care. Great numbers of patients are given inadequate examinations, told to return for an excessive number of visits, and often referred to other physicians for trivial reasons.

Others have also called attention to similar abuses or flaws in the health-care system that unnecessarily increase the cost of service. For example:

> For economic reasons, hospitals need to attract as many patients as they can handle. Since patients are referred to hospitals by physicians, hospitals must make themselves attractive to physicians. To do this usually means having the latest medical equipment. With the encouragement of equipment manufacturers, hospital administrators are often led to invest in equipment that will be rarely used. Its cost must eventually be borne by the consumer. Cooperation and sharing of equipment by hospitals would substantially reduce the need to buy equipment that would be used only infrequently.

> There are about twice as many surgeons per capita in the United States as there are in Great Britain. There are also about twice as many surgical procedures performed per capita. This suggests a great amount of unneeded surgery is being performed at considerable cost to the consumer.

Quite apart from various flaws in the way in which the health-care system operates, other factors having to do with a changing population and the state of medicine itself are no doubt responsible to some extent for increasing costs. Here are three of them:

As children born during the baby boom of the 1940s have reached adulthood, there has been an increase in the median age of the population. An aging population requires more medical care and more expensive medical care than a population with a lower median age.

Improvements in medical technology now make it possible to provide a greater number of services to hospitalized patients. This also means that more people are likely to be hospitalized in order to receive the services.

Improvements in medical treatments now make it possible to provide treatment for illnesses that once would not have been treated. The very availability of such treatments means increasing the hospital population, and the very success of such treatments means that more people will be alive who can benefit from additional care.

While the major item responsible for increasing the expense of health care in general is hospital costs, all of these factors significantly contribute to the overall costs.

Such considerations as the ones we have mentioned here have persuaded nearly everyone concerned with the formulation and implementation of health-care policies that the current state of affairs needs to be changed. There is a general belief that if it is not, the health-care system will become so economically unrealistic that it will collapse.

Health-Care Delivery

Despite the great economic investment in health care, some 12 percent of the population of this country (one out of eight people) receive no medical care at all. Others frequently lack access to care even when they can afford it, and a large number of people cannot receive the proper kind of care. Also, workers are hit particularly hard by the present system. Although they pay disproportionately higher taxes and expensive insurance premiums, they are not eligible for Medicare-Medicaid programs. Finally, there is some question as to whether health-care funds are really going to the programs that most need them.

The failures of the system to supply the amount and kind of required health care are often, although not always, closely connected with the same factors that make health care so expensive. Some factors frequently mentioned are the following:

Overspecialization by physicians leaves general social needs unsatisfied. We have already noticed that there seems to be an oversupply of surgeons. It has been claimed that this is also true of virtually every medical speciality. Specialists are more expensive to educate, and in practice they charge higher fees for what is often the same care as that given by nonspecialists. The financial and social incentives that encourage specialization are not only costly, they leave too few physicians in general-care practice.

Reductions in funding for community clinics, prenatal care centers, and pediatric clinics that were established in the 1960s have forced many to close or to cut back severely on services. This has deprived many people in the lower socioeconomic groups of a major source of health care.

Hospitals partially funded under the Hill-Burton Act were required to provide a "reasonable volume" of free or low-cost service for those unable to pay. Enforcement of this regulation by federal agencies has been lax. Often the interpretation has been taken to mean that a hospital must supply only emergency-room service.

In 1930 the ratio of family-care doctors was three for every two thousand patients. It is now one for every two thousand. This has led some critics to charge that there is a shortage of physicians. Some have also claimed that the shortage is artificially maintained through the political power of professional groups such as the American Medical Association because the shortage offers considerable economic advantages to the physician.

Others have asserted that there is no genuine shortage of physicians. There is, however, a serious problem caused by their distribution. Most have chosen to live and practice in major metropolitan areas. As a consequence, many rural areas and small towns have been left totally without professional medical care.

Factors such as these are often mentioned to support the claim that the American health-care system is not adequately serving the needs of the people. The charge is made that we live in a system in which there are still two kinds of medicine—one for the rich and one for the poor. And it often happens that the medicine for the poor is none at all.

The factors that we have discussed are much disputed. Both their truth and significance has been called into question. Yet virtually everyone is prepared to admit that the present system of health-care delivery requires immediate modification.

Possible Solutions

In 1974 Congress passed the National Health Planning and Resources Development Act. This established health systems agencies that were charged with developing guidelines for the planning and allocation of health care by municipal, state, and federal governments. These agencies have not yet produced significant results. Many hope, however, that such matters as hospital overbuilding and the duplication of equipment and services can be brought under control by the agencies. If this is so, then the cost of health care could be kept from increasing at its current rate.

A number of health planners have suggested that the United States should move toward the establishment of Health Maintenance Organizations (HMOs). An HMO is a medical plan in which an individual pays a fixed annual fee to an organized group of physicians. The group then undertakes to supply the individual with needed medical services, at no additional charge.

HMOs hold out the possibility of lowered medical costs. They avoid unnecessary tests and procedures because the profit of the group is determined by the money remaining after the expenses of patients have been paid. Better patient care may result because the HMO organization encourages patients to consult a physician at the beginning of an illness rather than waiting until it grows serious.

HMOs were part of the original general health plan developed by President Carter's administration. It was intended to be a way of providing health care to all citizens, while controlling the cost of such care. As such, the HMO plan would be a kind of national health insurance. However, the Carter proposals were never adopted by Congress.

Some form of national health insurance would be likely to guarantee wider access to health care. Yet some critics have pointed out that plans based on the HMO concept have potential weaknesses. Critics suggest that HMOs might well encourage physicians to provide inferior care in order to maximize the profits of their group. Furthermore, they believe that any form of national health insurance will infringe on the autonomy of the physician to practice medicine in the way he or she sees fit. The possibility of government regulations stipulating kinds of tests, procedures, and care that are legitimate and will be paid for, they argue, takes practicing medicine out of the hands of physicians and turns it over to bureaucrats. Patients, for their part, may be dissatisfied because physicians will be empowered to turn down their requests for medical services if the physician believes they are unnecessary.

In 1973 Congress passed legislation providing funds to establish HMO-type plans. So far they have not been very successful. But experiences in California suggest that HMOs can work quite well. The Kaiser plan, which was started in 1945, owns twenty-three hospitals, 158 clinics, and has as members 20 percent of the residents in the San Francisco area. Over six million people in California are members of either the Kaiser plan or the Ross-Loos plan.

Health insurance proposals recommended by President Reagan's administration essentially involve private insurance companies. Employers would be encouraged to present their employees with a choice of several different medical plans. Under the cheaper plans, larger shares of medical expenses would be paid by the individual. Those choosing the cheaper plans would receive tax-free cash rebates.

The theory behind this approach is basically the same as that mentioned earlier as an explanation for increasing costs in health care. Since people who are heavily insured do not spend their own money when they go to a physician, they go more frequently than they otherwise would. Furthermore, these people have no financial incentive to seek out lower-cost health care, for they are not paying for it directly. Thus, if people had to pay out more of their own money, they would have a motive to stay out of the health-care system and to reduce their demands for the highest-priced services.

At least one critic of the Reagan proposal, Toby Cohen, sees it as likely to weaken the whole medical-insurance system and thus to deprive many people of health care for financial reasons. Cohen points out that only 1 or 2 percent of the population have health insurance that covers 100 percent of their medical costs. Most people (60 percent) have insurance that requires them to pay at least 20 percent of their medical bills, and 38 percent have even less coverage for nonhospitalizable illnesses. It already costs people to see a physician (not to mention time lost from work and the need to pay bills before being reimbursed by the insurance company), and most people simply do not seek medical help frivolously.

More important, Cohen claims, the rebate plan poses a great danger to the whole purpose of health insurance. The basic idea behind insurance is spreading the risk within a large group. Since many in the group make no claims (or claims that are not substantial), money is available to pay costs for those who are forced to make claims because of accident or illness.

Under the rebate plan, however, those who are generally healthy would be likely to choose cheaper plans. As a result, the cost of medical treatment would no longer be spread over the entire insured population. Those who chose the more expensive plans would be in a group more likely to become ill. As a result, they would eventually have to start paying larger and larger premiums, ones coming close to matching the actual cost of the medical care they might receive. Under such a condition, there would be little point in having insurance. Even if there were, people would not be able to afford the premiums any more than they would be able to afford the cost of medical care. Thus a great number of people would be stranded in a situation in which they can neither pay for their medical needs nor pay for insurance to cover them.

In addition to various plans for providing health care on a national basis, efforts have also been made to reduce the amount spent on health care. In 1977, President Carter proposed a voluntary 9-percent limit on hospital cost increases. Despite attempts by hospitals to stay within that boundary, the voluntary effort is now regarded as not having worked very well. As the figures mentioned earlier indicate, hospital costs have continued to rise at a rate faster than the rise in consumer prices.

A new proposal to address this problem focuses on Medicare payments. Medicare, which is a federally funded program to provide medical expenses for the elderly, cost about 50 billion dollars in 1982.

Under a plan supported by the Reagan administration and developed by the Department of Health and Human Services, a "prospective payment," in the form of a single lump-sum of money, would be granted to each participating hospital to pay in advance for services provided to Medicare patients. Hospitals receiving the money would then be responsible for administering it. They would have the responsibility of cutting costs in order to avoid losing money on the Medicare patients treated by their institution. No additional federal money would be provided to pay them for any cost overruns.

Some who object to the advance-payment argue that the elderly would not be provided with high-quality health care under the scheme. To be sure that they do not lose money in caring for Medicare patients, hospitals would be tempted to forego ordering certain laboratory tests and treatments that might be helpful. Given an option, the hospitals would choose the least expensive method. Thus people who could afford to pay for all relevant tests and treatments would receive them, while those wholly dependent on Medicare would not.

Some have argued that more radical solutions to the health-care problems of the United States are required than would be provided by HMO-type national insurance, employee-option insurance, or particular cost-containment policies. Some claim that the entire medical-delivery system of the country needs to be totally altered. Only then, they say, can costs be controlled, medical needs met, and justice done. The following are among the many recommendations that have been made:

Issue health stamps to those whose income shows them to be in need. Health-stamp recipients could then shop around for medical services. This would introduce an element of competition among health-care providers and lead to a reduction in costs.

Place all pharmaceutical and medical-equipment manufacturers under public ownership. By eliminating excessive profits, the costs of drugs and equipment would come closer to reflecting their true development and production costs.

"Draft" physicians and assign them to work in rural areas or in inner-city neighborhoods where physicians are nonexistent or in short supply.

Limit by law the number of people allowed to enter a medical specialty. Or, alternatively, make it illegal to use public funds to finance specialty training.

Educate great numbers of additional physicians, nurses, and other health-care professionals and require that they put in a term of service in assigned areas.

Eliminate all fee-for-service transactions between physicians and patients and remove the profit motive from health care.

Place all hospital and clinics under community control.

Require that everyone pay premiums for a national health insurance program, but allow claims beyond a certain limit only by those who cannot afford to pay.

Not all of these proposals are equally sound, of course. Some are politically and socially unrealistic at the present time. They are suggestive, however, and they do provide alternative views about how a system that is almost universally regarded as dangerously unworkable might be modified. That such proposals should be made is itself evidence that the health-care system is indeed in crisis.

Introduction

It has been estimated that it was not until the middle 1930s that the intervention of a physician in the treatment of an illness was likely to affect the outcome in a substantial way. The change was brought about by the discovery and development of antibiotic agents such as penicillin and sulfa drugs. They made it possible, for the first time, both to control infection and to provide specific remedies for a variety of diseases. Additional advances in treatment modalities, procedures, and technology have helped establish contemporary medicine as an effective enterprise.

Before these dramatic changes occurred, there was little reason for anyone to be particularly concerned with the question of the distribution of medical care within society. The situation in the United States has altered significantly, and a number of writers have recently argued that everyone ought to be guaranteed at least some form of medical care. In part this is a reflection of the increased effectiveness of contemporary medicine, but it is also no doubt due to a growing awareness of the serious difficulties faced by disadvantaged groups within society.

In the last chapter we discussed one aspect of the problem of the distribution of medical resources—that of allocating limited resources among competing individuals in a particular situation. Here we need to call attention to some of the broader social issues. These are ones that transcend moral decisions about particular people and raise questions about the basic aims and obligations of society.

A great number of observers believe that the United States is currently faced with a health-care crisis. Some of the reasons supporting this belief, as well as some proposed solutions, are outlined in the Case Presentation of this chapter, and we need not repeat them here. But one element of the crisis is often said to be the lack of any program to provide health care for everyone in the society. That there should be people forced to do without needed health care for primarily financial reasons has seemed to some a morally intolerable state of affairs.

This point of view has frequently been based on the claim that everyone has a *right* to health care. Thus, it has been argued, society has a duty to provide that care, and if it does not, then it is sanctioning a situation that is inherently wrong. To remedy the situation requires redesigning the health-care system and present practices to see to it that all who need and want health care have access to it.

The language of "rights" is very slippery. To understand and evaluate arguments that involve claiming (or denying) rights to health care it is important to understand the nature of the claim. The word "rights" is used in several distinct ways, and a failure to be clear about the use in any given case leads only to unproductive confusion.

The following distinctions may help capture some of the more important sorts of things that people have in mind when they talk about rights.

Claim-Rights, Legal Rights, and Statutory Rights

Suppose I own a copy of the book *Anne of Green Gables*. If so, then I may be said to have a *right* to do with the book whatever I choose. Other people may be said to have a *duty* to recognize my right in appropriate ways. Thus, if I want to read the book, burn it, or sell it, others have a duty not to interfere with me. If I lend the book to someone, then he has a duty to return it.

It is generally agreed in the philosophy of law that a claim-right to something serves as a ground for other people's duties. A *claim-right*, then, always entails a duty or duties on the part of someone else. Right and duty thus go together like parent and child—one is not possible without the other.

Generally speaking, *legal rights* are claim-rights. Someone has a legal right when someone else has a definable duty, and legal remedies are available when the duty is not performed. Either the person can be forced to perform the duty or damages of some sort can be collected for failure to perform. If I pay someone to put a new roof on my house by a certain date, she has contracted a duty to perform the work we have agreed to. It the task is not performed, then I can turn to the legal system for enforcement or damages.

Statutory rights are claim-rights that are explicitly recognized in legal statutes or laws. They impose duties on certain classes of people under specified conditions. A hospital contractor, for example, has a duty to meet certain building codes. If he fails to meet them, he is liable to legal penalties. But not all legal rights are necessarily statutory rights. Such considerations as "customary and established practices" may sometimes implicitly involve a legally enforceable claim-right.

Moral Rights

Generally speaking, a *moral right* is one that is stated in or derived from the principles of a moral theory. More specifically, to say that someone has a moral right to certain goods or manner of treatment is to say that others have a moral duty to see to it that she receives what she has a right to. A moral right is a certain kind of claim-right. Here, though, the source of justification for the right and for the corresponding duty lies in moral principles and not in the laws or practices of a society.

According to Ross, for example, people have a right to expect benevolent treatment from others—we have a duty to treat other people benevolently. This is a right that is not recognized by our legal system. We may, if we wish, treat others in a harsh and unsympathetic manner and in doing so violate no law.

Of course many rights and duties that are based upon the principles of moral theories are also embodied in our laws. Thus, to take Ross again as an example, we have a prima facie duty not to injure or kill anyone. This duty, along with its correlative right to be free from injury or death at the hands of another, is reflected in the body of statutory law and common law that deals with bodily harm done to others and with killing.

The relationship between ethical theories and the laws of a society is complicated and controversial. The fundamental question is always the extent to which laws should reflect or be based upon an ethical theory. In a society such as ours, it does not seem proper that an ethical theory accepted by only a part of the people should determine the laws that govern us all. It is for this reason that some object to laws regulating sexual activity, pornography, and abortion. These are considered best regarded as a part of personal morality.

At the same time, however, it seems that we must rely upon ethical theories as a basis for evaluating laws. Unless we are prepared to say that what is legal is, in itself, what is right, we must recognize the possibility of laws that are bad or unjust. But what makes a law bad? A possible answer is that a law is bad when it violates a right derived from the principles of an ethical theory. Similarly, both laws and social practices may be criticized for failing to recognize a moral right. A moral theory, then, can serve as the basis for a demand for the reform of laws and practices.

Clearly there is no sharp line separating the moral and the legal. Indeed, virtually all of the moral theories we discussed in the introductory chapter have been used by philosophers and other thinkers as the basis for principles applying to society as a whole. Within such frameworks as utilitarianism, natural law theory, and Rawls's theory of a just society, legal and social institutions are assigned roles and functions in accordance with more general moral principles.

Political Rights

Not everyone attempts to justify claims to rights by referring such claims directly to a moral theory. Efforts are frequently made to provide justification by relying upon principles or commitments that are generally acknowledged as basic to our society. (Of course, to answer how these are justified may force us to invoke moral principles.) Our society, for example, is committed to individual autonomy and equality, among other values. It is by reference to commitments of this sort that we evaluate proposals and criticize practices.

From this point of view, to recognize health care as a right is to acknowledge it as a *political* right. This means showing that it is required by our political commitments or principles. Of course, this may also mean resolving any conflicts that may arise from other rights that also seem to be demanded by our principles. But this is a familiar state of affairs. We are all aware that the Constitutional guarantee of freedom of speech, for example, is not absolute and unconditional. It can conflict with other rights or basic commitments, and we look to the courts to provide us with guidelines to resolve the conflicts.

With the distinctions that we have discussed in mind, let us return now to the question of a general right to health care. What can those who make such a claim be asserting?

Obviously everyone in our society is free to seek health care and, when the proper arrangements are made, to receive it. That is, health care is a service available in society, and people may avail themselves of it. At the same time, however, no physician or hospital has a duty to provide health care that is sought. The freedom to seek does not imply that others have a duty to provide what we seek.

There is not in our society a legally recognized claim-right to health care. Even if I am sick, no one has a legal duty to see to it that I receive treatment for my illness. (A few states, such as New York, do impose legal duties on physicians and hospitals to treat people faced with life-threatening emergencies. Even this is not generally the case, however.) I may request care, or I may attempt to persuade a physician that it is his or her moral duty to provide me with care. But I have no legal right to health care, and if someone refuses to provide it, I cannot seek a legal remedy.

Of course I may contract with a physician, clinic, or hospital for care, either in general or for a certain ailment. If I do this, then the other party acquires a legally enforceable duty to provide me the kind of care that we agreed upon. In this respect, contracting for health care is not relevantly different from contracting for a new roof on my house.

Those who assert that health care is a right cannot be regarded as merely making the obviously false claim that there is a legal right to care. Their claim, rather, must be interpreted as one of a moral or political sort. They might be taken as asserting something like "Everyone in the society *ought* to be entitled to health care, regardless of his or her financial condition."

Anyone making such a claim must be prepared to justify it by offering reasons and evidence in support of it. The ultimate source of the justification is most likely to be the principles of a moral theory. For example, Kant's principle that every person is of inherent and equal worth might be used to support the claim that every person has an equal right to medical care, simply by virtue of being a person.

Justification might also be offered in terms of principles that express the aims and commitments of the society. A society that endorses justice and equality, it might be argued, must be prepared to offer health care to all if it offers it to anyone.

However justification is offered, it is clear that to claim that health care is a right is to go beyond merely expressing an attitude. It is to say more than something like "Everyone would like to have health care" or "Everyone needs health care." It is true that the language of "rights" is frequently used in a rhetorical way to encourage us to recognize the wants and needs of people—or even other creatures, such as animals and trees. This is a perfectly legitimate way of talking. But, at bottom, to urge that something be considered a right is to make a claim requiring justification in terms of some set of legal, social, or moral principles.

Why not recognize health care for all as a right? Certainly virtually everyone would admit that in the abstract it would be a good thing. If this is so, then why should anyone wish to oppose it? Briefly stated, arguments against a right to health care are most frequently of two kinds.

First, those who subscribe to a position sometimes called "medical individualism" argue that to recognize a right to health care would have the consequence of violating the rights of physicians and other medical practitioners. Physicians, they claim, would be required to employ their intelligence, knowledge, and skills in a way dictated by society. Thus, physicians would be deprived of their autonomy and, in a very real sense, made slaves of the state.

Second, some writers have pointed out that while it is possible to admit health care to the status of a right, we must also recognize that health care is just one social good among others. Education, transportation, housing, legal assistance, and so on are other goods that are also sought and needed by members of our society. It is impossible to admit all of these (and perhaps others) to the status of rights, for the society simply cannot afford to pay for them.

The first line of argument (medical individualism) is examined in some detail in the selections of this chapter. We need not attempt to evaluate it here. It should be kept in mind, however, that medical individualism fails to recognize that the health-care situation is perhaps best regarded as one in which there is a *conflict* of rights (between patients and providers) and not just one in which the rights of physicians are being restricted.

The second line of argument does not necessarily lead to the conclusion that we should not recognize a right to health care. It does serve to warn us that we must be very careful to specify just what sort of right—if any—we want to support. Do we want to claim, for example, that everyone has a right to a certain *minimum* of health care? Or do we want to claim that everyone has a right to *equal* health care (whatever anyone can get, everyone can demand)?

Furthermore, this line of argument warns us that we have to make decisions about what we, as a society, are willing to pay for. Would we, for example, be willing to give up all public support for education in order to use the money for health care? Probably not. But we might be willing to reduce the level of support for education in order to increase that for health care. Whatever we decide, we have to face up to the problem of distributing our limited resources. This is an issue that is obviously closely connected with what sort of right to health care (or really, the right to what sort of health care) we are prepared to endorse.

The Selections

Charles Fried's essay maintains that we cannot afford to accept the view that everyone has a right to equal health care. If everyone were given equal access to the *best* health care, Fried argues, this would absorb an intolerable portion of our gross national income. Fried is willing to grant a right to a "decent minimum" of health care to all. But, as he points out, this means that we have to face the problem of determining this minimum.

Furthermore, Fried recommends that we consider how to change the present "medical guild" so that highly paid and trained physicians might be replaced by people with less training who can provide a number of services more cheaply. Fried also suggests that we allow patients more choice in the "medical marketplace" by giving each person a certain amount of money to buy the medical services that he or she chooses. This might encourage the development of a variety of medical delivery systems suited to consumers' needs. Also those who want fancier or more individualized medical care could get it by paying additional money out of their own pocket.

The right to health care supported by Fried is a limited one. But Robert M. Sade in his essay rejects the claim to any right to health care. Sade argues that "from man's primary right—the right to his own life—derive all others." Among those that follow from this, Sade claims, is everyone's right to pursue his own values, and "the choice of the conditions under which a physician's services are rendered belongs to the physician as a consequence of his right to support his own life."

Sade attempts to show that if there were a right on the part of the patient to a physician's care, then this would lead to an immoral result. He argues that to guarantee a right, a government must use force; thus, a physician's professional judgment ("mind") is controlled through the threat of force. No one can survive as an individual without freedom of mind. "Thus," Sade concludes, "since the concept of medical care as the right of a patient entails the use or threat of violence against physicians, the concept is anti-mind—therefore, anti-life, therefore, immoral."

Sade's radical "medical individualism" is strenuously opposed by John D. Arras and Andrew Jameton. Arras and Jameton argue that medical individualists such as Sade are wrong to think that the right to life justifies an absolute control over property. Even if we grant that basic necessities cannot be taken from us, it does not follow that goods and services over and above those cannot be demanded for serious social purposes. Furthermore, Arras and Jameton claim the medical individualists fail to recognize that most rights are political rights, ones "claimed, argued for, and vindicated within the body politic." Society considers some rights more important than others, and for this reason may restrict certain ones in order to promote others. In particular, Arras and Jameton suggest, rights may be limited when they grant to some people "excessive control" over the lives of others, and the right to employ one's medical knowledge and skills may fall into this category.

Arras and Jameton also point out that the medical individualist ignores the fact that the knowledge and skills the physician has acquired represent more than individual effort. They also involve a considerable social investment through, among other things, public funds spent on education and training. Finally, Arras and Jameton attempt to show why the free-market economic model does not legitimately apply to health care.

Arras and Jameton then look at the other side of the issue by examining two arguments in support of the claim that everyone in our society has a right to health care. These arguments employ essentially the same principles as those of the medical individualist. Yet Arras and Jameton find that neither an argument based on the right to life nor an argument based on the use of public funds to support medical facilities and education is adequate to establish health care as a basic right.

The article concludes by briefly considering what the authors admit are very loose arguments favoring health care as a right. The strongest argument, they believe, is one that connects the right to health care with restoring health to individuals. Health is one of our social ideals because it is one element that is basic to the good life, whatever else it might involve. But, the authors point out, this argument does not support a health-care system as extensive as those who advocate a right to health care usually want.

None of the selections in this chapter attempts to provide detailed answers to the multitude of questions that swarm around the issue of a public health-care policy. Yet each of them calls attention to some of the fundamental issues of rights, values, and social goals that must be resolved before any practical policy can be accepted as legitimate. If medical individualists like Sade are correct, we would be acting immorally to recognize and implement a general right to health care. Since this view is likely to be a widespread one (particularly among health professionals), it is of crucial social importance to assess its worth. It is of equal importance to test the strength of the claim that there is a right to health care and to consider the steps our society would have to take to recognize and protect such a right.

The issues discussed in this chapter are of more than academic interest. And they concern more than just a handful of patients and physicians. How they are resolved will affect us all, both directly and indirectly, through the character of our society.

Equality and Rights in Medical Care

Charles Fried

In this article I present arguments intended to support the following conclusions:

1. To say there is a right to health care does not imply a right to equal access, a right that whatever is available to any shall be available to all.

2. The slogan of equal access to the best health care available is just that, a dangerous slogan which could be translated into reality only if we submitted either to intolerable government controls of medical practice or to a thoroughly unreasonable burden of expense.

3. There is sense to the notion of a right to a decent standard of care for all, dynamically defined, but still not dogmatically equated with the best available.

4. We are far from affording such a standard to many of our citizens and that is profoundly wrong.

5. One of the major sources of the exaggerated demands for equality are the pretensions, inflated claims, inefficiencies, and guild-like, monopolistic practices of the health professions.

I. Background

The notion of some kind of a right to health care is not likely to be found in any but the most recent writings, not to mention legislation. After all, even the much more well-established institution of free, universal public education has not achieved the status of a federal constitutional right, is not a constitutional right by the law of many states, and stands as a right more as an inference from the practices and legislation of states, counties, and municipalities. The federal constitutional litigation regarding rights in that area has been restricted to the provision *equally* of whatever public education is in fact provided. So it should not be surprising that the notion of a right to health care is something of a novelty. Moreover, it is only fairly recently that health care could deliver a product which was as unambiguously beneficial as elementary schooling. Nevertheless, if one looks to the laws, practices, and understandings of states, counties, and municipalities, one sees growing up through the last century, and certainly in the twentieth century, an understanding which might be thought of as the inchoate recognition of a right to health care. Indeed, there are those who might say that such an inchoate recognition might be discerned as far back as Elizabethan England.

As one considers this progress, one should not misrepresent history, for in that history lies an important lesson. For the progress may represent not simply a progress in our ideas of social justice, but a progress in what medicine could do. The fact is that the increasingly general provision of medical care may be correlated as well with what medical care could accomplish as with any changing social doctrines. What could medicine accomplish a hundred or even fifty years ago? It is well known that the improvements in health that were wrought in those days were largely the result of improved sanitation, working conditions, diet, and the like. Beyond that, specifically medical ministrations could do very little. They could provide ease, amenities, relief, but rarely a cure. So society may be forgiven if it did not provide elaborate medical care to the poor until recently, since provision of medical care in essence would have meant simply the provision of amenities and placebos. And since society appeared little concerned to assure the amenities to its poor generally, it is no great surprise that it had scant inclination to provide these amenities to the sick poor.

The detailed history of the extension of medical care to the poor, and indeed to those who were not poor but lived in out-of-the-way places, has yet to be written. The emergence of a notion of a right to health care and the embodiment of such a notion in legislation and court decisions must also await difficult historical research. Nevertheless, it is worth noting that, at least in American public discourse, the idea of a right to medical care developed into something which had the appearance of inevitability only recently, in what might be called the intermediate, perhaps golden, age of modern medicine. This was a period when advances in treating acute illness, advances such as the antibiotics, could really make a large difference in prolonging life or restoring health; but the most elaborate technologies which may make only marginal improvements in situations previously thought to be hopeless had not yet been generally developed. In this recent "Golden Age" we could unambiguously afford a notion of a general right to medical care because there were a number of clear successes available to medicine, and these successes were not unduly costly. Having conquered the infectious diseases, medical science has undertaken the degenerative diseases, the malignant neoplasms, and the diseases of unknown etiology; and one must say that the ratio between expense and benefit has become exponentially more unfavorable. So it is really only now that the notion of a right to health care poses acute analytical and social problems. It is for that reason that neither history nor legal analysis will much illuminate our future course. What we do now will be a matter of our choosing, and for this reason careful analysis of the notion of a right to health care is crucial.

II. Equality and Rights: Analytical Distinctions

First, something should be said by way of at least informal definition of this term "right." A right is more than just an interest that an individual might have, a state of affairs or a state of being which an individual might prefer. A claim of right invokes entitlements; and when we speak of entitlements, we mean not those things which it would be nice for people to have, or which they would prefer to have, but which they must have, and which if they do not have they may demand, whether we like it or not. Although I would not want to say that a right is something we must recognize "no matter what," nevertheless a right is something we must accord unless _____ and what we put in to fill in the unless clause should be tightly confined and specific.

This notion of rights has interesting and not altogether obvious relations to the concept of equality, and confusions about those relations are very likely to lead to confused arguments about the very area before us—rights to health care and equality in respect to health care.

First, it should be noted that equality itself may be considered a right. Thus, a person can argue that he is not necessarily entitled to any particular thing—whether it be income, or housing, or education, or health care—but that he is entitled to equality in respect to that thing, so that whatever anyone gets he should get, too. And this is a nice example of my previous proposition about the notion of rights generally. For to recognize a right to equality may very well be—I suppose it often is—contrary to many other policies that we may have, and particularly contrary to attempts to attain some kind of efficiency. Yet, by the very notion of rights, if there is a right to equality, then granting equality cannot depend on whether or not it is efficient to do so.

Second, there is the relation between rights and equality which runs the other way, too: to say that a class of persons, or all persons, have a certain right implies that they all have that right equally. If it is said that all persons within the jurisdiction of the United States have a constitutionally protected right to freedom of speech, whatever that may mean, one thing seems clear: that this right should not depend on what it is one wants to say, who one is, and the like. Indeed, if the government against whom this right is protected were to make such distinctions, for instance, subjecting to constraints the speech of "irresponsible persons," that would be the exact concept of denial of freedom of speech to those persons.

These relations between the notion of right and of equality suggest the great importance of being very clear and precise about how a particular right is conceived: confusions in this regard are rampant in respect to health, and are the source of much pointless controversy. But because the point is quite general, let me first take an example from another area. If we were sloppy in our thinking about what the right of freedom of speech is—and many people are as sloppy about that as they are about their definition of the rights in the area which is our immediate concern—if we were sloppy about that definition, we might, for instance, consider that there has been a denial of right because some people have access to radio or television in getting their ideas across, while others have only the street-corner soapbox to broadcast their views. Indeed, there are those who might find it unjust that even on the soapbox the timid or inarticulate are much less effective than the bold or eloquent. All of these disparities, of course, may or may not be regrettable but they have nothing to do with freedom of speech as a right, given the premise that there is a right to free speech and that this right must be an equal right. It seems clear to me that it is very different from the right to be heard, believed, admired, and applauded. The right to speak freely is just that: a right to be free of constraints and impositions on whatever speaking one might wish to do, should you be able to find someone to listen.

Now this analogy is offered as more than a distant irrelevance. Is it not very similar to many things that are said in the area of health? For analogous to the claim that the right to freedom of speech really implies a right to be heard by the multitude, is the notion that whatever rights might exist in respect to health care are rights to health, rather than to health *care*. And of course the claim is equally absurd in both instances. We may sensibly guarantee that all will be equally free of constraints on the speaking they wish to do, but we should not guarantee that all will be equally effective in getting their views across. Similarly, we may or may not choose to guarantee all equality of access to health care, but we cannot possibly guarantee to all equality of health.

Consider how these clarifications operate upon the historical development I alluded to at the beginning of this analysis. The right whose recognition might be said to have been implicit in social practices throughout the past hundred years was a right not to health care as such, nor yet a right to health, but rather a right to a certain standard of health care, which was defined in terms of what medicine could reasonably do for people. It is this notion which has become so difficult in our present situation, where the apparatus of medicine has become so much more elaborate, pretentious, and costly than it was in earlier times.

Bringing together the historical and the analytical sides, we might conclude that our present dilemma comes from the fact that there are very many expensive things that medicine can do which might possibly help. And if we commit ourselves to the notion that there is a right to whatever health care might be available, we do indeed get ourselves into a difficult situation where overall national expenditure on health must reach absurd proportions—absurd in the sense that far more is devoted to health at the expense of other important social goals than the population in general wants. Indeed, more is devoted to health than the population wants relative not only to important social goals—for example, education or housing—but relative to all the other things which people would like to have money left over to pay for. And if we recognize that it would be absurd to commit our society to devote more than a certain proportion of our national income to health, while at the same time recognizing a "right to health care," we might then be caught on the other horn of the dilemma. For we might then be required to say that because a right to health care implies a right to equality of health care, then we must limit, we must lower the quality of the health care that might be purchased by some lest our commitment to equality require us to provide such care to all and thus carry us over a reasonable budget limit.

Consider the case of the artificial heart. It seems to me not too fanciful an assumption that such a device is technically feasible within a reasonable time, and likely to be hugely expensive both in terms of its actual implantation and in terms of the subsequent care required by those benefiting from the device. Now if the right to health care is taken to mean the right to whatever health care is available to anybody, and if this entails that it is a right to an equal enjoyment of whatever care anyone else enjoys, then what are we to do with respect to the artificial heart? Might we decide not to develop such a device? Though the development and experimental use of it involves an entirely tolerable burden, the general provision of the artificial heart would be an intolerable burden, and since if we provide it to any we must provide it to all, therefore perhaps we should provide it to none.

This solution seems to me to be both uncomfortable and unstable. For surely there is something odd, if not perverse, about foregoing research on such devices, not because the research might fail, but because it might succeed. Might not this research then go on under some kinds of private auspices if such a governmental decision were made? Would we then go further and forbid even private research, rather than simply refusing to fund it? I can well imagine the next step, where artificial heart research and implantation would become like abortion or sex change operations in the old days: something one went to Sweden or Denmark for. Nor is a lottery device for distributing a limited number of artificial hearts likely to be more stable or satisfactory. For there, too, would we forbid people to go outside the lottery? Would it be a crime to cross national boundaries with the intent of obtaining an artificial heart? The example makes a general point about instituting an all-inclusive "right to health care," with the necessary concomitant of an equal right to whatever health care is available. For if we really instituted such a right and limited the provision of health care to a reasonable level, we would have to institute as well a degree of stringent state control, which it is both unlikely we can achieve and undesirable for us even to try to achieve. There is something that goes very deeply against the grain about any scheme which prohibits scientists from making discoveries which no one claims are harmful as such, but which will cause trouble because we can't give them to everybody. There is something which goes against the grain in a system which might forbid individual doctors to render a service, not because it is harmful, but because its benefits are not available to all.

Or take a much less dramatic case—dental care. It is said that ordinary basic prophylactic care is so lacking for tens of millions of our citizens that quite unnecessarily they do not have their own teeth while still in their prime. I take it that to provide the kind of elaborate dental care deployed on affluent suburban families to rural populations, and to all even poorer urban dwellers, would be a prodigiously expensive undertaking, one that would cost each of us quite heavily. But if we followed the slogan, "The best available made available to all," that is what is meant. My guess is the American people would not want to bear this burden and that as a form of transfer payment the poor would prefer just to have the money to spend on other things. But this shows the dangerousness of slogans, for perhaps the greatest part of the dental damage could be remedied at far less cost by fluoridation and by relatively routine care provided by a type of modestly trained person who is only now beginning to exist. Care of this sort can be afforded and should be provided. But this would mean abandoning the concept of equality and accepting the fact that the poor would be getting less elaborate care than those who are not poor.

Now it might be said that I am exaggerating. The case put forward is the British National Health Service, which is alleged to provide a model of high level care at reasonable costs with equality for all. But I would caution planners and enthusiasts from drawing too much from this example. The situation in Great Britain is very different in many ways. The country is smaller and more homogeneous. Moreover, even in Great Britain there are disparities between the care available between urban and rural areas; there are long waits for so-called "elective procedures"; and there is a small but significant and distinguished private sector outside of National Health which is the focus of great controversy and rancor. Finally, Great Britain is a country where a substantial portion of the citizenry is committed to the socialist ideal of equalizing incomes and nationalizing the provisions of all vital services. Surely this is a very different situation from that in the United States. Indeed, it may be that the cry for equality of access to health care bears to a general yearning for social equality much the same relation that the opposition to fetal research bears to the opposition to abortion. In each case it is a very large ideological tail wagging a relatively small and confused dog.

My point is analytical. My point is that apart from a rather general commitment to equality and, indeed, to state control of the allocation and distribution of resources, to insist on the right to health care, where that right means a right to equal access, is an anomaly. For as long as our society considers that inequalities of wealth and income are morally acceptable—acceptable in the sense that the system that produces these inequalities is in itself not morally suspect—it is anomalous to carve out a sector like health care and say that *there* equality must reign.

III. Towards a Better Definition of the Rights Involved

After all, is health care so special? Is it different from education, housing, food, legal assistance? In respect to all of these things, we recognize in our society a right, whose enjoyment may not be made wholly dependent upon the ability to pay. But just as surely in respect to all these things, we do not believe that this right entails equality of enjoyment, so that whatever diet one person or class of persons enjoys must be enjoyed by all. The argument, put forward for instance by some members of the Labor Party in Great Britain, that the independent schools in that country should be abolished because they offer a level of education better than that available in state schools, is an argument which would be found strange and repellent in the United States. Rather, in all of these areas—education, housing, food, legal assistance—there obtains a notion of a decent, fair standard, such that when this standard is satisfied all that exists in the way of *rights* has been accorded. And it is necessarily so; were we to insist on equality all the way up, that is, past this minimum, we would have committed ourselves to a political philosophy which I take it is not the dominant one in our society.

Is health care different? Everything that can be said about health care is true of food and is at least by analogy true of education, housing, and legal assistance. The real task before us is not, therefore, I think, to explain why there must be complete equality in medicine, but the more subtle and perilous task of determining the decent minimum in respect to health which accords with sound ethical judgments, while maintaining the virtues of freedom, variety, and flexibility which are thought to flow from a mixed system such as ours. The decent minimum should reflect some conception of what constitutes tolerable life prospects in general. It should speak quite strongly to things like maternal health and child health, which set the terms under which individuals will compete and develop. On the other hand, techniques

which will offer some remote relief from conditions that rarely strike in the prime of life, and which strike late in life because something must, might be thought of as too esoteric to be part of the concept of minimum decent care.

On the other hand, the notion of a decent minimum should include humane and, I would say, worthy surroundings of care for those whom we know we are not going to be able to treat. Here, it seems to me, the emphasis on technology and the attention of highly trained specialists is seriously mistaken. Not only is it unrealistic to imagine that such fancy services can be provided for everyone "as a right," but there is serious doubt whether these kinds of services are what most people really want or can benefit from.

In the end, I will concede very readily that the notion of minimum health care, which it does make sense for our society to recognize as a right, is itself an unstable and changing notion. As my initial historical remarks must have suggested, the concept of a decent minimum is always relative to what is available over all, and what the best which is available might be. I suppose (to revert to my parable of the artificial heart) that if we allowed an artificial heart to be developed under private auspices and to be available only to those who could pay for it, or who could obtain it from specialized eleemosynary institutions, then the time might well come when it would have been so perfected that it would be a reasonable component of what one would consider minimum decent care. And the process of arriving at this new situation would be a process imbued with struggle and political controversy. But since I do not believe in utopias or final solutions, a resolution of the problem of the right to health care having these kinds of tensions within it neither worries me nor leads me to suspect that I am on the wrong track. To my mind, the right track consists in identifying what it is that health care can and cannot provide, in identifying also the cost of health care, and then in deciding how much of this health care, what level of health care, we are ready to underwrite as a floor for our citizenry.

IV. Practical Proposals

Although the process of defining the decent minimum is inherently a political process, there is a great deal which analysis and research can do to make the process rational and satisfactory. Much of this is a negative service, clearing away misconceptions and fallacies. For instance, as I have already argued, to state that our objective is to provide the best medical care for all, regardless of the ability to pay, must be shown up for the misleading slogan that it is. But there are more subtle misconceptions as well. The most pervasive of these deal with the situation of the medical profession.

Many observers look at the medical profession, its history of resistance to social change, and the fact that doctors as a profession enjoy the highest incomes of any group in the nation—somewhere around $50,000 a year on the average—and they draw their own conclusions. They draw the conclusion that therefore what is needed is necessarily more regulation. They look at the oversupply of surgeons in this country. They note the obvious fact of over-recourse to surgery which seems to result, and they conclude that what is needed is more government regulation. For instance, the problems of supply would be met by a kind of doctors' draft, requiring service in underserviced rural areas. Now I would, for a moment, suggest that we consider some alternative explanations and alternative reforms. Perhaps, after all, the irrationalities in the supply of medical personnel, together with the high incomes earned, are the result not of market forces run wild, but the result of a guild system as tight and self-protective as any we know. It is, perhaps, an irony that the medical profession, having persuaded the public of the necessity of strictly limiting entry into the profession, having persuaded the public of the indispensability of highly trained specialists, is now faced with the threat of a kind of doctors' draft to make these rare specialists available to all. Perhaps clearer thinking might indicate that many of the things which highly paid and highly trained doctors do might be done by an army of less pretentious persons.

It is well known, of course, that doctors' fees as such represent the smaller portion of the total health care budget, so it might be thought that I am taking aim at an obvious, vulnerable, and somewhat irrelevant target. Yet this is not so. Though the fees of doctors represent the smaller portion of the medical budget, doctors themselves control almost all of the decisions—from the decision about hospitalization, to the decision whether to prescribe drugs by brand or generic name—which do influence the total cost of medical care.

And it is in this respect that doctors have resisted most attempts to make their behavior rational and cost-effective. In general, it is said that this is because no doctor would sacrifice the individual interests of his patient, and this may be a sincere claim. But a certain skepticism is in order. What choice do the patients have to choose more economical systems of delivery? What doctor, for that matter, even gives his patient the choice between a brand and a generic prescription drug?

But it is in the choice of delivery systems themselves that the consumer is most restricted. Most consumers do not have the choice between a variety of delivery systems from prepaid group plans to the present individual fee-for-service system, with each plan costing what it really costs. If the consumer did have this choice, we might soon find out whether the alleged advantages of the fee-for-service system were something the consumer was willing to pay for. But of course we will never find this out if we are committed to underwrite, out of general revenues, the cost of this most expensive possible delivery system. "The best available to all." That is what we tend to do today for those groups whose medical care we do underwrite. The result is that we are trying to drive down the cost of this most expensive delivery system not by changing its organization but by bureaucratic control. What if, instead, each person were assured a certain amount of money to purchase medical services as he chose? If the restrictive practices of the profession itself could be avoided, would this not help a vast variety of delivery systems to grow up, all competing for the consumer's federally assured dollar? And then those who would want what might be considered as fancier or more individualized services could get them, provided only that they were willing to pay more for them.

Finally, there is a feature of our modern situation which is responsible for the present crisis in health care, and for the impossible dilemma posed by the promise of a right to health care. This is a feature of the society and the culture as a whole. I refer to our culture's inability to face and cope with the persistent facts of illness, old age, and death. Because we are little able to come to terms with the hazards which illness proposes, because the old are a burden and an embarrassment, because we pretend that death does not exist, we employ elaborate ruses to put these things out of the ambit of our ordinary lives. The reason why we hospitalize so much more than is rationally required surely goes beyond the vagaries of the health insurance system. Is it not also the result of the fact that the ill are an embarrassment to us, and that we seek to put them away, so we do not have to care for them, while assuaging our consciences that those "best qualified" to care for them are doing so? And in order that the ruse will work, we greatly overstate what it is that these "qualified" people can do for the ill. Needless to say, they are our willing accomplices in this piece of deception. So it is with the mentally retarded, the aged, and the dying. All of these persons are defined as having an abnormal condition not only justifying but requiring their isolation from us and their care in the hands of "specialists." Perhaps it is time that we recognize that this is part of the neurosis of our age. And of course, those whom we hire to perform our proper human role toward the sick, the old, and the dying can get away with charging a very high price for relieving us of our ordinary human obligations. But is this medical care?

Finally, to avoid misunderstanding, a general theoretic point must be made. My argument must sound harsh and callous—unfeelingly, if not unerringly economic. I have elsewhere argued that it is of the essence of the physician's role and of the patient's expectations that the doctor faced with the patient's need will do everything in his power to alleviate that need.[1] I believe that. I believe that for the individual physician to do less than his best because of some economic calculation of equity or efficiency is a breach of trust. The doctor in his dealings with his patient must not act like a bureaucrat, policy maker, or legislator. But policy makers, voters, and legislators must think in different terms. It is monstrous if an individual doctor thinks like a budget officer when he cares for his patient in need; but it is chaotic and incoherent if budget officers and voters making general policy think like doctors at the bedside.

Note

1. In my book, *Medical Experimentations: Personal Integrity and Social Policy* (Amsterdam and New York: Associated Scientific Publishers/Elsevier, 1974).

Medical Care as a Right: A Refutation

Robert M. Sade

The current debate on health care in the United States is of the first order of importance to the health professions, and of no less importance to the political future of the nation, for precedents are now being set that will be applied to the rest of American society in the future. In the enormous volume of verbiage that has poured forth, certain fundamental issues have been so often misrepresented that they have now become commonly accepted fallacies. This paper will be concerned with the most important of these misconceptions, that health care is a right, as well as a brief consideration of some of its corollary fallacies.

Rights—Morality and Politics

The concept of rights has its roots in the moral nature of man and its practical expression in the political system that he creates. Both morality and politics must be discussed before the relation between political rights and health care can be appreciated.

A "right" defines a freedom of action. For instance, a right to a material object is the uncoerced choice of the use to which that object will be put; a right to a specific action, such as free speech, is the freedom to engage in that activity without forceful repression. The moral foundation of the rights of man begins with the fact that he is a living creature: he has the right to his own life. All other rights are corollaries of this primary one; without the right to life, there can be no others, and the concept of rights itself becomes meaningless.

The freedom to live, however, does not automatically ensure life. For man, a specific course of action is required to sustain his life, a course of

Reprinted by permission from the New England Journal of Medicine 285 (December 2, 1971): *pages 1288–1292. Editor's Note: The footnotes in this reading have been renumbered.*

action that must be guided by reason and reality and has as its goal the creation or acquisition of material values, such as food and clothing, and intellectual values, such as self-esteem and integrity. His moral system is the means by which he is able to select the values that will support his life and achieve his happiness.

Man must maintain a rather delicate homeostasis in a highly demanding and threatening environment, but has at his disposal a unique and efficient mechanism for dealing with it: his mind. His mind is able to perceive, to identify percepts, to integrate them into concepts, and to use those concepts in choosing actions suitable to the maintenance of his life. The rational function of mind is volitional, however; a man must *choose* to think, to be aware, to evaluate, to make conscious decisions. The extent to which he is able to achieve his goals will be directly proportional to his commitment to reason in seeking them.

The right to life implies three corollaries: the right to select the values that one deems necessary to sustain one's own life; the right to exercise one's own judgment of the best course of action to achieve the chosen values; and the right to dispose of those values, once gained, in any way one chooses, without coercion by other men. The denial of any one of these corollaries severely compromises or destroys the right to life itself. A man who is not allowed to choose his own goals, is prevented from setting his own course in achieving those goals and is not free to dispose of the values he has earned is no less than a slave to those who usurp those rights. The right to private property, therefore, is essential and indispensable to maintaining free men in a free society.

Thus, it is the nature of man as a living, thinking being that determines his rights—his "natural rights." The concept of natural rights was slow in dawning on human civilization. The first political expression of that concept had its beginnings in 17th and 18th century England through such exponents as John Locke and Edmund Burke, but came to its brilliant debut as a form of government after the American Revolution. Under the leadership of such men as Thomas Paine and Thomas Jefferson, the concept of man as a being sovereign unto himself, rather than a subdivision of the sovereignty of a king, emperor or state, was incorporated into the formal structure of government for the first time. Protection of the lives and property of individual citizens was the salient characteristic of the Constitution of 1787. Ayn Rand has pointed out that the principle of protection of the individual against the coercive force of government made the United States the first moral society in history.[1]

In a free society, man exercises his right to sustain his own life by producing economic values in the form of goods and services that he is, or should be, free to exchange with other men who are similarly free to trade with him or not. The economic values produced, however, are not given as gifts by nature, but exist only by virtue of the thought and effort of individual men. Goods and services are thus owned as a consequence of the right to sustain life by one's own physical and mental effort.

If the chain of natural rights is interrupted, and the right to a loaf of bread, for example, is proclaimed as primary (avoiding the necessity of earning it), every man owns a loaf of bread, regardless of who produced it. Since ownership is the power of disposal,[2] every man may take his loaf from the baker and dispose of it as he wishes with or without the baker's permission. Another element has thus been introduced into the relation between men: the use of force. It is crucial to observe who has initiated the use of force: it is the man who demands unearned bread as a right, not the man who produced it. At the level of an unstructured society it is clear who is moral and who immoral. The man who acted rationally by producing food to support his own life is moral. The man who expropriated the bread by force is immoral.

To protect this basic right to provide for the support of one's own life, men band together for their mutual protection and form governments. This is the only proper function of government: to provide for the defense of individuals against those who would take their lives or property by force. The state is the repository for retaliatory force in a just society wherein the only actions prohibited to individuals are those of physical harm or the threat of physical harm to other men. The closest that man has ever come to achieving this ideal of government was in this country after its War of Independence.

When a government ignores the progression of natural rights arising from the right to life, and agrees with a man, a group of men, or even a majority of its citizens, that every man has a right to a loaf of bread, it must protect that right by the passage of laws ensuring that everyone gets his loaf—in the process depriving the baker of the freedom to dispose of his own product. If the baker disobeys the law, asserting the priority of his right to support himself by his own rational disposition of the fruits of his mental and physical labor, he will be taken to court by force or threat of force where he will have more property forcibly taken from him (by fine) or have his liberty taken away (by incarceration). Now the initiator of violence is the government itself. The degree to which a government exercises its monopoly on the retaliatory use of force by asserting a claim to the lives and property of its citizens is the degree to which it has eroded its own legitimacy. It is a frequently overlooked fact that behind every law is a policeman's gun or a soldier's bayonet. When the gun and bayonet are used to initiate violence, to take property or to restrict liberty by force, there are no longer any rights, for the lives of the citizens belong to the state. In a just society with a moral government, it is clear that the only "right" to the bread belongs to the baker, and that a claim by any other man to that right is unjustified and can be enforced only by violence or the threat of violence.

Rights—Politics and Medicine

The concept of medical care as the patient's right is immoral because it denies the most fundamental of all rights, that of a man to his own life and the freedom of action to support it. Medical care is neither a right nor a privilege: it is a service that is provided by doctors and others to people who wish to purchase it. It is the provision of this service that a doctor depends upon for his livelihood, and is his means of supporting his own life. If the right to health care belongs to the patient, he starts out owning the services of a doctor without the necessity of either earning them or receiving them as a gift from the only man who has the right to give them: the doctor himself. In the narrative above substitute "doctor" for "baker" and "medical service" for "bread." American medicine is now at the point in the story where the state has proclaimed the nonexistent "right" to medical care as a fact of public policy, and has begun to pass the laws to enforce it. The doctor finds himself less and less his own master and more and more controlled by forces outside of his own judgment.

For instance, under the proposed Kennedy-Griffiths bill,[3] there will be a "Health Security Board," which will be responsible for administering the new controls to be imposed on doctors, hospitals and other "providers" of health care (Sec. 121). Specialized services, such as major surgery, will be done by "qualified specialists" [Sec. 22(b)(2)], such qualifications being determined by the Board (Sec. 42). Furthermore, the patient can no longer exercise his own initiative in finding a specialist to do his operation, since he must be referred to the specialist by a nonspecialist—i.e., a general practitioner or a family doctor [Sec. 22(b)]. Licensure by his own state will not be enough to be a qualified practitioner; physicians will also be subject to a second set of standards, those established by the Board [Sec. 42(a)]. Doctors will no longer be considered competent to determine their own needs for continuing education, but must meet requirements established by the Board [Sec. 42(c)]. The professional staff of a hospital will no longer be able to determine which of its members are qualified to perform which kinds of major surgery; specialty-board certification or eligibility will be required, with certain exceptions that include meeting standards established by the Board [Sec. 42(d)].

Control of doctors through control of the hospitals in which they practice will also be exercised by the Board by way of a list of requirements, the last of which is a "sleeper" that will by its vagueness allow the Board almost any regulation of the hospital: the hospital must meet "such other requirements as the Board finds necessary in the interest of quality of care and the safety of patients in the institution" [Sec. 43(i)]. Hospitals will also not be allowed to undertake construction without higher approval by a state agency or by the Board (Sec. 52).

In the name of better organization and coordination of services, hospitals, nursing homes and other providers will be further controlled through the Board's power to issue directives forcing the provider to furnish services selected by the Board [Sec. 131(a)(1),(2)] at a place selected by the Board [Sec. 131(a)(3)]. The Board can also direct these providers to form associations with one another of various sorts, including "making available to one provider the professional and technical skills of another" [Sec. 131(a)(B)], and such other linkages as the Board thinks best [Sec. 131(a)(4)(C)].

These are only a few of the bill's controls of the health-care industry. It is difficult to believe that such patent subjugation of an entire profession could ever be considered a fit topic for discussion in any but the darkest corner of a country founded on the principles of life and liberty. Yet the Kennedy-Griffiths bill is being seriously debated today in the Congress of the United States.

The irony of this bill is that, on the basis of the philosophic premises of its authors, it does provide a rationally organized system for attempting to fulfill its goals, such as "making health services available to all residents of the United States." If the government is to spend tens of billions of dollars on health services, it must assure in some way that the money is not being wasted. Every bill currently before the national legislature does, should, and must provide some such controls. The Kennedy-Griffiths bill is the closest we have yet come to the logical conclusion and inevitable consequence of two fundamental fallacies: that health care is a right, and that doctors and other health workers will function as efficiently serving as chattels of the state as they will living as sovereign human beings. It is not, and they will not.

Any act of force is anti-mind. It is a confession of the failure of persuasion, the failure of reason. When politicians say that the health system must be forced into a mold of their own design, they are admitting their inability to persuade doctors and patients to use the plan voluntarily; they are proclaiming the supremacy of the state's logic over the judgments of the individual minds of all concerned with health care. Statists throughout history have never learned that compulsion and reason are contradictory, that a forced mind cannot think effectively and, by extension, that a regimented profession will eventually choke and stagnate from its own lack of freedom. A persuasive example of this is the moribund condition of medicine as a profession in Sweden, a country that has enjoyed socialized medicine since 1955. Werkö, a Swedish physician, has stated: "The details and the complicated working schedule have not yet been determined in all hospitals and districts, but the general feeling of belonging to a free profession, free to decide—at least in principle—how to organize its work has been lost. Many hospital-based physicians regard their work now with an apathy previously unknown."[4] One wonders how American legislators will like having

their myocardial infarctions treated by apathetic internists, their mitral valves replaced by apathetic surgeons, their wives' tumors removed by apathetic gynecologists. They will find it very difficult to legislate self-esteem, integrity and competence into the doctors whose minds and judgments they have throttled.

If anyone doubts that health legislation involves the use of force, a dramatic demonstration of the practical political meaning of the "right to health care" was acted out in Quebec in the closing months of 1970.[5] In that unprecedented threat of violence by a modern Western government against a group of its citizens, the doctors of Quebec were literally imprisoned in the province by Bill 41, possibly the most repressive piece of legislation ever enacted against the medical profession, and far more worthy of the Soviet Union or Red China than a western democracy. Doctors objecting to a new Medicare law were forced to continue working under penalty of jail sentence and fines of up to $500 a day away from their practices. Those who spoke out publicly against the bill were subject to jail sentences of up to a year and fines of up to $50,000 a day. The facts that the doctors did return to work and that no one was therefore jailed or fined do not mitigate the nature or implications of the passage of Bill 41. Although the dispute between the Quebec physicians and their government was not one of principle but of the details of compensation, the reaction of the state to resistance against coercive professional regulation was a classic example of the naked force that lies behind every act of social legislation.

Any doctor who is forced by law to join a group or a hospital he does not choose, or is prevented by law from prescribing a drug he thinks is best for his patient, or is compelled by law to make any decision he would not otherwise have made, is being forced to act against his own mind, which means forced to act against his own life. He is also being forced to violate his most fundamental professional commitment, that of using his own best judgment at all times for the greatest benefit of his patient. It is remarkable that this principle has never been identified by a public voice in the medical profession, and that the vast majority of doctors in this country are being led down the path to civil servitude, never knowing that their feelings of uneasy foreboding have a profoundly moral origin, and never recognizing that the main issues at stake are not those being formulated in Washington, but are their own honor, integrity and freedom, and their own survival as sovereign human beings.

Some Corollaries

The basic fallacy that health care is a right has led to several corollary fallacies, among them the following:

That health is primarily a community or social rather than an individual concern.[6] A simple calculation from American mortality statistics[7] quickly corrects that false concept: 67 per cent of deaths in 1967 were due to diseases known to be caused or exacerbated by alcohol, tobacco smoking or overeating, or were due to accidents. Each of those factors is either largely or wholly correctable by individual action. Although no statistics are available, it is likely that morbidity, with the exception of common respiratory infections, has a relation like that of mortality to personal habits and excesses.

That state medicine has worked better in other countries than free enterprise has worked here. There is no evidence to support that contention, other than anecdotal testimonials and the spurious citation of infant mortality and longevity statistics. There is, on the other hand, a good deal of evidence to the contrary.[8,9]

That the provision of medical care somehow lies outside the laws of supply and demand, and that government-controlled health care will be free care. In fact, no service or commodity lies outside the economic laws. Regarding health care, market demand, individual want, and medical need are entirely different things, and have a very complex relation with the cost and the total supply of available care, as recently discussed and clarified by Jeffers et al.[10] They point out that " 'health is purchaseable,' meaning that somebody has to pay for it, individually or collectively, at the expense of foregoing the current or future consumption of other things." The question is whether the decision of how to allocate the consumer's dollar should belong to the consumer or to the state. It has already been shown that the choice of how a doctor's services should be rendered belongs only to the doctor: in the same way the choice of whether to buy a doctor's service rather than some other commodity or service belongs to the con-

sumer as a logical consequence of the right to his own life.

That opposition to national health legislation is tantamount to opposition to progress in health care. Progress is made by the free interaction of free minds developing new ideas in an atmosphere conducive to experimentation and trial. If group practice really is better than solo, we will find out because the success of groups will result in more groups (which has, in fact, been happening); if prepaid comprehensive care really is the best form of practice, it will succeed and the health industry will swell with new Kaiser–Permanente plans. But let one of these or any other form of practice become the law, and the system is in a straightjacket that will stifle progress. Progress requires freedom of action, and that is precisely what national health legislation aims at restricting.

That doctors should help design the legislation for a national health system, since they must live with and within whatever legislation is enacted. To accept this concept is to concede to the opposition its philosophic premises, and thus to lose the battle. The means by which nonproducers and hangers-on throughout history have been able to expropriate material and intellectual values from the producers has been identified only relatively recently: the sanction of the victim.[11] Historically, few people have lost their freedom and their rights without some degree of complicity in the plunder. If the American medical profession accepts the concept of health care as the right of the patient, it will have earned the Kennedy–Griffiths bill by default. The alternative for any health professional is to withhold his sanction and make clear who is being victimized. Any physician can say to those who would shackle his judgment and control his profession: I do not recognize your right to my life and my mind, which belong to me and me alone; I will not participate in any legislated solution to any health problem.

In the face of the raw power that lies behind government programs, nonparticipation is the only way in which personal values can be maintained. And it is only with the attainment of the highest of those values—integrity, honesty and self-esteem—that the physician can achieve his most important professional value, the absolute priority of the welfare of his patients.

The preceding discussion should not be interpreted as proposing that there are no problems in the delivery of medical care. Problems such as high cost, few doctors, low quantity of available care in economically depressed areas may be real, but it is naïve to believe that governmental solutions through coercive legislation can be anything but shortsighted and formulated on the basis of political expediency. The only long-range plan that can hope to provide for the day after tomorrow is a "nonsystem"—that is, a system that proscribes the imposition by force (legislation) of any one group's conception of the best forms of medical care. We must identify our problems and seek to solve them by experimentation and trial in an atmosphere of freedom from compulsion. Our sanction of anything less will mean the loss of our personal values, the death of our profession, and a heavy blow to political liberty.

Notes

1. Rand, A. Man's rights, Capitalism: The unknown ideal. New York, New American Library, Inc., 1967, pp 320–329.
2. Von Mises, L. Socialism: An economic and sociological analysis. New Haven, Yale University Press, 1951, pp 37–55.
3. Kennedy, E. M. Introduction of the Health Security Act. Congressional Record 116:S 14338–S 14361, 1970.
4. Werkö, L. Swedish medical care in transition. N Engl J Med 284:360–366, 1971.
5. Quebec Medicare and Medical Services Withdrawal. Toronto, Canadian Medical Association, October 19, 1970.
6. Millis, J. S. Wisdom? Health? Can society guarantee them? N Engl J Med 283:260–261, 1970.
7. Department of Health, Education, and Welfare, Public Health Service: Vital Statistics of the United States 1967. Vol II, Mortality. Part A. Washington, DC, Government Printing Office, 1969, pp 1–7.
8. Financing Medical Care: An appraisal of foreign programs. Edited by H. Shoeck. Caldwell, Idaho, Caxton Printers, Inc, 1962.
9. Lynch, M. J.; Raphael, S. S. Medicine and the State. Springfield, Illinois, Charles C. Thomas, 1963.
10. Jeffers, J. R.; Bognanno, M. F.; Bartlett, J. C. On the demand versus need for medical services and the concept of "shortage." Am J Publ Health 61:46–63, 1971.
11. Rand, A. Atlas Shrugged. New York, Random House, 1957, p 1066.

Medical Individualism and the Right to Health Care

John Arras and Andrew Jameton

If the basic rights of life, liberty, and the pursuit of happiness seem uncontroversial to us, this is in part because they don't appear to cost very much. These and other so-called "negative rights" merely demand that others leave us alone to pursue our respective visions of the good life. To be sure, this requirement of forebearance places limits on the freedom of others—they cannot act on desires to violate our persons or property—but it doesn't compel others to render us any positive services. The purported right to health care differs from these other basic rights in that it imposes positive obligations on some persons to provide others with the benefit of health services. The right to health care thus entails greater costs both in terms of dollars and human freedom. If we have a right to health care, it necessarily follows that others are obligated to provide us with it. Precisely who these others are is not specified in political slogans concerning the right to health care, but *someone* must be charged with providing it, lest the slogan turn out to be completely vacuous.

The right to health care is problematic because it seems to conflict with the basic rights of others to liberty and to the pursuit of their own happiness. This apparent conflict of rights has set the stage for a remarkably acrimonious debate between the champions of social equality and the defenders of personal liberty. The purpose of this essay is to assess the respective arguments of these warring factions in order to arrive at a clearer understanding of the purported right to health care and its ethical justifications.

Some preliminary remarks are in order before we can get to the arguments. Any careful and responsible discussion of the right to health care must distinguish clearly between health and health care. Unfortunately, few discussions do. Proponents of this right often overlook the important difference between the value to be achieved (health) and one institutional means for securing it (health care). Although it could conceivably be argued that the benefits of greater social equality are a sufficient reason to institute a right to health care—whether or not this would actually improve people's health—we presume for most of this discussion that health care is good only insofar as it effectively promotes, protects, or restores health.

Even if we define "health" inclusively as the mere absence of disease, health care is neither a necessary nor a sufficient condition of health. If we rightly insist on a narrower definition of health —whether as rational free agency,[1] the well-working of the organism as a whole,[2] or the ability to adapt[3]—we notice immediately that health care can play only a relatively minor role in affecting public health. This intuitive impression has been confirmed by medical sociologists and public health researchers whose studies demonstrate that health is a function of many different variables including public hygiene, stress, speed limits, social change, working conditions, and personal habits such as sleep, exercise, diet, and the consumption of tobacco and alcohol.[4]

We must realize that even if the proponents of a right to health care get everything they want, they will not necessarily give us a healthy or safe culture. If we are serious about health as a basic human *virtue*, then we must abandon the illusion that it can be guaranteed by health care. The achievement of genuine health will require profound changes both in our social practices and personal living habits. The task is immense.

In spite of the limited effectiveness of health care in achieving overall public health, we must not forget that, in individual cases, medical care often plays an indispensable role in preserving life and health through the treatment of disease and injury. Health care does accomplish a great deal, even though it cannot do everything. Should it then be equally available to all, regardless of ability to pay, or should it be bought and sold in the marketplace like any other commodity? Should we recognize a right to health care?

I. Medical Individualism

Western medical practice has always been highly individualistic. An exclusive concern for the well-being of the patient defines the core of the venerable Hippocratic tradition. The physician pledges to devote his or her skills and confidence to the patient alone—not to society, the state, or the greatest happiness of the greatest number. This single-minded emphasis on the integrity of the doctor-patient relationship has tended to insulate physicians from the larger problems of health care allocation. It has also predisposed them to interpret the right to health care as a threat to the individualism upon which their profession is based.

Responding to this threat, a number of physicians and likeminded philosophers have challenged the very notion of a right to health care.[5] Their criticisms are remarkably similar, and thus can be easily subsumed into a reconstructed "model" of medical individualism. The individualist's argument goes something like this: We begin with the undeniable fact that all humans are unique individuals. From this natural fact we can infer that all human beings *own* their respective minds and bodies. Human beings belong to themselves, not to each other or to abstract entities such as the state. Two important corollaries are then derived from the natural right to control our own lives. First, the individualist asserts that we have a right to engage in the production of commodities or values that sustain our lives. Second, we have the right to control or dispose of these commodities or values in any way we see fit. Each of us is morally entitled to whatever we can create by ourselves or acquire through exchanges, gifts, inheritance, and so on.

The individualist claims that all of the above rights are natural rights—that is, they derive their authority from human nature itself, rather than from society or the state. The rights to life and property cannot be conferred or abrogated by the state since, according to the individualist, it is precisely these rights that provide the state with its only reason for being. On this account, the only legitimate function of the state is to safeguard and enforce our natural rights to life and property. Thus, the only morally justified state is the minimal or "night watchman" state of classical libertarian political theory—a state charged only with the protection of private citizens from violence, theft, fraud, and breach of contract.[6]

The individualist describes the violation of these alleged natural rights—by either greedy individuals or benevolent governments—in terms of coercion, theft, and enslavement. Our rights to life and property cannot justly be overridden in the name of social justice—they are inviolable and absolute vis-à-vis all social goals, no matter how important or pressing these may seem. Individual rights are incommensurate with appeals to social utility or distributive justice, so that all attempts to redistribute wealth (without the consent of the parties involved) amount to theft, whether the responsible agent is a burglar in the night or the county tax collector. In spite of Robin Hood's good intentions, the individualist would insist that he was still a thief: he *stole* from the rich to give to the poor, as does the modern welfare state.

The medical individualist is now ready to apply his theory of property rights to the issue at hand—the purported right to health care. His first move is to define health care as property—that is, as a commodity or value produced by individuals in order to sustain life. Health care is neither a right nor a mere privilege; rather, it is a *service* rendered by the physician to the patient. Health services are the exclusive private property of those who create them.

The adherents of a right to health care ignore this basic fact. According to the medical individualist, health services do not fall like manna from heaven;[7] on the contrary, they always come already attached to those individuals who produce them. In this respect, health services are more like bread produced by a baker—a favorite medical individualist analogy.[8] Manna rains down from the skies ready for immediate distribution; bread goes through a process of production that transforms it (precisely *how* is never made entirely clear) into the private property of the baker. By focusing all of their attention on the problem of redistribution, the advocates of a right to health care have overlooked the crucial processes of production through which goods such as health care come to be and to be owned. Once we place health services in the category of private property we can conclude with

the individualist that a right to health care makes no more sense than a right to a loaf of bread. Both of these rights supposedly lay claim to goods produced and justly controlled by others and thus amount to a right to theft.

From the individualist's perspective, the notion of a right to health care contradicts the natural and inalienable rights to life and to free action in support thereof. Health care providers have a right to dispense their services as they see fit, free from governmental interference. For the medical individualist, this right is the fundamental moral issue at stake in the debate over the right to health care.

II. Critique of Medical Individualism

The medical individualist's theory of rights and subsequent denial of a right to health care are vulnerable to devastating criticisms. In this section, we shall argue that the individualist misconceives the nature and scope of rights, the social status of the medical profession, and the probable fate of freedom and autonomy in a free medical market.

Rights: Their Social Nature and Scope

Rights promote and guarantee certain values or interests, and these values are the natural reason for having certain rights. A complete theory of rights must include an account of the human interests or values that prompt us to claim certain rights. Faced with the argument of medical individualism, we first need to inquire about the values that support the individualist's theory of rights. To be more specific, we must know whether the individualist's supreme values can support an absolute right to private property.

The fundamental value animating the entire individualistic theory of rights is the interest of the individual in sustaining his or her own life. This interest grounds a corresponding right to life. The case against health care rights ultimately rests on the alleged connection between this absolute right to life and a derivative, but equally absolute, right to the ownership of property. We shall argue that there is no such connection, and that the individualist's case against health care rights founders on this glaring non sequitur.

Suppose that we grant the existence of a right to life and a derivative right to produce goods in support of life. Does it follow that we also have an absolute and inviolable right to dispose of these goods in any way we see fit? No, it doesn't. At the very most, the individualist's argument shows that we have a right to control those goods that are necessary for life, such as food, shelter, clothing, and so on. But supposing that these basic needs were met and that we had enough to live on, would we have an absolute right to control whatever *surplus* goods we happened to accumulate by dint of hard work, gifts, inheritance, or dumb luck? The answer is no—not if the right to *life* is advanced as the sole justification of property rights. Any surplus goods we produced could justly be alienated from us in order to secure a worthwhile social purpose.

Because the individualist focuses exclusively on the isolated individual and his or her life, he does not appreciate the importance of social relations for the theory of rights. Although there may be some so-called natural rights that can be understood apart from a social context, most rights are best described as social or political—that is, as rights that are claimed, argued for, and vindicated within the body politic. Such rights are based on appeals to liberties and values that people consider essential for leading a good life.[9] Of course, the goods necessary for a full, satisfactory life will vary from society to society. Take the value of privacy, for example. In our society we tend to value privacy very highly—so much so that we have trouble imagining what friendship and love would be like if we couldn't exclude others from our company or prevent them from knowing certain things about us.[10] But we can nevertheless imagine societies that would be much more open than our own, wherein privacy would have much less importance.

This example nicely illustrates the socially relative origin and nature of rights. Whether or not we assign people rights over certain goods will depend on the role played by these goods in the life of our society. Since we value privacy as the cornerstone of social relations, we grant it the status of a right; but a society that had little use for privacy could make little or no sense of a right to have it. Thus, rights are generated within a social context, and systems of rights should be viewed as mechanisms for adjusting the competing claims of individuals for certain forms of liberty and control over certain goods. Because medical individualism sees only the isolated individual and his or her life,

it cannot account for the way rights come to be recognized within society.

Likewise, the individualist's omission of social relations prevents him from establishing a criterion for limiting the scope of rights. How far should rights extend? How much control over goods should people be allowed to have? As long as the individualist ignores the social nature of rights, he cannot begin to answer these questions, since they necessarily involve adjusting and reconciling the competing claims of many individuals on limited resources. The individualist's only available move is simply to declare that "rights cannot exist in conflict,"[11] that his rights to property are absolute—that is, not subject to limitation by any conceivable social goal. Once we deprive the individualist of this gambit by revealing the gaping hole in his argument for absolute property rights, we see that he can be of no help in determining the legitimate extent or scope of rights.

For purposes of discussion (not proof) we will advance the notion that rights should be limited if they grant some persons excessive control over the lives and well-being of others.[12] Admittedly, this criterion requires considerable refinement, not to mention an argument. We certainly would have to know more about what would constitute "excessive" control. Yet some such criterion surely lies behind the stock Lockean example of someone gaining complete control of a formerly public water supply in a desert community.[13] Would such an acquisition be just? Does the new owner have the right to dispense the water as he or she sees fit? Most of us would deny the owner that right, even if he or she acquired title to the water supply fairly and squarely, without coercing or defrauding anyone. And we would most likely base our denial on the fact that such a right to control the water supply would give the owner excessive or unacceptable control over the lives of others who depend on the water for their life and health.

This, of course, brings us to the status of physicians in a libertarian paradise. It is likely that a system of absolute property rights over medical services would have the effect of protecting the liberties of physicians in such a way that it would also give them an excessive degree of power over the lives and health of others. If this turned out to be the case, then the individualist's claim to complete control over the allocation of medical care would run afoul of our suggested criterion for limiting the scope of rights.

Social Realities of the Medical Profession

As we have seen, the medical individualist claims that medical skills and services should be considered the private property of physicians. Since individuals obtain these skills through their own efforts, so the argument runs, they should be able to dispose of them as they see fit. What is true for the baker and candlestick maker is also true for the doctor.

The trouble with this claim is that it is simply preposterous. His head buried securely in the sand, the individualist refuses to acknowledge the massive *public* investment in medical education, hospital construction, and research. Because of the enormous price tags attached to each of these items, public support has assumed an indispensable role in the allocation of health care. These economic facts of life are so well known that we will not dwell on them. Suffice it to say that they are impossible to square with the individualist's romantic portrait of the rugged physician doing it all on his own and then claiming it all as his own private property. Were it not for the infusion of tax dollars into our medical system, our rugged medical individualist would never have gotten an education, would have no hospital in which to practice, and would have substantially less knowledge on which to base his practice. Whether he admits it or not, the individualist physician is caught up in a web of social and economic entanglements, apart from which he could neither develop nor practice his medical skills.

These social and economic facts effectively refute the medical individualist's attempt to classify his medical skills and services as his private property. Those skills were developed with public assistance and are thus not properly subject to the exclusive control of physicians.

Freedom and Autonomy in the Medical Marketplace

Our third criticism of medical individualism concerns the fate of freedom and autonomy in the free medical market. As we have seen, freedom and autonomy are the individualist's supreme values. He contends that these values can flourish only in the atmosphere of a free-market economy—one in which sellers are free to dispose of their goods and services as they see fit, and buyers are free to spend their money on the kind of services they explicitly desire. We will argue that the individualist overestimates the liberating potential of the free market concept and that the economic system favored by medical individualists would actually pose a grave threat to the individualist's own ideals of freedom and autonomy.

The individualist advocates a laissez-faire, free-market version of capitalism because he wants to maximize the individual's control over his or her own life. The maximization of autonomy thus demands the minimization of imposed obligations and restrictions on financial transactions. Individualists often argue that a right to health care would unjustifiably curtail the physician's right to treat whomever he or she pleases, at whatever price he or she chooses to exact. Such a right would also limit the patients' right to spend health care dollars the way they see fit without governmental interference. According to individualism, the right to health care poses a threat to the freedom of physicians and patients alike. A system of absolute property rights maximizes the values of liberty and autonomy and is thus morally preferable to alternative systems that, in varying degrees, limit freedom and violate human dignity.

The most objectionable feature of this free-market approach to health care allocation is that it makes our freedom and autonomy completely contingent upon the strength of our bargaining position within the free market.[14] Our competitive ability can be severely compromised or entirely wiped out by factors beyond our control. Negligent parents, for example, can fail to shield their children from the effects of catastrophic disease. If the parents are unable to pay for medical costs, and if no one else is willing to donate money or medical services, there would be no remedy in a free-market economy. The sins or negligence of parents would be visited upon their children. Through no fault of their own, many children would enter the game of exchange and acquisition with irremedial inequalities. Justice would seem to require some mechanism for neutralizing the transmission of familial advantages and disadvantages to children.

The freedom and autonomy of adults would also be vulnerable in the free market. A drastic shift in the balance of supply and demand for certain services could easily destroy our bargaining position. Through no fault of our own, we could be rendered destitute and unable to pay for basic medical care. At such a juncture, we would obviously exercise precious little control over our own lives. We would not find much consolation reflecting on the alleged maximization of freedom and autonomy on the free market, for our freedom would be nonexistent. In a market governed only by free competition, the liberty and autonomy of the individual would be threatened constantly by events beyond his or her control. Once our bargaining position was undermined, our ability to control our lives would be imperiled. Since freedom and autonomy are worth little without health, the individualist's preferred economic system would thus tend to undermine his own supreme values.

The libertarian paradise would thus enhance the freedom of some while destroying the freedom of others. If the medical individualist is honestly concerned with the maximization of freedom, he would have to compare the extent to which freedom would be limited by a right to health care *and* by a free market. He would then have to explain why the loss of liberty in a free market would be preferable to that incurred within a system guaranteeing the right to health care.[15] The failure of medical individualists even to consider this question prompts us to suspect that their spirited defense of freedom is, at bottom, a mere smoke screen for the vested interests of a privileged class of physicians.

In any case, we doubt that the loss of freedom entailed by a right to health care would be quite as great as the medical individualists would have us believe. Just as they underestimate the costs to freedom inherent in their conception of laissez-faire capitalism, so they overestimate the probable constraints on physicians in a regime guaranteeing the right to health care. Recall that the individualist defines the right to health care as the right to control the skills and services of a physician. From this flawed definition, he correctly infers that the right to health care is a threat to his liberty, autonomy, and human dignity. But does the right to health care necessarily violate the physician's rights? Is the embattled individualist's talk of enslavement a genuine cause for concern, or is it rather a red herring drawn across our path?

We smell red herring. There is no necessary conflict between the right of persons to health care and the right of physicians to liberty. Those who insist on the inevitability of conflict between these rights misplace the duty to provide care. Opponents of the right to health care often assume that the duty corresponding to this right must reside in the individual physician. But we need not assume this. We can just as easily assume that the duty to provide care would reside in the political organs of society. On this view, society, not the individual physician, should bear the cost of realizing the right to health care. If we displace the duty to provide care in this fashion, the alleged conflict between the right to health care and the physician's right to liberty disappears. A public system guaranteeing the right to health care would obtain the services of qualified providers, not by enslaving doctors, but rather by providing them with pay and other incentives—the same way we attract teachers for our system of public education.

III. False Starts Toward a Right to Health Care

Ironically, two separate arguments in favor of a right to health care can be discerned amid the rubble of the individualist's model. One is based on the right to life, the other on physicians' acceptance of public funds. Although there is something to be said for each approach, we shall see that neither suffices to establish an adequate standard of health care as a basic right to all persons.

Rights to Life and Health Care

The individualist's first and most important argument hinged on the fact that each person is a living human individual and, as such, deserves the right to live. From this basic right followed the right to produce and control values necessary to sustain life. This argument can be turned around to produce a limited right to health care. It can be argued that if we have a right to life, then we should have rights to those things that are necessary for life. Since food (bread?), shelter, clothing—and health care—are all values necessary for life, then, according to the individualist's logic, we should have the right to obtain these goods regardless of our ability to pay for them.

Similar objections from two different quarters can be lodged against this argument. First, advocates of a right to health care will object that it does not go far enough. At most, arguments premised on the right to *life* can only secure a right to *lifesaving* medical care. Such a right would guarantee treatment for the critically ill and injured, but it would exclude the vast majority of patients whose medical needs are serious, but not absolutely critical. Thus, the limits of the right-to-life gambit cut both ways: the medical individualist used it to establish absolute property rights, but all he got in the end was a right to property necessary for life. Advocates of the right to health care could likewise ground their proposals for comprehensive health services on the right to life, but they would salvage only a right to lifesaving care. Both approaches are subverted by their reliance on a common premise—the right to life—that simply cannot carry the required freight.

A second, related objection comes from the medical individualist, who argues that having a right to life does not give us a right to whatever we need in order to live—especially if the goods we require are already *owned* by others. Suppose you are subdued and kidnapped by the society of music lovers in order to save the life of a famous violinist suffering from end-stage kidney failure.[16] You wake up to discover the violinist sitting next to you in bed, his kidneys plugged into yours. Granted, the violinist has a right to life, but does he have a right to the use of your kidneys? If we consult our moral intuitions, most people would probably reply, "No, this violinist might well have the right to life, but he certainly doesn't have the right to use *my* kidneys—even if he cannot live without them." Likewise, even supposing we have a right to life, and that health care is necessary for continued life, we do not have a right to health services that belong as a matter of right to others.

But as we have seen, the individualist's claim that health services are the private property of physicians is itself vulnerable to attack. In our critique of medical individualism we noted the extent to which the institutions of modern medicine are subsidized by the taxpayer. The moral significance of the physician's acceptance of public funds is twofold. We have already shown how the individualist physician's economic dependency on the

public negates his contention that health skills and services are his exclusive private property. We will now investigate a more constructive interpretation of the physician's economic dependency.

Health Care as a Special Right

It can be argued that the physician's acceptance of public aid generates a set of corresponding rights and obligations.[17] The recipients of the public investment in medical education, research, and hospital construction owe a debt of some kind to the public. In spite of the protests of the medical individualist, this debt has not been foisted on physicians in violation of their moral autonomy. On this account, the physician's obligation to the public derives from his or her free decision to accept the benefits of public support. This *act* of the health professional creates the duty to the public.

Conversely, it can be maintained that the providers of this public support—the taxpayers—have a *right* to medical services corresponding to the physician's *obligation*. If the taxpayers contribute vast sums of money to underwrite our health care system, it follows that they have a right to expect something in return. In the parlance of contemporary social philosophers,[18] this is a "special right" that exists not simply by virtue of one's status as a human being—as do "general rights"—but rather by virtue of the fact that specific individuals have entered into a particular kind of social relationship. The physician's obligation to provide health services to the public, and the public's corresponding right to those services, is thus grounded on the fact that both parties have freely entered into certain economic and social relations of interdependence. If the public decided to cash in on its right by claiming the services of physicians, it could do so without violating their moral integrity and autonomy. Provided such claims are not excessive, physicians would have no right to complain since they voluntarily accepted the benefits and corresponding burdens of public assistance.

This is an attractive and popular argument. The claim that the acceptance of social benefits imposes social obligations appeals to our sense of justice and fair play. On closer inspection, however, this relationship between social benefits and burdens becomes increasingly obscure. In the first place, we note that accepting public assistance generates no clear-cut duties. To what extent would individual physicians be obligated to society? Should they devote their services to the public for one year? Two? Three? Would wealthy physicians and nurses who pay their own way through school incur less of a public obligation than their less well-heeled colleagues? Would they be allowed to pay off their public debt in cash, instead of in medical services? Suppose that physicians owned all the hospitals and financed their own educations. Would defenders of the right to health care simply sputter "Pardonnez-moi" and desert the field? We think not.

Conversely, the extent of this special right to health care is equally obscure and problematic. If health care is a special right, then it must be generated by the voluntary acts of definite persons. Who are these individuals entitled to health care, and what must they do to deserve it?

The argument under consideration asserts that the *public* is entitled to the services of physicians because it pays the bills for modern medicine. But precisely who is the public? According to the theory of special rights, would not the public consist only of those who actually contribute in some way to the medical enterprise? If so, it would follow that the poor who pay no taxes (except on sales) would have less right to health care than those wealthy and middle income families that bear the brunt of public support for medicine. This would certainly be an ironic outcome for the advocates of health care rights. Those who needed this right the most would have the least claim to it, while those who needed it least would have the strongest right. Obviously, an unacceptable result.

IV. Positive Approaches to a Right to Health Care

The position that there is a right to health care turns out to be intricate and difficult to defend on the basis of positive arguments in its favor. Most arguments in defense of a right to health care treat it as a means to achieve an end. It may be seen as a means to realize a right to health,[19] or a duty to care for one's health.[20] Other ends sought by a right to health care are normally seen as linked to its role in maintaining and restoring health, which is seen as directed to even further ends, such as autonomy,[21] equal opportunity,[22] or one's duty to

labor for social good.[23] At first, this means-to-end approach seems natural. Few see physicians for pleasure; health care is not ordinarily desired as an end in itself. The well-established rights—to life, liberty, food, shelter, pursuit of happiness—seem more directly valuable because they are satisfying in themselves. But, we do not list any of these as rights simply because they are deeply enjoyable, or because they are ends in themselves. We defend them as rights because they also have a place in a scheme of life. For the overwhelming majority of people, a full spectrum of these rights must be realized in order to lead a good or happy life, however much that conception may vary from person to person in other respects.

Talk of "rights" helps us to set a standard by which we assess the ability of a social organization to support or encourage a good life for each of us in a just way. Being part of a short list of elements necessary to leading a good life is the main reason for treating health care as a right. But rights have a way of proliferating. In certain circumstances additional things are needed (such as transportation) to get what we have a right to (such as pursuit of happiness). Since we tend to think that if I have a right to something, it follows that I have a right to the means to obtain it, the list of rights has a potential for explosive growth. However, we have argued earlier in this paper that this is not a sound principle. Thus, we think that a fairly clear area of rights can be distinguished from a fairly clear area of nonrights. To take this position plausibly, however, one must recognize its vagueness. We would expect there to be a broad disputable gray area of goods that may or may not be seen as basic.

Moreover, not every element basic to a good life should appear on such lists. Only if the needed item is subject to distribution and control by organized social means in a developed society should we have occasion to mention it. For example, although breathing is important to a good life, we do not list a "right to breathe," partly because we have no effective means of allocating breathing, and partly because it is usually well-managed on an individual basis. What appears on the basic list need not be seen as fixed by nature; new forms of production and new forms of living may change its content. Lest the list cease to characterize anything basic, however, it is important that it be a short one.

From this perspective on what we should say we have a right to, there is no difficulty about placing a right to health, as contrasted with a right to health care, on the list of desiderata. One can find many authorities who defend the cliché that health is a basic good in life. As health declines, so does the appeal of autonomy, property, and the pursuit of happiness. Nevertheless, two objections must be met: first, that people often act as though they do not really desire health, and second, that people desire many things, among them health, so that health must compete with a wide range of desires to be called a "right." These objections are worth considering, but only because the psychology of health management is important to understanding how best to support health. The desire for health is not like the desire for other goods, especially consumer goods. Even though people weaken their health for other ends, they can rarely be charged with *desiring* ill health or seeking it out. For most consumer goods, there are times we desire to be without them. Although worth exploring, these objections are largely irrelevant. To commit oneself to a set of rights is not to choose a set of "more valued" desires in competition with others. It is to choose those that interact in an important way with other desires, such that were the objects of these desires absent, most other desires that people have would be unrealizable because their objects would be either unobtainable or undesirable.

In saying that a right to health falls squarely in the realm of basic rights, we should not be misunderstood. Health is not a good or commodity that can be provided by society. It is a condition—like life, liberty, or happiness. Society cannot make people healthy; much depends on their personal life styles. A right to health simply creates an obligation to produce social conditions conducive to health and to personal health maintenance. Society need make people healthy no more than it need make people morally virtuous. Indeed, health as a virtue or duty[24] represents an ideal of health beyond the lesser standard on which a wide range of goods depend. It is unclear whether we should make sacrifices to encourage this virtue, but we should not make the mistake of assuming that a society in which it is easy to be unhealthy, such as one in which it is difficult to exercise and easy to consume a poor diet, is necessarily more liber-

tarian than one in which it is easy to maintain healthy personal habits. Moreover, a right to health ought to protect us from conditions destructive to health created by social activities.

There is a deeper problem with the arguments for the rights to health and to health care. Rights talk confuses allocation of goods with allocation of power to obtain goods. Usually, two things are being said when I claim a "right to X": that "X should be available to me," and that "I am entitled to control X." These are partially independent considerations. It would be possible to guarantee health care to all who need it, but to have someone else determine who needs it. We are entitled to own property, but the uses to which we may put it are subject to limitation. A person may be put in a position to control a good, but be required to control it for public benefit, as in professional licensure.

This lack of clarity creates difficulties for arguments in defense of the rights to health and to health care, by restricting too much our conceptions of what social institutions might be used to realize these rights. Depending on how they are organized, social factors affecting health may emphasize benefits to whole populations, or benefits to individuals. They may consist in services over which individuals have much control, such as physicians' services, or which may be widely distributed without much individual attention, such as clean air. Health maintenance need not be seen as a service at all, but as a set of social conditions making it easy to lead a healthy life consistent with other satisfactions. The use of rights language makes it hard to see these possibilities because it assumes that individuals ought to control these goods, when many of the most important social goods, such as basic production, cannot be readily controlled by individuals.

The argument for the right to health care, being one step more complex, is even more problematic than the argument for a right to health. To the medical individualist, health care is an oddity on the list of rights because it costs money—it must be *provided*, while life and liberty are merely *protected* and not actively provided. This, however, should not distress us. Although it must be provided, health care may nevertheless still be necessary to any form of good life. Moreover, the monetary differences between provided and protected goods is not so sharp as it first seems. Liberty is protected by laws, political processes, the police, and the courts. These jobs are done by people with marketable skills in need of survival, just like physicians. In some sense, liberty must be provided like any other social good.

The strongest argument for a right to health care, as modeled on the present system of delivery, does not rest on its role in maintaining overall public health status. As we argued above, health care is not a dominant factor in public health status. Indeed, we should avoid sacrificing other health factors in order to provide health care. For example, it would be ironic, as well as harmful and unjust, for us to be unable to afford adequate nutrition in order to maintain a complex health care system. Instead, the argument for a right to health care services rests mainly on the benefit they provide to particular individuals in particular need. When an individual gets sick, that person's autonomy and welfare are threatened. Like the protective functions of fire departments and police, the right to health care can be defended in relationship to individual health restoration.[25]

This argument does not support an extensive health care system. We get well from most ailments anyway, and do not need health services in recovering from them. The incurable illnesses likewise pass from the scope of the right to health care. The argument has an unfortunately strong focus on the "cure" functions of medicine. Unfortunate, because health care services do many things. Apart from cure, they play a minor role in health maintenance and disease prevention (for example, polio vaccination); palliate, aid, comfort, and protect during illness (for example, morphine for pain, nursing care); and restore function without restoring health (for example, dialysis, eyeglasses, prosthetics).

The last two functions deserve more attention in right to health care arguments than they usually get. Functional restoration and protection can be defended by means-end arguments in a manner analogous to a defense of a right to health. Palliation and comfort—the "care" functions—could also be defended as part of our conception of basic goods, and therefore be treated as things to which we have a right. As goods in themselves, they fall squarely under a humane conception of social life and can be defended as rights more readily than many liberties and consumer goods. Many of them

need not even be provided by professionals, and some may be better managed outside the health care system.[26] However, since it is unclear whether other goods depend on these, it is unclear whether we can defend a right to these by the means-ends arguments. An uncomforted illness could be a psychologically incapacitating disaster for some; others may prefer to be ill alone. Insofar as these goods are independent of other goods, the defense of a right to them is weakened, unless a commitment to humane care of the ill and helpless is so widespread as to make it an important part of almost any conception of a good life. We take comfort in thinking that aid in extremity seems desirable even to those willing to risk their health for other ends.

In this quick look at positive arguments in defense of a right to health care, we have tried to stick closely to the question of what we have a right to. We think these arguments are too loose at this point to require, or to bear, a carefully calculated exposition. In order to keep the outline clear, we have avoided some of the issues we think important in understanding the right to health care argument, such as questions as to the extent of health care services,[27] standards of public health, appropriate principles of justice for distributing health care,[28] and the extent to which other things ought to be sacrificed for the sake of health care. These, however, must also be developed in order to give a full defense of a right to health care. It is an irony of the debate over medical individualism that if health is to be our goal, it may be easier to establish a right to a decent standard of living than to establish a right to health care.

Notes

An earlier draft of this paper was read by John Arras and criticized by Andrew Jameton at the "Symposium on Medicine, Morals, and Society," California State University, Chico, in April 1977. We thank Robert Hunt and Richard Wasserstrom for helpful discussion and the University of Redlands Research Committee for a Wilcox Fund award.

1. H. Tristram Engelhardt, Jr., "Human Well-being and Medicine: Some Basic Value-Judgments in the Biomedical Sciences," in H. Tristram Engelhardt, Jr. and Daniel Callahan, eds., Science, Ethics and Medicine (Hastings-on-Hudson, N.Y.: Institute of Society, Ethics, and the Life Sciences, 1976), pp. 120–39.

2. Leon R. Kass, "Regarding the End of Medicine and the Pursuit of Health," *The Public Interest* 40 (1975): 11—41. Reprinted in Robert Hunt and John Arras, eds., *Ethical Issues in Modern Medicine* (Palo Alto, California: Mayfield Publishing Company, 1977).

3. Ivan Illich, *Medical Nemesis* (New York: Pantheon, 1976).

4. See Nedra B. Belloc and Lester Breslow, "Relationship of Physical Health Status and Health Practices," *Preventive Medicine* 1 (1972): 409–21 and Thomas McKeown, *The Role of Medicine: Dream, Mirage, or Nemesis* (London: Nuffield Provincial Trust, 1976).

5. Robert M. Sade, "Medical Care as a Right: A Refutation," *New England Journal of Medicine* 285 (1971): 1288–92; Thomas S. Szasz, "The Right to Health," *Georgetown Law Journal* 57 (1969): 734–51. Garvan F. Kuskey, "Health Care, Human Rights and Government Intervention: A Critical Appraisal," *California Dental Association Journal* (July 1973); Robert Nozick, *Anarchy, State, and Utopia* (New York: Basic Books, 1974), especially pp. 232–35. Sade and Szasz are reprinted in Samuel Gorovitz, et al., eds., *Moral Problems in Medicine* (Englewood Cliffs, New Jersey: Prentice-Hall, 1976). Kuskey is reprinted in Hunt and Arras, *Ethical Issues in Modern Medicine*.

6. For a contemporary defense of the "minimal state," see Nozick, *Anarchy, State, and Utopia.*

7. Nozick, p. 198.

8. Sade explores the implications of this analogy in "Medical Care as a Right: A Refutation."

9. For a useful discussion on the relationship between rights and our notion of a good life, see Charles Fried, *Medical Experimentation: Personal Integrity and Social Policy* (New York: American Elsevier, 1974), pp. 89–94.

10. The relationship between privacy and love is discussed in Charles Fried, *An Anatomy of Values: Problems of Personal and Social Choice* (Cambridge, Mass.: Harvard University Press, 1970), ch. IX.

11. Kuskey, "Health Care, Human Rights and Government Intervention: A Critical Appraisal," reprinted in Hunt and Arras, p. 467.

12. This limitation on rights receives fuller treatment in Thomas Scanlon's excellent article, "Nozick on Rights, Liberty, and Property," *Philosophy and Public Affairs* 6 (Fall 1976): 3–25.

13. John Locke, *The Second Treatise of Government* (Cambridge: Cambridge University Press, 1967), Ch. V.

14. This point is cogently argued by Scanlon in "Nozick on Rights, Liberty, and Property."

15. For a defense of the view that, from a purely *libertarian* point of view, it is better for a government to coercively transfer property from some citizens to others, see Ernest Loevinsohn, "Liberty and the Redistribution of Property," *Philosophy and Public Affairs* 6 (Spring 1977): pp. 226–39.

16. Judith Jarvis Thomson's example. See "A Defense of Abortion," *Philosophy and Public Affiars* 1 (1971): 47–66. [See above, pp. 76–86.]

17. Typical statements of this argument can be found in B. B. Page, "Who Owns the Professions?" *Hastings Center Report* 5 (October 1975): 7–8 and in correspondence addressed to Sade's "Medical Care as a Right: A Refutation" in the *New England Journal of Medicine* 286 (1972): 488–93. These letters are conveniently reprinted in Stanley Joel Reiser, Arthur J. Dyck, and William J. Curran, eds., *Ethics in Medicine: Historical Perspectives and Contemporary Concerns* (Cambridge, Mass.: The MIT Press, 1977), pp. 577–80.

18. The distinction between special and general rights figures prominently in H. L. A. Hart's influential article, "Are There Any Natural Rights?" reprinted in A. I. Melden, *Human Rights* (Belmont, California: Wadsworth Publishing Company, 1970), pp. 61–75. William Nelson attempts to ground redistributive principles of social justice on a similar conception of special rights. See his article "Special Rights, General Rights, and Social Justice," *Philosophy and Public Affairs* 3 (Summer 1974): 410–30.

19. Albert R. Jonsen, "Right to Health Care Services," *Encyclopedia of Bioethics,* ed. Warren Reich (New York: Macmillan Publishing Co., 1978).

20. Leon R. Kass, "Regarding the End of Medicine and the Pursuit of Health."

21. Albert R. Jonsen, "Right to Health Care Services."

22. John Arras, "Medical Individualism and the Right to Health Care." An earlier version of this paper, read at the "Symposium on Medicine, Morals, and Society," California State University, Chico, April 15, 1977.

23. T. H. Green, "Liberal Legislation and Freedom of Contract," in *Works of Thomas Hill Green,* ed. R. L. Nettleship (London: Longmans, Green and Co., 1891), p. 372.

24. Leon R. Kass, *op. cit.,* pp. 38–39.

25. Our argument is similar to that of Henry Sigerist: "The chief cause of disease is poverty. If we are unable to provide work for everybody and to guarantee a decent standard of living to every individual willing to work, whatever his intelligence may be, we are collectively responsible for the chief cause of disease. The least we can do is

to make provision for the protection and restoration of the people's health. They have an undeniable right to such provisions." (Henry E. Sigerist, "Socialized Medicine," reprinted in Gorovitz, *et al.*, *Moral Problems in Medicine*, p. 468.) Our argument is different in that it focuses clearly on individuals, rather than on aggregate public health. Moreover, we believe that a right to health care can be defended in cases of disease or injury lacking social causes. Even in a just society, people would have the right to services needed to restore health, because no one would be duly deprived of the basic means necessary to lead a good life, with certain exceptions, such as sacrifice of one right for another in order to allocate scarce resources.

26. Is a good death a firm part of most everyone's conception of a good life? We should claim a right to health care services for the dying only insofar as they support a humane conception of dying, but much terminal health care is invested in aggressive attempts at cure or postponement of death, while other options, such as hospice care, appear to be more humane in some cases. Insofar as the right to health care is rooted in a conception of the good life, it places a claim on society for services different from some of those now provided by our existing health care services.

27. Charles Fried, "Equality and Rights in Medical Care," *The Hastings Center Report* 6 (1976): 29–34. [See above, pp. 530–36.]

28. Robert M. Veatch, "What is a 'Just' Health Care Delivery?" *Ethics and Health Policy,* ed. R. M. Veatch and Roy Branson (Cambridge, Mass.: Ballinger Publishing Co., 1976). Gene Outka, "Social Justice and Equal Access to Health Care," *The Journal of Religious Ethics* 2 (1974): 11–32.

Decision Scenario 1

The Cashier's Office of Archway Memorial Hospital is, even for the wealthy and best educated, a place of frustration. Bills are presented in the form of long computer printouts, covered with unfamiliar names referring to supplies, medical treatment, and diagnostic tests. Associated with each item is a price that seems absurdly high.

For someone without any form of medical insurance, being faced with such a bill can be more than confusing. It can be frightening. And that is just the situation that Marvin Baldesi found himself in.

"Your age makes you ineligible for Medicaid," said Ms. Kearney, the Archway billing officer. "And you say you aren't covered by Blue Cross or a private insurance plan."

"That's right," said Mr. Baldesi. "I own my own business. My wife and me, we run a small upholstery shop. We decided we couldn't afford to keep up our insurance."

"Normally we wouldn't have admitted you," said Ms. Kearney. "It's only because you came in as an acute emergency that you were allowed to run up such a bill."

Mr. Baldesi looked down to keep from meeting Ms. Kearney's eyes. He felt embarrassed. He had always paid his bills, and now this woman didn't bother to disguise the fact that she saw him as a deadbeat.

"I don't guess you have any money in savings?" Ms. Kearney asked.

"About fifty dollars. Just enough to keep the account open."

"Then it looks to me like you've only got two choices," Ms. Kearney said.

"You've got to borrow the money or you've got to declare yourself bankrupt. If you do that, then you'll be eligible for Medicare payments and the hospital may be able to collect from the government. I'm not sure of the legal process."

"But the bill is almost three thousand dollars," Mr. Baldesi said. "I can't borrow money like that. My family and friends don't have it, and no bank would loan it to me without collateral."

"Then you'll just have to get a lawyer and get yourself declared bankrupt."

"But if I do that, I'll lose my business. My credit will be ruined, and I won't be able to get the materials I need from suppliers. Isn't there any other way?"

"I don't know of any," said Ms. Kearney. "But that's not really my problem. All I know is that Archway has to be paid. You received our services and we have to have the money for them."

Is Mr. Baldesi's situation possible in the U.S. today?

How might the health-care proposal outlined by Fried apply to such a case?

Archway Hospital (in the person of Ms. Kearney) is asserting its claim as a participant in a free-market economy. Can this case be used to support the Arras-Jameton contention that health care should not be considered a free-market commodity?

Would Kant's moral principles support the view that Mr. Baldesi is entitled to health care, even if he cannot pay for it?

If Sade's position is accepted, how should our society deal with cases like Mr. Baldesi's?

Suppose you know that Mr. Baldesi's illness is connected with his failure to give up smoking and drinking, even though advised to do so by his physician. Would this lead you to view his situation any differently?

Decision Scenario 2

"I'm pleased to tell you," said Mr. Ching, "that both your academic record and your financial state qualify you for the new Federal Health Care Fellowship."

"I'm delighted!" Emily Rosenhans said. "These first two years of medical school have really been hell for me. Not only am I up to my ears in debt, but I've had to work twenty-five hours a week as an admitting clerk to pay my board bill."

"The HCF will cover your tuition and expenses for the next two years," said Mr. Ching. "But if you accept the fellowship, you'll be committing yourself to three years in the Health Corps after you finish your internship and get your degree."

"What exactly does that mean?" Emily asked.

"It means that you will have to go and practice medicine at a federal or state clinic. You'll either be sent to some rural area where physicians are needed or to some city where you'll be a part of an urban medicine program."

"Will I have a choice about where I go?"

"I'm afraid not," said Mr. Ching.

"And do I really have to leave right after my internship? I'd planned to stay on and do a residency in neurology for a couple of years. My father died of multiple sclerosis, and that's one of the things that got me interested in medicine in the first place."

"You could come back and do a residency," said Mr. Ching. "But the conditions of the fellowship require immediate service."

Emily shook her head. "I really don't know what to do," she said. "I need that fellowship. And I'm even sympathetic with the aims of the program. I think physicians owe something to society, and we should do something to help people who don't have access to doctors."

"That's one of the purposes of the program. The government wants to encourage more people to be family practitioners and to go where they are needed."

"But," Emily said, "that means changing everything I've planned to do. I want to be a neurologist, and if I accept the fellowship, the chances are very good that I will never become one. At best I'll have to interrupt my education for three years. That would make it very hard for me to pick up where I left off."

"I understand your predicament," said Mr. Ching.

"I just don't know what to do," Emily said. "I feel like I'm being blackmailed. And just because I can't afford to pay for my medical education."

> *On what grounds might Sade support Emily's claim that she is being "blackmailed"?*
>
> *What arguments might Arras and Jameton offer in reply?*
>
> *Do such fellowship conditions violate the autonomy of the individual as conceived by Kant?*
>
> *How might such a program be justified on utilitarian grounds?*
>
> *Would Rawls's principles of justice be violated (necessarily) by the fellowship requirements? Might the requirements actually satisfy the principles?*

Decision Scenario 3

Frank Clemet disliked medical administrators, and he felt that those in universities were the worst. They were all so arrogant, so certain that they knew what was best for both the medical profession and the country. It was a shame his job required him to spend most of his working hours with them.

"It's flatly ridiculous," Dr. Snyder said. "We are the ones best qualified to choose candidates for medical schools. And if we rejected these people before, it's because we didn't think they had the education, or the grades, or the qualities to make good medical students."

"I'm sure that's true," Clemet said. "Assuming that you have a fixed number of places available in the entering class, you would obviously take those students you considered best. But HHS is not asking you to take unqualified students."

"I don't see why not. We are forced to accept transfer students from foreign medical schools or give up our federal grants."

"But they are not necessarily unqualified," Clemet said patiently.

"Of course they are. That's why we turned them down in the first place. That's why they went to Italy, Mexico, Puerto Rico, and places like that."

"They went there because you didn't have enough space for them. You might have accepted more of them if you were able to do so. Isn't that right?"

"Some of them we might have," Dr. Snyder admitted. "There is an element of judgment in the selection process. And had there been more places available, we would probably have given some the benefit of the doubt."

"I'm glad you agree even to that extent. Now HHS isn't making the rules. We're only following the requirements in the bill approved by Congress. And that says you've got to take your quota of transfer students or give up your grants. It's really that simple."

"But what you don't understand," Dr. Snyder said, "is that that means that we have no control over the selection of students. Let's grant that some are qualified—not all of them are, but let's grant that some are. Now we have to take our chances on getting students that we think are capable of doing the work and becoming good physicians."

"That's right," Clemet said.

"But that runs counter to the accepted notion that scholars and scientists are those best able to select qualified students. It takes away the autonomy of universities and makes them appendages of the government. The government is now telling us who to educate."

"To a certain extent you are right," Clemet said. "But you seem to forget that universities are a part of society. If nothing else, the vast amount of public money that has been poured into them is proof of that. If the universities don't voluntarily help the society, then they have to be encouraged to do so."

"Help the society! We do it all the time. But what we're talking about here is just a political payoff. Senators and Congressmen are just responding to pressure from middle-class parents whose children couldn't get into medical school through the front door. They now want to force open the back door."

"Maybe they wouldn't have to force open the door if groups like the AMA didn't hold it so tightly closed that only a trickle of people can get past it." Clemet was speaking out of turn and he knew it. But the righteousness of Snyder was practically unbearable.

"Are you suggesting that the AMA controls our policies?"

"Indirectly and directly. Not only are you all members, but medical associations also control licensing in every state. It's certainly to the advantage of physicians to limit the supply."

"I can show you figures to prove that there are more than enough physicians to meet the health needs of this country," Snyder said.

"I'm sure you can. But that's not the point. One point, at least, is that not everyone who wants to get a medical education can get one. And that's control."

"I don't see any point in arguing with you about this," Snyder said. "But I just want to make it clear to you why this university is seriously considering giving up its federal funds so that it can continue to base its admissions on the professional judgment of the faculty."

"I think I understand," Clemet said. "But I think you are wrong."

Can an argument like Sade's be used to support the position taken by Snyder?

Is the issue of requiring the admission of transfer students the same—in principle—as that of requiring physicians to locate in certain geographical areas?

Can arguments like those of Arras and Jameton be employed to justify forced admission to medical schools? Do you think that their arguments can be used to justify requiring the admission of transfer students in the present situation?

Decision Scenario 4

"There's more than one way to get to Rome," Dr. Kenton said. "And we've got a couple of options to offer you."

"I'll take anything that will make the pain stay away," Mr. Czahz said.

"We can do a surgical procedure that we call a coronary-artery bypass. In your case, there are two arteries involved so it would be a double bypass."

"This is not something experimental, is it?'

"No, it's a well-established procedure with a pretty good safety record. Now something like 80 percent of the people who have the bypass get rid of their angina pains."

"I don't much like the idea of being cut, but I'd do most anything to stop those chest pains."

"Let me tell you the other option. We can treat you medically instead of surgically. That is, we can try you on some drugs and see how you do, put you on a diet, and keep a close watch on you. Now people we treat this way do a little bit better in terms of living longer than those treated surgically do. That's a little misleading, though, because those who have surgery usually have worse cases of the disease."

"What about the angina pains?" Mr. Czahz asked.

"There's the problem. Medical treatment can do something about the pains, but it's really not as effective as surgery."

"So I'll take the surgery."

"Aren't you on health stamps?" Dr. Kenton asked.

"That's right."

"We've got a problem then. You see, health stamps won't cover the cost of bypass surgery. It's an optional procedure under the HHS guidelines, and they won't kick in the extra money to pay for it."

"So I have to make up the difference myself?"

"That's right," Dr. Kenton said. "You're going to have to come up with about two thousand in cash."

"Dr. Kenton, there's no way I can do that."

"Okay, then. I just wanted you to know what the possibilities were. We can put you on a treatment program, and I'm sure you'll do just fine."

"But what about the angina pain?"

"We'll do what we can," Dr. Kenton said.

Of course, there is not at present a health-stamp program. What might be the advantages of such a program? What might be some of its drawbacks?

According to Fried, should Mr. Czahz be entitled to anything more than medical treatment for his heart condition?

Would a health-stamp program change the status of health care from its current one of being a free-market commodity?

Would such a program be likely to promote equality in health care?

Would Sade be likely to oppose a health-stamp program? If so, on what grounds?

Decision Scenario 5

"I've decided to do something that may cause me a lot of trouble," Dr. Miles Burgone said.

Alan Warfard took a sip of his drink and sat back in his chair. He had known Miles for a long time and knew he could be counted on to see most things in a novel way. Sometimes Miles could be annoying, but he always made you think.

"I'm not going to accept women as patients anymore," Burgone said. "I don't like dealing with them, and there's nothing that says I have to. From now on, I'm restricting my practice to men only."

"I don't think you can do that," Warfard said. "I suspect that involves civil rights violations of some sort. You know, discriminating on the basis of race or sex or something like that."

"Then I'll get a lawyer and show that the government can't force me to treat women without violating my own rights."

"I don't follow you."

"Look at it this way," Burgone said. "My medical knowledge and skills belong to me. I acquired them through the exercise of my own mind, and I have a constitutional right to privacy and freedom of expression. Therefore, I have a right to exercise my knowledge and skills in the way I see fit. Therefore, if I don't want to treat women, then I don't have to."

"That's an argument I've never heard," Warfard said.

"The government can't force me to do what I don't want to do without violating my rights and being despotic."

"I suspect you'll have to prove that in court."

"I'm prepared to," Burgone said.

State explicitly (and more fully if it seems necessary) the argument presented by Dr. Burgone.

Is the argument the same as Sade's argument? If not, how do the two differ?

Burgone's argument might be construed as one supporting what is sometimes called "medical individualism." Do the objections to medical individualism made by Arras and Jameton also apply to Burgone's argument?

NOTES AND REFERENCES
FOR INTRODUCTIONS,
CASES, AND SCENARIOS

Ethical Theories and Medical Decisions:
An Introduction

I learned much about medical ethics and about presenting it to a general audience from those who have gone before me. I have benefitted from the example (among others) of Samuel Gorovitz, et al., eds., *Moral Problems in Medicine* (Englewood Cliffs, N.J.: Prentice-Hall, 1976), Robert Hunt and John Arras, eds., *Ethical Issues in Modern Medicine* (Palo Alto, Ca.: Mayfield Publishing Co., 1977), and Richard W. Wertz, ed. *Readings on Ethical and Social Issues in Biomedicine* (Englewood Cliffs, N.J.: Prentice-Hall, 1973). All three have informative introductions, but the one by Hunt and Arras I found most helpful and most philosophically interesting.

"The Declaration of Geneva" and the American Medical Association "Principles of Medical Ethics" are reprinted in Milton D. Heifetz and Charles Mangel, *The Right to Die* (New York: G. P. Putnam, 1975). The Oath of Hippocrates and the Oath of Maimonides are also reprinted there. For an examination of difficulties of applying codes to cases, see Robert M. Veatch, "Codes of Medical Ethics in Medical Education," in *The Teaching of Medical Ethics*, edited by Willard Gaylin and Councilman Morgan (Hastings-on-Hudson, New York: Hastings Institute, 1973), pp. 144–147. For an understanding of the Hippocratic Oath in its historical context, see "Hippocratic Oath: Text, Translation, and Interpretation," Ludwig Edelstein, *Ancient Medicine*, edited by Oswei Temkin and C. L. Temkin (Baltimore: Johns Hopkins University Press, 1967), pp. 3–63. On Maimonides and Jewish medical ethics, see Immanuel Jakobovits, *Jewish Medical Ethics* (New York: Bloch Publishing Company, 1959) and Fred Rosner, *Modern Medicine and Jewish Law* (New York: Yeshiva University Press, 1972). "Ethical and Religious Directives for Catholic Hospitals" is reprinted in Charles J. McFadden, *Medical Ethics,* 6th ed. (Philadelphia: F. A. Davis, 1967). For a guide to other oaths and codes, see Cheryl Calhoun, *Annotated Bibliography of Medical Oaths, Codes, and Prayers* (Washington, D.C.: Kennedy Institute, 1975).

My discussion of ethical relativism owes something to James W. Cornman and Keith Lehrer, *Philosophical Problems and Arguments,* 2d ed. (New York: Macmillan, 1974), pp. 432–439 and to Carl Wellman, *Morals and Ethics* (New York: Scott, Foresman, 1975), 290–293.

My discussion of ethical theories is generally indebted to Richard B. Brandt, *Ethical Theory* (Englewood Cliffs, New Jersey: Prentice-Hall, 1959) and William K. Frankena, *Ethics,* 2d ed. (Englewood Cliffs, New Jersey: Prentice-Hall, 1973). My treatment of utilitarianism owes much to the excellent introductory essay by Paul W. Taylor in his anthology *Problems of Moral Philosophy* (Belmont, California: Dickenson Publishing Company, 1971), pp. 137–151. The John Stuart Mill statement of the principle of utility is from *Utilitarianism* (Indianapolis: Bobbs-Merrill, 1971), p. 18; the second quotation is from the same work, p. 24. The work was first published in 1863 and is currently available in many reprints. See Taylor for selections from Mill and from Jeremy Bentham's *An Introduction to the Principles of Morals and Legislation* (1869). The whole work is available, edited by L. J. Lafleur (New York: Hafner Press, 1948).

The statements of Kant's categorical imperative are more paraphrases than literal translations. They are from his *Groundwork of the Metaphysics of Morals,* translated by H. J. Paton (New York: Harper and Row, 1964). Other translations and editions are easily available. Some of the criticisms of Kant are based on those of Brandt (*Ethical Theory,* pp. 27–35) and Frankena (*Ethics,* pp. 30–33).

The quotation from Ross is from his *The Right and the Good* (New York: Oxford University Press, 1930), p. 24. The prima facie duties are found on pp. 21–22 and the "rules" for resolving conflict on pp. 41–42. My exposition is indebted, in part, to G. J. Warnock, *Contemporary Moral Philosophy* (New York: St. Martin's Press, 1967).

Rawls's theory is presented in *A Theory of Justice* (Cambridge, Massachusetts: Harvard University Press, 1971). The principles are quoted from p. 203; "natural duties" are discussed on pp. 340–350. My statement of the theory is indebted to Norman Daniels's introduction to his anthology *Reading Rawls* (New York: Basic Books, 1976). The first criticism is one made by Thomas Nagel, "Rawls on Justice" (Daniels, pp. 1–16) and Ronald Dworkin, "The Original Position" (Daniels, pp. 16–53). The second criticism is urged by R. M. Hare, "Rawls's Theory of Justice" (Daniels, 81–108) and David Lyons, "Nature and Soundness of the Contract and Coherence Arguments" (Daniels, 141–169). A relatively easy entrance into Rawls's theory is provided by the general reviews of the book that are listed in the Bibliography.

For Aquinas's view on "man," see his *Summa Theologica,* Part II (First Part), vol. 6, translated by Fathers of the English Dominican Province (London: Burns Oates and Washbourne, 1914). For his views on natural law and law in general, see vol. 8, "Treatise on Law." For an interpretation of Aquinas, see Frederick Copleston, *A History of Philosophy,* vol. 2, part 2 (New York: Doubleday,

1962), pp. 126–131, to which my account is indebted. For the presentation of the current Catholic natural law view I am indebted to Charles J. McFadden, *Medical Ethics*, 6th ed. (Philadelphia: F. A. Davis, 1967). The doctrine of double effect is treated on pp. 121–155; euthanasia, extraordinary means, and medical experimentation, pp. 239–270. The quotations from the Directives are from the appendix in McFadden: abortion, p. 441, euthanasia, p. 442.

Anyone who wishes to deal with ethics in more depth than has been possible in this chapter should use the Bibliography as a further guide.

Chapter 1: Abortion and Infanticide

The Case Presentation has been fictionalized to protect the privacy of the individuals involved. It is, however, a close parallel to an actual case with identical medical and moral issues. For a similar case, see the United Press International story "Court Orders Abortion for a Rape Victim, 12," (Oklahoma City, 29 September 1981).

Information on fetal development is to be found in Arthur J. Vender, J. H. Sherman, and D. S. Luciano, *Human Physiology*, chapter 15 (New York: McGraw-Hill, 1970). I am also indebted to Joel Feinberg's introduction to his anthology *The Problem of Abortion* (Belmont, California: Wadsworth Publishing Company, 1973).

The Finkbine case in the Case Retrospective is based on the report in Allan F. Guttmacher, *The Case for Legalized Abortion* (Berkeley, California: Diablo Press, 1977), pp. 15–17.

Information about possible changes in Medicaid that may influence the current funding for abortion is presented by Nadine Brozan in a story in the *New York Times*, 5 February 1982.

Chapter 2: Treating or Terminating: The Problem of Birth Defects

The fictional Case Presentation is similar to an actual case presented in James M. Gustafson, "Mongolism, Parental Desires, and the Right to Life," *Perspectives in Biology and Medicine* 16 (1973): 529–557 and in Milton D. Heifetz and Charles Mangel, *The Right to Die* (New York: G. P. Putnam's, 1975), pp. 59–60.

For a discussion of the medical and biological aspects of birth defects, see E. P. Volpe, *Human Heredity and Birth Defects* (New York: Pegasus, 1971). On prenatal diagnosis, see Theodore Friedman, "Prenatal Diagnosis of Genetic Disease," *Scientific American* 225 (November 1971): 34–42.

The R. S. Duff and A. G. M. Campbell article referred to is "Moral and Ethical Dilemmas in the Special-Care Nursery," *New England Journal of Medicine* 289 (1973): 75–78.

The "Juli" Decision Scenario is based on a case reported in B. D. Colen, *Karen Ann Quinlan: Dying in the Age of Eternal Life* (New York: Nash Publishing Company, 1976), pp. 130–137. The "Susan Roth" scenario is based on a case reported in Richard Trubo, *An Act of Mercy* (Los Angeles: Nash Publishing Company, 1973), pp. 149–150. The "Irene Towers" scenario is based on a Chicago case reported by the Associated Press, 18 May 1981.

Chapter 3: Euthanasia

For a discussion of covert and unilateral decisions made about euthanasia by physicians, see Milton D. Heifetz and Charles Mangel, *The Right to Die* (New York: G. P. Putnam's Sons, 1975). The information about and the criticisms of the California Natural Death Act are from Karen Lebacqz, "On 'Natural Death,' " *Hastings Center Report* 7 (1977): 14. An excellent discussion of the history and practice of euthanasia and of euthanasia legislation is O. Ruth Russell, *Freedom to Die: Moral and Legal Aspects of Euthanasia* (New York: Dell Publishing Company, 1976).

By far the most detailed account of the Karen Quinlan case is Joseph and Julia Quinlan with Phyllis Battelle, *Karen Ann Quinlan* (New York: Doubleday, 1977). The facts in the case presentation are mostly from Phyllis Battelle, "The Story of Karen Quinlan," *Ladies' Home Journal* 93 (September 1976): 69–76, 172–180. Direct quotations are from Battelle. I have also drawn from B. D. Colen, *Karen Ann Quinlan: Dying in the Age of Eternal Life* (New York: Nash Publishing Company, 1976) and *In the Matter of Karen Quinlan: The Complete Legal Briefs, Court Proceedings, and Decisions* (Arlington, Virginia: University Publications of America, 1975).

No philosophical or legal analysis has so far been made of the J. K. Collums case. The facts and quotations in the Case Presentation are from the account by William K. Stevens, *New York Times*, 9 December 1981. The facts and quotations about the punishment hearing are from a United Press International news story of 5 February 1982. Information about the sentencing is from a United Press International story of 5 March 1982.

The "Virginia Crawford" Decision Scenario is based on a Baltimore case reported by United Press International on 25 February 1979.

Chapter 4: Paternalism, Truth Telling, and Confidentiality

For an account of the physician-patient relationship and the development of licensing procedures for physicians in the United States, see John Duffy, *The Healers: The Rise of the Medical Establishment* (New York: McGraw-Hill, 1977). Duffy also deals with American medical quackery, but the classic works in this area are James Harvey Young, *The Toadstool Millionaires: A Social History of Patent Medicines in America before Federal Regulation* (Princeton, New Jersey: Princeton University Press, 1961) and *The Medical Messiahs* (Princeton, New Jersey: Princeton University Press, 1971). An influential sociological account of the nature of the doctor-patient relationship as a social role is Talcott Parsons, "Illness and the Role of the Physician: A Sociological Perspective," in Clyde Kluckhohn and H. A. Murray, eds., *Personality in Nature, Society, and Culture* (New York: Alfred A. Knopf, 1961).

The facts in the first Case Presentation are taken almost exclusively from the excellent article "Laetrile: The Political Success of a Scientific Failure," *Consumer Reports* 42 (August 1977): 444–447. The quotation from the *FDA Drug Bulletin* and that attributed to the American Cancer Society are from this source. The story of the Laetrile controversy can be traced by following the *New York Times Index* and consulting the relevant articles. See the Bibliography for a listing of related works.

The final report of the National Cancer Institute study appeared in the *New England Journal of Medicine* (February 1982). The quotations from DeVita and Bradford about the study, as well as additional facts, are from *Time* (11 May 1981).

The facts and quotations that appear in the second Case Presentation, on contraception and the notification rules, are from Nadine Brozan, "Adolescents, Parents, and Birth Control," *New York Times*, 8 March 1982. For well-considered editorial opinions on the topic, see those in the same newspaper, 5 February and 26 February 1982.

For an account of the V.D. inspection program mentioned in the Decision Scenario concerning it, see Clyde Haberman, "New York Testing Prostitutes for V.D.," *New York Times*, 5 March 1982.

Chapter 5: Medical Experimentation and Informed Consent

The description of Nazi medical experiments is from the indictment in *United States* v. *Karl Brandt,* a selection from which is reprinted in *Hastings Center Report,* "Special Supplement: Biomedical Ethics and the Shadow of Nazism," 6 (August 1976): 5.

The description of drug testing is based on the account by Ross J. Baldessarini, *Chemotherapy in Psychiatry* (Cambridge, Massachusetts: Harvard University Press, 1977), pp. 4–11.

For a discussion of some of the problems of providing information, testing understanding, and getting consent I am indebted to William Shebar's unpublished paper "Understanding and Informed Consent in Psychiatric Research." The paternalistic view that physicians must decide because patients can never understand is expressed in Eugene G. Laforet, "The Fiction of Informed Consent," *Journal of the American Medical Association* 235 (12 April 1976): 1579–85. Problems with placebos are discussed in Sissela Bok, "The Ethics of Giving Placebos," *Scientific American* 231 (November 1974): 17–23. The discussion of research and children is indebted to Jean D. Lockhart, "Pediatric Drug Testing," *Hastings Center Report* 7 (June 1977): 8–10. Prisoners and research is discussed at length in Jessica Mitford, *Kind and Usual Punishment* (New York: Alfred A. Knopf, 1973). The historical cases of research on the poor are from M. H. Pappworth, *Human Guinea Pigs* (Boston: Beacon Books, 1961), pp. 61–62. The details of the Tuskegee case are from the "Final Report of the Tuskegee Syphilis Study Ad Hoc Advisory Panel," U.S. Public Health Service (Washington, D.C.: 1973), part of which is reprinted in S. J. Reiser, *et al., Ethics in Medicine* (Cambridge, Massachusetts: MIT Press, 1977), pp. 316–321. I am indebted to the letter by Jay Katz, in particular. In the discussion of fetal experimentation, I am indebted to "Individual Risks vs. Societal Benefits: The Fetus," a forum appearing in *Experiments and Research with Humans: Values in Conflict* (Washington, D.C.: National Academy of Sciences, 1975), pp. 59–90.

The details of the experiments in the Willowbrook Case Presentation are taken from Saul Krugman and Joan P. Giles, "Viral Hepatitis: New Light on an Old Disease," *Journal of the American Medical Association* 212 (1970): 1019–21.

The case of Ms. Mink presented in the Decision Scenario is based on a report in *Time*, 9 May 1977, p. 44 and on Marlene Cimons's article in the *Los Angeles Times*, 16 May 1977. The quotations are from these sources.

A report on the charges of so-called "guinea-pig" surgery involving mental patients in Chicago is to be found in the *New York Times*, 19 April 1979. Additional information is from *Time*, 23 April 1979.

Chapter 6: Behavior Control and Psychosurgery

The information on ESB and Delgado's dramatic experiment is from Thomas Meehan, "The Brain Manipulators," *Cosmopolitan Magazine* 174 (April 1973): 168–171, 203; and from José M. R. Delgado, "Psychocivilized Direction of Behavior," *The Humanist* 32 (March 1972): 10–15. The quotation about the use of implanted electrodes in released prisoners is from Barton L. Ingrahm and Geral W. Smith, "The Use of Electronics in the Observation and Control of Human Behavior and Its Possible Use in Rehabilitation and Control," *Issues in Criminology* 7 (Fall 1972), 35–53.

The general discussion of psychosurgery is based on the facts presented in Constance Holden, "Psychosurgery: Legitimate Therapy or Laundered Lobotomy," *Science* 179 (4 March 1973): 1109–12; Virginia Snodgrass, "Debate over Benefits and Ethics of Psychosurgery Involves the Public," *Journal of the American Medical Association* 225 (20 August 1973): 913–920; the criticisms by George J. Annas are in "Psychosurgery," *Hastings Center Report* 7 (April 1977): 11–13; the Coleman and Seeley quotations are from Pacific News Service, "Federal Commission Endorses the Pursuit of Psychosurgery," 10 April 1977. See also the "Recommendations of the National Commission for the Protection of Human Subjects of Biomedical Research," February 1977 (Washington, D.C.: United States Government Printing Office). The most influential work in the area is the Mark and Ervin book *Violence and the Brain* (New York: Harper and Row, 1970). The controversial letter by Mark, Sweet, and Ervin is in the *Journal of the American Medical Association* 201 (1967): 895.

See Meehan's article mentioned above for a discussion of aversive conditioning. The materials on psychotherapy are both numerous and well known, but for a general review of all forms of behavior alteration see Perry London, *Behavior Control* (New York: Harper and Row, 1969) and Seymour Halleck, *The Politics of Therapy* (New York: Science House, 1971).

The Kaimowitz Case Presentation is based on the opinion of the Wayne County Circuit Court (references cited in the selection). (The quotation from the consent form is from the notes of the opinion.) But it is most indebted to the excellent account by Ronald S. Gass, "Kaimowitz v. Department of Mental Health," W. M. Gaylin and J. S. Meister, eds., *Operating on the Mind* (New York: Basic Books, 1975), pp. 73–87. Anyone seriously concerned with the Detroit case should read Gass's article. The full opinion is reprinted as an appendix to the book.

The Case Presentation entitled "The Agents" is wholly fictional. However, it has been written in such a way that the character portrayed exhibits features that satisfy the criteria of schizophrenic disorder, paranoid type that are contained in the American Psychiatric Association's *Diagnostic and Statistical Manual of Mental Disorders*, third edition (DSM-III) (Washington, D.C.: American Psychiatric Association, 1980), pp. 189–191.

Chapter 7: Genetics: Intervention, Control, and Research

The sources most heavily relied on were Clifford Grobstein, "The Recombinant-DNA Debate," *Scientific American* 237 (July 1977): 22–33 and Bernard D. Davis, "Threat and Promise in Genetic Engineering," in Preston Williams, ed., *Ethical Issues in Biology and Medicine* (Cambridge, Mass.: Schenkman Publishing Company, 1973), pp. 17–32. Also used were "The Transfer of Genes That Make Insulin," *New York Times*, 28 May 1977; "DNA Research," *Time*, 15 August 1977, p. 56; and Joshua Lederberg, "DNA Splicing: Will Fear Rob Us of Its Benefits?" *Prism* 2 (November 1975): 33–37. The Dobzhansky quotation is from his "Changing Man," *Science* 155 (27 January 1967): 409–415.

The Case Presentation is based heavily on the information in "Tinkering," *Time*, 18 April 1977, pp. 32–45. (This is particularly so for the historical aspects of the debate. The Sinsheimer, Califano, and Zinder quotations are also from this source.) Other sources used include Paul Berg, *et al.*, "Asilomar Conference on Recombinant DNA Molecules," *Science* 188 (6 June 1975): 991–994; the Grobstein article cited above; and Daniel Callahan, "Recombinant DNA: Science and the Public," *Hastings Center Report* 7 (1977): 20–23.

Responses to federal research guidelines and comments by scientists about the problems and prospects of recombinant-DNA research are to be found in a series of news stories. See the *New York Times* (1, 13, 14, and 15 December 1981). For issues in business applications and the problems caused by potential conflicts of interest within universities, see the *New York Times* (19 August and 16 November 1981).

Several books on the problems and prospects of recombinant-DNA research are well worth consulting. Michael Rogers, in *Biohazard* (New York: Alfred A. Knopf, 1977), concentrates on the nature of the dangers and the difficulties of control. The book is generally reliable and is written in an engaging style. A book devoted to the potential benefits as well as the dangers is June Goodfield, *Playing God* (New York: Random House, 1977). A concise account of both the scientific issues and the public controversy is Clifford Grobstein, *A Double Image of the Double Helix* (San Francisco: W. H. Freeman, 1979).

For an account of diseases currently screened for and their relation to legal and social issues, see George Annas and B. Coyne, "Fitness for Birth and Reproduction: Legal Implications of Genetic Screening," *Family Law Quarterly* 9 (Fall 1975): 463–490. A general survey of the types of screening that are current and the ethical problems they pose is presented by Tabitha M. Powledge, "Genetic Screening," in Warrent T. Reich, ed., *Encyclopedia of Bioethics*, vol. 2 (New York: Free Press, 1978), pp. 567–573. The account of the experiences and problems (social and scientific) in PKU screening is found in National Academy of Sciences, *Genetic Screening: Programs, Principles, and Research* (Washington, D.C.: National Academy of Sciences, 1975). For an account of alpha-fetoprotein screening, see Barbara Gastel, et al., eds., *Maternal Serum Alpha-Fetoprotein: Issues in the Prenatal Screening and Diagnosis of Neural Tube Defects* (U.S. Department of Health and Human Services Publication HE 20.2: M41, 1981). For a discussion of social problems caused by PKU laws and sickle-cell screening, see Philip Reilly, "There's Another Side to Genetic Screening," *Prism* (January 1976): 55–57. A popular survey of fetal surgery is Robin Marantz Henig, "Saving Babies Before Birth," *New York Times Magazine* (28 February 1982), pp. 18ff. For a report of early attempts at gene therapy, see the *New York Times*, 8 September 1981.

Chapter 8: Reproductive Control: In Vitro Fertilization, Artificial Insemination, and Sterilization

The basic information for the Louise Brown Case Presentation is from *Newsweek*, 7 August 1978; *Time*, 7 August 1978; and *U.S. News and World Report*, 7 August 1978. For a discussion of the techniques and issues of in vitro fertilization, in addition to the popular accounts cited above, see R. G. Edwards, "Fertilization of Human Eggs In Vitro: Morals, Ethics, and the Law," *Quarterly Review of Biology* 49 (March 1974): 3–26. I am also indebted for information to George H. Kieffer, "Reproductive Technology: The State of the Art," in Thomas A. Mappes and Jane S. Zembaty, eds., *Biomedical Ethics* (New York: McGraw-Hill Book Company, 1981), pp. 485–490.

The historical background on artificial insemination is presented in R. Snowden and G. D. Mitchell, *The Artificial Family* (London: George Allen and Unwin, 1981). The technical aspects of the process and the statistics mentioned are discussed in Ronald P. Goldstein, "Artificial Insemination by Donor—Status and Problems," in Aubrey Milunsky and George J. Annas, eds., *Genetics and the Law* (New York: Plenum Press, 1976), pp. 197–202. I am also indebted for information to Donald A. Goss, "Current Status of Artificial Insemination with Donor Semen, *American Journal of Obstetrics and Gynecology* 122 (May 1975): 246–249. For general objections to artificial insemination and other forms of reproductive technology, see Paul Ramsey, *Fabricated Man* (New Haven: Yale University Press, 1970), particularly Chapter 3.

The information about the Relf case and the federal sterilization guidelines prompted by it is from the *New York Times*, 4 December 1977. Additional information about the federal guidelines and the response to them is from Patricia

Donovan, "Sterilizing the Poor and Incompetent," *Hastings Center Report* 6 (1976): 7–8. The account of *Buck v. Bell*, as well as the quotation from the opinion, is from "Eugenic Sterilization: A Biomedical Intervention," in Jonas Robitscher, ed., *Eugenic Sterilization* (Springfield, Illinois: Charles C. Thomas, 1973), pp. 10–12. The account of the Hartford sterilization case is based on information in the *New York Times*, 2 October 1978.

The account of the new proposal by Edwards and Steptoe to freeze embryos and the public reactions to it are from an Associated Press news story datelined London, 28 January 1982.

Chapter 9: Competition and Allocation

For an account of how dialysis takes place and of what it is like from a personal point of view, see Lee Foster, "Man and Machine: Life without Kidneys," *Hastings Center Report* 6 (June 1976): 5–8. I have drawn heavily from Foster's account. The statistics concerning the number of people receiving dialysis and its cost are from Carol Levine, "Home Dialysis and the Medicare Gap," *Hastings Center Report* 6 (December 1976): 5–6.

The lifeboat analogy is discussed by Paul Ramsey in *The Patient as Person* (New Haven, Conn.: Yale University Press, 1970).

An important sociological study on dialysis and transplants is Renée C. Fox, "A Sociological Perspective on Organ Transplantation and Hemodialysis," *New Dimensions in Legal and Ethical Concepts for Human Research, Annals of the New York Academy of Sciences* 169 (1970): 406–428. A volume that concentrates on the transplant issue is G. W. Wostenholme and M. O'Connor, eds., *Ethics in Medical Progress: With Special Reference to Transplantation* (Boston: Little, Brown, and Company, 1966). See also the relevant chapters in Paul Ramsey, *The Patient as Person* (New Haven, Conn.: Yale University Press, 1970). The ethical issues involved in transplants go beyond the question of distribution, of course.

There is no Brattle County, Texas, and the Case Presentation is wholly fictional. It does represent, however, the problem that was faced by some dialysis centers when programs were just starting. For a fine account of the workings of a real committee (the one at Swedish Hospital, Seattle, Washington, in 1961), see Shana Alexander, "They Decide Who Lives, Who Dies." The piece first appeared in *Life* magazine in 1962, but it is usefully reprinted in Robert Hunt and John Arras, eds., *Ethical Issues in Modern Medicine* (Palo Alto, California: Mayfield Publishing Company, 1977), pp. 409–424.

The second Case Presentation is also fictional. However, it is based on an actual event, which took place in a Florida hospital in 1982.

Chapter 10: The Claim to Health Care

The discussion of rights in the introduction is indebted to Joel Feinberg, "The Nature and Value of Rights," *Journal of Value Inquiry* 4 (1970): 243–257. For a discussion of the legal status of claims to health care, see Edward V. Sparer, "The Legal Right to Health Care: Public Policy and Equal Access," *Hastings Center Report* 6 (1976): 39–47.

The Case Presentation is most closely indebted to Stanley Hwang, "Dissecting the Health Care Beast," *Harvard Political Review* 6 (Fall 1977): 12–15. (Many of the criticisms of the current system and the description of the operation of HMOs are from Hwang.) I am also indebted to Bernard Winter, "The Problem is Profits," *The Progressive* 41 (October 1977): 16–19. (Criticisms, statistics, and some of the proposals for radical change came from Winter.) More general information is from Victor R. Fuchs, *Who Shall Live?: Health, Economics, and Social Change* (New York: Basic Books, 1974).

Increases in the costs of health care are described in an Associated Press story of 3 September 1981. Discussion of the proposed lump-sum Medicare payment plan and more recent statistics about costs are to be found in the *New York Times*, 2 February 1982. The Reagan administration's health plan is outlined and criticized by Toby Cohen, "Reagan's Health Plan," *New York Times*, 19 March 1982. A potential health-stamp plan is discussed by Gordon K. MacLeod, "Health Stamps, Maybe?" *New York Times*, 8 April 1980.

BIBLIOGRAPHY

The number of books and articles dealing with medical ethics is staggering, and it is growing larger at a rapid rate. The materials listed here are no more than a sample of those currently available. Thus, this bibliography is best thought of as a guide to further reading. The general and special bibliographies listed below—some book-length works—will provide guides for those who are looking for comprehensiveness.

I have tried to select works with substantial philosophical content. Thus, with a few exceptions, I have not listed publications that are primarily medical, biological, sociological, or otherwise scientific. Furthermore, I have not attempted to duplicate the references given in the selections or in the chapter introductions, and for the most part, I have restricted this bibliography to works that have appeared in the last five to ten years.

The Reference Center (Behavioral Science Section) of the University of Missouri Libraries kindly provided me with some assistance.

General Works and Anthologies

Augenstein, Leroy. *Come, Let Us Play God.* New York: Harper and Row, 1969.

Bandman, Elsie and Bertram Bandman, eds. *Bioethics and Human Rights: A Reader for Health Professionals.* Boston: Little, Brown, 1978.

Beauchamp, Tom L. and LeRoy Walters, eds. *Contemporary Issues in Bioethics*, 2nd ed. Belmont, Calif. Wadsworth Publishing Company, 1982.

Beauchamp, Tom L. and James F. Childress. *Principles of Biomedical Ethics.* New York: Oxford University Press, 1979.

Brody, Howard. *Ethical Decisions in Medicine.* Boston: Little, Brown, 1976.

Chapman, Carleton, B. "The Importance of Being Ethical." *Perspectives in Biology and Medicine* 24 (Spring 1981): 422–439.

Clouser, K. Danner. "Medical Ethics: Some Uses, Abuses, and Limitations." *Arizona Medicine* 33 (January 1976): 44–49.

Curran, William J. "The Proper and Improper Concerns of Medical Law and Ethics." *New England Journal of Medicine* 259 (4 November 1976): 1057–58.

Cutler, Donald R., ed. *Updating Life and Death.* Boston: Beacon Press, 1969.

Duncan, A. S. et al., eds. *Dictionary of Medical Ethics.* London: Darton, Longman, and Todd, 1975.

Englehardt, H. Tristram, Jr., and Daniel Callahan, eds. *Science, Ethics and Medicine.* Hastings-on-Hudson, N.Y.: Institute of Society, Ethics and the Life Sciences, 1976.

Fletcher, Joseph. *Morals and Medicine*. Boston: Beacon Press, 1954. A classic book stating the Christian "situation ethics" view of euthanasia, truth telling, contraception, etc.

Glover, Jonathan. *Causing Death and Saving Lives*. New York: Penguin Books, 1977.

Gorovitz, Samuel, et al., eds. *Moral Problems in Medicine*. Englewood Cliffs, N.J.: Prentice-Hall, 1976.

Humber, James M. and Robert F. Almeder, eds. *Biomedical Ethics and the Law*. New York: Plenum Publishing Corporation, 1976.

Hunt, Robert and John Arras, eds. *Ethical Issues in Modern Medicine*. Palo Alto, Calif.: Mayfield Publishing Company, 1977. Good selections and good introductions.

Kunz, Robert M., and Hans Fehr, eds. *The Challenge of Life: Biomedical Progress and Human Values*. Basel: Birkhauser Verlag, 1972.

Labby, Daniel H., ed. *Life or Death: Ethics and Options*. Seattle: University of Washington Press, 1968.

Mappes, Thomas A., and Jane S. Zembaty, eds. *Biomedical Ethics*. New York: McGraw-Hill, 1980.

Mendelsohn, Everett, Judith P. Swazey, and Irene Taviss, eds. *Human Aspects of Biomedical Innovation*. Cambridge, Mass.: Harvard University Press, 1971.

Ostheimer, Nancy and John Ostheimer, eds. *Life or Death—Who Controls?* New York: Springer Publishing Company, 1976.

Peters, Karl E., ed. "Is Ethics A Science?" *Zygon* 15 (March 1980). Articles by Abraham Edel, R. B. Brandt, and Marcus Singer.

Rachels, James. "Can Ethics Provide Answers?" *Hastings Center Report* 10 (1980): 32–40.

Ramsey, Paul. *Ethics at the Edges of Life: Medical and Legal Intersections*. New Haven: Yale University Press, 1978.

———. *The Patient as Person*. New Haven: Yale University Press, 1970. A classic work by a Christian theologian that presents influential views on experimentation, transplantation, allocation of resources, etc.

Reich, W. T., ed. *Encyclopedia of Bioethics*. New York: Macmillan, 1978. A wide-ranging collection of articles by many scholars. Good for a quick survey of major issues.

Reidy, Maurice. *Foundations for a Medical Ethic*. New York: Paulist Press, 1979.

Reiser, S. J., A. J. Dyck, and W. J. Curran, eds. *Ethics in Medicine: Historical Perspectives and Contemporary Concerns*. Cambridge, Mass.: M.I.T. Press, 1977. A large book, strong on historical writings and documents but not on philosophy.

Rivlin, Alice M., and P. Michael Timpane, eds. *Ethical and Legal Issues of Social Experimentation*. Washington, D.C.: The Brookings Institution, 1975. See in particular "Ethical Principles in Medical Experimentation" by Robert M. Veatch.

Shannon, Thomas A., ed. *Bioethics*. New York: Paulist Press, 1981

Spicker, Stuart F. and H. Tristram Engelhardt, Jr., eds. *Philosophical Medical Ethics: Its Nature and Significance*. Boston: D. Reidel, 1977.

Torrey, E. Fuller, ed. *Ethical Issues in Medicine*. Boston: Little, Brown and Company, 1968.

Trial 16 (December 1980). An issue devoted to bioethical and biolegal issues.

Varga, Andrew C., S. J. *The Main Issues in Bioethics*. New York: Paulist Press, 1980.

Vaux, Kenneth. *Biomedical Ethics: Morality for the New Medicine*. New York: Harper and Row, 1974.

Veatch, Robert M. *Case Studies in Medical Ethics*. Cambridge: Harvard University Press, 1977.

———. *Death, Dying, and the Biological Revolution*. New Haven, Conn.: Yale University Press, 1976. Deals with dying patients, euthanasia, birth defects, defining death, and transplant organs. Contains much information.

———. *A Theory of Medical Ethics*. New York: Basic Books, 1981.

Wertz, Richard W., ed. *Readings on Ethical and Social Issues in Biomedicine*. Englewood Cliffs, N.J.: Prentice-Hall, 1973.

Williams, Granville. *The Sanctity of Life and the Criminal Law*. New York: Alfred Knopf, 1957.

Williams, Preston, ed. *Ethical Issues in Biology and Medicine*. Cambridge, Mass.: Schenkman Publishing Company, 1973. Original papers, several with a theological orientation.

Williams, Robert H., ed. *To Live and to Die: When, Why, and How*. New York: Springer-Verlag, 1973.

Wojcik, Jan. *Muted Consent: A Case Book of Modern Medical Ethics*. West Lafayette, Ind.: Purdue University Press, 1978.

Yezzi, Ronald. *Medical Ethics: Thinking About Unavoidable Questions*. New York: Holt, Rinehart, and Winston, 1980.

Bibliographies

American Nurses' Association, Committee on Ethics. *Ethics in Nursing: References and Resources*. Kansas City, Mo.: American Nurses' Association, 1979.

"Bioethics and the Law: A bibliography, 1974–1976."

American Journal of Law and Medicine 2 (Winter 1976–1977): 263–281.

A Comprehensive Set of Bibliographies on Voluntary Sterilization. New York: The International Project of the Association for Voluntary Sterilization, January 1976.

Calhoun, Cheryl. *Annotated Bibliography of Medical Oaths, Codes, and Prayers*. Washington, D.C.: Kennedy Institute, 1975.

Carmody, James. *Ethical Issues in Health Services: A Report and Annotated Bibliography*. Washington, D.C.: U.S. Department of Health, Education, and Welfare, 1974.

Clouser, K. Danner and Arthur Zucker. *Abortion and Euthanasia: An Annotated Bibliography*. Philadelphia: Society for Health and Human Values, 1974.

Euthanasia: An Annotated Bibliography. New York: Euthanasia Educational Fund, 1970.

Goldstein, Doris M. *Bioethics: A Guide to Information Sources*. Detroit: Gale Research Company, 1982.

Kalish, Richard A. "Death and Dying: A Briefly Annotated Bibliography." In *The Dying Patient*. Edited by Orville G. Brim, Jr., et al. New York: Russell Sage Foundation, 1970, pp. 323–380.

Kutscher, A. *Bibliography of Books on Death, Bereavement, Loss, and Grief: 1955–1968*. New York: Health Sciences Publishing Corporation, 1969.

Lineback, Richard H., ed. *Philosopher's Index*. Vols. 1–. Bowling Green, Ohio: Philosophy Documentation Center, Bowling Green State University. Issued quarterly.

Nevins, Madeline M., ed. *Annotated Bibliography of Bioethics: Selected 1976 Titles*. Rockville, Md.: Information Planning Associations, 1977.

Sollitto, Sharmon and Robert M. Veatch. Revised by Ira D. Singer. *Bibliography of Society, Ethics and the Life Sciences: 1979–1980*. Hastings-on-Hudson, N.Y.: Institute of Society, Ethics and the Life Sciences, 1978. This is the best general bibliography and also the best guide to philosophical articles on medical ethics. It is partially annotated and brought up to date periodically.

Sorenson, James R. *Social and Psychological Aspects of Applied Human Genetics: A Bibliography*. Washington, D.C.: Department of Health, Education, and Welfare, 1973.

Vernick, Joel J. *Selected Bibliography on Death and Dying*. Washington, D.C.: U.S. Department of Health, Education, and Welfare, National Institute of Health, n.d.

Walters, LeRoy, ed. *Bibliography of Bioethics*. Vols. 1,2. Detroit: Gale Research Company, 1975, 1976.

Ethical Theories and Medical Decisions: An Introduction

A. General Works on Ethics

Brandt, Richard B. *Ethical Theory*. Englewood Cliffs, N.J.: Prentice-Hall, 1959.

Ewing, A. C. *Ethics*. New York: Free Press, 1965.

Feinberg, Joel. *Doing and Deserving: Essays in the Theory of Responsibility*.

———. *Social Philosophy*. Englewood Cliffs, N.J.: Prentice-Hall, 1973.

———. *Rights, Justice, and the Bounds of Liberty*. Princeton, N.J.: Princeton University Press, 1980.

Frankena, William K. *Ethics*. 2d ed. Englewood Cliffs, N.J.: Prentice-Hall, 1973.

Gert, Bernard. *The Moral Rules*. New York: Harper and Row, 1970.

Ladd, John. *Ethical Relativism*. Belmont, Calif.: Wadsworth Publishing Company, 1973.

Rachels, James. *Understanding Moral Philosophy*. Encino, Calif.: Dickenson Publishing Company, 1976. A short, readable introduction.

Taylor, Paul W., ed. *The Moral Judgment: Readings in Contemporary Meta-Ethics*. Englewood Cliffs, N.J.: Prentice-Hall, 1963.

———, ed. *Problems of Moral Philosophy*. Belmont, Calif.: Dickenson Publishing Company, 1971. Clear and sophisticated introduction.

Warnock, Geoffrey James. *Contemporary Moral Philosophy*. New York: St. Martin's Press, 1967.

Wellman, Carl. *Morals and Ethics*. New York: Scott, Foresman, 1975.

Williams, Bernard. *Morality: An Introduction to Ethics*. New York: Harper and Row, 1972.

B. Utilitarianism

Bayles, Michael D., ed. *Contemporary Utilitarianism*. New York: Doubleday, 1968.

Bentham, Jeremy. *A Fragment on Government and An Introduction to the Principles of Morals and Legislation*. Edited by Wilfried Harrison. Oxford: Blackwell, 1967.

Hodgson, D. H. *Consequences of utilitarianism: A Study in Normative Ethics and Legal Theory*. Oxford: Clarendon Press, 1967.

Lyons, David. *Forms and Limits of Utilitarianism*. New York: Oxford University Press, 1965.

———. *In the Interest of the Governed: A Study in Bentham's Philosophy of Utility and Law*. Oxford: Oxford University Press, 1973.

Mill, John Stuart. *Utilitarianism: With Critical Essays*. Edited by Samuel Gorovitz. Indianapolis: Bobbs-Merrill, 1971.

Quinton, A. M. *Utilitarian Ethics.* New York: St. Martin's Press, 1973.

Regan, Donald H. *Utilitarianism and Co-operation.* New York: Oxford University Press, 1980.

Smart, J. J. C. and Bernard Williams. *Utilitarianism: For and Against.* New York: Cambridge University Press, 1973.

C. Kant

Beck, L. W. *Studies in the Philosophy of Kant.* Indianapolis: Bobbs-Merrill, 1965.

Kant, Immanuel. *Foundations of the Metaphysics of Morals: Text and Critical Essays.* Edited by Robert P. Wolff. New York: Bobbs-Merrill, 1969.

———. *Lectures on Ethics.* New York: Harper and Row, 1963.

Paton, H. J. *The Categorical Imperative: A Study of Kant's Moral Philosophy.* New York: Harper and Row, 1967.

Singer, Marcus G. *Generalization in Ethics: An Essay in the Logic of Ethics, with the Rudiments of a System of Moral Philosophy.* New York: Atheneum, 1971.

Wolff, R. P., ed. *Kant: A Collection of Critical Essays.* Garden City, New York: Doubleday, 1967.

D. Ross

Ross, W. D. *Foundations of Ethics.* Oxford: Oxford University Press, 1963. A reissue of the 1939 edition.

Ross, W. D. *The Right and the Good.* Oxford: Clarendon Press, 1930. (For evaluations of Ross, see relevant sections of Frankena, Brandt, Ewing, Rachels, and Taylor listed above.)

E. Rawls

Barry, Brian. *The Liberal Theory of Justice.* New York: Oxford University Press, 1974. An exposition and criticism of Rawls.

Chen, Marshall. "The Social Contract Explained and Defended." *New York Book Review,* 16 July 1972, p. 1.

Daniels, Norman, ed. *Reading Rawls.* New York: Basic Books, 1976. This volume has a helpful introduction and contains some of the more important critical articles.

F. Aquinas and Natural Law

Copleston, F. C. *Aquinas.* Baltimore: Penguin Books, 1965.

Gilson, Etienne. *The Philosophy of St. Thomas Aquinas.* 3d ed. Translated by Edward Bullough. St. Louis: Herder Book Company, 1937.

Kelly, Gerald. *Medico-Moral Problems.* St. Louis: Catholic Hospital Association, 1958.

McFadden, Charles J. *Medical Ethics.* 6th ed. Philadelphia: F. A. Davis, 1967.

O'Connor, D. J. *Aquinas and Natural Law.* New York: St. Martin's Press, 1969.

Pegis, Anton, ed. *Basic Writings of St. Thomas Aquinas.* New York: Random House, 1945.

Part I: Termination
Chapter 1: Abortion and Infanticide

Altman, Andrew. "Abortion and the Indigent." *Journal of Social Philosophy* 11 (1980): 5–9. Favors the Supreme Court decision that states need not fund abortions.

Annis, David. "Self-Consciousness and the Right to Life." *Southwestern Journal of Philosophy* 6 (1975): 123–128.

Bagley, C. "On the Sociology and Social Ethics of Abortion." *Ethics in Science and Medicine* 3 (1976): 21–32.

Becker, Laurence C. "Human Being: The Boundaries of the Concept." *Philosophy and Public Affairs* 4 (1975): 334–359. Attempts to develop a biological concept relevant to abortion and euthanasia.

Bok, Sissela. "Ethical Problems of Abortion." *Hastings Center Report* 2 (1974): 33–52.

———. "Who Shall Count as a Human Being? A Treacherous Question in the Abortion Discussion." In Robert L. Perkins, ed. *Abortion: Pro and Con.* Cambridge, Mass.: Schenkman, 1974, pp. 91–105.

Brandt, R. B. "The Morality of Abortion." *Monist* 56 (1972): 503–526.

Brody, Baruch. *Abortion and the Sanctity of Human Life.* Cambridge, Mass.: MIT Press, 1975. Brody's several papers are embodied here.

———. "Thomson on Abortion." *Philosophy and Public Affairs* 1 (1972): 335–340.

Callahan, Daniel. *Abortion: Law, Choice and Morality.* New York: Macmillan, 1970.

Camenisch, Paul F. "Abortion: For the Fetus's Own Sake?" *Hastings Center Report* 6 (1976): 38–41.

———. "Abortion Analogies and the Emergence of Value." *Journal of Religious Ethics* 4 (1976): 131–158.

Cohen, Marshall, et al., eds. *The Rights and Wrongs of Abortion.* Princeton: N.J. Princeton University Press, 1974.

Connery, John R. *Abortion: The Development of the Roman Catholic Perspective.* Chicago: Loyola University Press, 1977.

Daniels, Charles B. "Abortion and Potential." *Dialogue* 18 (June 1979): 220–223.

Engelhardt, H. Tristram. "The Ontology of Abortion." *Ethics* 84 (April 1974): 217–234.

Feinberg, Joel. "Abortion." In Tom Regan, ed. *Matters of Life and Death.* New York: Random House, 1980, pp. 183–217.

———. "Is There a Right to Be Born?" In James Rachels, ed. *Understanding Moral Philosophy.* Belmont, Calif.: Dickenson Publishing Company, 1976.

———, ed. *The Problem of Abortion.* Belmont, Calif.: Wadsworth Publishing Company, 1973.

Finnis, John, Judith Thomson, Michael Tooley, and Roger Wertheimer. *The Rights and Wrongs of Abortion.* Princeton, N.J.: Princeton University Press, 1974. A collection of influential articles.

Fletcher, Joseph. "Four Indicators of Humanhood— The Enquiry Matures." *Hastings Center Report* 4 (December 1974): 4–7.

Foot, Phillippa. "The Problem of Abortion and the Doctrine of Double Effect." *Oxford Review* 5 (1967): 5–15.

Gerber, D. "Abortion: The Uptake Argument." *Ethics* 83 (1972): 80–83.

Gerber, R. J. "Abortion: Parameters for Decision." *Ethics* 82 (1972).

Gillespie, Norman C. "Abortion and Human Rights." *Ethics* 87 (April 1977): 237–243.

Goldman, Alan H. "Abortion and the Right to Life." *Personalist* 60 (October 1979): 402–406.

Goodrich, T. "The Morality of Killing." *Philosophy* 44 (1969): 127–139.

Gordon, Robert M. "The Abortion Issue." In Eugene Freeman, ed. *The Abdication of Philosophy: Essays in Honor of Paul A. Schilpp.* Chicago: Open Court, 1974, pp. 267–277.

Granfield, David. *The Abortion Decision.* New York: Doubleday, 1971. A Catholic point of view.

Hall, Robert E., ed. *Abortion in a Changing World.* New York: Columbia University Press, 1970.

Hare, R. M. "Abortion and the Golden Rule." *Philosophy and Public Affairs* 4 (1975): 201–222.

Harrison, S. M. "The Unwilling Dead." *Proceedings of the Catholic Philosophical Association* 46 (1972): 199–208. Argues that the concept of a person is central to the abortion issue and offers one based on C. S. Peirce.

Herbewick, Raymond M. "Remarks on Abortion, Abandonment, and Adoption Opportunities." *Philosophy and Public Affairs* 5 (Fall 1975): 98–104.

Humber, James M. "The Case against Abortion." *The Thomist* 39 (1975): 65–84. A criticism of major arguments.

Jaffee, Frederick, Barbara Lindheim, and Philip Lee. *Abortion Politics: Private Morality and Public Policy.* New York: McGraw-Hill, 1981.

Kohl, Marvin. "Abortion and the Argument from Innocence." *Inquiry* 14 (1971): 147–151.

———, ed. *Infanticide and the Value of Life.* Buffalo, N.Y.: Prometheus Books, 1978.

Langham, Paul. "Between Abortion and Infanticide." *Southern Journal of Philosophy* 17 (1979): 465–471.

Levy, Steven R. "Abortion and Dissenting Parents: A Dialogue." *Ethics* 90 (1980): 162–163.

Manier, Edward, William Liu, and David Solomon. *Abortion: New Directions for Policy Studies.* Notre Dame, Ind.: University of Notre Dame Press, 1977.

Margolis, Joseph. "Abortion." *Ethics* 84 (1973): 51–61.

Moore, E. C., et al. "Abortion: The New Ruling." *Hastings Center Report* 3 (1973): 4–7.

Moore, Harold F. "Abortion and the Logic of Moral Justification." *Journal of Value Inquiry* 9 (1975): 140–151.

Noonan, John T. *A Private Choice: Abortion in America in the Seventies.* New York: Free Press, 1979.

Pole, Nelson. "To Respect Human Life." *Philosophical Context* 2 (1973): 16–22. Argues that a right to abortion promotes human dignity.

Regan, Tom. *Matters of Life and Death.* New York: Random House, 1980.

Rorty, Amelie O. "Persons, Policies, and Bodies." *International Philosophical Quarterly* 13 (March 1973): 63–80.

Schneider, Carl E. and Maris A. Vinouskis, eds. *The Law and Politics of Abortion.* Lexington, Mass.: D. C. Heath and Company, 1980.

Sher, George. "Hare, Abortion and the Golden Rule." *Philosophy and Public Affairs* 6 (Winter 1977): 185–190.

Sumner, L. W. *Abortion and Moral Theory.* Princeton, N.J.: Princeton University Press, 1981.

Talmage, R. S. "Utilitarianism and the Morality of Killing." *Philosophy* 47 (1972): 55–63.

Thomson, Judith Jarvis. "Rights and Deaths." *Philosophy and Public Affairs* 2 (1973): 146–159.

Tietze, Christopher. *Induced Abortion: A World Review, 1981.* New York: The Population Council, 1981.

Vandever, Donald. "Justifying Wholesale Slaughter." *Canadian Journal of Philosophy* 5 (1975): 245–258.

Wade, Francis C. "Potentiality in the Abortion Discussion." *Review of Metaphysics* 29 (December 1975): 239–255.

Warren, Mary Anne. "Do Potential People Have Moral Rights?" *Canadian Journal of Philosophy* 7 (June 1977): 275–289.

Wasserstrom, Richard. "The Status of the Fetus." *Hastings Center Report* 5 (June 1975): 18–22.

Weiss, Roslyn. "The Perils of Personhood." *Ethics* 89 (October 1978): 66–75.

Werner, Richard. "Abortion: The Moral Status of the Unborn." *Social Theory and Practice* 3 (Fall 1974): 201–222.

———. "Abortion: The Ontological and Moral Status of the Unborn." In Richard A. Wasserstrom, ed. *Today's Moral Problems*, 2nd ed. New York: Macmillan, 1979, pp. 51–74.

Wertheimer, Roger. "Understanding the Abortion Argument." *Philosophy and Public Affairs* 1 (1971): 67–95. A clear statement of issues.

Zaitchik, Alan. "Viability and the Morality of Abortion." *Philosophy and Public Affairs* 10 (Winter 1981): 18–26.

Chapter 2: Treating or Terminating: The Problem of Birth Defects

Augenstein, Leroy. "Birth Defects, The Ethical Problem." *Humanist* 28 (1968): 18–20.

A Children's Physician. "Non-Treatment of Defective Newborn Babies." *Lancet* 2 (24 November 1979): 1123–1124.

Coburn, Robert C. "Morality and the Defective Newborn." *Journal of Medicine and Philosophy* 5 (December 1980): 340–357.

Darling, Rosalyn Benjamin. "Parents, Physicians, and Spina Bifida." *Hastings Center Report* 7 (August 1977): 10–13.

Duff, R. S. and A. G. M. Campbell. "Moral and Ethical Dilemmas in the Special Care Nursery." *New England Journal of Medicine* 289 (1973): 890–894.

Engelhardt, H. T. "Euthanasia and Children: The Inquiry of Continued Existence." *Journal of Pediatrics* 83 (1973): 170–171.

Fletcher, John C. "Abortion, Euthanasia, and Care of Defective Newborns." *New England Journal of Medicine* 292 (1975): 75–78.

———. "Attitudes toward Defective Newborns." *Hastings Center Studies* 2 (1974): 21–32.

———. "Choices for Life or Death in the Case of Defective Newborns." *Social Responsibility: Journalism, Law, Medicine*. Program on Society and the Professions: Studies in Applied Ethics. Lexington, Va.: Washington and Lee University, 1975, pp. 62–78.

Freeman, J. M. "To Treat or Not to Treat: Ethical Dilemmas of Treating the Infant with a Myelomeningocele." *Clinical Neurosurgery* 20 (1973): 134–146.

Gustafson, James M. "Mongolism, Parental Desires, and the Right to Life." *Perspectives in Biology and Medicine* 16 (1973): 529–557.

Hemphill, M., et al. "Ethical Aspects of Care of the Newborn with Serious Neurological Disease." *Clinical Perinatology* 4 (March 1977): 201–209.

Hetmann, Philip B., and Sara Holtz. "The Severely Defective Newborn: The Dilemma and the Decision Process." *Public Policy* 23 (Fall 1975): 381–418.

Jonsen, A.R., et al. "Critical Issues in Newborn Intensive Care: A Conference Report and Policy Proposal." *Pediatrics* 55 (1975): 756–768.

——— and Michael J. Garland, eds. *Ethics of Newborn Intensive Care*. Berkeley: University of California, Institute of Governmental Studies, 1976.

Kelly, S., et al., eds. *Birth Defects*. New York: Academic Press, 1976.

Kelsey, Beverly. "Which Infants Shall Live? Who Shall Decide?" *Hastings Center Report* 5 (April 1975): 5–7.

Kohl, Marvin, ed. *Infanticide and the Value of Life*. Buffalo, N.Y.: Prometheus Books, 1978. See in particular papers by Richard Brandt and R. S. Duff.

Lorber, John. "Selective Treatment of Myelomeningocele." *Pediatrics* 53 (1974): 307–308.

McCormick, Richard A. "To Save or Let Die: The Dilemma of Modern Medicine." *Journal of the American Medical Association* 229 (1974): 172–76.

Sherlock, Richard. "Selective Non-Treatment of Defective Newborns: A Critique." *Ethics in Science and Medicine* 7 (1980): 111–117.

Smith, David H. "On Letting Some Babies Die." *Hastings Center Studies* 2 (1974): 37–46.

Smith, G. and E. D. Smith. "Selection for Treatment in Spina Bifida Cystica." *British Medical Journal* 27 (October 1973): 189–204.

Swinyard, Chester A., ed. *Decision Making and the Defective Newborn*. Springfield, Ill.: Charles C. Thomas, 1978.

Veatch, Robert M. "The Technical Criteria Fallacy." *Hastings Center Report* 7 (August 1977): 15–16.

Waldman, A. M. "Medical Ethics and the Hopelessly Ill Child." *Journal of Pediatrics* 88 (1976): 890–892.

Chapter 3: Euthanasia

Annas, George J. "In re Quinlan: Legal Comfort for Doctors." *Hastings Center Report* 6 (1976): 29–31. A criticism of the grounds of the New Jersey Supreme Court decision.

Anscombe, G. E. M. "Reply to Bennett's 'Whatever the Consequences.' " *Analysis* 26 (1966): 16–17.

Barnard, Christian. *Good Life/Good Death: A Doctor's Case for Euthanasia and Suicide*. Englewood Cliffs, N.J.: Prentice-Hall, 1980.

Bayles, Michael D. "The Value of Life—By What Standard?" *American Journal of Nursing* 80 (December 1980): 2226–2230.

Baylor Law Review 27 (Winter 1975). Entire issue on euthanasia.

Beauchamp, T. L. and S. Perlin, eds. *Ethical Issues in Death and Dying*. Englewood Cliffs, N.J.: Prentice-Hall, 1978.

Beauchamp, Tom L. "The Moral Justification for Withholding Heroic Procedures." In Nora K. Bell, ed. *Who Decides? Conflicts of Rights in Health Care*. Clifton, N.J.: Humana Press, 1982.

———. "A Reply to Rachels on Active and Passive Euthanasia." In Wade L. Robinson and Michael S. Pritchard, eds. *Medical Responsibility*. Clifton, N.J.: Humana Press, 1979, pp. 182–195. See also Rachels below.

Behnke, John A. and Sissela Bok. *The Dilemmas of Euthanasia*. New York: Doubleday Anchor, 1975.

Benjamin, Martin. "Moral Agency and Negative Acts in Medicine." In Wade L. Robinson and Michael S. Pritchard, eds. *Medical Responsibility*. Clifton, N.J.: Humana Press, 1979, pp. 170–181.

Bennett, Jonathan. "Whatever the Consequences." *Analysis* 26 (1966): 83–102.

Beresford, H. Richard. "Who Should Decide to Withhold Care in Chronic Coma?" *Archives of Neurology* 33 (1976): 371.

Bernat, James L., et al. "On the Definition and Criterion of Death." *Annals of Internal Medicine* 94 (March 1981): 389–394.

Black, Peter M. "Focusing on Some Ethical Problems Associated with Death and Dying." *Geriatrics* 31 (1976): 138–141.

———. "Three Definitions of Death." *Monist* 60 (January 1977): 136–146.

Bok, Sissela. "Personal Directions for Care at the End of Life." *New England Journal of Medicine* 295 (12 August 1976): 367–369.

Cahill, L. S. "A 'Natural Law' Reconsideration of Euthanasia." *Linacre Quarterly* 44 (February 1977): 47–63.

Cantor, Norman L. "A Patient's Decision to Decline Lifesaving Medical Treatment." *Rutgers Law Review* 26 (1973): 228.

Cassem, Ned. "When Illness Is Judged Irreversible: Imperative and Elective Treatments." *Man and Medicine* 5 (1980): 154–166.

Childress, James F. "To Live or Let Die," In his *Priorities in Biomedical Ethics*. Philadelphia: Westminster Press, 1981, pp. 34–50.

Collins, V. J. "Limits of Medical Responsibility in Prolonging Life: Guides to Decision." *Journal of the American Medical Association* 206 (1968): 389–392.

Devine, Philip E. *The Ethics of Homicide*. Ithaca, N.Y.: Cornell University Press, 1978.

Dinello, Daniel. "On Killing and Letting Die." *Analysis* 31 (1971): 83–86. A criticism of Jonathan Bennett's "Whatever the Consequences."

Downing, A. B., ed. *Euthanasia and the Right to Die: The Case for Voluntary Euthanasia*. London: Peter Owen, 1969. See in particular the article by Anthony Flew.

Elkinton, J. R. "When Do We Let the Patient Die?" *Annals of Internal Medicine* 68 (1968): 695–700.

Feinberg, Joel. "Voluntary Euthanasia and the Inalienable Right to Life." *Philosophy and Public Affairs* 7 (Winter 1978): 93–123.

Fitzgerald, P. J. "Acting and Refraining." *Analysis* 27 (1974): 133–139.

Fletcher, Joseph. "Elective Death." In E. F. Torrey, ed. *Ethical Issues in Medicine*. Boston: Little, Brown, 1968.

———. "Ethics and Euthanasia." In Robert H. Williams, ed. *To Live and To Die: When, Why, and How*. New York: Springer Verlag, 1973, pp. 113–122.

———. "The 'Right' to Live and the 'Right' to Die." *The Humanist* 34 (1974): 12–15.

Fried, Charles. "Terminating Life Support: Out of the Closet." *New England Journal of Medicine* 295 (12 August 1976): 390–391.

Geddes, Leonard. "On the Intrinsic Wrongness of Killing Innocent People." *Analysis* 33 (1974): 93–97. A criticism of Jonathan Bennett's "Whatever the Consequences."

Gillick, Muriel. "The Ethics of Cardiopulmonary Resuscitation: Another Look." *Ethics in Science and Medicine* 7 (1980): 161–169.

Goodrich, T. "The Morality of Killing." *Philosophy* 44 (1969): 127–129. Euthanasia and abortion.

Green, Michael B. and Daniel Wikler. "Brain Death and Personal Identity." *Philosophy and Public Affairs* 9 (Winter 1980): 105–133.

Grisez, Germain and Joseph M. Boyle, Jr. *Life and Death with Liberty and Justice: A Contribution to the Euthanasia Debate*. Notre Dame, Ind.: University of Notre Dame Press, 1979.

Hare, R. M. "Euthanasia: A Christian View," *Proceedings of the Center for Philosophic Exchange* 2 (1975): 43–52.

Hausman, David B. "On Abandoning Life Support: An Alternative Proposal." *Man and Medicine* 2 (Spring 1977): 169–177. Also see 178–188 for commentaries.

Horan, Dennis J. and David Mall, eds. *Death, Dying, and Euthanasia*. Washington, D.C.: University Publications of America, 1977.

Human Life Review 2 (Spring 1976): 27–70. Three articles on euthanasia.

Institute of Society, Ethics and the Life Sciences, Task Force on Death and Dying. "Refinements in Criteria for the Determination of Death." *Journal of the American Medical Association* 221 (3 July 1972): 48–53.

Jonsen, Albert R. "Dying Right in California: The Natural Death Act." *Clinical Research* 26 (February 1978): 55–60

Kamisar, Yale. "Some Non-Religious Views against Proposed 'Mercy-Killing' Legislation." *Minnesota Law Review* 42 (1958): 969–1042.

Kelly, Gerald. "The Duty of Using Artificial Means of Preserving Life." *Theological Studies* 11 (1950): 203–220.

———. "The Duty to Preserve Life." *Theological Studies* 12 (1951): 550–556.

Kohl, Marvin, ed. *Beneficent Euthanasia.* Buffalo, N.Y.: Prometheus Books, 1975. Contains several interesting philosophical articles.

———. "Beneficent Euthanasia." *The Humanist* 34 (1974): 9–11.

———. "Understanding the Case for Beneficent Euthanasia." *Science, Medicine and Man* 1 (1973): 111–121.

———. "The Word 'Mercy' and the Problem of Euthanasia." *The American Rationalist* 9 (1965): 5–7.

Ladd, John, ed. *Ethical Issues Relating to Life and Death.* New York: Oxford University Press, 1979.

Lombardi, Joseph L. "Killing and Letting Die: What is the Moral Difference?" *New Scholasticism* 54 (1980): 200–212.

Long, P. H. "On the Quantity and Quality of Life: Fruitless Longevity." *Physician* 6 (1960): 69–70.

McIntyre, R. V. "Voluntary Euthanasia: The Ultimate Perversion." *Medical Counterpoint* 2 (1970): 26–29.

Maguire, Daniel C. "A Catholic View of Mercy Killing." *The Humanist* 34 (1974): 16–18.

———. *Death by Choice.* New York: Doubleday, 1974.

Margolis, Joseph. "On Being Allowed to Die." *The Humanist* 36 (1976): 17–19.

Meilaender, Gilbert. "The Distinction between Killing and Allowing to Die." *Theological Studies* 37 (September 1976): 467–470.

Menzel, Paul T. "Are Killing and Letting Die Morally Different in Medical Contexts?" *Journal of Medicine and Philosophy* 4 (September 1979): 269–293.

Middleton, Carl L., Jr. "Principles of Life-Death Decision Making." *Linacre Quarterly* 42 (1975): 268–278.

Monagle, John F. "Living Will Does Not Resolve Medical-Ethical-Legal Dilemma." *Hospital Progress* 57 (1976): 76–79.

Moore, F. D. "Medical Responsibility for the Prolongation of Life." *Journal of the American Medical Association* 206 (1968): 384–386.

Morrison, Robert and Leon Kass. "Death—Process or Event?" *Science* 173 (20 August 1971): 694–702.

Potter, Ralph B. "The Paradoxical Preservation of a Principle." *Villanova Law Review* 13 (1968): 874–892.

Rachels, James. "Euthanasia." In Tom Regan, ed. *Matters of Life and Death.* New York: Random House, 1980, pp. 28–66.

———. "Euthanasia, Killing, and Letting Die," in Wade L. Robinson and Michael S. Pritchard, eds. *Medical Responsibility.* Clifton, N.J.: Humana Press, 1979, pp. 153–169. See also Beauchamp.

———. "Killing and Starving to Death." *Philosophy* 54 (1979): 159–171.

Rhodes, Jonathan E. "The Right to Die and the Chance to Live." *Journal of Medical Ethics* 6 (1980): 53–54.

Robertson, John A. and Norman Fost. "Passive Euthanasia of Defective Newborn Infants: Legal Considerations." *Journal of Pediatrics* 88 (May 1976): 883–889.

Russell, O. Ruth. *Freedom to Die: Moral and Legal Aspects of Euthanasia.* New York: Human Sciences Press, 1975 (also New York: Dell Publishing Co., 1976). Contains a clear review of objections.

Strong, Carson. "Euthanasia: Is the Concept Really Nonevaluative?" *Journal of Medicine and Philosophy* 5 (December 1980): 313–325.

Suckiel, Ellen K. "Death and Benefit in the Permanently Unconscious Patient: A Justification of Euthanasia." *Journal of Medicine and Philosophy* 3 (March 1978): 38–52.

Sullivan, Thomas D. "Active and Passive Euthanasia: An Impertinent Distinction?" *Human Life Review* 3 (Summer 1977): 40–47.

Trammell, Richard L. "The Presumption Against Taking Life." *Journal of Medicine and Philosophy* 3 (March 1978): 53–67.

Vanderpool, H. Y. "The Ethics of Terminal Care." *Journal of the American Medical Association* 239 (27 February 1978): 850–852.

Veatch, Robert M. "Choosing Not to Prolong Dying." *Medical Dimensions* 1 (1972): 8–10.

Walton, Douglas N. "Omissions and Other Negative Actions." *Metamedicine* 1 (1980): 305–324.

———. *On Defining Death: An Analytic Study of the Concept of Death in Philosophy and Medical Ethics.* Montreal: McGill-Queen, 1979.

Weir, Robert F., ed. *Ethical Issues in Death and Dying.* New York: Columbia University Press, 1977.

White, R. J. "Medical and Ethical Problems of Long-Term Profound Unconsciousness." *Resuscitation* 5 (1976): 1–4.

Williams, Glanville. "Mercy-Killing Legislation—A Rejoinder." *Minnesota Law Review* 43 (1958): 1–12.

Williams, Peter C. "Rights and the Alleged Rights of Innocents to be Killed." *Ethics* 87 (July 1977): 383–394.

Wolstenholme, Gordon, et al. "Euthanasia." *Proceedings of the Royal Society of Medicine* 63 (1970): 659–670.

Young, Robert. "Voluntary and Involuntary Euthanasia." *Monist* 59 (April 1976): 264–283.

Chapter 4: Paternalism, Truth Telling, and Confidentiality

Annas, George J. "Confidentiality and the Duty to Warn." *Hastings Center Report* 6 (December 1976): 6–8.

Barber, Barry, et al. "Some Problems of Confidentiality in Medical Computing." *Journal of Medical Ethics* 2 (June 1976): 71–73.

Basson, Marc, ed. *Rights and Responsibilities in Modern Medicine.* New York: Alan R. Liss, 1981.

Beigler, Jerome (American Psychiatric Association Committee on Confidentiality). "Statement of the American Psychiatric Association Before the Subcommittee on Government Information and Individual Rights." *New York State Journal of Medicine* 79 (December 1979): 2088–2092.

British Medical Association. "New Horizons in Medical Ethics: Confidentiality." *British Medical Journal* (23 June 1973): 700–705.

Brody, Howard. "The Physician-Patient Contract: Legal and Ethical Aspects." *Journal of Legal Medicine* 4 (1976): 25–29.

Byrn, Robert M. "Compulsory Life-Saving Treatment for the Competent Adult." *Fordham Law Review* 44 (1975): 1–36.

Cantor, Norman L. "A Patient's Decision to Decline Life-Saving Medical Treatment: Bodily Integrity vs. the Preservation of Life." *Rutgers Law Review* 26 (1972): 228–264.

"Compulsory Medical Treatment: The State's Interest Re-evaluated." *Minnesota Law Review* 51 (1966): 293–305.

"The Confidentiality of Health Records." *Psychiatric Opinion* 12 (January 1975). Entire issue on confidentiality and society.

Cousins, Norman. "A Layman Looks at Truth-Telling in Medicine." *Journal of the American Medical Association* 244 (24 October 1980): 1929–1930.

Curran, W. J. "Ethical and Legal Problems in Medical Participation in Criminal Investigations." *New England Journal of Medicine* 249 (1976): 764–765.

———, et al. "Protection of Privacy and Confidentiality." *Science* 182 (1973): 797–802.

Davies, Edmund. "The Patient's Right to Know the Truth." *Proceedings of the Royal Society of Medicine* 66 (1973): 533–536.

Eck, Marcel. *Lies and Truth.* New York: Macmillan, 1970.

Everstine, Louis, et al. "Privacy and Confidentiality in Psychotherapy." *American Psychologist* 35 (September 1980): 828–840.

Ford, John C. "Refusal of Blood Transfusions by Jehovah's Witnesses." *Catholic Law* 10 (1964): 212–226.

Freedman, Alfred. "Threats to Confidentiality." *Journal of the American Academy of Psychoanalysis* 7 (January 1979): 1–5.

Fry, John. *A New Approach to Medicine: Principles and Priorities in Health Care.* Baltimore: University Park Press, 1978.

Gaylin, Willard and Daniel Callahan. "The Psychiatrist as Double Agent." *Hastings Center Report* 4 (February 1974): 11–14.

Gazza, B. A. "Compulsory Medical Treatment and Constitutional Guarantees: A Conflict?" *University of Pittsburgh Law Review* 33 (1972): 628–637.

Gewirth, Alan. "Human Rights and the Prevention of Cancer." *American Philosophical Quarterly* 17 (April 1980): 117–125.

Gibbs, R. F. "Money and Medical Ethics." *Journal of Legal Medicine* 4 (1976): 3–4.

Gilbert, Richard M. "Ethical Considerations in the Prevention of Smoking in Adults and Children." *Medicolegal News* 8 (June 1980): 4–7.

Gordis, Leon and Ellen Gold. "Privacy, Confidentiality, and the Use of Medical Records in Research." *Science* 207 (11 January 1980).

Grossman, M. "Confidentiality in Medical Practice." *Annual Review of Medicine* 28 (1977): 43–55.

Gurevitz, Howard. "Tarasoff: Protective Privilege Versus Public Peril." *American Journal of Psychiatry* 134 (March 1977): 289–292.

Journal of Medical Ethics 2 (1976): 28–33. "Limits of Confidentiality."

Kelsey, Jennifer L. "Privacy and Confidentiality in Epidemiological Research Involving Patients." *IRB: A Review of Human Subjects Research* 3 (February 1981): 1–4.

Litin, E. M. "Should the Cancer Patient be Told?" *Postgraduate Medicine* 28 (November 1960): 470–475.

Mahowald, Mary B. "Against Paternalism: A Developmental View." *Philosophy Research Archives* 6, no. 1386 (1980).

Marsh, Frank. "The 'Deeper Meaning' of Confidentiality within the Physician-Patient

Relationship." *Ethics in Science and Medicine* 6 (1979): 131–136.

Meyer, B. C. "Truth and the Physician." *Bulletin of the New York Academy of Medicine* 45 (January 1969): 59–71.

Nesbitt, Nancy A. "Tarasoff v. Regents of the University of California: Psychotherapist's Obligation of Confidentiality Versus the Duty to Warn." *Tulsa Law Journal* 12 (1977): 747–757.

Noll, John O. and Mark J. Hanlon. "Patient Privacy and Confidentiality at Mental Health Centers." *American Journal of Psychiatry* 133 (November 1976): 1286–1289.

Oken, Donald. "What to Tell Cancer Patients." *Journal of the American Medical Association* 175 (1961): 1120–1128.

Pemberton, L. B. "Diagnosis: Can/Should We Tell the Truth?" *Bulletin of the American College of Surgeons* (May 1971): 7–13.

Perr, I. N. "Confidentiality and Consent in the Psychiatric Treatment of Minors." *Journal of Legal Medicine* 4 (1976): 9–13.

Phillips, William R. "Patients, Pills, and Professionals: The Ethics of Placebo Therapy." *The Pharos* 44 (Winter 1981): 21–25.

Richardson, J. A. and Patricia Griffin. *Laetrile Case Histories*. New York: Bantam books, 1977.

Roth, L. H., et al. "Dangerousness, Confidentiality, and the Duty to Warn." *American Journal of Psychiatry* 134 (March 1977): 508–511.

Samuels, Alec. "The Duty of the Doctor to Respect the Confidence of the Patient." *Medicine, Science, and the Law* 20 (January 1980): 58–66.

Sissons, P. L. "The Place of Medicine in the American Prison: Ethical Issues in the Treatment of Offenders." *Journal of Medical Ethics* 2 (1976): 173–179.

Stein, Eugene J. "Doctors and Patients: Partners or Adversaries?" *Bioethics Quarterly* 2 (Summer 1980): 118–122.

Standard, Samuel and Helmuth Nathan, eds. *Should the Patient Know the Truth?* New York: Springer, 1955.

Thomson, Judith J. "The Right to Privacy." *Philosophy and Public Affairs* 4 (1975): 295–314.

Van de Veer, Donald. "Autonomy Respecting Paternalism." *Social Theory Practice* 6 (Summer 1980): 187–208.

———. "The Contractual Argument for Withholding Medical Information." *Philosophy and Public Affairs* 9 (Winter 1980): 198–205.

———. "Paternalism and Subsequent Consent." *Canadian Journal of Philosophy* 9 (1979): 631–642.

Wangenstein, O. H. "Should Patients Be Told They Have Cancer?" *Surgery* 27 (1950): 944–947.

Weir, Robert. "Truthtelling in Medicine." *Perspectives in Biology and Medicine* 24 (Autumn 1980): 95–112.

Wexler, David B. "Patients, Therapists, and Third Parties: The Victimological Virtues of Tarasoff." *International Journal of Law and Psychiatry* 2 (1979): 1–28.

Zimmerman, David R. "An Ethical Dilemma: Patient Privacy vs. His Insurability." *Modern Medicine* 42 (1974): 18–24.

Chapter 5: Medical Experimentation and Informed Consent.

AAP Task Force on Pediatric Research, Informed Consent and Medical Ethics. "AAP Code of Ethics for the Use of Fetuses and Fetal Material for Research." *Pediatrics* 56 (August 1975): 304–305.

Abrams, Natalie. "Justice in Fetal Experimentation." *Journal of Value Inquiry* 13 (1979): 103–113.

Annas, George J. *Informed Consent to Human Experimentation: The Subject's Dilemma*. Cambridge, Mass.: Ballinger Publishing Company, 1977.

———. "Report on the National Commission: Good as Gold." *Bioethics Quarterly* 2 (Summer 1980): 84–93. On the protection of human subjects.

———. *The Rights of Hospital Patients*. New York: Avon Books, 1975. Ayd, Frank J., Jr. "Fetology: Medical and Ethical Implications of Intervention in the Prenatal Period." *Annals of the New York Academy of Sciences* 169 (1970): 376–381.

Berber, Bernard. "The Ethics of Experimentation with Human Subjects." *Scientific American* 234 (1976): 25–31.

———, et al. *Research on Human Subjects: Problems of Social Control in Medical Experimentation*. New York: Russell Sage Foundation, 1973 (reprinted New Brunswick, N.J.: Transaction Books, 1979).

Bartholome, William G. "Parents, Children, and the Moral Benefits of Research." *Hastings Center Report* 6 (December 1976): 44–45.

Beauchamp, Tom L. and Ruth R. Faden. "Decision-Making and Informed Consent: A Study of the Impact of Disclosed Information." *Social Indicators Research* 7 (1980): 313–336. An empirical and normative study.

Beecher, H. K. "Ethics and Clinical Research." *New England Journal of Medicine* 274 (1966): 1354–1360.

———. "Experimentation in Man." *Journal of the American Medical Association* 169 (1959): 461–478.

———. *Research and the Individual: Human Studies*. Boston: Little, Brown, 1970.

Bloomberg, Seth Allan and Leslie Wickins. "Ethics of Research Involving Human Subjects in Criminal Justice." *Crime and Delinquency* (October 1977): 435–444.

Bogomolny, Robert L., ed. *Human Experimentation.* Dallas: Southern Methodist University Press, 1976.

British Medical Association. "New Horizons in Medical Ethics: Research Investigation and the Fetus." *British Medical Journal* (26 May 1973): 464–468.

Capron, Alexander. "Informed Consent in Catastrophic Disease Research." *University of Pennsylvania Law Review* 123 (1974): 340–438.

———. "Medical Research in Prisons." *Hastings Center Report* 3 (1973): 4–6. *Case Western Reserve Law Review* 24 (Spring 1975). A symposium on human experimentation.

Childress, James. "A Response to 'Conferred Rights and the Fetus.'" *Journal of Religious Ethics* 2 (1974): 27–33.

Cooke, Robert E. "An Ethical and Procedural Basis for Research on Children." *Journal of Pediatrics* 90 (April 1977): 681–682.

Cowles, Jane. *Informed Consent.* New York: Coward, McCann and Geoghegan, 1976.

Curran, W. J. "The Tuskegee Syphilis Study." *New England Journal of Medicine* 289 (4 October 1973): 730–731.

Eisenberg, Leon. "The Social Imperatives of Medical Research." *Science* 198 (December 1977): 1105–1110.

Experiments and Research with Humans: Values in Conflict. Washington, D.C.: National Academy of Sciences, 1975.

Federal Proceedings 36 (September 1977): 2344–2364. Special section on drugs and human research.

Fletcher, John. "Human Experimentation: Ethics in the Consent Situation." *Law and Contemporary Problems* 32 (1967): 620–649. A good general review.

Forssman, Werner. *Experiments on Myself: Memoirs of a Surgeon in Germany.* New York: St. Martin's Press, 1974. An experimenter who used himself as a research subject for cardiac catheterization.

Freund, Paul A. "Ethical Problems in Human Experimentation." *New England Journal of Medicine* 273 (1965): 687–692.

———, ed. *Experimentation with Human Subjects.* New York: George Braziller, 1970. An influential collection of twenty articles.

Fried, Charles. *Medical Experimentation: Personal Integrity and Social Policy.* New York: American Elsevier, 1974.

Gardner, E. Clifton. "Ethical Issues in the Testing of New Drugs in Man." *Journal of Drug Issues* 7 (Summer 1977): 275–286.

Gaylin, Willard and Marc Lappé. "Fetal Policies: The Debate on Experimenting with the Unborn." *Atlantic Monthly* 235 (May 1975): 66–71.

Goldiamond, Israel. "Protection of Human Subjects and Patients: A Social Contingency Analysis of Distinctions between Research and Practice and Its Implications." *Behaviorism* 4 (1976): 1–41.

Graham, John B. "Ethical and Social Issues Posed by Genetic Studies of Cardiovascular Disease." *Perspectives in Biology and Medicine* 20 (Winter 1977): 260–270.

Guttentag, O. E. "Ethical Problems in Human Experimentation." In E. F. Torrey, ed. *Ethical Issues in Medicine.* Boston: Little, Brown, 1968.

Halper, Thomas. "Ethics and Medical Experimentation: Some Unconfronted Problems." *Connecticut Medicine* 40 (1976): 267–268.

Hastings Center Report 5 (June 1975): 13–46. Special issue on fetal research. Hatfield, Frank. "Prison Research: The View from Inside." *Hastings Center Report* 7 (February 1977): 11–12.

Heller, P. "Informed Consent and the Old-Fashioned Conscience of the Physician-Investigator." *Perspectives in Biology and Medicine* 20 (Spring 1977): 434–438.

Hilton, Bruce and Daniel Callahan, eds. *Ethical Issues in Human Genetics: Genetic Counseling and the Use of Genetic Knowledge.* New York: Plenum Publishing Corporation, 1976.

The Human Life Review 1 (Fall 1975). "A Symposium: Fetal Research."

Katz, Jay. *Experimentation with Human Beings.* New York: Russell Sage Foundation, 1972.

Kidd, Alexander M. "Limits of the Right of a Person to Consent to Experimentation on Himself." *Science* 117 (1953): 211–212.

Ladimer, Irving, ed. "New Dimensions in Legal and Ethical Concepts for Human Research.' *Annals of the New York Academy of Sciences* 169 (1970): 293–593.

——— and R. W. Newman, eds. *Clinical Investigation in Medicine: Legal, Ethical and Moral Aspects.* Boston: Boston University Press, 1963.

Langer, E. "Human Experimentation: New York Verdict Affirms Patients' Rights." *Science* 151 (1966): 663–666. On the Sloan-Kettering case.

Lebacqz, Karen and Robert Levine. "Respect for Persons and Informed Consent to Participate in Research." *Clinical Research* 25 (April 1977): 101–107.

Laforet, Eugene G. "The Fiction of Informed Consent." *Journal of the American Medical Association* 235 (12 April 1976): 1579–1585.

Lower, Charles U. et al. "Nontherapeutic Research on Children: An Ethical Dilemma." *Journal of Pediatrics* 84 (April 1974): 468–473.

Ludlum, James E. *Informed Consent.* Chicago: American Hospital Association, 1978. McCormick, Richard A. "Proxy Consent in the Experimentation Situation." *Perspectives in Biology and Medicine* 18 (Autumn 1974): 2–20.

———. "A Reply to Paul Ramsey— Experimentation in Children: Sharing in Sociality." *Hasting Center Report* 6 (December 1976): 41–46.

Macklin, Ruth. "Consent, Coercion, and Conflicts of Rights." *Perspectives in Biology and Medicine* 20 (Spring 1977): 360–371.

——— and Susan Sherwin. "Experimenting on Human Subjects: Philosophical Perspectives." *Case-Western Reserve Law Review* 25 (1975): 434–471. A good review of issues with respect to Mill, Kant, and Rawls. Part of a symposium on human experimentation.

Margolis, Joseph. "Conceptual Aspects of a Patient's Bill of Rights." *Journal of Value Inquiry* 11 (Summer 1977), 126–135.

Martin, Michael M. "Ethical Standards for Fetal Experimentation." *Fordham Law Review* 43 (1975): 548–570.

Meisel, Alan. "Informed Consent—The Rebuttal." And Mills, Don Harper. "Informed Consent—the Rejoinder." *Journal of the American Medical Association* 234 (1975): 615–616.

——— and Lisa Kabnick. "Informed Consent to Medical Treatment: An Analysis of Recent Legislation." *University of Pittsburgh Law Review* 41 (Spring 1980): 407–564.

Meyers, David W. *The Human Body and the Law.* Chicago: Aldine Publishing, 1970.

Miller, Leslie J. "Informed Consent: I, II, III, IV." *Journal of the American Medical Association* 244 (7 November 1980–12 December 1980): 2100–2103, 2347–2350, 2556–2558, 2661–2662.

Mills, D. H. "Whither Informed Consent?" *Journal of the American Medical Association* 229 (1974): 305–310.

Montange, C. H. "Informed Consent and the Dying Patient." *Yale Law Journal* 83 (1974): 1632–1664.

Murphy, Jeffrie G. "Therapy and the Problem of Autonomous Consent." *International Journal of Law and Psychiatry* 2 (1979): 415–430.

———. "Total Institution and the Possibility of Consent to Organic Therapies." *Human Rights* 5 (Fall 1975): 25–45.

Norton, Martin L. "When Does an Experimental/ Innovative Procedure Become an Accepted Procedure?" *Pharos* 38 (October 1975): 161–165.

Ramsey, Paul. "Children as Research Subjects— A Reply." *Hastings Center Report* 7 (April 1977): 40–41.

———. "A Reply to Richard McCormick—The Enforcement of Morals: Nontherapeutic Research on Children." *Hastings Center Report* 6 (August 1976): 21–30.

———. "The Enforcement of Morals: Nontherapeutic Research on Children." *Hastings Center Report* 6 (1975): 21–30.

———. "The Ethics of a Cottage Industry in an Age of Community and Research Medicine." *New England Journal of Medicine* 284 (1971): 700–706.

———. *The Ethics of Fetal Research.* New Haven: Yale University Press, 1975.

Ratnoff, O. D. and M. F. Ratnoff. "Ethical Responsibilities in Clinical Investigation." *Perspectives in Biology and Medicine* 11 (1967): 82–90.

Robinson, Wade L. and Michael S. Pritchard, eds. *Medical Responsibility: Paternalism, Informed Consent, and Euthanasia.* Clifton, N.J.: Humana Press, 1979. See in particular articles by Abrams, Browne, and Toulmin.

Schreiner, G. E. "The Ethics of Human Experimentation." *Pharos* 29 (1966): 78–83.

Science 198 (18 November 1977): 677–705. "Medical Research: Statistics and Ethics."

Varley, A. B. "Protection of Human Research Subjects: Are Ethics Necessary?" *Journal of Legal Medicine* 4 (1976): 23–26.

Veatch, Robert M. "Human Experimentation: The Crucial Choices Ahead." *Prism* 2 (1974): 58ff.

———. "'Experimental' Pregnancy." *Hastings Center Report* 1 (1971): 2–3. About the Goldzieher experiment, in which placebos were used instead of contraceptive pills.

Visscher, Maurice B. *Ethical Constraints and Imperatives in Medical Research.* Springfield, Ill.: Charles C. Thomas, 1975.

Walters, LeRoy. "Ethical Issues in Experimentation on the Human Fetus." *Journal of Religious Ethics* 2 (1974): 33–54.

———. "Some Ethical Issues in Research Involving Human Subjects." *Perspectives in Biology and Medicine* 20 (Winter 1977): 193–211.

Wecht, C. H. "Medical, Legal and Moral Considerations in Human Experiments Involving Minors and Incompetent Adults." *Journal of Legal Medicine* 4 (1976): 27–30.

Welt, L. G. "Reflections on the Problems of Human Experimentation." *Connecticut Medicine* 25 (1961): 75–78.

White, L. P. "Biomedical Experimentation on Prisoners." *Western Journal of Medicine* 124 (1976): 514–516.

Wolfenberger, W. "Ethical Issues in Research with Human Subjects." *Science* 155 (1967): 47–51.

Part III: Controls
Chapter 6: Behavior Control and Psychosurgery

American Behavioral Scientist 18 (May–June 1975). "New Technologies and Strategies for Social Control:

Ethical and Practical Limits." A special issue on psychosurgery, behavior control, etc. See in particular the articles by H. A. Bedau and Frank Ervin.

Annas, George. "Psychosurgery: Procedural Safeguards." *Hastings Center Report* 7 (April 1977): 11–13.

"Anthropotelemetry: Dr. Schwitzgebel's Machine." *Harvard Law Review* 80 (December 1966): 403–421. See the Schwitzgebel book below.

Bandura, A. *Principles of Behavior Modification.* New York: Holt, Rinehart, and Winston, 1969.

Beauchamp, Tom L. "The Regulation of Hazards and Hazardous Behaviors." *Health Education Monographs* 6 (Summer 1980): 242–257.

Bedau, Hugo Adam. "Physical Interventions to Alter Behavior in a Punitive Environment." *American Behavioral Scientist* 18 (1975): 657–678.

Black, Peter McL. "Psychiatric Diseases, Informed Consent, Psychosurgery: A Reply to Dr. Thomas Szasz." *The Humanist* (January–February 1978): 45–47.

——— and Thomas Szasz. "The Ethics of Psychosurgery." *The Humanist* (July–August 1977): 6–11.

Boorse, Christopher. "What A Theory of Mental Health Should Be." *Journal for the Theory of Social Behavior* 6 (April 1976): 61–84.

Boston University Law Review 54 (March 1974). "Symposium on Psychosurgery." A special issue. See in particular articles by Stephan Chorover, Vernon Mark, and John Mason.

Breggin, Peter. "The Return of Lobotomy and Psychosurgery." *Congressional Record* 118 (24 February 1972): E1602–E1612. The best known critic of psychosurgery reviews its history and offers objections.

Brock, Dan W. "Involuntary Commitment of the Mentally Ill: Some Moral Issues." In John W. Davis, et al., eds. *Contemporary Issues in Biomedical Ethics.* Clifton, N.J.: Humana Press, 1978, pp. 213–226.

California Supreme Court, 1 July 1976. 131 California *Reporter* 14. West Publishing Company. Opinion on Tarasoff.

Carrera, Frank and P. L. Adams. "An Ethical Perspective on Operant Conditioning." *Journal of the American Academy of Child Psychiatry* 9 (1970): 607–623.

Chodoff, Paul. "The Case for Involuntary Hospitalization of the Mentally Ill." *American Journal of Psychiatry* 133 (May 1976): 496–501.

Chorover, Stephan L. "Big Brother and Psychotechnology." *Psychology Today.* 43 (October 1973): 47–48.

Culver, Charles M. and Bernard Gert. "The Morality of Involuntary Hospitalization." In Stuart F. Spicker, et al., eds. *The Law-Medicine Relation: A Philosophical Exploration.* Boston: D. Reidel, 1981, pp. 159–175.

Curran, William J. "The Supreme Court and Madness: A Middle Ground on Proof of Mental Illness for Commitment." *New England Journal of Medicine* 301 (9 August 1979): 317–318.

Dalton, Elizabeth, et al. "Ethical Issues in Behavioral Control: A Preliminary Examination." *Man and Medicine* 2 (Autumn 1976): 1–40.

"Debate over Psychosurgery." *Journal of the American Medical Association* 225 (20 August 1973): 913–920.

Delgado, José M. R. "Psychocivilized Direction of Behavior." *Humanist* 32 (March–April 1972): 10–15.

Duquesne Law Review 13 (Summer 1975): 673–936. "Medical Experimentation on Behavior Control."

Ennis, Bruce J. and Richard D. Emery. *The Rights of Mental Patients.* New York: Avon Books, 1978.

Field, L. H., Henry Rollin, and C. A. H. Watts. "New Horizons in Medical Ethics: Changing the Patient's Personality." *British Medical Journal* 2 (1973): 594–598.

Flew, Antony. *Crime or Disease?* New York: Barnes and Noble, 1973.

Gardner, C. Q. "Deliberate Efforts to Control Human Behavior and Modify Personality." *Deadalus* 96 (Summer 1967).

Gaylin, Willard. "On the Borders of Persuasion: A Psychoanalytic Look at Coercion." *Psychiatry* (February 1974): 1–9.

———, J. S. Meister, and Robert C. Neville, eds. *Operating on the Mind.* New York: Basic Books, 1975. Six essays on history, technique, and social and ethical issues. See in particular discussion on the Kaimowitz case.

Greenblatt, Steven J. "The Ethics and Legality of Psychosurgery." *New York Law School Law Review* 12 (1977): 961–980.

Hartmann, H. *Psychoanalysis and Moral Values.* New York: International University Press, 1960.

Harvard Law Review 85 (1972): 1489–1498. "Violence and the Brain."

Hasker, William. "The Critique of 'Mental Illness' Conceptual and/or Ethical Crisis?" *Journal of Psychology and Theology* 5 (Spring 1977): 110–124.

Holden, Constance. "Psychosurgery: Legitimate Therapy or Laundered Lobotomy?" *Science* 179 (1973): 1109–1112. A survey of current practices and a recent Congressional hearing.

Kittrie, Nicholas N. *The Right to be Different: Deviance and Enforced Therapy.* Baltimore: Johns Hopkins University Press, 1971.

Klerman, Gerald L. "Behavior Control and the Limits of Reform." *Hastings Center Report* 5 (1975): 40–45.

London, Perry. *Behavior Control.* New York: Harper and Row, 1969.

——. "Legislating the Brain: The Citizen as Patient." *Columbia Forum* 1 (1972): 2–7.

——. "Personal Liberty and Behavior Control Technology." *Hastings Center Report* 2 (1972): 4–7.

Macklin, Ruth. "Mental Health and Mental Illness: Some Problems of Definition and Concept Formation." *Philosophy of Science* 39 (September 1972): 341–365.

Mark, V. H. and F. R. Ervin. *Violence and the Brain.* New York: Harper and Row, 1970.

Mearns, E. A., Jr. "Law and the Physical Control of the Mind: Experimentation in Psychosurgery." *Case-Western Reserve Law Review* 25 (1975).

Michels, Robert. "Ethical Issues of Psychological and Psychotherapeutic Means of Behavior Control." *Hastings Center Report* 3 (1973): 11–13.

Murphy, Jeffrie G. "Total Institutions and the Possibility of Consent to Organic Therapies." *Human Rights* (Fall 1975): 24–25.

Narvard, Vincente. "Justice, Social Policy, and the Public's Health." *Medical Care* 15 (May 1977): 363–370.

Noll, John O. "The Psychotherapist and Informed Consent." *American Journal of Psychiatry* 133 (December 1976): 1451–1453.

Peszke, Michael. *Involuntary Treatment of the Mentally Ill: The Problem of Autonomy.* Springfield, Ill.: Charles C. Thomas, 1975.

Reiss, S. "A Critique of Thomas S. Szasz's 'Myth of Mental Illness.'" *American Journal of Psychiatry* 28 (March 1972): 1080–1084.

Rokeach, Milton. "Long Range Experimental Modification of Values, Attitudes and Behavior." *American Psychologist* 26 (1971): 453–459.

Rothman, David J. "Behavior Modification in Total Institutions." *Hastings Center Report* 5 (1975): 17–24.

Rozycki, Edward G. "Rewards, Reinforcers, and Voluntary Behavior." *Ethics* (1973): 38–47.

Salter, Andrew. "Psychosurgery vs. Political Psychiatrists." *Medical Opinion* 1 (1972): 46–51.

Schleifer, Michael. "Instrumental Conditioning and the Concept of the Voluntary." *Ethics* 82 (1972): 163–170. Concern is mostly epistemological.

Schrag, Peter. *Mind Control.* New York: Pantheon Books, 1978.

Schwitzgebel, Robert L. and Ralph K. Schwitzgebel, eds. *Psychotechnology: Electronic Control of Mind and Behavior.* New York: Holt, Rinehart, and Winston, 1973.

Shuman, Samuel I. *Psychosurgery and the Medical Control of Violence: Autonomy and Deviance.* Detroit: Wayne State University Press, 1977.

Skinner, B. F. *Beyond Freedom and Dignity.* New York: Alfred A. Knopf, 1971.

Smith, J. Sydney and L. G. Kiloh, eds. *Psychosurgery and Society.* Oxford: Pergamon Press, 1977.

Smith, W. Lynn and Arthur King, eds. *issues in Brain/Behavior Control.* New York: Spectrum Publications, 1976.

Spoonhour, J. M. "Psychosurgery and Informed Consent." *University of Florida Law Review* 26 (Spring 1974): 432–452.

Szasz, Thomas. *Law, Liberty, and Psychiatry: An Inquiry into the Social Uses of Mental Health Practices.* New York: Macmillan, 1963.

——. *The Myth of Mental Illness.* New York: Harper and Row, 1974.

——. *The Theology of Medicine: The Political-Philosophical Foundations of Medical Ethics.* New York: Harper and Row, 1977.

U.S. Senate Subcommittee on Constitutional Rights of the Committee on the Judiciary. *Individual Rights and the Federal Role in Behavior Modification.* Washington, D.C.: Government Printing Office, 1974.

Valenstein, Elliot S. *Brain Control: A Critical Examination of Brain Stimulation and Psychosurgery.* New York: John Wiley, 1973. See pp. 336–353 in particular.

Vispo, Paul H., ed. "The Dangerous Patient." *Psychiatric Quarterly* 52 (Summer 1980). A special issue on the topic. Includes discussions of the Tarasoff case.

Wheeler, Harvey, ed. *Beyond the Punitive Society: Operant Conditioning—Social and Political Aspects.* San Francisco: W. H. Freeman, 1973.

Winter, Arthur. *Surgical Control of Behavior.* Springfield, Ill.: Charles C. Thomas, 1971.

Zakowski, Phil. "Psychosurgery." *Journal of Legal Medicine* 4 (April 1976): 26–31.

Chapter 7: Genetics: Intervention, Control, and Research

The Ann Arbor Science for the People Editorial Collective. *Biology as a Social Weapon.* Minneapolis: Burgess Publishing Company, 1977.

Annas, George J. and Brian Cogne. "Fitness for the Birth and Reproduction: Legal Implications of Genetic Screening." *Family Law Quarterly* 9 (Fall 1975): 463–489.

Ausubel, F., J. Beckwith, and K. Janssen. "The Politics of Genetic Engineering: Who Decides Who's Defective." *Psychology Today* 7 (June 1974): 30–43. The authors are members of Science for the People.

Baker, Robert. "Protecting the Unconceived." In John W. Davis, Barry Hoffmaster, and Sarah Shorten, eds. *Contemporary Issues in Biomedical Ethics.* Clifton, N.J.: Humana Press, 1978, pp. 89–100.

Bass, I. Scott. "Governmental Control of Research in Positive Eugenics." *Journal of Law Reform* 8 (Spring 1974): 615–630.

Bayles, Michael D. "Harm to the Unconceived." *Philosophy and Public Affairs* 5 (Spring 1976): 292–304.

Beckwith, Jon and Jonathan King. "The XYY Syndrome: A Dangerous Myth." *New Scientist* 14 (November 1974): 474–476.

Beers, Roland F., Jr., and Edward G. Bassett, eds. *Recombinant Molecules: Impact on Science and Society.* New York: Raven Press, 1977.

Berg, Paul, et al. "Asilomar Conference on Recombinant DNA Molecules." *Science* 188 (1975): 991–994.

Breyer, Stephan and Richard Zeckhauser. "The Regulation of Genetic Engineering." *Man and Medicine* 1 (Winter 1976): 1–9.

Buckley, John J., Jr., ed. *Genetics Now: Ethical Issues in Genetic Research.* Washington, D.C.: University Press of America, 1978.

Bulletin of the Atomic Scientists 33 (May 1977): 10–33. Issue on recombinant DNA research.

Capron, Alexander. *Genetic Counseling: Facts, Values and Norms.* New York, Alan R. Liss, 1979.

———. "Reflections on Issues Posed by Recombinant DNA Molecule Technology." *Annals of the American Academy of Sciences* 265 (1976): 71–81. Entire issue is devoted to genetic issues.

Curran, William J. "The Questionable Virtues of Genetic Screening Laws." *American Journal of Public Health* 64 (1974): 1003–1004.

Daedalus 90 (1961). "Evolution and Man's Progress." See in particular the articles by Muller and Crow.

Danielli, James F. "Industry, Society, and Genetic Engineering." *Hastings Center Report* 2 (December 1972): 5–7.

Davidson, Michael D. "First Amendment Protection for Biomedical Research." *Arizona Law Review* 19 (1977): 893–918.

Davis, Bernard D. "Prospects for Genetic Intervention in Man." *Science* 170 (1970): 1279–1283.

Dobzhansky, Theodosius. "Changing Man." *Science* 155 (1967): 409–415.

Edwards, Robert G. "Fertilization of Human Eggs in Vitro: Morals, Ethics, and the Law." *Quarterly Review of Biology* 49 (March 1974): 3–26.

Ellison, Craig W., ed. *Modifying Man.* Washington, D.C.: University Press of America, 1978. A "Christian evangelical" view.

Etzioni, Amitai. "Amniocentesis: A Case Study of the Management of 'Genetic Engineering.'" *Ethics in Science and Medicine* 2 (May 1975): 13–24.

———. *Genetic Fix: The Next Technological Revolution.* New York: Harper and Row, 1975.

———. "Sex Control, Science and Society." *Science* 161 (1968): 1107–1112.

Ferguson, James R. "Scientific Inquiry and the First Amendment." *Cornell Law Review* 64 (April 1979): 639–665.

Fletcher, John C. "Ethics and Amniocentesis for Fetal Sex Identification." *Hastings Center Report* 10 (1980): 15–17.

———. "Moral and Ethical Problems of Pre-Natal Diagnosis." *Clinical Genetics* 8 (1975): 251–257.

Fletcher, Joseph. "Ethical Aspects of Genetic Controls." *New England Journal of Medicine* 285 (1971): 776–783.

Frankel, Charles. "The Specter of Eugenics." *Commentary* 57 (1974): 25–33.

Frankel, Mark S. "The Application of Genetic Technology: Ethics and Pitfalls." *Impact of Science on Society* 25 (1975): 85–90.

Friedman, Theodore. "The Future of Gene Therapy: A Reevaluation." *Annuals of the American Academy of Sciences* 265 (1976): 141–152.

Fudenberg, H. Hugh and Vijaya Melnick, eds. *Biomedical Scientists and Public Policy.* New York: Plenum Press, 1978.

Gastel, Barbara. *Maternal Serum Alpha-Fetoprotein: Issues in the Prenatal Screening and Diagnosis of Neural Tube Defects.* Washington: Government Printing Office, 1981.

Gaylin, Willard. "Genetic Screening: The Ethics of Knowing." *New England Journal of Medicine* 286 (22 June 1972): 1361–1362.

Georgia Law Review II (Summer 1977): 785–878. "Recombinant DNA and Technology Assessment." Special issue.

Golding, Martin. "Obligations to Future Generations." *The Monist* 56 (January 1972): 85–99.

Goodfield, June. *Playing God: Genetic Engineering and the Manipulation of Life.* New York: Random House, 1977.

Green, Harold P. "The Boundaries of Scientific Freedom." *Newsletter on Science, Technology, and Human Values* 20 (June 1977): 17–21.

Grobstein, Clifford. *A Double Image of the Double Helix: The Recombinant-DNA Debate.* San Francisco: W. H. Freeman, 1979.

Harris, Maureen, ed. *Early Diagnosis of Human Genetic Defects: Scientific and Ethical Considerations.* Fogarty International Center Proceedings, no. 6, 1972.

Hilton, Bruce, et al., eds. *Ethical Issues in Human Genetics: Genetic Counseling and the Use of Genetic Knowledge.* New York: Plenum Press, 1973.

Hoffman, John C. *Ethical Confrontation in Counseling.* Chicago: University of Chicago Press, 1979.

Holton, Gerald, ed. "Limits of Scientific Inquiry." *Daedalus* 107 (Spring 1978): 1–234. Special issue.

Hull, R. T. "Philosophical Considerations in the Growing Potential for Human Genetic Control." *Annals of the American Academy of Sciences* 265 (1976): 118–126.

Humber, James M. and Robert F. Almeder, eds. *Biomedical Ethics and the Law.* New York: Plenum Press, 1976.

Ingle, D. J. "Ethics of Genetic Intervention." *Medical Opinion Review* 3 (1967): 54–61.

Institute of Society, Ethics and the Life Sciences: Research Group on Ethical, Social and Legal Issues in Genetic Counseling and Genetic Engineering. "Ethical and Social Issues in Screening for Genetic Disease." *New England Journal of Medicine* 286 (25 May 1972): 1129–1132.

Jackson, David A. and Stephen P. Stich, eds. *The Recombinant DNA Debate.* Englewood Cliffs, N.J.: Prentice-Hall, 1979.

Kass, Leon. "Implications of Prenatal Diagnosis for the Human Right to Life." In Bruce Hilton, et al., eds. *Ethical Issues in Human Genetics.* New York: Plenum Press, 1973.

———. "Making Babies: The New Biology and the 'Old' Morality." *Public Interest* 26 (1972): 18–56.

———. "New Beginning in Life." In Michael Hamilton, ed. *The New Genetics and the Future Man.* Grand Rapids, Mich.: Eerdmans, 1972, pp. 15–63. On in vitro fertilization.

Kelly, Patricia T. *Dealing with Dilemma: A Manual for Genetic Counselors.* New York: Springer Verlag, 1977.

Klein, David. "Genetic Manipulations." *Impact of Science on Society* 23 (1973): 21–27.

Kolata, Gina B. "Prenatal Diagnosis of Neural Tube Defects." *Science* 209 (12 September 1980): 1216–1218.

Kopelman, Loretta. "Genetic Screening in Newborns: Voluntary or Compulsory?" *Perspectives in Biology and Medicine* 22 (Autumn 1978): 83–89.

Lakoff, Sanford A. "Moral Responsibility and the 'Galilean Imperative.'" *Ethics* 91 (October 1980): 100–116.

Lappé, Marc and Robert S. Morrison, eds. "Ethical and Scientific Issues Posed by Human Uses of Molecular Genetics." *Annals of the New York Academy of Sciences* 265 (1976): 1–208.

Lappé, Marc, et al. "Ethical and Social Issues in Screening for Genetic Disease." *New England Journal of Medicine* 286 (1972): 1129–1132. Problems and guidelines in social programs.

———. *Genetics Politics: The Limits of Biological Control.* New York: Simon and Schuster, 1979.

———. "Moral Obligations and the Fallacies of Genetic Control." *Theological Studies* 33 (1972): 411–427.

——— and Peter Steinfels. "Choosing the Sex of Our Children." *Hastings Center Report* 4 (1974): 1–4.

Lederberg, Joshua. "DNA Splicing: Will Fear Rob Us of Its Benefits?" *Prism* 2 (November 1975): 33–37.

———. "Experimental Genetics and Human Evolution." *American Naturalist* 100 (1966): 519–531.

———. "Orthobiosis: The Perfection of Man." In Nicholas Rescher, ed. *The Place of Value in a World of Facts.* New York: John Wiley, 1970.

Leiser, Burton M. "The New Genetics and Lives Not Worth Living." In John J. Buckley, Jr. ed. *Genetics Now: Ethical Issues in Genetic Research.* Washington, D.C.: University Press of America, 1982, pp. 41–58.

Leonard, C. O., et al. "Genetic Counseling: A Consumer's View." *New England Journal of Medicine* 287 (1972): 433–449. An empirical survey of consumer attitudes and information.

Lenzer, Gertrud. "Gender Ethics." *Hastings Center Report* 10 (1980): 18–19.

Lipkin, Mack, Jr., and P. T. Rowley, eds. *Genetic Responsibility: On Choosing Our Children's Genes.* New York: Plenum Press, 1974.

Ludmerer, Kenneth M. *Genetics and American Society.* Baltimore: Johns Hopkins University Press, 1972. A history of the eugenics movement.

McCormick, Richard. "Genetic Medicine: Notes on the Moral Literature." *Theological Studies* 33 (September 1972): 531–532.

Man and Medicine 2 (Winter 1977): 78–132. Special issue on recombinant DNA.

Mercola, Karen and Martin Cline. "The Potentials of Inserting New Genetic Information." *New England Journal of Medicine* 303 (27 November 1980): 1297–1300.

Milunsky, A. and G. J. Annas, eds. *Genetics and the Law.* New York: Plenum Press, 1976.

Muller, H. J. "The Guidance of Human Evolution." *Perspectives in Biology and Medicine* 3 (1959): 1–43.

———. "What Genetic Course Will Man Steer?" In J. F. Crow and J. V. Neel, eds. *Proceedings of the Third International Congress of Human Genetics.* Baltimore: Johns Hopkins University, 1967.

National Academy of Sciences. *Genetic Screening: Programs, Principles, and Research.* Washington, D.C.: National Academy of Sciences, 1975.

———. *Research with Recombinant DNA: An Academy Forum, 7–9 March 1977.* Washington, D.C.: National Academy of Sciences, 1977.

National Research Council, Committee for the Study of Inborn Errors of Metabolism. *Genetic Screening: Programs, Principles, and Research.* Washington, D.C.: National Academy of Sciences, 1975.

Neville, Robert. "Gene Therapy and the Ethics of Genetic Therapeutics." *Annals of the New York Academy of Sciences* 265 (1976): 153–161.

Omenn, Gilbert. "Genetics and Epidemiology: Medical Interventions and Public Policy." *Social Biology* 26 (Summer 1979): 117–125.

Osborn, Frederick. "The Emergence of a Valid Eugenics." *American Scientist* 61 (1973): 425–429.

Powledge, Tabitha and John Fletcher. "Guidelines for the Ethical, Social, and Legal Issues in Prenatal Diagnosis." *New England Journal of Medicine* 300 (January 1979): 168–172.

Powledge, Tabitha. "The New Ghetto Hustle." *Saturday Review of the Sciences* (February 1973): 38–47.

———. "There's Another Side to Genetic Screening." *Prism* 3 (1976): 55–57.

Ramsey, Paul. *Fabricated Man: The Ethics of Genetic Control.* New Haven: Yale University Press, 1970.

———. "Genetic Engineering." *Bulletin of the Atomic Scientists* 29 (December 1972): 14–17.

Reed, Sheldon. *Counseling in Medical Genetics.* New York: Alan R. Liss, 1980.

Reilly, Philip. *Genetics, Law and Social Policy.* Cambridge: Harvard University Press, 1977.

Richards, John, ed. *Recombinant DNA: Science, Ethics and Politics.* New York: Academic Press, 1978.

Robitscher, Jonas. *Eugenic Sterilization.* Springfield, Ill.: Charles C. Thomas, 1973.

Rogers, Michael. *Biohazard.* New York: Alfred A. Knopf, 1977.

Ruse, Michael. "Genetics and the Quality of Life." *Social Indicators Research* 7 (January 1980): 419–441.

Sinsheimer, Robert. "An Evolutionary Perspective for Genetic Engineering." *New Scientist* 73 (20 January 1977): 150–152.

———. "Troubled Dawn for Genetic Engineering." *New Scientist* 68 (1975): 148–151. An excellent review of problems.

Southern California Law Review 51 (September 1978): 969–1573. "Biotechnology and the Law: Recombinant DNA and the Control of Scientific Research." Special issue.

Stetten, DeWitt. "Freedom of Enquiry." *Genetics* 81 (November 1975): 415–425.

Thomas, Lewis. "The Hazards of Science." *New England Journal of Medicine* 296 (10 February 1977): 324–328.

Tormey, Judith F. "Ethical Considerations of Prenatal Genetic Diagnosis." *Clinical Obstetrics and Gynecology* 19 (1976): 957–963.

Tsuang, Ming T. and Randall VanderMey. *Genes and the Mind: Inheritance of Mental Illness.* New York: Oxford University Press, 1980.

Twiss, S. B., Jr. "Ethical Issues in Priority Setting for the Utilization of Genetic Technologies." *Annals of the New York Academy of Sciences* 265 (1976): 22–45.

Ulrich, Lawrence P. "Reproductive Rights and Genetic Disease." In James M. Humber, ed. *Biomedical Ethics and the Law.* New York: Plenum Press, 1976, pp. 351–360.

Veatch, Robert M. "Ethical Issues in Genetics." Arthur G. Steinberg and Alexander G. Bearn, eds. *Progress in Medical Genetics*, vol. X. New York: Grune and Stratton, 1974.

Wade, Nicholas. "Genetics: Conference Sets Strict Controls to Replace Moratorium." *Science* 187 (1975): 931–935.

———. *The Ultimate Experiment.* New York: Walker and Company, 1977.

Walters, LeRoy. "Genetics, Reproductive Biology, and Bioethics." In Marguerite Neumann, ed. *The Tricentennial People: Human Applications of the New Genetics.* Ames, Iowa: Iowa State University Press, 1978, pp. 66–80.

Wautz, Jon R., and Carol R. Thigpen. "Genetic Screening and Counseling: The Legal and Ethical Issues." *Northwestern University Law Review* 68 (September–October 1973): 696–767.

Watson, James D. "Moving toward Clonal Man: Is That What We Want?" *Atlantic Monthly* 227 (1971): 50–53.

Westoff, Charles F. and R. R. Rindfuss. "Sex Preselection in the U.S.: Some Implications." *Science* 184 (1974): 633–636.

Chapter 8: Reproductive Control: In Vitro Fertilization, Artificial Insemination and Sterilization.

Amicus. 2 (February 1977): 33–47. "Society's Right to Sterilize: What are the Limits?" A special issue.

Beck, William W., Jr. "A Critical Look at the Legal, Ethical, and Technical Aspects of Artifical Insemination." *Fertility and Sterility* 27 (January 1976): 1–8.

Bellotis, Raymond A. "Morality and *in Vitro* Fertilization." *Bioethics Quarterly* 2 (1980): 6–19.

Burgdorf, Robert and Marcia Burgdorf. "The Wicked Witch Is Almost Dead: Buck vs. Bell and the Sterilization of Handicapped Persons." *Temple Law Quarterly* 50 (1977): 995–1034.

Burt, Robert and Monroe E. Price. "Sterilization, State Action and the Concept of Consent." *Law and Psychology Review* (Spring 1975): 57–78.

Callahan, Daniel, et al. "In Vitro Fertilization: Four Commentaries." *Hastings Center Report* 8 (October 1978): 7–14.

Davis, Morris E. "Involuntary Sterilization: A History of Social Control." *Journal of Black Health* 1 (August–September 1974).

Donovan, Patricia. "Sterilization and the Poor: Two Views on the Need for Protection from Abuse." *Family Planning/Population Reporter* 5 (April 1976): 28–30.

Edwards, Robert G. "Fertilization of Human Eggs in Vitro: Morals, Ethics, and the Law." *Quarterly Review of Biology* 49 (March 1974): 3–26.

―――― and D. J. Sharpe. "Social Values and Research in Human Embryology." *Nature* 231 (14 May 1971): 87–91.

Frankel, Mark S. "Human Semen Banking: Social and Public Policy Issues." *Man and Medicine* 1 (Summer 1976): 289–309.

Hellegers, Andre and Richard A. McCormick. "Unanswered Questions on Test-Tube Life." *America* 139 (August 1978): 74–78.

Holder, A. R. "Voluntary Sterilization." *Journal of the American Medical Association* 225 (24 September 1973): 1743–1744.

Horne, Herbert, Jr. "Artificial Insemination Donor: An Issue of Ethical and Moral Values." *New England Journal of Medicine* 293 (23 October 1975): 873–874.

Kass, Leon R. "Babies by Means of In Vitro Fertilization: Unethical Experiments on the Unborn?" *New England Journal of Medicine* 285 (18 November 1971): 1174–1179.

―――――. "Making Babies: The New Biology and the Old Morality." *Public Interest* 26 (Winter 1972): 18–56.

Law and Ethics of A.I.D. and Embryo Transfer. CIBA Foundation Symposium 17. New York: Associated Scientific Publishers, 1973.

McGarrah, Robert E., Jr., and Susan L. Peck. "Voluntary Female Sterilization." *Hastings Center Report* 4 (June 1974): 5–10.

Macklin, Ruth and William Gaylin, eds. *Mental Retardation and Sterilization: A Problem of Competency and Paternalism.* New York: Plenum Press, 1981.

Marsh, Frank H. and Donnie L. Self. "In Vitro Fertilization: Moving from Theory to Therapy." *Hastings Center Report* 10 (January 1980): 5–6.

Marx, Jean L. "Embryology: Out of the Womb—Into the Test Tube" and "In Vitro Fertilization of Human Eggs: Bioethical and Legal Considerations." *Science* 182 (23 November 1973): 811–814.

Meyers, David. *The Human Body and the Law.* Chicago: Aldine Publishing Company, 1970.

Peckins, David M. "Artificial Insemination and the Law." *Journal of Legal Medicine* (July–August 1976): 17–22.

Perrin, J. C., et al. "A Considered Approach to Sterilization of Mentally Retarded Youths." *American Journal of Diseases of Children* 130 (March 1976): 288–290.

Ramsey, Paul. "Shall We Reproduce?" *Journal of the American Medical Association* 220 (5 June 1972): 1346–1350.

Robitscher, Jonas, ed. *Eugenic Sterilization.* Springfield, Ill.: Charles C. Thomas, 1973.

Rosoff, Jennie. "Sterilization: The Montgomery Case." *Hastings Center Report* 3 (September 1973): 6.

Schima, Marilyn and Ira Lumbell, eds. *Advances in Voluntary Sterilization.* New York: Elsevier, 1974.

Smith, George P., II. "Through a Test Tube Darkly: Artificial Insemination and the Law." *Michigan Law Review* 67 (1968): 127–150.

Snowden, R. and G. D. Mitchell. *The Artificial Family: A Consideration of Artificial Insemination by Donor.* London: George Allen and Unwin, 1981.

Veatch, Robert M. "Sterilization: Its Socio-Cultural and Ethical Determinants." In Marilyn E. Schima and Ira Lumbell, eds. *Advances in Voluntary Sterilization.* New York: Elsevier, 1974, pp. 138–150.

Wadlington, Walter. "Artificial Insemination: The Dangers of a Poorly Kept Secret." *Northwestern University Law Review* 64 (January–February): 777–807.

Walters, LeRoy, "Human In Vitro Fertilization." *Hastings Center Report* 9 (August 1979): 23–43.

Part IV: Resources
Chapter 9: Competition and Allocation

American Medical Association Judicial Council. "Ethical Guidelines for Organ Transplantation." *Journal of the American Medical Association* 25 (1968): 341–342.

Anscombe, G. E. M. "Who Is Wronged?" *Oxford Review* 5 (1967): 16–17. A general argument relating to distribution.

Beecher, Henry K. "Scarce Resources and Medical Advancement." In Paul Freund, ed. *Experimentation with Human Subjects.* New York: George Braziller, 1970.

Bermant, Gordon, Peter Brown, and Gerald Dworkin. "Of Morals, Markets, and Medicine." *Hastings Center Report* 5 (1975): 14–16.

Daniels, Norman. "Cost-Effectiveness and Patient Welfare." In Marc Basson, ed. *Rights and Responsibilities in Medicine.* New York: Alan R. Liss, 1981, pp. 159–170.

Dukeminier, J., Jr., and D. Sanders. "Organ Transplantation: A Proposal For Routine Salvaging of Cadaver Organs." *New England Journal of Medicine* 279 (22 August 1968): 413–419.

Ezorsky, Gertrude. "How Many Lives Shall We Save?" *Metaphilosophy* 3 (1972): 156–162. Includes a criticism of Anscombe's "Who Is Wronged?"

Fellner, Carl H. "Altruism in Disrepute." *New England Journal of Medicine* 284 (1973): 589–592.

———. "Kidney Donors—the Myth of Informed Consent." *American Journal of Psychiatry* 126 (1970): 9.

———. "Organ Donation: For Whose Sake?" *Annals of Internal Medicine* (October 1973): 589–592.

Fox, R. C. and J. P. Swazey. *The Courage to Fail: A Social View of Organ Transplants and Dialysis.* Chicago: University of Chicago Press, 1974.

Gorovitz, Samuel. "Ethics and the Allocation of Medical Resources." *Medical Research Engineering* 5 (1966): 5–7.

Hanink, J. G. "On the Survival Lottery." *Philosophy* 51 (1976): 223–225. Criticism of John Harris's "The Survival Lottery."

Harris, John. "The Survival Lottery." *Philosophy* 50 (1975): 81–87. Argues that perfection of transplants would make it right to sacrifice a healthy person chosen by lottery to save lives of several people needing organs.

Havighurst, Clark C. "The Ethics of Cost Control in Medical Care." *Soundings* 60 (Spring 1977): 22–39.

Hiatt, H. "On the Distribution of Resources." *New England Journal of Medicine* 293 (1975).

Jinks, Robert W. "California's Response to the Problems of Procuring Human Remains for Transplantation." *California Law Review* 57 (May 1969): 671–693.

Kaplan, M. B. "The Case of the Artificial Heart Panel." *Hastings Center Report* 5 (1975): 41–48.

Katz, Jay and Alexander Morgan Capron. *Catastrophic Diseases: Who Decides What? A Psychological and Legal Analysis of the Problems Posed by Hemodialysis and Organ Transplantation.* New York: Russell Sage Foundation, 1975.

Knutson, A. L. "Body Transplants and Ethical Values." *Social Science and Medicine* 2 (1968–1969): 393–414.

Leake, C. D. "Technical Triumph and Moral Muddle." In T. E. Sturzl, ed. *Experience in Renal Transplantation.* Philadelphia: W. B. Saunders Company, 1964.

Leenen, H. J. J. "The Selection of Patients in the Event of a Scarcity of Medical Facilities—An Unavoidable Dilemma." *International Journal of Medicine and Law* (1980): 161–180.

Lyons, Catherine. *Organ Transplants: The Moral Issues.* Philadelphia: Westminister Press, 1970.

Mack, Eric. "Bad Samaritanism and the Causation of Harm." *Philosophy and Public Affairs* 9 (Spring 1980): 230–259.

Mechanic, David. *Future Issues in Health Care: Social Policy and the Rationing of Medical Sources.* New York: Free Press, 1979.

Miller, George W. *Moral and Ethical Implications of Human Organ Transplants.* Springfield, Ill.: Charles C. Thomas, 1971.

Mooney, Gavin. "Cost-Benefit Analysis and Medical Ethics." *Journal of Medical Ethics* 6 (December 1980): 177–179.

Plant, Raymond. "Gifts, Exchanges and the Political Economy of Health Care." Part 1: "Should Blood be Bought and Sold?" *Journal of Medical Ethics* 3 (December 1977): 166–173; and Part 2: "How Should Health Care be Distributed?" (March 1978): 5–11.

Ramsey, Paul. "Choosing How to Choose: Patients and Sparse Medical Resources." In *The Patient as Person.* New Haven: Yale University Press, 1980, chapter 7.

Rhoads, Steven E. "How Much Should We Spend to Save a Life?" *Public Interest* 51 (Spring 1978): 74–92.

"The Sale of Human Body Parts." *Michigan Law Review* 72 (1974): 1182–1264.

"Scarce Medical Resources." *Columbia Law Review* 69 (1969): 620–692.

Schiffer, R. M. and Benjamin Freedman. "Case Studies in Bioethics: The Last Bed in the ICU." *Hastings Center Report* 7 (December 1977): 21–22.

Shapiro, M. H. "Who Merits Merit? Problems in Distributive Justice and Utility Posed by the New Biology." *California Law Review* 48 (1974): 318–370.

Simmons, Roberta G., et al. *Gift of Life: The Social and Psychological Impact of Organ Transplantation.* New York: John Wiley and Sons, 1977.

Smith, Harmon L. "Distributive Justice and American Health Care." In W. M. Finnin, Jr., ed. *The Morality of Scarcity.* Baton Rouge: Louisiana State University Press, 1977, pp. 67–80.

Taurek, John M. "Should the Numbers Count?" *Philosophy and Public Affairs* 6 (Summer 1977): 293–316.

Westervelt, B., Jr., "The Selection Process Viewed from Within: A Reply to Childress." *Soundings* 53 (1970): 154–158.

Chapter 10: The Claim to Health Care

Alford, Robert R. *Health Care Politics: Ideological Interest Group Barriers to Reform.* Chicago: University of Chicago Press, 1975.

Arrow, Kenneth J., et al. "Government Decision Making and the Preciousness of Life." In Lawrence R. Ranoredi, ed. *Ethics of Health Care.* Washington D.C.: National Academy of Sciences, 1974, pp. 33–64.

Bayles, Michael D. "National Health Insurance and Non-Covered Services." *Journal of Health Politics, Policy and Law* 2 (Fall 1977): 335–348.

Birnbaum, Morton. "The Right to Treatment." *American Bar Association Journal* 46 (1960): 499–505.

Black, M. M. and C. Riley. "Moral Issues and Priorities in Biomedical Engineering." *Science, Medicine and Man* 1 (1973): 67–74.

Blackstone, William T. "On Health Care as a Legal Right: Philosophical Justifications, Political Activity, and Adequate Health Care." *Georgia Law Review* 10 (Winter 1976): 391–418.

Brown, Lawrence D. "The Scope and Limits of Equality as a Normative Guide to Federal Health Care Policy." *Public Policy* 26 (Fall 1978): 481–532.

Buxton, M. J. and R. R. West. "Cost-Benefit Analysis of Long-Term Hemodialysis for Chronic Renal Failure." *British Medical Journal*, 17 (May 1975): 376–379. A caution about instituting similar programs for other diseases.

Cairl, R. E., et al. "National Health Insurance Policy in the United States: A Case of Non-Decision-Making." *International Journal of Health Services* 7 (1977): 167–178.

Callahan, Daniel. "How Much Is Enough? A National Perspective." *Alabama Journal of Medical Sciences* 17 (January 1980): 76–80.

Childress, James F. *Priorities in Biomedical Ethics*. Philadelphia: Westminster Press, 1981.

Cleverly, W. "Cost Containment in the Health Care Industry." *Topics in Health Care Financing* 3 (Spring 1977): 1–17.

Curran, William J. "The Right to Health in National and International Law." *New England Journal of Medicine* 284 (1971): 1258.

Devries, Andre. "Health Care Responsibility." *Metamedicine* 1 (Fall 1980): 95–106.

"Due Process in the Allocation of Scarce Lifesaving Medical Resources." *Yale Law Journal* 84 (1975): 1734–1749.

Edwards, Marvin Henry. *Hazardous to Your Health: A New Look at the "Health Care Crisis" in America*. New York: Arlington House, 1972.

Ehrenreich, Barbara and John Ehrenreich. *The American Health Empire: Power, Profits and Politics*. New York: Random House, 1970.

Falk, I. S. "Proposals for National Health Insurance in the USA: Origins and Evolution, and Some Perceptions for the Future." *Milbank Memorial Fund Quarterly: Health and Society* (Spring 1977): 161–191.

Fein, Rashi. "On Achieving Access and Equity in Health Care." *Milbank Memorial Fund Quarterly* 50 (1972): 157–190.

Feldstein, Paul J. "National Health Insurance: An Approach to the Redistribution of Medical Care." In *Health Care Economics*. New York: John Wiley & Sons, 1979, chapter 19.

Freedman, Benjamin. "The Case for Medical Care: Inefficient or Not." *Hastings Center Report* 7 (April 1977): 31–39.

Fried, Charles. "Rights and Health Care—Beyond Equity and Efficiency." *New England Journal of Medicine* 293 (31 July 1975): 241–245.

Fromer, Margot Joan. *Ethical Issues in Health Care*. St. Louis: C. V. Mosby Company, 1981.

Fuchs, Victor. *Who Shall Live?* New York: Basic Books, 1974.

Garfield, Sidney. "The Delivery of Medical Care." *Scientific American* 222 (1970): 15–23.

Ginzberg, Eli. *The Limits of Health Reform: The Search for Realism*. New York, Basic Books, 1977.

——— and Miriam Ostow. *Men, Money and Medicine*. New York: Columbia University Press, 1969.

Greenberg, Selig. *The Quality of Mercy*. New York: Atheneum, 1971.

Hiatt, Howard H. "Protecting the Medical Commons: Who Is Responsible?" *New England Journal of Medicine* 293 (31 July 1975): 235–241.

Halberstam, Michael. "Liberal Thought, Radical Theory and Medical Practice." *New England Journal of Medicine* 284 (1971): 1180–1185.

Hodgson, Godfrey. "The Politics of American Health Care." *Atlantic* (October 1973): 45–61.

Illich, Ivan. *Medical Nemesis*. New York: Pantheon, 1976.

Journal of Medicine and Philosophy 4 (1979). Special issue on the right to health care.

Kass, Leon R. "Reading the End of Medicine and the Pursuit of Health." *The Public Interest* 40 (1975): 11–42.

Knowles, John H., ed. *Doing Better and Feeling Worse: Health Care in the United States*. New York: Norton, 1977.

Krizay, John and Andrew Wilson. *The Patient as Consumer: Health Care Financing in the United States*. Lexington, Mass.: D.C. Heath and Company, 1974.

Lesser, Paul B. "A Right to Health?" *Forum on Medicine* 3 (October 1980): 667–669.

Lewis, Charles E., et al. *A Right to Health—The Problem of Access to Medical Care*. New York: John Wiley and Sons, 1976.

Lomasky, Loren E. "Medical Progress and National Health Care." *Philosophy and Public Affairs* 10 (Winter 1981): 65–88.

McCreadie, Claudine. "Rawlsian Justice and Financing of the National Health Service." *Journal of Social Policy* 5 (April 1976): 113–130.

MacLeon, Gordon and Jeffrey A. Prussin. "Continuing Evolution and Health Maintenance Organizations." *New England Journal of Medicine* 288 (1973): 439–443.

Mechanic, David. "Approaches to Controlling the Costs of Medical Care: Short-Range Alternatives." *New England Journal of Medicine* 298 (2 February 1978): 249–254.

————. *The Growth of Bureaucratic Medicine: An Inquiry into the Dynamics of Patient Behavior and the Organization of Medical Care.* New York: John Wiley and Sons, 1976.

————. "Rationing Health Care: Public Policy and the Medical Marketplace." *Hastings Center Report* 6 (1976): 34–37.

Morison, Robert S. "Rights and Responsibilities: Redressing the Uneasy Balance." *Hastings Center Report* 4 (1974): 1–4.

Navarro, Vicente. "Justice, Social Policy, and the Public's Health." *Medical Care* 15 (May 1977): 363–370.

New England Journal of Medicine 293 (31 July 1975). A large part of this issue is devoted to health-care delivery. See, in particular, the articles by Hiatt and Fried.

Northwestern University Law Review 70 (1975). "Current Problems in Health Care: A Symposium."

Outka, Gene. "Social Justice and Equal Access to Health Care." *Journal of Religious Ethics* 2 (1974): 11–32.

Pilpel, Harriet F. "Minors' Rights to Medical Care." *Albany Law Review* 36 (1972): 462–487.

Review of Radical Political Economics 9 (Spring 1977). A special issue entitled "The Political Economy of Health."

Sade, R. "Concepts of Rights: Philosophy and Application to Health Care." *Linacre Quarterly* 46 (November 1979): 330–344.

Schwartz, William B. "Policy Analysis, Politics and the Problems of Health Care." *New England Journal of Medicine* 286 (1972): 1057–1058.

Seham, Max. *Blacks and American Medical Care.* Minneapolis: University of Minnesota Press, 1973.

Shelp, Earl, ed. *Justice and Health Care.* Boston: D. Reidel, 1981.

Slaby, Andrew E. and Laurance R. Tancredi. "The Economics of Moral Values: Policy Implications." *Journal of Health Politics, Policy, and Law* 2 (Spring 1977): 20–31.

Soble, Alan. "On Health Care as a Right: More on the Right to Health Care." *Georgia Law Review* 10 (Winter 1976): 525–544.

Sparer, Edward V. "The Legal Right to Health Care: Public Policy and Equal Access." *Hastings Center Report* 6 (October 1976): 39–47.

Stevens, Rosemary. *American Medicine and the Public Interest.* New Haven: Yale University Press, 1971.

Steiner, Hillel. "The Just Provision of Health Care: A Reply to Elizabeth Telfer." *Journal of Medical Ethics* 2 (December 1976): 185–189.

Taylor, Vincent. "How Much is Good Health Worth?" *Policy Sciences* 1 (1970): 49–72.

Tancredi, Laurence, ed. *Ethics of Health Care.* Washington, D.C.: National Academy of Sciences, 1975.

Telfer, Elizabeth. "Justice, Welfare and Health Care." *Journal of Medical Ethics* 2 (September 1976): 107–111.

Veatch, R. M. and Roy Branson, eds. *Ethics and Health Policy.* Cambridge, Mass.: Ballinger Publishing Company, 1976.

Weaver, Jerry L. *National Health Policy and the Underserved: Ethnic Minorities, Women, and the Elderly.* St. Louis: C. V. Mosby Company, 1976.